Comprehensive Perioperative Nursing

The Jones and Bartlett Series in Nursing

Adult Emergency Nursing Procedures, Proehl

Basic Steps in Planning Nursing Research, Fourth Edition, Brink/Wood

Cancer Chemotherapy, Barton Burke et al.

Cancer Nursing: Principles and Practice, Third Edition, Groenwald et al.

A Challenge for Living, Corless et al.

Chemotherapy Care Plans, Barton Burke et al.

Chronic Illness: Impact and Intervention, Third Edition, Lubkin

Comprehensive Cancer Nursing Review, Groenwald et al.

A Comprehensive Curriculum for Trauma Nursing, Bayley/Turcke

Comprehensive Perioperative Nursing Review, Fairchild et al.

Crisis Counseling, Second Edition, Janosik

Desk Reference for Critical Care Nursing, Wright/Shelton

Drugs and Protocols Common to Prehospital and Emergency Care, Cummings

Drugs and the Elderly, Swonger/Burbank

Essential Medical Terminology, Stanfield

Essentials of Oxygenation, Ahrens/Rutherford

Ethics Consultation, LaPuma/Schiedermayer

Fundamentals of Nursing Research, Second Edition, Brockopp/Hasting-Tolsma

Grant Application Writer's Handbook, Reif-Lehrer

Handbook of Oncology Nursing, Second Edition, Gross/Johnson

Health Assessment in Nursing Practice, Third Edition, Grimes/Burns

Health Policy and Nursing: Crisis and Reform in the U.S. Health Care Delivery System, Harrington/Estes

Healthy People 2000, U.S. Department of Health and Human Services

Human Aging and Chronic Disease, Kart et al.

Human Development, Fourth Edition, Freiberg

Intravenous Therapy, Nentwich

Introductory Management and Leadership for Clinical Nurses, Swansburg

Management and Leadership for Nurse Managers, Swansburg

Management of Spinal Cord Injury, Second Edition, Zejdlik

Medical Ethics, Veatch

Medical Instrumentation for Nurses and Allied Health-Care Professionals, Aston/Brown

Memory Bank for Chemotherapy, Second Edition, Preston/Wilfinger

Memory Bank for Critical Care, Third Edition, Ervin

Memory Bank for Hemodynamic Monitoring, Second Edition, Ervin/Long

Memory Bank for HIV Medications, Wilkes

Memory Bank for Intravenous Therapy, Second Edition, Weinstein

Memory Bank for Medications, Second Edition, Kostin/Sieloff

The Nation's Health, Fourth Edition, Lee/Estes

New Dimensions in Women's Health, Alexander/LaRosa

Nursing and the Disabled, Fraley

Nursing Assessment and Diagnosis, Second Edition, Bellack/Edlund

Nursing Research with Basic Statistical Applications, Dempsey/Dempsey

Nursing Staff Development, Swansburg

Oncology Nursing Drug Reference, Wilkes et al.

Oncology Nursing Society's Instruments for Clinical Nursing Research, Frank-Stromborg

Oxygen Administration, National Safety Council

Pediatric Emergency Nursing Procedures, Bernardo/Bove

Perioperative Nursing: Principles and Practice, Fairchild

Perioperative Patient Care, Third Edition, Kneedler/Dodge

Perspectives on Death and Dying, Fulton/Metress

Primary Care of Women and Children with HIV Infection: A Multi-Disciplinary Approach, Kelly et al.

Ready Reference for Critical Care, Strawn/Stewart

Working with Older Adults, Third Edition, Burnside/Schmidt

Comprehensive Perioperative Nursing

VOLUME 2   PRACTICE

BARBARA J. GRUENDEMANN, RN, MS, FAAN
Director, Professional Education & Services
Johnson & Johnson Medical Inc.
Arlington, Texas

BILLIE FERNSEBNER, RN, MSN, CNOR
Perioperative Clinical Nurse Specialist
Massachusetts General Hospital
Boston, Massachusetts

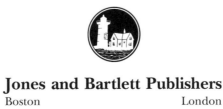

Jones and Bartlett Publishers
Boston   London

The material contained in this book is endorsed by AORN as a useful component in the ongoing education process of perioperative nurses.

Editorial, Sales, and Customer Service Offices
Jones and Bartlett Publishers
One Exeter Plaza
Boston, MA 02116
617-859-3900
800-832-0034

Jones and Bartlett Publishers International
7 Melrose Terrace
London W6 7RL
England

Library of Congress Cataloging-in-Publication Data

Gruendemann, Barbara J.
    Comprehensive perioperative nursing / Barbara J. Gruendemann.
    Billie Fernsebner.
        p.   cm. — (Jones and Bartlett series in nursing)
    Includes bibliographical references and index.
    Contents: v. 1. Principles — v. 2. Practice.
    ISBN 0-86720-719-1
    1. Operating room nursing.   I. Fernsebner, Billie.   II. Title.
III. Series.
    [DNLM: 1. Operating Room Nursing.   WY 162 G886c 1995]
RD32.3.G78   1995
610.73′677—dc20
DNLM/DLC
for Library of Congress   94-46726
                                                        CIP

Acquisitions Editor: Jan Wall
Assistant Production Manager/Coordination: Judy Songdahl
Manufacturing Buyer: Dana L. Cerrito
Editorial Production Service: Ruttle, Shaw & Wetherill, Inc.
Typesetting: Weimer Graphics, Inc.
Cover Design: Hannus Design Associates
Printing and Binding: Courier-Westford

Printed in the United States of America
99 98 97 96 95   10 9 8 7 6 5 4 3 2 1

To Warren and Luke,
our other partners

Brief Contents

VOLUME 1
Principles

VOLUME 2
Practice

Contents

PART I
Instrumentation for Surgery

PART II
Surgical Procedures

PART III
Special Information

Foreword

Comprehensive Perioperative Nursing is an essential resource with much to commend it. This two-volume text does great service to a dynamic and important field of nursing care.

I am frequently asked to forecast the future of health care and nursing, but I generally decline to do so because the technology-driven changes in the world are too dramatic to predict. Science fiction has become reality. However, I do believe it is very possible to prepare persons for an uncertain future. *Comprehensive Perioperative Nursing* well capitalizes on that approach and successfully bridges today and tomorrow. The first volume is one of universal and enduring principles, concepts, and fundamental skills that will serve today's novice and experienced practitioners now and throughout their careers. The second volume—equally practical—is firmly rooted in contemporary surgical procedures. To achieve such richness and scope, the author-editors have enlisted and coordinated the work of more than 65 expert contributors.

The past twenty years have witnessed the pushing out of the borders of operating room nursing and the technical skills required therein to the extended field of perioperative nursing, embracing psychosocial, managerial, legal, ethical, and educational dimensions. *Comprehensive Perioperative Nursing* both reflects and supports this evolution from operating room to perioperative nursing.

Moreover, beyond the growing dimensions of the specialty, *Comprehensive Perioperative Nursing* reaches out internationally to touch on the practice of colleagues in other nations. Again, it extends vision and expands horizons, encouraging readers to prepare for "the global village" described by futurists.

The authors have planned this work to be useful as a text for students and teachers as well as a reference for practicing nurses and others with an interest within the broad range of perioperative nursing. Therefore, the content and style will be found to appeal to a wide audience.

With such enormous and unequaled breadth, *Comprehensive Perioperative Nursing* has very deservedly been titled "comprehensive" in its field.

Margretta Madden Styles, RN, EdD, FAAN

Preface

Why a new book on perioperative nursing? We believe that you, as perioperative nurses, need a textbook that combines the newest theories and behavioral aspects of perioperative nursing with the traditional technical skills. This text contains the critical elements of contemporary perioperative nursing.

The roots of the specialty are in operating room nursing and in the scrubbing and circulating roles for surgical procedures. These roots are nurtured by futuristic thinking about perioperative nursing as we continue to identify the scope and patterns of practice and the increasing knowledge base.

While once operating room nurses were primarily concerned with the care of the patient during surgical procedures, the perioperative nurse's world now extends much further. In today's health care environment, perioperative nurses must be multiskilled. They have finely honed skills in such areas as education, research, quality management, and operating room safety. As managers of the operating room, they are knowledgeable about budgeting, staffing and scheduling, materials management, and management information systems. Perioperative nurses are customer-oriented to the needs of both patients and physicians who come to the surgical suite. They are leading efforts to provide high-quality care that is also cost-effective. As they fill managerial and leadership roles, they are visionary, meeting new opportunities that arise.

Volume 1 is entitled Principles; Volume 2 is entitled Practice. This two-volume text meets the growing needs of today's perioperative nurse. It moves beyond the procedural aspects of traditional operating room nursing to a comprehensive approach to perioperative nursing. The text describes the skills, technical and behavioral, that will prepare you, as a perioperative nurse, for a future that is both exciting and uncertain. Two volumes were necessary to incorporate perioperative principles and practice and the ever-widening scope of the global specialty. The two volumes complement each other and, together, encompass the full scope of perioperative nursing. Each volume, however, stands alone and is a text unto itself.

Although the book is intended primarily for novice and experienced perioperative nurses as well as students, others may find useful information. Clinical nurses in other areas, surgical technologists, physicians, government officials, hospital executives, and medical products representatives may use this text as a reference. Even patients who want to know more about their procedures may find it a valuable resource.

The book's contents are applicable to the care of the patients wherever surgical procedures are performed—in hospital operating rooms, same-day surgery centers, physicians' offices, and clinics. The emphasis is on consistency of standards and guidelines for all patients regardless of setting.

This text is not a traditional "recipe" book or encyclopedia but, rather, a carefully planned and coordinated source. Whether you are a professional nurse or a student, you can choose the information you need. A beginning student, for example, might select the chapters on asepsis and presurgical assessment as starting points. The advanced practitioner might turn first to sections on performance management or research. Chapters such as "The Art of Surgery" are essential reading for all perioperative clinicians. This book does not always tell you what to do, but gives you an understanding of our options and guides your problem-solving.

The scope of this book is broad. Emphasizing both technical skills and behavioral aspects of perioperative nursing, it has the information you need as a staff nurse, an educator, a researcher, or manager in the operating room. Although Volume 1 includes discussion of some hands-on skills, it focuses mainly on behaviors and theories. These behavioral skills, which support the technical skills, are the "why" of perioperative nursing—the knowledge and ways of thinking that are the broader dimensions, or "templates," of routine actions. Carrying out Universal Precautions, for example, can be taught and practiced by memory and rote. A list of procedures for which eyewear is required can be memorized. But knowing the reasons for Universal Precautions adds judgment to the nurse's thought and action. Decision-making is more accurate and professional, and patients receive better care. In Volume 1, Part I, "Perioperative Constructs and Behaviors" covers leadership, communications, risk management, legal and ethical aspects, and research, common threads running through all of perioperative nursing. Part II, "Resource Planning," discusses budgets, management information systems, staffing and scheduling, performance management, materials management, and operating room suite design. Part III, "The Surgical Environment," considers infection prevention and control, sterilization and disinfection, safety, and waste management. "Technology Management," covers lasers, electrosurgery, and radiology. A section on "Global Perioperative Nursing" expands our vision of perioperative nursing through the practices of colleagues in other nations. In the final part, "Concepts of Perioperative Care," presurgical assessment, positioning, surgical incisions, wound closure, anesthesia, same-day surgery, and postanesthesia nursing care are discussed.

Technical skills are an important component of perioperative nursing. Being technically skilled assistants and partners at the sterile field—knowing anatomy, anticipating procedural steps, and being highly competent "scrubbed" personnel—expedites a positive outcome for both the surgeon and the patient. Surgical procedures have been placed in one convenient volume (Volume 2), which can be used as a complete clinical reference.

Volume 2, "Practice," focuses on the technical component, or the "what" and "how" of perioperative nursing. The core of perioperative nursing is to be able to anticipate the flow of events in each surgical procedure, taking into consideration alterations due to patient characteristics, surgeon expectations, and normal versus abnormal outcomes. Volume 2 opens with a chapter on instrumentation and then moves to detailed descriptions of sixteen surgical specialties. Discussion of one of the newer developments, minimally invasive surgery, is included, as are trauma, oncologic surgery, and pediatric surgery.

At the beginning of each chapter, key concepts summarize the salient points. For consistency, perioperative nurses are referred to as "she," although we are aware that it could just as well have been "he." In addition, "anesthesia provider" is used throughout the text to describe the nurse anesthetists and physician anesthesiologists who administer anesthesia to surgical patients.

The term "surgery" is used throughout the book to depict invasive and less invasive procedures. Although terminology may change in the future, the word "surgery" is still used by both medical and nursing professionals and is commonly understood.

A section at the end of each volume, "Yellow Pages of Resources," lists associations and organizations relevant to the practice of perioperative nursing.

We, as the authors, have written many of the chapters and coordinated and edited others. We have assembled a distinguished group of contributors with invaluable expertise. We thank these professionals for providing us with different perspectives and thought-provoking chapters. We hope that both volumes of the textbook will guide and challenge each of you in your professional growth as a perioperative nurse.

Barbara J. Gruendemann
Billie Fernsebner

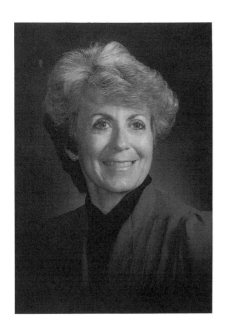

Barbara J. Gruendemann, RN, MS, CNOR, FAAN, is an active professional speaker and consultant in nursing and health care issues in the United States and abroad. She has extensive experience as a staff nurse, clinical specialist, manager, and educator. She is one of the first perioperative nurses in the United States to be inducted as a Fellow into the American Academy of Nursing.

Gruendemann is a noted nursing leader, having authored seven textbooks, numerous journal articles and videotapes, as well as having served as President of the Association of Operating Room Nurses, Inc. (AORN). She was the first recipient of AORN's Award for Excellence in Perioperative Nursing.

In her present position, Gruendemann is integrating professional education into a medical products corporation, domestically and internationally. She is Director of Professional Education & Services at Johnson & Johnson Medical Inc., in Arlington, Texas. Her forte is "spreading the gospel" about the value of education and perioperative nursing.

Billie Fernsebner, RN, MSN, CNOR, is Education Coordinator and Consulting Editor for *OR Manager* Inc., in Boulder, Colorado. Before that, she was Perioperative Clinical Nurse Specialist at Massachusetts General Hospital in Boston, Massachusetts.

Fernsebner has authored many journal articles, book chapters, and videotapes, and wrote the book *Core Curriculum for Perioperative Nursing*. She has developed and taught courses for perioperative nurses and RN first assistants and has lectured nationally and internationally on topics of interest to perioperative nurses.

She is a member of ANA, AORN, and Sigma Theta Tau International and has held offices and served on numerous committees of these associations. In 1990, Fernsebner received AORN's most prestigious award, The Award for Excellence in Perioperative Nursing. She is widely recognized for her contributions to perioperative nursing education and research.

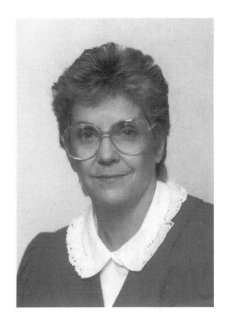

Contributors

Christine Donahue Annese, RN, MSN
Staff Specialist
Massachusetts General Hospital
Boston, Massachusetts

Renée Duérr Bailey, RN, BSN, CNOR
Clinical Program Coordinator
Baylor University Medical Center
Dallas, Texas

Dina Bardel, RN, BSN
Operating Room/Surgical ICU Staff Nurse
Henry Ford Hospital
Detroit, Michigan

Cheryl Barratt, RN, MHA
Managing Associate
Coopers & Lybrand
Chicago, Illinois

Carolyn Bartlett, RN, MS
Consultant
Bartlett Enterprises
Rowley, Massachusetts

Jeannie Botsford, RN, MS, CNOR
Administrative Director
Surgical and Ambulatory Services
Scripps Memorial Hospital
La Jolla, California

Pola Brenner, RN, CIC
Head of Nosocomial Infection Program
Ministry of Health—Chile
Associate Professor, University of Chile
Santiago, Chile

Cindy L. Bata Brumley, RN, CNOR
Operating Room Educator
Baylor University Medical Center
Dallas, Texas

Judith A. Brumm, RN, CNOR
Clinical Nurse III
Operating Room Education
Baylor University Medical Center
Dallas, Texas

Linda Callahan, CRNA, MA
Assistant Director/Education
Kaiser Permanente School of Nurse Anesthesia
Pasadena, California

Tim Cambridge, RN, BS, BSEd
Staff Nurse and Educational Coordinator
Casey Eye Institute
Portland, Oregon

Mary Chiweshe, RN, SCM, OT Diploma
Operating Room Supervisor
Harare Central Hospital
Harare, Zimbabwe

Helen Cluett, RN, MS
Perioperative Nurse Educator
Brigham and Women's Hospital
Boston, Massachusetts

Edward E. Coakley, RN, MSN, MEd, MA
Chief, Operating Room Nursing Services and
Deputy Chief Nurse Executive
Massachusetts General Hospital
Boston, Massachusetts

Barbara J. Crim, RN, MBA, CNOR
Director, Value Management and Education
Methodist Hospitals of Dallas
Dallas, Texas

Nancy B. Davis, BSN, NP, CNOR, CRNFA
Nurse Practitioner, RNFA
Cardiovascular and Chest Surgical Associates, PA
Boise, Idaho

Judith A. Eagan, RN, BS, CNOR
Manager of Clinical Education
Valleylab Inc.
Boulder, Colorado

Anita Earl, RN, BSN
Infection Control Coordinator
Loyola University Medical Center
Maywood, Illinois

Barba J. Edwards, BSN, MA
Nurse Consultant
Corporate Strategies 2001, Inc.
Omaha, Nebraska

Billie Fernsebner, RN, MSN, CNOR
Perioperative Clinical Nurse Specialist
Massachusetts General Hospital
Boston, Massachusetts

Constance Fleming, RN, MA
Nurse Manager Operating Room
Brigham and Women's Hospital
Boston, Massachusetts

Anne Mercurio Fogarty, RN
Staff Nurse Operating Room
Massachusetts General Hospital
Boston, Massachusetts

Kristine M. Gilberg, RN, CNOR
OR Educator/Laser Coordinator
Henry Ford Hospital
Detroit, Michigan

Mary T. Gilley, RN, MS, CNOR
Clinical Coordinator
Section of Colon and Rectal Surgery
Washington University
St. Louis, Missouri

Valarie Giordamo, RN, BSN
Nurse Management Consultant
Concepts in Healthcare Inc.
Ashland, Massachusetts

Nancy J. Girard, PhD, RN, CS
Associate Professor
University of Texas Health Science Center at San
  Antonio
School of Nursing
San Antonio, Texas

Barbara J. Gruendemann, RN, MS, FAAN
Director, Professional Education and Services
Johnson & Johnson Medical Inc.
Arlington, Texas

Diane Gulczynski, RN, MS, CNOR
Nursing Director for Critical Care and Surgical Services
New England Deaconess Hospital
Boston, Massachusetts

Jackie L. Hamblet, RN, MS, CNOR
Coordinator General, Genitourinary, Otorhinolaryngeal
  and Eye Surgeries
Children's Hospital
Boston, Massachusetts

C. Rollins Hanlon, MD, FACS
Professor of Surgery, Emeritus, Northwestern University
Executive Consultant, American College of Surgeons
Chicago, Illinois

Eddie Hedrick, BS, MT (ASCP), CIC
Manager Infection Control, Staff Health, and Safety
University Hospitals and Clinics
Columbia, Missouri

Narelle Hines, RN, RMN, COTN, DNA, M. Admin.
President, Australian Confederation of Operating Room
  Nurses
Deputy Director Surgical Nursing, Operating Theatres
Royal Prince Alfred Hospital
Sydney, Australia

Ann W. Hood, RN, MEd
Value Management Coach
Methodist Medical Center
Dallas, Texas

Mark F. Hulse, RN
Trauma Team Leader
Massachusetts General Hospital
Boston, Massachusetts

Jeanette R. Ives, RN, MS, CNA
Chief, Orthopaedic and Neuroscience Nursing Services
Director, Nursing Support Services
Massachusetts General Hospital
Boston, Massachusetts

Munna Kachhal, PhD
Professor and Chair, Department Industrial and
  Manufacturing Systems Engineering
University of Michigan
Dearborn, Michigan

Aileen R. Killen, RN, MS, CNOR
Doctoral Student
Boston College
Boston, Massachusetts

Frances Koch, RN, MSN, CNOR
Patient Care Director, Operating Room
Presbyterian Hospital of Dallas
Dallas, Texas

Helen Rosen Kotilainen, MA, MT (ASCP), CIC
Manager Infection Control Program
The Medical Center of Central Massachusetts
Worcester, Massachusetts

Dina A. Krenzischek, BSN, RN, MAS, CPAN
Nurse Manager, Same Day Surgery Prep Unit and Post
  Anesthesia Care Unit
The Johns Hopkins Hospital
Baltimore, Maryland

Scott Leavell, BIE
Hamilton K.S.A.
Atlanta, Georgia

Margaret C. Lewis, MSN, RN, CNOR
Clinical Instructor, Surgical Services
Lahey Clinic
Burlington, Massachusetts

Jeffrey S. Mark, AIA
Managing Associate
Herman Smith Associates/Coopers & Lybrand
Chicago, Illinois

Brenda McKonly, RN, MS, CNOR
Nurse Manager, Operating Room
Beth Israel Hospital
Boston, Massachusetts

Elise Michau, Diploma—General Nurse, Midwife,
    Operating Theatre Technique, Nursing Education,
    Nursing Administration
Former Operating Room Inspectress, Cape Provincial
    Administration
Former Operating Room Instructor, Panorama Hospital
    and Medical Clinic
Past President and Honorary Life President, South
    African Theatre Sisters
Panorama, Republic of South Africa

Anne Jenks Micheli, RN, MS
Director, Perioperative Program
Children's Hospital
Boston, Massachusetts

Barbara Miele, RN, BS, CNOR
Nurse Manager, Surgical Services
Grady Memorial Hospital
Delaware, Ohio

Sharon Morselander, RN, MBA, CNAA
Healthcare Management Consultant
Atlanta, Georgia

Ellen K. Murphy, MS, JD, CNOR, FAAN
Associate Professor
University of Wisconsin—Milwaukee
Milwaukee, Wisconsin

Suzan W. New, BSN, RN, CNOR
Program Coordinator, Continuous Quality Improvement
Baylor University Medical Center
Dallas, Texas

Patricia Patterson
Editor, *OR Manager* Newsletter
Denver, Colorado

Judith I. Pfister, RN, MBA
President, Education Design
Denver, Colorado

Clarice J. Powers, RN, PhD
Director of Patient Care—Surgery
St. Joseph Medical Center
Wichita, Kansas

Susan Puterbaugh, MBA, RN, CNOR
Account Executive
Management Recruiters of Monterey
Monterey, California

Barbara J. Randolph, RN, MSN, CNOR
Supervisor, Operating Rooms, PACU, and Ambulatory
    Surgery Programs
Veterans Administration Medical Center
Affiliate Professor, School for Health Care Professions
Regis University
Denver, Colorado

Mary E. Roddick, RN, CNOR
Nurse-In-Charge, Gynecologic Surgery
Brigham and Women's Hospital
Boston, Massachusetts

Monica C. Rupp, RN, BSN, CNOR
Nurse Consultant
Beltsville, Maryland

Jeaney Savickis, RN
Clinical Program Coordinator
Operating Room Services
Baylor University Medical Center
Dallas, Texas

Beta L. Smith, RN
Staff Nurse, Gynecologic Surgery
Brigham and Women's Hospital
Boston, Massachusetts

Maureen P. Spencer, RN, MEd, CIC
Director Infection Control Unit
Massachusetts General Hospital
Boston, Massachusetts

Cynthia Spry, RN, MA, MSN, CNOR
Director of Surgical Services
United Hospitals Medical Center
Newark, New Jersey

Gloria Stephens, RN
Nurse Clinician—Operating Room
St. Paul's Hospital
Vancouver, British Columbia, Canada
Past President, Operating Room Nurses Association
    of Canada

Jody M. Thompson, RN, BSN, CNOR, CNRN
Head Nurse, Neurosurgery and Transplant
Operating Room
Henry Ford Hospital
Detroit, Michigan

Joan A. Uebele, RN, MS, CNOR
Practitioner/Teacher Operating Room
Rush Presbyterian St. Luke's Medical Center
Instructor, Rush University College of Nursing
Chicago, Illinois

Brenda Cole Ulmer, RN, BS, CNOR
Clinical Educator
Valleylab Inc.
Stone Mountain, Georgia
Staff Nurse
Eastside Medical Center
Snellville, Georgia

Carolyn Volpicello, RN, MA, CNOR
Senior Staff Nurse
St. Vincent's Hospital and Medical Center of New York
New York, New York

Kenneth S. Weinberg, PhD
Director of Safety
Massachusetts General Hospital
Boston, Massachusetts

John Wheeler, RN, BSN, CNOR
Clinical Program Coordinator
Baylor University Medical Center
Dallas, Texas

PART I

Instrumentation for Surgery

Chapter 1

Surgical Instrumentation

Key Concepts

- Surgical instruments, which may be considered as actual extensions of the hands, can be classified according to use: cutting, clamping, grasping, and retracting.

- Most instruments are made of stainless steel, an alloy composed of iron, carbon, and chromium. Others are made of titanium. Instruments are designed to be durable and easily cleaned, and are of simple, functional designs that allow sterilization. Some are designed so that they can be disassembled.

- Knowing the names and functions of instruments permits the perioperative nurse to be thoroughly prepared for each procedure, surgeon, and patient. The nurse can then anticipate certain instrument use for specific steps in the surgical procedure.

- Powered instruments make working with bone easier and quicker than working by hand. These instruments cut, drill, or shape bone and drive screws or pins into bone.

- Some rules of thumb for the scrub person handling instruments are: use instruments only for their intended purpose; standardize instrument set-ups; handle instruments sparingly; inspect instruments and identify those needing attention; prepare instruments in order of their use; and count the instruments.

- Care in the decontamination and reprocessing of instruments is essential.

INTRODUCTION

A surgical instrument is an extension of the surgeon's hands. The instrument enables the surgeon to manipulate or excise tissue to create a positive outcome for the surgical patient.

This chapter is a discussion of instrument manufacturing, classification, uses, handling, and processing. The role of the perioperative nurse in organizing, using, handling, and caring for instruments is also covered. The proper care of instruments cannot be overemphasized.

HISTORICAL PERSPECTIVE

Earliest Found Instruments

The earliest known instrument used for a surgical procedure dates back 350,000 years to the Stone Age, when Neanderthal man sharpened a piece of flint to use in trephining (Riall, 1981). Until the middle of the nineteenth century, only about 200 different instruments were being made. By 1900, around 1,000 instruments were identified; today, one manufacturer may have more than 4,500 products in one catalogue and more than 7,500 instruments (Riall, 1983).

Early Composition and Design

Between the Stone Age and the beginning of the "modern period" (Riall, 1982b) in 1865, instruments changed little. They were originally made of materials found in nature: stone, bone, ivory, and wood. Later, different metals were used, including iron, bronze, steel, tin, silver, and gold. A surgeon contracted with a cutler or armorer to make instruments to desired individual specifications. The artisan made instruments as a sideline to the regular work of making knives or guns.

The instrument was a personal statement for the surgeon. Each instrument reflected the nature of the user. During the sixteenth and seventeenth centuries, instruments were ornate and were made of several precious metals. In the sixteenth century, Henry III of England owned an amputation knife with the carved figure of a winged female as the handle (Riall, 1982b).

Anesthesia and Asepsis (The Modern Period)

Two major advances in the medical field affected the design of surgical instruments. The first, in 1846, was the discovery of anesthesia. The ability to perform pain-free surgery on any part of the body led to the need for more variety in instrumentation. Surgeons looked for instruments that could be used inside the chest and abdomen. As a result, the manufacture of instruments increased tremendously.

The advent of asepsis in 1865 was the second major advance affecting instrumentation. Three changes in instrument design resulted. First, a single component, metal, replaced the multiple materials formerly used to construct one instrument. Second, instruments were designed so that the pieces could be taken apart for thorough cleaning. Finally, the ornate designs of previous years gave way to simple, functional designs that could be sterilized.

Traditional materials used to make instruments could not withstand sterilization. New materials were needed so that surgeons could perform aseptic surgery without repeatedly having to replace instruments. Carbon steel with an electroplated finish of silver, platinum, or chrome to prevent rust was the metal of choice. Because of the high cost of the precious metal finishes, nickel plating became more common.

Instruments lasted longer than in the past, but a major problem still existed. Debris collected in the joints of the instruments, making cleaning and sterilization difficult. The instruments needed to be made in two parts so that they could be taken apart, necessitating a reliable connection, a lock, between the two parts.

After several changes in design and several patents, the Aesculap lock emerged as the aseptic lock of choice among surgeons. This lock, patented in Germany, permitted easy disassembly and cleaning of two-part instruments. The two parts were sterilized and reassembled before the surgical procedure. The lock was also easily produced by machine. With the advent of machine manufacturing of the Aesculap lock in 1900, the number of instruments that could be forged in a day rose from 60 to 75 per day to 1,500 (Edmonson, 1991).

Stainless Steel Composition

World War II brought the next major change in surgical instruments. Carbon steel composition gave way to stainless steel manufacturing, developed in Germany. The electroplating that covered carbon steel would chip off, leaving steel exposed to the steam used in sterilization. Water droplets picked up carbon from the instrument and deposited it on other instruments in that set, causing black spots and deterioration of the entire kit.

Stainless steel is an alloy composed of iron, carbon, and chromium. The chromium provides resistance to heat and corrosion, and the carbon provides hardness for sharp edges. Other metals, such as nickel, can be added to the alloy, each addition changing the characteristics of the final product.

Current Trends

Today's trend toward minimally invasive surgery is having a major impact on the development of instrumentation. Many instruments must function through narrow lumens that permit access to closed body cavities. The lumens are often only 5 to 10 mm in diameter. Instruments for endoscopic surgery have a long shaft with handles at one end

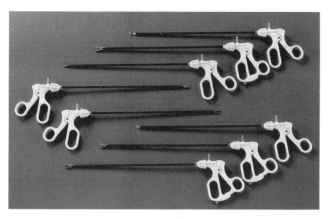

FIGURE 1-1 Various endoscopic surgical instruments. (Photograph courtesy of Ethicon Endo-Surgery, Cincinnati, Ohio.)

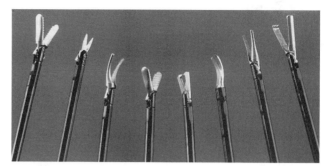

FIGURE 1-2 Tips of endoscopic surgical instruments. (Photograph courtesy of Ethicon Endo-Surgery, Cincinnati, Ohio.)

to control the working tips at the other end (Figs. 1-1 and 1-2). Several endoscopic instruments are shown in this chapter in their respective categories. Although these instruments may look unique, most fall into the traditional categories of cutting, clamping, grasping, and retracting.

INSTRUMENT MANUFACTURING

Physical Properties

Today, most surgical instruments are made from stainless steel. Stainless steel has strength, resists rust, and will hold a sharp edge. Stainless steel is identified by a series number based on the amount of each component metal present. The 400 series has a greater carbon content than found in the 300 series. Depending on its use, a single instrument may be made of more than one type of steel. For example, the cup and shank of a curette are made of a 400 series stainless steel, whereas the handle is produced from a 300 series. The greater amount of carbon in the 400 series permits stainless steel to be ground to a sharper edge, making it hold that edge longer. As in fine cutlery, the knives that are sharpest have the highest carbon content.

Titanium, another metal used in surgical instruments, is 43% lighter in weight than stainless steel, making it suitable for microsurgical instruments. When surgeons operate for hours looking through a microscope, the lighter weight of titanium instruments causes less fatigue. General instruments are not normally made of titanium because of the high cost of the material and labor required in their manufacture.

Process Related to Cost

Manufacturing surgical instruments is an art. Only a few authentic instrument makers remain in business today, working for large instrument-manufacturing companies. An instrument maker is a person skilled in the entire process of designing and creating an instrument. Today, the

process is broken down into specialized steps. These specialists are tool and die makers, forgers, machinists, grinders, and finishers, to name only a few. One instrument will usually be worked on by 25 individuals before it is ready for sale.

Although methods are constantly being improved in the manufacture of surgical instruments, the final steps involve the expertise of the hand craftsmen. The labor-intensive nature of the process, coupled with increased regulatory control of medical devices, creates a product with additional cost implications that guarantee high quality and traceability.

The instrument inventory of an operating room represents an enormous investment over which the perioperative nurse has great control. With proper care and handling, an instrument should last indefinitely and its material and workmanship are guaranteed by reputable manufacturers.

Manufacturing Process

The manufacturer buys stainless steel in long rods or bars. The long lengths are cut into short pieces. Several rough outlines of the instrument are cut, using a pattern. These outlines, called blanks, have only the general shapes of the instrument pieces into which they will be made. Each blank is heated to glowing red in a flame, much the same way a blacksmith heated metal in colonial days. The heated piece is forged with a forging hammer, creating an impression of the instrument piece. The hammer falls onto the steel, forcing it to fill a mold. A three-dimensional form takes shape, with the excess steel flattened around it.

The forged piece, now hardened or tempered from the heating, must be softened (annealed) again so it can be worked. After the softening process has been completed, the precision process of finishing begins. Many of the finishing steps are performed by hand. Machining makes each edge smooth, corners precise, and curves curved. The tips of scissors or clamps must be created by machine. A grinding wheel is used to fine tune the shape and sharpen the edges of sharp instruments.

Scissors and needle holders have inserts made of stellite or tungsten carbide. The inserts withstand the extra wear and contact with harder metal instruments, adding to the life of the instrument. Inserts on needle holders can be replaced to prolong their use.

The various pieces are assembled into a recognizable instrument and given their proper finish. The three common finishes for surgical instruments are bright, dull, and ebonized or blackened. The bright finish is the hardest and longest lasting finish, but it can glare under the operating lights and lead to eyestrain. The dull finish, created with sand blasting, is most popular because of its decreased glare. The ebonized finish is found on specialty instruments, mostly instruments used with a laser. The black finish prevents reflection of laser light to an unintentional target. Gold plating is an additional finish given to the handles of instruments to identify that the instrument has inserts in the tips. The finished instrument is hardened (tempered) again by exposing it to heat. Each instrument is inspected, stamped, or etched with manufacturer and identifying lot number, and put into inventory for sale.

Quality Issues in Manufacturing

The U.S. Food and Drug Administration has become more involved in regulating the manufacturing of surgical instruments to be used in the United States. It requires that the information stamped or etched on each instrument include the name of the manufacturer, the country of origin, and a lot number.

The country of origin refers to the country where the product was finished but does not necessarily mean that the entire instrument was made in that country. Manufacturers may send the forged pieces to another country, such as Hungary or Pakistan, for finishing. The names of these countries are also stamped on the instrument even when the manufacturer is a United States–based company using United States or German steel and forgings. An instrument forged and finished in the United States does not need a country stamp.

The lot number permits the manufacturer to track the entire manufacturing process of each instrument. The origin and composition of the steel, date of manufacture of the instrument, and the persons involved in making it can be determined through the lot number.

The issue of quality must be addressed when evaluating instruments for purchase. Can the manufacturer ensure the purity of the steel used? Does the steel meet the American Society of Testing Materials (ASTM) standards for stainless steel? Is the entire manufacturing process monitored by the company even when some work is done outside the country? Where was the product made and finished? If the company is reputable, this information should be available to the potential buyer.

INSTRUMENT CLASSIFICATION

Importance of Instrument Identification

When the new perioperative nurse begins working in the operating room setting, the seemingly endless array of surgical instruments may seem overwhelming. Identifying the instruments is a fundamental technical skill in perioperative nursing.

Knowing the name (including any nicknames) and use of each instrument is necessary for good communication and a positive patient outcome. Having the correct instrument ready for the surgeon contributes to safe and efficient tissue handling and minimizes trauma. The surgeon need not take his or her attention from the wound when the scrub person is ready with the instruments needed. This level of competence comes with experience, but even the novice can contribute to the efficiency of the procedure by quickly providing the instrument requested. Imagine the outcome of an emergency procedure if the scrub person fumbled for the correct clamp or placed the wrong instrument in the surgeon's hand.

Knowing the names and functions of instruments permits the nursing team to be thoroughly prepared for each patient. When the nurse assesses the patient and develops the plan of care, the need for additional instruments may be determined. When the nurse does not know the range of instruments available, the needs of the patient may not be recognized, resulting in a possible delay at the patient's expense.

Classifications

The four basic categories of instruments are cutting, clamping, grasping, and retracting. Each type serves a specific purpose during the surgical procedure and will be discussed separately.

Cutting

The cutting instruments are used to incise, dissect, or divide tissue. Instruments of this type include scalpels, scissors, rongeurs, and osteotomes.

Scalpels are used to incise the skin and cut through internal structures to expose other structures or to separate tissue for removal. Scalpels usually have two parts: a reusable handle made of stainless steel and a disposable blade. Both knife handle and blade come in a variety of styles and sizes (Fig. 1-3). Not all blades are compatible with every handle. The blade must be attached to a handle before use and may become dull and need to be replaced during the procedure. When a blade is attached or removed, an assistive device, not fingers, is used, to protect the fingers from cuts (Fig. 1-4).

Scissors are used to cut through tissue. They come in a variety of styles (Fig. 1-5) and may be curved or straight, heavy or fine, with a blunt or sharp tip, and long or short. The characteristics of the scissors determine their proper use. Straight scissors are used for cutting suture material, whereas curved scissors are used to cut tissue because the curve enables the surgeon to see the tips of the scissors without the hand getting in the line of sight. Heavy scissors cut strong or tough tissue, such as fascia, but the delicate tissue around a nerve or vessel requires fine scissors. Blunt tips protect surrounding tissue when gross dissection is being performed, but when fine dissection is being performed, sharp tips are needed for precision.

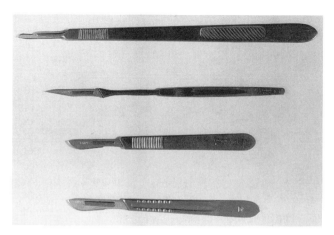

FIGURE 1-3 Knife handles with disposable blades attached. *Top to bottom*, #3 long handle with #15 blade, #7 handle with #11 blade, #3 handle with #10 blade, and #4 handle with #20 blade.

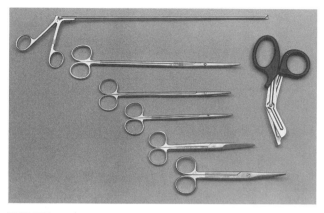

FIGURE 1-5 Various scissors. *Top to bottom*, endoscopic, 10-inch Metzenbaum, 7-inch Metzenbaum, 5-inch Metzenbaum, straight Mayo, and curved Mayo; *right*, utility shears.

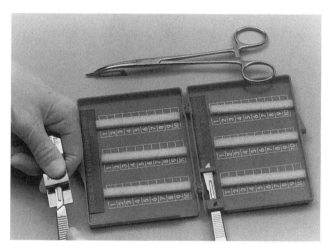

FIGURE 1-4 Assistive devices for attaching and removing blades.

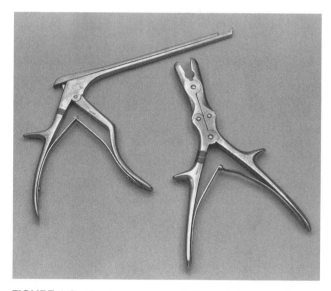

FIGURE 1-6 Kerrison rongeur (*left*), and double-action bone rongeur (*right*).

Long scissors are necessary in deep cavities; short scissors are more appropriate when working with surface tissues.

Rongeurs cut through tissue with a biting action (Fig. 1-6). When the surgeon squeezes the handles together, two sharp cuplike ends come together to bite into the tissue and remove a small section. These are most commonly used on bone or heavy ligament.

An osteotome cuts through bone with a chisel-like action. It is flat with one tapered, sharpened end and comes in several widths (Fig. 1-7). It may be used to scrape tissue off bone or, when tapped with a mallet, it will cut bone.

Clamping

The next major category of instruments is the clamp (Fig. 1-8). These instruments grasp and hold onto tissue. Ratchets on the handles lock together as the surgeon squeezes the handles (Fig. 1-9). When the surgeon lets go of the handles, a clamp will remain closed and stay in place by means of its box-lock action. The closer the han-

dles are locked together, the tighter the tips of the clamp will hold the tissue.

Tips (or jaws) of clamps come in many variations (Fig. 1-10). They are straight, curved, or angled; heavy or fine; and manufactured with or without teeth. The tips also have serrations to produce a firm grip on tissue without crushing it as two smooth tips coming together would do. The characteristics of each clamp determine its proper use.

Clamps are also commonly known as hemostats. Hemostasis is provided in one of two ways. A blood vessel that has been cut and is actively bleeding is controlled by sealing the cut ends between the tips of a clamp. The vessel is then cauterized, tied with a suture (ligated), or left with the clamp acting as a source of pressure, causing natural clotting. Another method of producing hemostasis is ligation and division. As the surgeon encounters a vessel while dissecting tissue, two clamps are placed on the vessel, and the vessel is cut between the clamps. Each end is ligated with a suture.

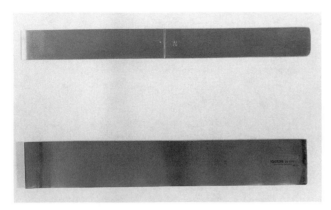

FIGURE 1-7 Curved and straight osteotomes.

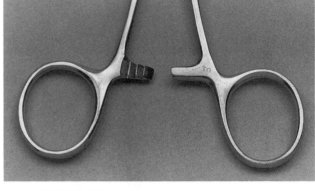

FIGURE 1-9 Ratchets on handles of a clamp.

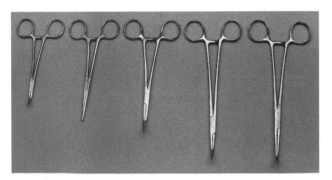

FIGURE 1-8 Various clamps (forceps). *Left to right*, curved mosquito, straight and curved Kelly, Schnidt (tonsil), and right angle.

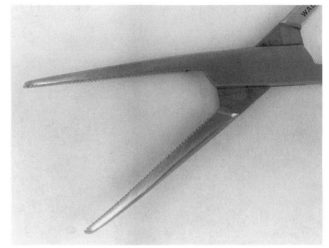

FIGURE 1-10 Serrations on the tips (jaws) of a clamp.

For assistance in hemostasis, ligating clips may be used. Ligating clips are made of metal or are absorbable. The clips are available in several sizes in prepackaged, single-use units.

When "loaded" into ligating appliers (Figs. 1-11,*A* and *B*), ligating clips are a rapid and secure method of hemostasis. The clips can also be used to ligate other small structures such as ducts and tissue. Ligating clips are available in several sizes (each size designed for specific appliers). Clip appliers come in long and short lengths.

Clamps may also be used for holding tissue or sutures for retraction or identification. For retraction, the surgeon places "stay" sutures in the tissue. Attaching clamps to the stay sutures provides retraction to hold the tissue in place. For identification, clamps are attached to tissue or sutures, identifying them for a specific purpose.

A clamp should never be used to attach items to the surgical drapes. Heavy drape material can bend the tips and strain the box lock. If a damaged clamp is used on a vessel, it may spring open unexpectedly and cause unnecessary bleeding.

Grasping

The third basic category of instruments is grasping (Fig. 1-12). Graspers enable the surgeon to pick up and hold tissue. The most common type of grasper is the forceps, but some instruments in the clamping category also

grasp. Another type of grasping instrument is the needle holder, which is designed to grasp needles. Graspers for endoscopic use resemble clamps in that they have a locking mechanism to hold the tips firmly in place.

Tissue forceps are similar to tweezers. Two metal pieces are fused at one end and shaped so that the opposite ends come together when the surgeon squeezes the instrument (Fig. 1-13). The tips of the forceps have several variations (Fig. 1-14). Smooth forceps have simple serrations for holding delicate tissue; toothed forceps have teeth to improve the grip for holding heavier tissue. Another variation is the atraumatic DeBakey tip that holds a blood vessel with minimal trauma.

Several clamps will grasp tissue (Fig. 1-15). The Babcock clamp is especially suited for grasping bowel because its smooth edges and bowed shape will not penetrate or crush the delicate tissue. The Allis clamp will hold slightly heavier tissue because it has serrations along its edges, and the Lahey triple hook and Kocher clamps will hold the heaviest tissue.

The needle holder is designed to hold needles, not tissue. The jaws of the needle holder have inserts etched with a diamond pattern that prevent the needle from rotating or slipping while passing through tissue (Fig. 1-16).

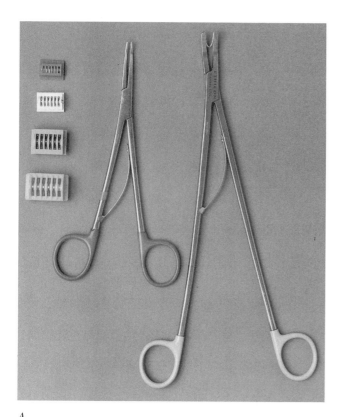

A

FIGURE 1-11 *A,* Ligating clip appliers and various sizes of clips. *B,* Close-up of "loaded" ligating clip appliers.

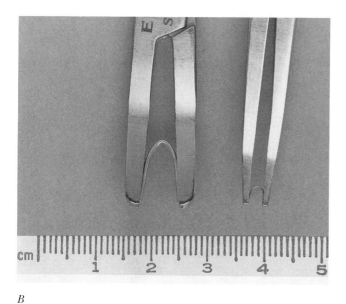

B

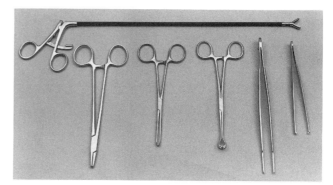

FIGURE 1-12 Various grasping instruments. *Top,* endoscopic grasper. *Left to right,* needle holder, Allis forceps, Babcock forceps, DeBakey tissue forceps, and tissue forceps with teeth.

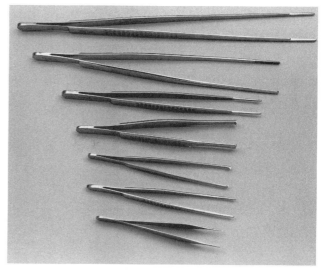

FIGURE 1-13 Various tissue forceps.

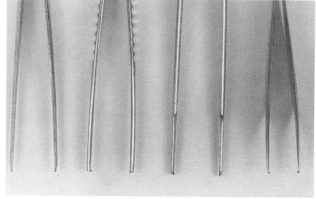

FIGURE 1-14 Tips of forceps. *Left to right,* tissue forceps without teeth, tissue forceps with teeth, DeBakey forceps, and Adson forceps with teeth.

Retracting

The last major category of instruments is the retractor. Retractors expose the surgical field by holding intervening structures out of the way. Some are held by hand (Fig. 1-17); other "self-retaining" retractors will hold themselves in place with ratchets (Fig. 1-18).

Retractor tips vary according to the fragility of tissue and the depth within the body of the structures being

retracted. Some retractors have short blades for surface retraction, whereas other retractors have long blades for deep organ retraction. Retractors meant for holding

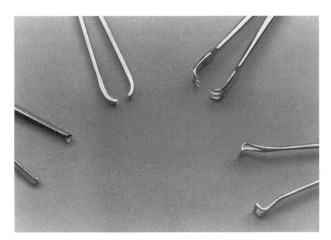

FIGURE 1-15 Tips of grasping clamps. *Left to right*, Kocher, Allis, Lahey, and Babcock.

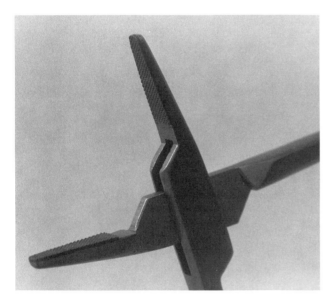

FIGURE 1-16 Tips of needle holder showing inserts.

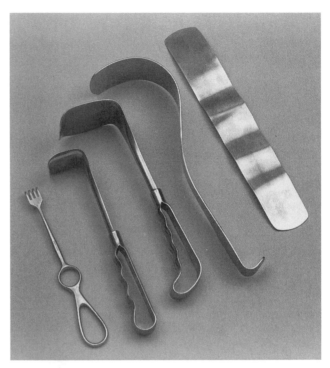

FIGURE 1-17 Hand-held retractors. *Left to right*, rake, Richardson, Kelly, Deaver, and ribbon (malleable).

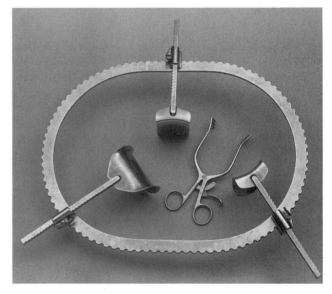

FIGURE 1-18 Self-retaining retractors: Bookwalter and (*on the inside*) Weitlaner.

tough tissue, such as skin or bone, have sharp points. Retractors that hold delicate tissue, such as bowel or liver, have smooth tips and edges.

Powered Instruments

Surgical instrumentation entered the industrial age in the early 1900s when the air motors used since 1800 in industry were made small enough to fit into a hand-held device. Dr. Luck created a circular saw for cutting bone, and the era of powered surgical instruments began (Walling, 1992). Stryker then created an oscillating saw that would cut bone but resist cutting soft tissue (Walling, 1992). These early models had limited use because they were powered from an electrical motor attached to a stand.

In the 1960s, industry began to increase its share in the medical market with the development of the small pneumatic motor. This motor, which works with nitrogen gas, is contained in the handpiece itself and is the standard motor used today (Walling, 1992). Battery-operated motors are becoming increasingly common. The battery pack is charged when not in use and is sterilized immediately before the powered instrument is used. This technique eliminates the need for air power and thus the cord going from the sterile field to the nitrogen source.

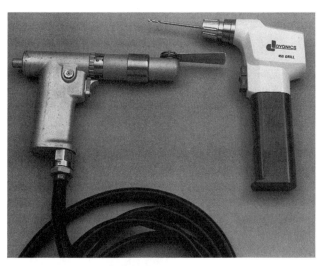

FIGURE 1-19 Air-powered saw (*left*) and battery-powered drill (*right*).

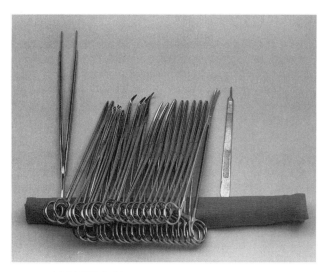

FIGURE 1-21 Deep basic instrument set.

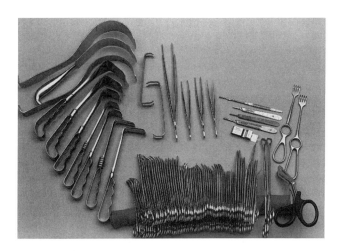

FIGURE 1-20 Major basic instrument set.

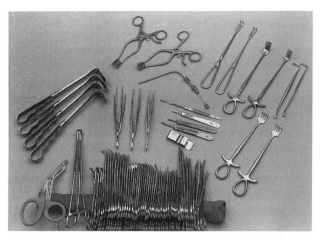

FIGURE 1-22 Minor basic instrument set.

Powered instruments make working with bone easier and quicker than working by hand. Powered instruments cut, drill, or shape bone and drive screws or pins into bone. They consist of a handpiece with an attached saw blade, drill bit, burr, or driver and a source of power (Fig. 1-19). Again, the power source may be nitrogen gas delivered through a cord/hose or electricity generated from a battery pack.

ORGANIZING INSTRUMENTS FOR USE

Assembled into Sets

Instruments are not usually gathered individually for a surgical procedure. This task would be time consuming and could lead to errors. To provide all the instruments routinely used for a specific procedure, they are orga-

nized into sets. The following are some common general surgery sets found in most operating rooms. (1) The major basic set is a general one with instruments that can be used in a major body cavity, such as the abdomen or chest (Fig. 1-20). Additional special instruments can be used with the basic set. (2) The deep set contains longer versions of scissors, forceps, and clamps for use in deep areas, such as the pelvis, or for the obese patient (Fig. 1-21). (3) The minor kit is similar to the major basic kit but has fewer instruments and smaller retractors (Fig. 1-22). This set is for procedures such as repair of a hernia or biopsy of the breast.

Many more instrument sets are available. Each surgical specialty has a variety of sets designed for their basic procedures. For example, the neurosurgical service may have a laminectomy set and a craniotomy set. The ophthalmology service may have a cataract set and a retinal set. Learning the instruments and sets of each service is part of the orientation process for that service. In addition, each surgeon may have a special set of instruments designated specifically for that surgeon.

Creating Standardized Sets

To promote a positive patient outcome from surgery and to ensure that no retained instrument injures the patient, an instrument count is performed for every surgical procedure. To make counting more efficient and accurate, sets of instruments must be standardized. Each set must always have the same type and number of instruments. When the sets are standardized, the scrub person and circulating nurse can count quickly and avoid delays in the surgical procedure.

AT THE STERILE FIELD

Use Only for Intended Purpose

Each surgical instrument must be used only for its intended purpose. Each instrument is used in a precise manner and if used or handled incorrectly could cause injury to the patient or a team member. Scissors for cutting delicate human tissue are not meant to cut sutures or drapes. Using scissors improperly will dull the blades. Dull scissors can cause unnecessary damage to tissue by pulling instead of cutting the tissue. A clamp meant for clamping a blood vessel must not be used to clamp something in place on the drapes. The bulkiness of the drape material can damage the locking action of the clamp.

Setting Up

Standardized set-ups

Many institutions have standardized layouts for the back table and Mayo stand in each surgical specialty. Standardization makes orientation easier and counting smoother and contributes to continuity of care when relieving a team member. The Mayo stand holds the instruments and supplies currently in use (Fig. 1-23). The back table holds items that must be ready but not immediately available (Fig. 1-24).

Handle sparingly

When the back table and Mayo stand are set up, the instruments should be handled the fewest times possible. When an instrument is taken out of the pan or from the circulator, it is put immediately where it belongs on the set-up. A knife blade is attached to the appropriate handle and is placed directly on the Mayo stand. Moving items around unnecessarily adds to preparation time and may delay the start of the operation.

Inspect

While setting up the back table and Mayo stand, the scrub person inspects each instrument for proper function. The instrument should operate smoothly and the box locks hold securely. Ensure that forceps and clamp

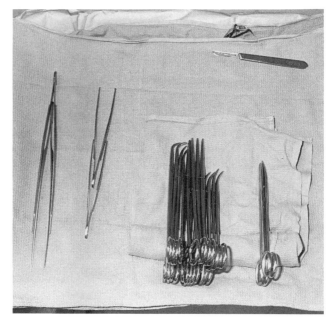

FIGURE 1-23 Mayo stand set-up for a general surgical procedure.

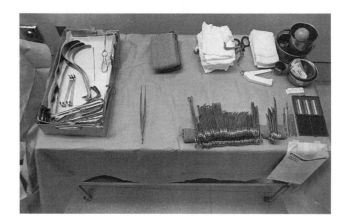

FIGURE 1-24 Back table set-up for a general surgical procedure.

tips meet accurately, screws are secure, and no pieces are missing or parts broken. No light should be visible through the closed tips of a clamp, but closed scissors should allow light to pass through when only the tips are touching.

Identify instruments needing attention

Before or during a procedure, an instrument that needs repair or lubrication is tagged with a label stating the problem (Fig. 1-25). When it is brought to the decontamination area, it can be processed separately and sent for the needed work. Any item sent out for repair must be decontaminated and sterilized before it leaves the institution to protect the person who will be making the repair.

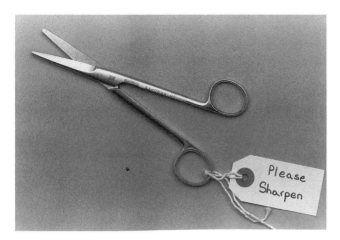

FIGURE 1-25 Instrument tagged for repair.

Prepare in order of use

Preparing the instruments in the order they will be used is a good habit to acquire. Most procedures begin with an incision so the first item needed will be a scalpel followed by clamps or the electrosurgical pencil for hemostasis. Having these ready ensures that the procedure will begin with minimal set-up time. Adequate time is available to prepare for scheduled procedures, but setting up in the order of the procedure enhances readiness for an emergency situation.

Count

Counting the instruments is an essential part of setting up for any procedure. *AORN Recommended Practices* (1994) state "Instruments should be counted on all procedures." Counting helps safeguard against a retained instrument. The scrub person and the circulating nurse count each instrument opened for the procedure before the operation begins. It is helpful to follow a preprinted count sheet for the instrument set(s) (Fig. 1-26). The count sheet can be sterilized in the pan with the instruments so it will be readily available.

Subsequent instrument counts should be taken:

* Of additional instruments added to the sterile field
* Before closure of a cavity or incision that might contain an instrument
* At the time of permanent relief of scrub and/or circulating person(s)
* At the completion of the surgical procedure (AORN, 1994)

During the Procedure

Passing instruments

During the procedure, the scrub person provides the necessary instruments by continually observing the surgical field to anticipate the instrument that will be needed next. An instrument should be in the hand, ready to pass at all times. Passing instruments correctly is a basic skill in scrubbing. Each instrument is passed so that the surgeon can use it immediately with little or no adjustment.

The scrub person should be able to handle and pass instruments with either hand. Often two persons will ask for instruments simultaneously or an instrument is returned at the same time another needs to be delivered. Working with both hands makes handling of instruments easier and more efficient in these situations. With practice, this technique will feel less awkward than relying on only the dominant hand.

Scalpels are passed to and from the neutral zone or directly hand to hand; there are times, however, when hand to hand passing of a scalpel is necessary. When the instrument is passed directly, the knife handle is held from the top and the handle end is placed firmly into the surgeon's hand. The sharp edge of the blade is down (Fig. 1-27). When the surgeon returns the scalpel, be sure the blade is in sight before taking it back to avoid injury.

Use of a neutral zone can eliminate some risk involved in passing sharp instruments. The neutral zone is a designated area on the sterile field where the scrub person and the surgeon place sharp instruments instead of passing them directly hand to hand. Many institutions are making the use of a neutral zone standard practice. The zone may be a magnetic pad, a basin, or a disposable pad with a specifically designated area built in (Fig. 1-28).

Curved instruments, such as scissors, clamps, or clip appliers, are passed with the curve in the same direction as the curve of the surgeon's hand unless otherwise requested (Fig. 1-29). The tips are always visible for safety. These instruments are held at the joint so that the surgeon receives the handles, ready for use.

When the instrument has a box lock, such as a clamp, it is passed with the lock secured so that it does not open before the surgeon has control of the handles. The surgeon will release the lock before using the clamp.

For needle holders or other instruments with ringed handles, the thumb and ring finger are placed into the rings (Fig. 1-30). The ring finger or fourth finger, not the third finger, provides greater control of the instrument. The jaws can be opened farther, and the index finger is free to control the tips. It sometimes takes a conscious effort to learn this skill, but it will make loading needles and cutting sutures more precise.

To prepare needles and suture material for passing, the needle should be loaded on the needle holder so that the tip of the needle will point to the surgeon's thumb (Fig. 1-31). When the surgeon receives it, the needle can be passed directly into the tissue. The surgeon may be left-handed or ask for the needle to be reversed. In this situation, the needle should be loaded on the needle holder in the opposite direction.

Safety

Safety is a high priority when passing instruments at the sterile field. Because the surgeon rarely looks up from the site, the scrub person must use careful and deliberate motions. The instrument is held so that all team members are protected from sharp edges or tips. The instrument is

LAHEY CLINIC MEDICAL CENTER
INSTRUMENT COUNT RECORD

Major Basic

DATE: _____
COUNT #1 CSS TECH: _____
COUNT #2 SURGERY: _____
COUNT #3 SURGERY: _____
RE:MBAS

QUANTITY & INSTRUMENT		COUNT				QUANTITY & INSTRUMENT		COUNT			
		1	2	3	M			1	2	3	M
	Retractors						**Strung Instruments**				
1	Narrow Deaver					2	7" Needle Holders				
1	Wide Deaver					2	8" Needle Holders				
1	Medium Deaver					6	Str. Snaps				
2	Sm.6 Prong Rakes(Shp)					12	Kellys				
1	Narrow Ribbon					6	Allis'				
1	Wide Ribbon					2	Babcocks				
1	Sm. Right Angle					2	Triple Hooks				
1	Med. Right Angle					6	Str. Kochers				
2	Lg. Right Angle					4	Schnidts				
2	McBurneys					6	Rt. Angle Clamps				
2	Richardsons					2	Long Allis'				
2	Strattles					4	Dull Towel Clips				
	Knife Handles					2	Prep Sticks				
2	#3						**Scissors**				
1	#4					1	Str. Mayo				
1	#7					1	Cvd. Mayo				
1	Long Probe					2	7" Metz				
1	Blade Safe					1	5" Metz				
	Forceps					1	10" Metz				
2	Short Smooth					1	Utility Scissor				
2	Short Toothed										
2	Rat Toothed										
2	Toothed Adsons										
2	Long Dressing										

FIGURE 1-26 Standardized instrument count sheet. (Courtesy of Lahey Clinic Medical Center, Burlington, Massachusetts).

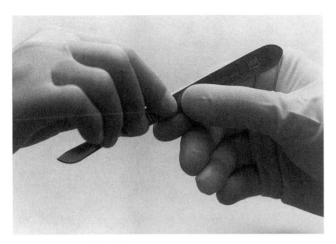

FIGURE 1-27 Passing a scalpel.

passed with firm pressure, and the nurse should be sure the surgeon has control of it before letting go. When the instrument is passed back from the surgeon, the nurse should wait until the motion stops before reaching to take it. Reaching for it too soon can lead to injury from misjudged motions.

Keeping the instruments clean

AORN Recommended Practices (1994) state "Instruments should be kept free of gross soil during the surgical procedure." Debris building up on the instrument can impair its function, making it unsafe for use. Drying blood can cause pitting and damage to the instrument. A radiopaque sponge moistened with sterile water helps to keep the instruments clean. Saline solution should not be used because it can cause pitting and damage. The opposing edges of clamps, forceps, and scissors and external visible areas are cleaned.

Keeping the field organized

Throughout the procedure, it is important to keep the sterile field organized. Place an instrument back in the same location each time it is returned from the surgeon. Knowing where each item is prevents unnecessary rearranging of the Mayo stand or back table, which draws the scrub person's attention from the surgical field. When the surgeon is using a particular instrument frequently, it may be left near the surgical field so that he or she may reach for it without having to ask. Be careful that this instrument is accounted for at all times and that it does not slide off the field. This technique should not be followed with a sharp instrument that could cause injury.

POSTOPERATIVE CARE AND HANDLING

Immediate Postoperative Period

After the surgical procedure, the scrub person is responsible for disassembling the sterile field and preparing the

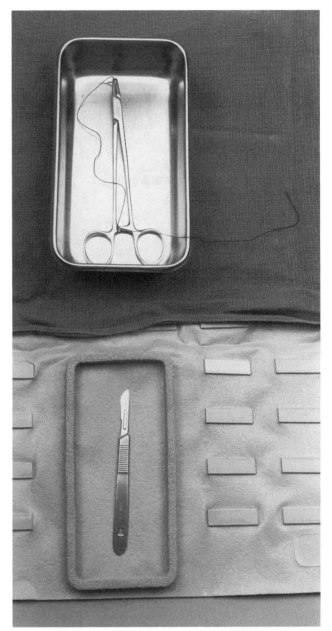

FIGURE 1-28 *Top,* Basin used as a neutral zone. *Bottom,* Disposable magnetic pad with a built-in neutral zone.

instruments for reprocessing. This process should not begin until the patient has left the room. Emergence from anesthesia is a critical time for the patient, and a quiet environment is essential to avoid unnecessary stimulation. The scrub person must also continue to be ready for any emergency.

Confine and contain

The basic principle in dealing with contaminated instruments is to confine and contain. Contaminated items should be confined to a small area and contained in a closed system until ready for reprocessing or disposal. When a case cart system is used, the dirty instruments,

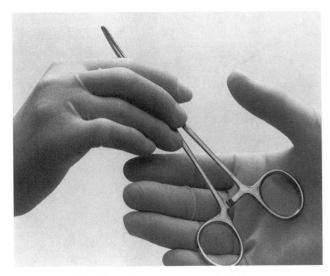

FIGURE 1-29 Passing a curved clamp.

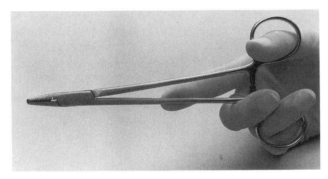

FIGURE 1-30 Holding a ringed instrument.

trash, and linen can be confined within the case cart until the cart arrives in the decontamination area.

Decontamination

AORN Recommended Practices (1994) state "Decontamination of instruments should occur immediately after completion of the surgical procedure." Decontamination renders the instruments safe to handle without personal protective equipment. The four components to decontamination are precleaning, washing, rinsing, and sterilizing. These steps occur before the instruments are reassembled into a set, wrapped or replaced into an instrument container, and sterilized.

The scrub person begins precleaning (or prerinsing) the instruments while still in the operating room. Kneedler and Darling (1990) state that this phase can be accomplished adequately with an enzymatic cleaner. An enzymatic cleaner contains an enzyme that breaks down the organic debris and a detergent that lifts the debris off the instrument. The scrub person places the dirty instruments in a basin containing water and the enzymatic cleaner. As the instruments travel to the decontamination area, the cleaner is working to remove the

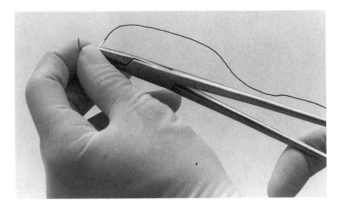

FIGURE 1-31 Loading a needle onto a needle holder (for a right-handed person).

soil. The enzyme is usually effective in 2 minutes, thus eliminating the need for cleaning by hand and added exposure of personnel.

Certain principles apply when the instruments are placed in trays for decontamination. All box locks are opened to permit full exposure to the cleaning agent. All removable parts are removed for exposure. The instruments are handled with care. Heavier items should be on the bottom and lighter items on top to prevent damaging the more delicate instruments.

In the Processing Department

Washing and rinsing

Washing and rinsing are accomplished with an ultrasonic washer, a washer/decontaminator, or a washer/sterilizer. The ultrasonic washer cleans with detergent and sound waves that loosen and remove debris from the instruments, including the locks and joints. After the rinse, the instruments are removed and sterilized before handling. Ultrasonic cleaners do not disinfect or sterilize instruments, only remove debris.

The washer/sterilizer performs a washing/rinsing cycle followed by a sterilization cycle. When the instruments are heavily soiled, both an ultrasonic washer and a washer/sterilizer may be used.

Lubrication

After decontamination, the instruments are lubricated. *AORN Recommended Practices* (1994) state "Instruments with movable parts should be lubricated after every cleaning and according to the manufacturers' written instructions." Lubricating the instruments helps protect them from rust and bacterial growth and keeps them functioning properly. The lubricating solution, "instrument milk," is antimicrobial and water-soluble to permit the steam to penetrate it during sterilization. The instruments are soaked in the lubricant and are dried without rinsing.

Reassembly

Each instrument is inspected as it is being reassembled into proper order in the set. Any instrument that needs repair is replaced. The instruments are assembled according to the standardized count sheet for that particular set. When any instrument is missing, it is replaced from a stock supply. Every attempt should be made to complete the set. When an item cannot be replaced, the set is held from use or a label is attached to the outside indicating what is missing. When an item is missing, it is noted on the count sheet so that the nurses can adjust for the missing item when performing the counts.

Sterilization

When the instruments are assembled into sets and wrapped or sealed in a rigid sterilization container with a chemical sterilization indicator, they are ready for sterilization. Sets that have only metal instruments are steam sterilized in a gravity-displaced or vacuum-type autoclave. Delicate instruments, such as microsurgical sets, endoscopic equipment, or electrical equipment, are gas sterilized with ethylene oxide. A new technology using peracetic acid sterilizes in less time than is required with gas sterilization. This method may be used with items that cannot be steam sterilized between surgical procedures such as endoscopic lenses. The manufacturers' instructions for each type of instrument dictate which method of sterilization to use.

Storage

Sterilized instruments must be stored so that their sterility is protected. Wrapped or containerized sets are stored on open wire racks protected from dust, humidity, and damage. Smaller items are stored in well-labeled containers to prevent overhandling and damage when someone is looking for a particular item.

Outside Instrument Processing

Dorsey (1988) described off-site processing, a new concept in instrument handling. The hospital contracts with an off-site company for the complete process of decontamination, repackaging, and sterilization of its standard instrument kits. The contracting agency uses large-scale industrial equipment in processing and sterilizing, making the service timely and cost-effective. Dorsey reported many benefits with use of this service: Sets are standardized; fewer scheduling and nonavailability problems have occurred; instrument loss is tracked; and better maintenance of instruments and better use of professional staff have been realized.

SUMMARY

Knowledge of the historical background, development, and manufacture of surgical instruments helps the nurse understand their care and handling. Specific instruments are described in relation to their use in the operative techniques of cutting, clamping, grasping, and retracting. How and when powered instruments are used and their sterilization requirements are important factors to know. Perioperative nurses must know how to organize instruments for use, what each instrument is used for and when it will be used during the operation, when and how to hand instruments to the surgeon and take them back, and the postoperative care and handling of surgical instruments. Competence in the identification and handling of surgical instruments is basic to the practice of perioperative nursing and should be a priority for both the new and the advanced perioperative nurse.

REFERENCES

Association of Operating Room Nurses, Inc. (1994). 1994 *AORN Standards and Recommended Practices.* Denver: The Association.

Dorsey, R. (1988). Off-site instrument sterilizing: A new concept. *AORN Journal, 47,* 975–988.

Edmonson, J. M. (1991). Asepsis and the transformation of surgical instruments. *Transactions and Studies of the College of Physicians of Philadelphia, 13,* 75–91.

Groah, L. K. (1983). Surgical instruments. In L. K. Groah, *Operating room nursing: The perioperative role* (pp. 281–296). Reston, VA: Reston Publishing Co.

Gruendemann, B. J., & Meeker, M. H. (1987). Sutures, needles, and instruments. In B. J. Gruendemann & M. H. Meeker (Eds.), *Alexander's care of the patient in surgery* (8th ed., pp. 114–137). St. Louis: C. V. Mosby.

Kneedler, J. A., & Darling, M. H. (1990). Using an enzymatic detergent to prerinse instruments. *AORN Journal, 51,* 1326–1332.

Kneedler, J. A., & Dodge, G. H. (1994). Instruments and equipment. In J. A. Kneedler & G. H. Dodge, *Perioperative patient care: The nursing perspective* (3rd ed., pp. 249–295). Boston: Jones and Bartlett Publishers.

Riall, C. T. (1981). Surgical and medical devices and their origins. Chapter VI: Surgical instruments: Introduction. *Journal of the Operating Room Research Institute, 1,* 52–56.

Riall, C. T. (1982a). Surgical and medical devices and their origins. Chapter VII: Surgical instruments in Greek and Roman times. *Journal of the Operating Room Research Institute, 2,* 81–88.

Riall, C. T. (1982b). Surgical and medical devices and their origins. Chapter IX: Instruments of the London period, 1800–1865. *Journal of the Operating Room Research Institute, 2,* 28–33.

Riall, C. T. (1982c). Surgical and medical devices and their origins. Chapter X: Surgeons and their instruments 1600–1800 AD. *Journal of the Operating Room Research Institute, 2,* 22–24, 61–63.

Riall, C. T. (1983). Surgical and medical devices and their origins. Chapter XVII: Surgical instrument manufacturers. *Journal of the Operating Room Research Institute, 3,* 33–42.

Thro, E. (1983). Surgical instruments: Their care and characteristics. *Journal of the Operating Room Research Institute, 3,* 3–8.

Walling, T. L., Jr. (1992). A brief history of power instrumentation. *Advances in Surgical Power Instrument Technologies, 1,* 7.

PART II

Surgical Procedures

Chapter 2

Ophthalmic Surgery

Key Concepts

- The eye is a highly specialized, complex organ. Therefore, a good understanding of eye anatomy is essential to planning and executing specialty perioperative patient care.

- Pathology of the eye creates visual impairment, with all of its associated problems.

- The development and use of operating microscopes and a wide variety of complex microsurgical equipment have made every part of the eye accessible to the surgeon. The microscopic nature of the equipment and the tissue on which it is used create special problems in the care and handling of this delicate and expensive equipment.

- Because of the protein and other nutrients in the eye's structure and fluids, it is a good growth medium for bacteria, leading to endophthalmitis, which can be life threatening. For this reason, there is a need for strict adherence to asepsis.

- Since even minor movement by the patient can be catastrophic during microsurgical procedures, accurate preoperative assessment and teaching, comfort measures, and pain control are major considerations.

- Many of the medications used in ophthalmology are specific to the eye and are rarely used in other areas of health care, so like the ophthalmic terminology, the medication used requires more effort on the part of the health care professional to learn and understand.

- Correcting children's vision requires early, sometimes emergent, intervention and ongoing evaluation. Because repeated procedures, examinations, and surgeries are often needed, usually with anesthesia, the child may become sensitized to the hospital environment.

- There is as yet no replacement for the eye, but many of the problems associated with the eye and vision can now be treated.

- Ophthalmic surgery is becoming primarily an outpatient procedure, with a majority of procedures done under local anesthesia with minimal sedation.

- Much of the terminology used in ophthalmology is based on Greek, and not on Latin, which creates a language interpretation problem for most medical professionals because of their Latin foundation.

INTRODUCTION

This chapter deals with eye disorders that are amenable to surgical intervention. Included are anatomy, perioperative nursing considerations, instrumentation, and surgical procedural steps.

Because sight is one of the most precious of senses, the perioperative nurse must be vigilant to orientation of the patient, explanation of happenings, and gentle touch and movements. Prevention of infection and adherence to asepsis are prime considerations in ophthalmic nursing.

Historical Background

Eye diseases have plagued mankind from the very beginning of time. Most eye problems lay beyond medicine until the mid 1700s, when doctors began using the scientific method to investigate various medical problems. It was during the mid 1800s that several useful developments in medicine came about that assisted in the treatment of eye problems: the use of anesthetic agents (chloroform and cocaine), the development of antisepsis, and the advent of the ophthalmoscope (to examine the eye and assist in treatment). It was from this time that ophthalmology had its modern beginning, but there were several important landmarks in ophthalmology prior to this period.

The earliest ophthalmic treatment programs were related to people who had normal sight for a period of their lives but had lost it. The two areas of the eye that were easiest to treat and that were directly related to a loss of sight were the cornea and the crystalline lens. According to David Paton (1974) the oldest documented surgical procedure was "couching" of an opacified crystalline lens, known as a cataract, 2500 years ago by a Hindu surgeon named Shusruta. The procedure consisted of striking the crystalline lens with a sharp probe, which pushed the lens into the posterior vitreous cavity. Although the procedure was initially successful, most patients lost their sight and probably their eye and/or their lives, due to infection.

The next major development in cataract surgery had to wait until 1748 when J. Daviel first successfully extracted the crystalline lens. Since this time many other methods have been developed with continually improving results (see section on cataracts).

The other area where early treatment programs were attempted was the cornea. According to Thomas A. Casey and Daniel J. Mayer (1984), documented treatment for corneal scarring dates back to the Egyptians around 1500 B.C., and consisted of rubbing soot in the eye. Another important landmark in corneal surgery was the earliest performed organ transplant, a cornea (between a pig and a human in 1838), which was unsuccessful. The first successful organ transplant, a cornea between two humans, was done in 1905 by Edward Zirm from Czechoslovakia.

From the mid 1800s until the mid 1900s, progress in ophthalmology was slow but steady. The mid 1900s saw the development of operating microsurgical instrumentation and the use of the microscope in the operating room. From the 1950s to the present there has been an explosion in the surgical treatment of eye disorders. Currently there is no area of the eye that cannot be reached and treated surgically.

ANATOMY

The primary function of the eye, a specialized and complex organ, is to focus light waves on the sensory nerve endings of the optic nerve, producing sight (Fig. 2-1). The principal organ of sight is called the globe. It is supported, in the orbit, by the ocular muscles (which are responsible for eye movement) and fatty tissue. The six extraocular muscles are the superior, inferior, lateral, and medial rectus muscles and the superior and inferior oblique muscles. The outer area of the globe is the sclera, which is contiguous with the cornea at the junction of the limbus. The conjunctiva, a mucous membrane, lines the eyelids and the exposed area of the sclera.

The globe is divided into two sections by the lens, the anterior segment and the posterior segment. The posterior segment is further divided into the anterior vitreous area and the posterior vitreous area by the pars plana. The anterior segment of the eye contains the cornea, anterior chamber filled with aqueous humor (fluid), posterior chamber, iris (pupil), lens, ciliary body, and zonules (Fig. 2-2). The posterior segment contains the vitreous body, retina, choroid, sclera, optic nerve, and central retinal artery.

The eye functions like a camera with a compound lens system. Light waves reflected off an object are focused by the cornea, through the transparent aqueous fluid of the anterior chamber and pupil onto the lens, which further focuses the image on the retina, after it passes through the transparent vitreous. The retina acts like a film, recording the image, transforming it from a photochemical reaction to an electrical chemical impulse, which is transmitted by the optic nerve to the occipital portion of the brain, where the impulses are interpreted.

Lids and Lacrimal Duct System

The eyelid consists of the concentric orbicularis oculi muscle, which interdigitates with the frontalis muscle and, along with the oblique-oriented corrugator muscle, gives us our facial expression (Fig. 2-3). The function of the orbicularis muscles is to close the lids.

In the upper lid, the levator muscle comes forward and splits at Whitnall's ligament. The anterior levator aponeurosis connective tissue attaches to the tarsus and sends slivers of connective tissue out to the skin to hold the skin tightly to the tarsus. Its function is to elevate the lid. Just above where this occurs is the eyelid crease. In Asians, connections of the levator slivers to the skin occur further down on the lid and fat slides in behind the orbicularis muscle, eliminating this crease and producing a fuller upper lid.

Behind the levator attachments is the tarsus, which is dense connective tissue, not cartilage. Its function is to

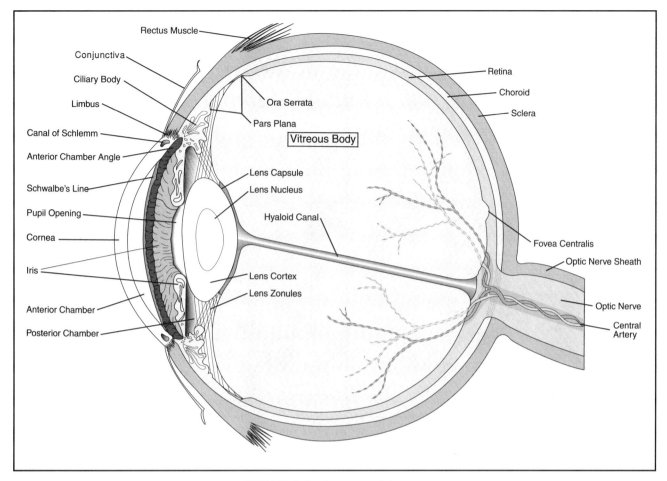

FIGURE 2-1   Anatomy of the eye.

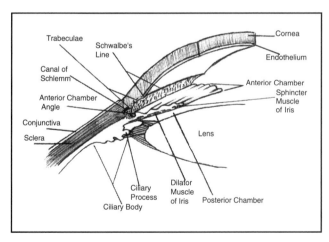

FIGURE 2-2   Anterior segment of the eye.

provide form to the lid and protection for the globe. Behind the tarsus are three types of glands in the lid; the sebaceous meibomian gland, which creates an oily layer on the surface of the tear, thereby preventing the tear from evaporating too fast; the sebaceous glands of Zeis, which are connected to the eyelash follicles; and the sweat glands of Moll.

The inferior layer of the lid is covered by the palpebral conjunctiva. The conjunctiva contains goblet cells that produce a mucin layer that makes the tear spread out over the eye.

Tears are produced by the lacrimal gland and moved across the surface of the eye by the blinking action of the lids (tear pump) where they are drained into the lacrimal duct system (Fig. 2-4) through the puncta and canaliculus. They exit the lacrimal duct system at the valve of Hasner in the nose under the inferior turbinate. The lubricating tear contains lysozyme, which inhibits the growth of bacteria, but the major antibacterial function of the tear is washing conjunctival debris and bacteria into the lacrimal duct system for excretion into the nasal passages. The lids close from the outer canthus to the inner canthus.

The orbit is formed from the junction of the maxillary, temporal, and ethmoid bone plates and the frontal bone.

Cornea

The main refracting surface of the eye is the cornea. It provides a tough outer protective covering along with the sclera. The cornea is composed of four distinct layers: the epithelium; stroma, which includes Bowman's membrane; Descemet's membrane; and endothelium. The epithelium is 5 to 6 cell layers thick and is bordered by Bowman's membrane. Its upper surface is shed and replaced daily. The epithelium will repair itself without scar in a few days because of its high metabolism. It derives its nutrition from the tears, aqueous humor, limbal capillaries, and oxygen diffused across the tear film. The stroma com-

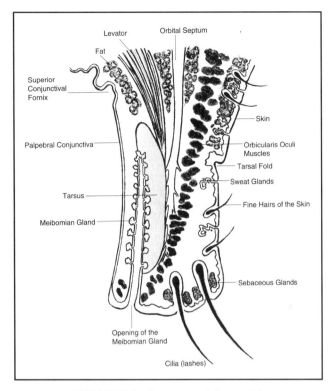

FIGURE 2-3   Anatomy of the eyelid.

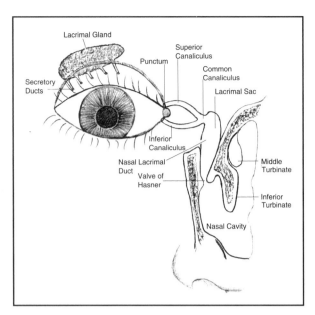

FIGURE 2-4   Anatomy of the lacrimal duct system.

prises 90% of the cornea. It is bordered anteriorly by Bowman's membrane, which is highly resistant to trauma, and inferiorly by Descemet's membrane. The collagen fibrils in the stroma are arranged in layers, or lamellae, which makes split-thickness keratoplasty possible. Trauma to Bowman's membrane or the stroma results in a scar. Descemet's membrane is elastic and increases in thickness with age. It is permeable to solutes but impermeable to chemicals. The innermost layer is the endothelium. It is in direct contact with aqueous fluid.

Uveal Tract

Three structures comprise the uveal tract: the iris, the ciliary body, and the choroid. The iris is an elastic tissue that regulates the amount of light entering the posterior chamber of the eye. It can open as large as $1/3$ of an inch and constrict to .01 of an inch. The ancient Greeks called the opening the pupil, which means "doll," because of the reflection of themselves in the pupil. The color of the iris is caused by melanin and its impurities. Iris colors progress in degrees of color from gray to blue to green to brown. When the iris is cut it seldom bleeds, and the wound may not heal. The iris is innervated by the third cranial nerve, and pain can be felt if the iris is manipulated. It is the anterior extension of the ciliary body and forms the dividing line between the anterior and posterior chambers of the eye. The ciliary body consists of a ciliary process and three ciliary muscles: the meridional fibers, which are longitudinal; the radial fibers; and the circular fibers. The ciliary body performs several functions: the production of aqueous fluid in the ciliary pro-

cess and the contraction and relaxation of the suspensory ligaments of the lens, called zonula. The contraction and relaxation of the lens help to fine focus the light image on the retina.

Lens

The lens of the eye is biconvex, avascular, usually colorless, and almost completely transparent. It is made up of a long concentric lamellar capsule, similar in structure to the stroma of the cornea, called the cortex, and the nucleus. It is 4 mm thick and 9 mm in diameter and consists of 65% water and 35% protein and trace minerals. The lens has no nerve fibers or blood vessels. Its epithelial cells get their nutrients from the aqueous fluid and continue to produce new fibers throughout life. The lens is suspended and manipulated in its position by the zonule ligaments that connect the lens equator to the ciliary body. The ciliary body and the zonules alter the anteroposterior diameter of the lens, which accounts for the focusing power of the lens, called accommodation. The lens receives a focused image from the cornea and further focuses the image on the retina. As the eye ages, the accommodating power of the lens is reduced and the lens acquires impurities that make it opaque. This opacity is called a cataract.

Retina

The retina of the eye is likened to the film in a camera. The chief function of the retina is to record the images focused on it by the cornea and the lens. The retina is the most important part of the eye, with all of the other structures playing a supportive role. It covers the entire inner portion of the posterior segment of the globe, from the ora serrata anteriorly to the optic nerve posteriorly. The ora serrata and the optic nerve are the only two points where the retina is attached to the choroid.

The retina is held in place by the normally transparent vitreous humor, which consists of 99% water, collagen, and hyaluronic acid. The choroid is the inner structure of the sclera, which is composed largely of blood vessels that supply nourishment to the sclera and the entire outer one-third layer of the retina. The inner two-thirds of the retina is nourished by the central retinal artery, which originates from the optic nerve disc. The retina consists of 10 distinct layers, with an average thickness of only 0.4 mm. It is thinnest at the macula and the ora serrata. The macula is a round area, temporally to the optic disc, which is in direct visual axis from the pupillary opening. It consists of cone cells, which are used for detailed vision and color perception. The remainder of the retina consists of both cones and rod cells (used to detect movement and for night vision). The retina is highly developed nerve tissue that is normally transparent but appears gray when it is detached. It leaves the eye as the optic nerve.

NURSING CONSIDERATIONS

General Information

Ophthalmologic surgery once required patients to be in the hospital for weeks, where they were required to lie in bed with both eyes patched and allowed little or no movement. This treatment was necessary to protect the postsurgical eye from rupture and evisceration caused by straining. Many of the early corneal transplants were not even sutured in place. Today, this process has been totally reversed and now virtually all ophthalmologic surgery patients are outpatients and can return to normal activities of daily living (ADL) within days and frequently on the same day as the surgery. The advent of microsurgical suturing, microinstrumentation, and new advances in equipment and techniques has made this possible. This presents the perioperative nurse with a different set of challenges.

The preoperative assessment is an essential tool in evaluating ophthalmologic surgery patients. A review of the patient's chart helps the perioperative nurse to plan nursing actions based on individual nursing diagnoses and patient goals. Baseline laboratory, radiologic, and electrocardiographic data and the patient's current physical status, surgical history, and any preexisting medical conditions must be considered. Because most eye surgery is done under local anesthesia with sedation (except in children), it is important that the surgical team evaluate the patient's ability to lie still under drapes for periods of 1 to 3 hours. Factors involved in this decision might be chronic cough or airway difficulties, claustrophobia, or involuntary motions.

The patient interview provides an opportunity for the perioperative nurse, in cooperation with the surgeon and anesthesia provider, to give the patient valuable information regarding the impending surgery and to obtain additional information for the plan of care.

Preoperatively the patient will receive intravenous fluids and eye drops for pupil dilation. Occasionally a pressure device will be placed on the operative eye prior to surgery to reduce intraocular pressure. Patients should be observed for any untoward reactions to all medications.

Information from the preoperative and intraoperative phases gives the postoperative nurse a baseline for the recovery phase of eye surgery. In addition to monitoring vital signs carefully, the nurse must consider the patient's pain and discomfort as well as nausea. This varies a great deal, depending on efficacy of anesthesia and sedation as well as complexity and location of surgery. Intraoperatively the patient will have to lie still and flat for an hour or longer. Postoperatively the patient may feel stiff and sore. Additionally certain procedures require specific positioning requirements postoperatively. Patients will have less postoperative pain if the head of the bed is slightly elevated. Pain is frequently controlled with acetaminophen or acetaminophen #3.

The manipulation of the eye and the eye muscles during surgery may cause postoperative nausea, which can be treated with medication. Because of the medication used during surgery and the visual impairment from the surgery, all patients will need support help at home upon discharge, so these arrangements should be made prior to admission and verified on discharge.

Ophthalmic Anesthesia

Most ophthalmologic surgery is done under a local anesthesia block. The exceptions to this are patients that would have difficulty lying still and children; these patients may be given a general anesthetic. Most operations are done under intravenous conscious sedation or monitored anesthesia care.

The anesthesia typically begins with the instillation of topical anesthetic drops. The drugs commonly used are 0.5% proparacaine hydrochloride, 0.5% tetracaine hydrochloride, or 2% lidocaine hydrochloride.

The optic nerve can be blocked like all other nerves. Eye blocks are done in two stages. The first stage blocks the eyelid. There are three basic methods to block the lid: the Van Lint method, which blocks peripheral branches of cranial nerve VII in the orbicularis oculi muscle; the Atkinson method, which blocks temporal arborization of cranial nerve VII to the orbicularis oculi muscle; and the O'Brien method, which blocks the main trunk of cranial nerve VII near the temporomandibular joint (Fig. 2-5). The second stage is the retrobulbar block (Fig. 2-6). Local anesthetic agents are injected into the retrobulbar space, effecting anesthesia to the globe and muscular attachments by blocking the branches of cranial nerves III, IV, V, and VI (Paton, 1974). Drugs commonly used for the blocks are 2% or 4% lidocaine hydrochloride mixed in equal parts with 0.75% bupivacaine hydrochloride with hyaluronidase, which is used for diffusing the local anesthetic into the surrounding tissue. Epinephrine hydrochloride may be added to prolong the effectiveness of the agents. As much as 6 ml of these agents may be used in

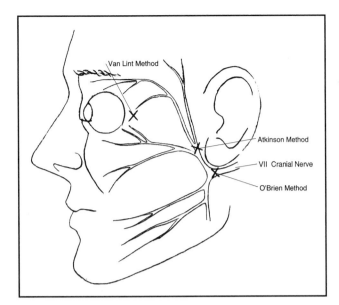

FIGURE 2-5 Methods of facial nerve blocks (lid) in eye surgery.

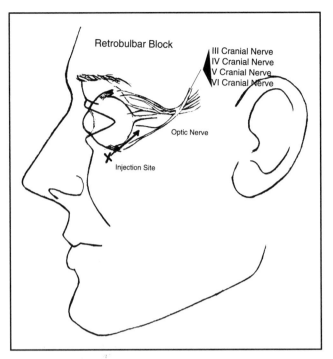

FIGURE 2-6 Retrobulbar block.

the retrobulbar block, and as much as 10 ml may be used in the peripheral tissue. The patient should be informed of a burning sensation, which will pass quickly, and a pressure sensation behind the eye during the retrobulbar injection. The patient's eye is usually massaged after the injection to decrease intraocular pressure and aid in diffusing the agents. The patient is frequently given intravenous medications to aid relaxation and toleration of the discomfort of the block. The patient's vital signs must be monitored throughout the blocks and the surgery. Since the patient is in a semiawake state throughout the procedure, room noise must be kept to a minimum in order to avoid a startled response from the patient.

There are several complications that can accompany the administration of the blocks:

1. The insertion of the retrobulbar needle through the globe, resulting in retinal detachment
2. The injection of the anesthetic agent into the optic nerve, causing irreparable damage
3. Retrobulbar hemorrhage, the most frequent complication

Retrobulbar hemorrhage is controlled with pressure to the globe. Cancellation of surgery should be seriously considered if any of these complications occur.

Medications

Prior to surgery the pupil is dilated to permit the surgeon to see the surgical site behind the iris. Mydriatic (pupil-dilating) drops, cycloplegic (paralysis of accommodation) drops, and scopolamine hydrobromide (iris-constricting and paralysis of accommodation) drops are the most frequently used. Frequently used mydriatic drops are 2.5% or 10% phenylephrine hydrochloride. Mydriatic–cycloplegic drops frequently used are 1% to 2% cyclopentolate hydro-

chloride, 1% atropine, and 0.25% scopolamine hydrobromide. Miotic (pupil-constricting) drops are used to constrict the pupils by the flattening out of the iris; these drops are primarily used in the treatment of glaucoma. Postoperatively, anti-inflammatory agents and antibiotic agents are administered. The most frequently used anti-inflammatory drug is the naturally occurring celestone. The antibiotic is injected between the tenon and the sclera and is used topically as an ointment. The anti-inflammatory drug is injected into the subconjunctiva and is sometimes used as a topical ointment.

Instillation of eyedrops is done by having the patient look upward (to avoid contact with the sensitive cornea), gently retracting the lower lid, and instilling the drops into the cul-de-sac. Blinking aids the dispersion of the medication.

Prepping

Ophthalmologic prepping is different than prepping of other areas of the body. The area to be prepped includes a mucous membrane; soap products should not be used. A 5% iodophor may be the best broad-spectrum, nonreactive agent available, but it needs to be diluted in half with saline. If other agents are used, the eye needs to be cleansed first with the lids closed and then flushed with saline when they are open to prevent the soap from entering the eye.

The eyelashes may or may not be trimmed to prevent them from entering the wound during surgery and/or to reduce postoperative crustation around the eyelid, causing them to adhere together. The lashes should be trimmed if no adhesive drape that adheres the lashes to the eyelid is used during surgery.

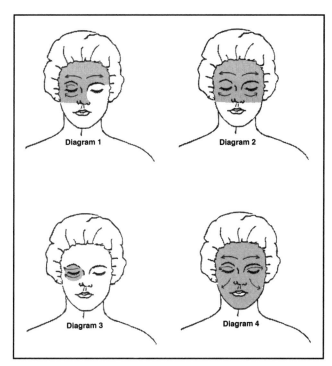

FIGURE 2-7 Eye prepping. (1) Area prepped with prep sponges for surgery on one eye. (2) Area prepped with prep sponges for surgery for Pediatric and for both eyes. (3) Area prepped with cotton tipped applicators. (4) Area prepped with prep sponges for Ocular Plastic procedures.

The prep is primarily painting of the lids, orbital area, and the face (Fig. 2-7). Cotton-tipped applicators are used to prep the eyelashes, the lash margins, and the eyelids, one applicator per sweep of the lashes. Patients should be reminded to remove eye makeup prior to admittance. The eye may or may not be flushed after the prep, depending on the surgeon's preference. A burning sensation is felt if the prep solution is instilled into the fornix of the eye, but no harm is done as long as a soap solution was not used. If a soap solution should get into the eye, the eye should be flushed with copious amounts of saline solution. Soap or alkaline solutions can cause corneal clouding, which may lead to scarring and a loss of vision.

Draping

To prevent the physician from resting a hand on the patient's head, a wrist rest should be employed. The wrist rest should attach to the bed and be adjusted to the level of the patient's ears or to the surgeon's preference.

A head drape is placed just above the eyebrows and folded to cover the ears. A Mayo stand is placed over the patient's upper chest, as close to the patient's chin as possible, to keep the drapes away from the patient's mouth, permitting breathing room. A split sheet is placed on top of the Mayo stand with the splits placed just under the operative eye, across the ridge of the nose, and to the lateral aspect of the operative eye between the drape covering the ear and the operative eye. To hold the lashes

back and to open the eyelids as wide as possible, a plastic drape is applied to the eye using two 6-inch cotton applicators to roll the eyelids back. A disposable plastic Mayo or a sterilized metal Mayo tray is placed on top of the Mayo drape with the instrumentation.

Equipment and Instrumentation

General equipment should include but not be restricted to the following:

Operating microscope

Physician's wrist rest

Direct ophthalmoscope

Schotz tenometer

An ocular pressure measuring device, i.e., a tonopen or Perkins tenometer

Indirect ophthalmoscope

Bipolar wetfield cautery

Headlight

Nikon lenses

General instrumentation should include (Figs. 2-8, *A*, *B*, and *C*):

Tenotomy scissors

Tying forceps

Castroviejo forceps

Serrated forceps

Graefe hook

Beaver knife handle

Eyelid speculum

Vannas scissors

Westcott scissors

Nonlocking needle holder

Locking needle holder

Specialized instruments are introduced later in this chapter. Due to the delicate nature of these instruments great care should be taken when handling them. A container system should be used to protect the instruments when not in use. Periodic inspection of the instruments should be done under magnification to ensure their working order.

An adult intravenous tubing with extension and a 18-gauge blunt needle can be used for suction. Micro eye spears are used to absorb any serous fluid, keeping the incisional site dry. A bipolar wetfield cautery should be available to control bleeding. The bipolar cautery should be used in a wet field with irrigation to reduce charring and adhesions and to reduce thermal damage to the eye.

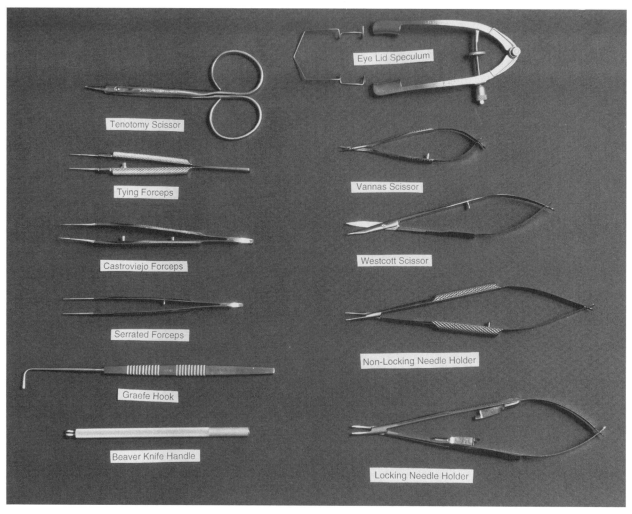

A **FIGURE 2-8** *A, B, C:* Basic instrumentation for ophthalmic surgery.

Dressings

Eye dressings are used to protect the eye and absorb any drainage or tears. Eye pads (occasionally with metallic shields for extra protection) are the most common eye dressings and are secured with tape.

OCULOPLASTIC PROCEDURES

Oculoplastic surgery involves the eyelids, lacrimal duct system, and the orbit.

Lid Disorders

Perioperative nursing considerations

Lid disorders are among the most common of all ocular problems. Fortunately, most of these problems can be corrected in the physician's office. Bacterial inflammation of the glands of the lid rarely requires surgery but is the most common eye problem.

Closely associated with bacterial infection is the chalazion, which is a sterile granulomatous inflammation of the meibomian gland. Most chalazions are surgically removed in the physician's office but occasionally will require an operating room setting.

Other eyelid problems are related to positional defects of the lids, which are entropion, ectropion, and ptosis. *Entropion* is defined as the inward turning of the lid. It usually affects the lower lid but can also affect the upper lid. When the lids turn inward the lashes scrape across the cornea with each blink of the eye, eventually causing a corneal ulcer. Surgery is performed on the skin and orbicularis oculi muscle to pull the lashes outward, and/or cryotherapy is used to freeze and remove the lashes. The freezing of the lash margin destroys the lash follicle, preventing regrowth of the lashes, and is the preferred method of treatment.

Ectropion is the turning outward of the lid. It is usually caused by relaxation of the orbicularis oculi muscle following Bell's palsy or as a result of the normal aging process. Exposure of the underlying conjunctiva will lead to

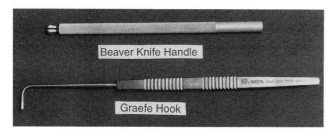

B

keratitis. Marked ectropion is surgically treated by shortening the lid horizontally. Mild ectropion can be treated by deep electrocautery 4 to 5 mm from the lid margins. The resulting scar formation will draw the lid up to its normal position. This treatment program is usually done in the physician's office.

Ptosis is the drooping of the lid and may be congenital or acquired. Congenital ptosis is usually caused by the failure of the levator muscle to develop. Acquired ptosis can be caused by mechanical failure, such as the weight of the lid or trauma; myogenic by disease, such as muscular dystrophy or myasthenia gravis; or by neurogenic factors, such as the interference of the third cranial nerve that innervates the levator muscle. The treatment program will be based on the cause of the ptosis and the severity of the problem. Acquired ptosis has been associated with loss of the superior visual field in primary gaze. Many patients complain of difficulty reading or performing other visual functions in the reading gaze. Patients with ptosis exhibit the clinical sign whereby the ptotic upper eyelid goes further down than normal in reading gaze (Patipa, 1992).

The patient with ptosis is evaluated by measuring the marginal reflex distance (MRD) and the edge of the lid. The marginal reflex distance is determined by shining a light on the cornea; where it reflects back is called the marginal reflex. If the marginal reflex distance is 12 to 15 mm, a brow fixed levator procedure is performed. When the MRD is 5 to 8 mm, a levator resection is performed. If the MRD is less than 4 mm, a fascia lata sling is performed. And if the patient is under the age of 3, a suture sling is used temporarily until the child is 3 or older and has produced the fascia needed to do the sling. If the levator muscle is not completely paralyzed, resection or shortening of the muscle is the procedure of choice. For absence of the levator muscle or complete paralysis, a substitute is necessary. The procedure to correct this problem is called a fascia lata sling or, in children under the age of 3, a suture sling. The fascia connects the tarsus to the frontalis muscle, so when the eyebrow is raised, the lid will elevate.

Ptosis repair

Key steps

1. Fascia lata is harvested from the patient's leg or abdomen with a fascia lata stripper, or a free graft is dissected free with a toothed forceps and scissors.

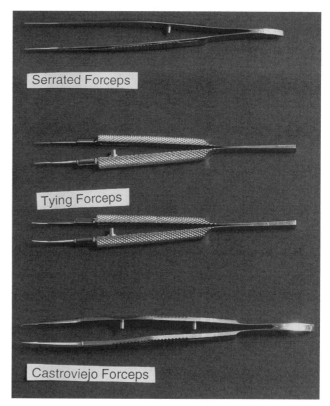

C

2. The incision is usually made just superior to the lashes. Blunt and sharp dissection is used to reach and clear the tarsus.
3. A free needle with an eye large enough to feed the fascia lata or suture is used to feed the sling material through the tarsus and the frontalis muscle at the same time.
4. A heavy nonabsorbable suture is substituted for the fascia lata in children under the age of 3 because their fascia is not well developed yet and a long enough strip cannot be taken. This procedure is called a suture sling. Tissue bank fascia is not used because it is not strong enough and because of the possible problems with hepatitis, HIV, and tissue rejection.
5. Absorbable suture is used to close the wound in two or three layers.

Lacrimal Duct Disorders

Perioperative nursing considerations

The lacrimal duct system begins at the lateral superior aspect of the orbit with the lacrimal gland, which secretes the tears, through the superior conjunctival fornix (see Fig. 2-4). The tears are squeezed across the cornea by the blinking of the lids and are drained into the superior and inferior canaliculus from the superior and inferior punctum. The canaliculi join and drain into the lacrimal sac. The lacrimal sac drains into the inferior meatus beneath the inferior turbinate bone, where the tear is absorbed (see Fig. 2-4). Infections, both chronic and acute, most commonly occur in infants and in adults over age 40. The infections cause a blockage of the canaliculus, which is cleared with lacrimal duct probing and topical antibiotics. If the infections are not treated or chronic infections cause a scarring of the lacrimal duct system, more extensive surgery is needed (dacryocystorhinostomy, or DCR).

Dacryocystorhinostomy

Key steps

1. A 20-cm incision is made on the nasal side of the orbital rim.
2. Blunt and sharp dissection is carried down to the periosteum, which is then scraped off the lacrimal bone with a semisharp periosteal elevator.
3. The anterior lacrimal bone crest is opened with a drill or chisel and enlarged with bone punches or rongeurs.
4. The lacrimal sac is probed and opened, usually with a number 11 knife blade.
5. The opening of the lacrimal sac can be sutured to the nasal mucosa with absorbable suture or left as is.
6. If the lacrimal sac is completely closed, it can be bypassed and an opening of the tear sac higher into the nasal cavity is made.
7. A stent is placed through the lacrimal duct drainage system to keep the system open while epithelium forms around it, creating a new opening. The stent will remain in place for about 6 weeks.
8. The wound is closed in three or more layers with absorbable suture.

A variation of this procedure is the conjunctivodacryocystorhinotomy (CDCR). This procedure becomes necessary because the lacrimal sac has been destroyed and must be recreated, or the canaliculi are absent.

Conjunctivodacryocystorhinotomy

Key steps

1. Conjunctiva is taken from the lower lid and sutured to the nasal mucosa after the DCR is completed to form the lacrimal sac.
2. The conjunctiva is closed with a rapidly absorbing suture.
3. If the canaliculus cannot be kept open or is absent, a permanent stent in the form of a Pyrex tube must be placed. If the Pyrex tube is used, the patient will need to be instructed on how to put the tube back in if it falls out, how to clean the tube, and how to hold the tube in case of sneezing.

A new approach to a DCR is the use of an endonasal laser to open a new pathway into the lacrimal sac and the use of endoscopic equipment to do the procedure intranasally. This eliminates the external incision and scar, decreases the amount of discomfort, provides hemostasis, and increases the healing time, for less cost. A 20-gauge fiberoptic light pipe is passed through the canaliculi into the medial lacrimal sac. Using a nasal endoscope, the transilluminated area is then treated with an argon laser that is delivered through a 300-μm quartz fiberoptic laser catheter (Christenbury, 1992).

Orbital Disorders

Perioperative nursing considerations

The wall of the orbit is composed of thin bone plates of the sphenoid, maxilla, ethmoid, and frontal bones. The two leading causes of problems to these bones are traumatic fracture of the orbit and tumor growth, usually originating from the sinuses. In both cases the support structure of the bones must be reconstructed or the globe will sag. If, as in the case of a traumatic fracture, the bones are present, they are generally reapproximated and wired back together. If the bone is missing, it must be replaced with bone taken from another area of the body and sculpted, or a wire mesh covered in fascia is used. Care must be taken during this surgery that excessive pressure is not applied to the globe for better visualization of the surgical site and that the rectus muscles that control eye movement are not severed.

Orbital surgery

The surgical treatment of the bones of the orbit usually entails a multidiscipline approach with the otorhinolaryngologists doing the sharp and blunt dissection down to the bones and closure from the nasal side. If the problem is small and can be done from the orbit, the oculoplastic surgeon will do it. A decompression of the orbit may be necessary for severe cases of exophthalmos caused by Graves' disease.

Key steps

1. The ethmoid and sphenoid bones at the back of the eye are fractured and the sinus behind them is cleaned out with a Takahashi rongeur.
2. The lateral orbit of the frontal process of the zygomatic bone is fractured, removed, reshaped, and reinserted superiorly to its original position.
3. The bones are plated in place, and the skin is closed.

Postoperatively, patients frequently develop diplopia, both horizontal and vertical, which is induced by restrictive extraocular myopathy. This problem is due to the prolapse of the orbital soft tissue into the opened antral and ethmoidal sinuses (Garrity et al., 1992). These patients will usually return for strabismus surgery.

Optic Nerve Sheath Decompression

Perioperative nursing considerations

Patients with progressive nonarteritic ischemic optic neuropathy (NAION) (occurring most commonly in middle-aged overweight females) or who have pseudotumor cerebri may need decompression of the optic nerve. NAION typically presents with sudden, often profound visual loss from anterior optic nerve infarction. In up to 25% of affected patients' visual acuity continues to worsen 1 to 4 weeks after onset of symptoms. The dynamics of evolving vision loss seen in progressive NAION may relate to progressive ischemia and blocked axoplasmic transport (Kelman & Elman, 1991).

In pseudotumor cerebri, the basic underlying problem is increased pressure on the optic nerve created by increased cerebrospinal fluid (CSF) pressure.

Key steps

1. An incision is made in the lateral conjunctiva with Westcott scissors and a small-toothed forceps.
2. The lateral rectus muscle is isolated and a suture is placed and cut to provide a clear view of the posterior orbit.
3. The optic nerve is located with Desmarres retractors, and cotton-tipped applicators are used to retract the orbital fat.
4. Blood vessels are removed from the optic nerve with a blunt nerve hook.
5. The optic nerve sheath is incised with a new pointed knife blade and permitted to drain.
6. The rectus muscle is reattached to the globe, and the conjunctiva is closed with an absorbable suture.

All patients show marked improvement in visual acuity following surgery, according to Kelman and Elman (1991). The mechanism by which optic nerve sheath fenestration produces resolution of papilledema in pseudotumor cerebri remains controversial. The two main hypotheses are that it (1) creates a CSF drainage site, or (2) it causes scar tissue proliferation at the incisional site, which occludes the subarachnoid space in the area and forms a barrier that "protects" the optic disc from elevated CSF pressure (Hamed et al., 1992). Complications associated with optic nerve decompression include central retinal artery occlusion, tonic pupils, intraoperative bleeding from trauma to posterior ciliary arteries, and transient diplopia (Kelman & Elman, 1991).

Removal of the Globe

The removal of the globe may become necessary because of painful blind eyes, tumors, or trauma. Three methods for dealing with these problems are: exenteration, evisceration, and enucleation.

Exenteration is done for evasive tumor of the lids or globe that extend into the orbital area. The entire contents of the orbit are removed, with extensive plastic reconstruction required. *Evisceration* is the removal of the contents of the globe while preserving the sclera and its muscular attachments. Specialized evisceration spoons are used for this procedure. A prosthesis is placed in the wound to maintain the shape of the eye. The sclera is closed over the prosthesis, with the conjunctiva closed over the sclera. A conformer is placed under the eyelids to maintain the space until the swelling subsides and an

artificial eye is created. The advantage of this method is the natural attachment of the eye muscles, thereby causing normal eye movement. *Enucleation* is the total removal of the diseased globe along with a portion of the optic nerve.

Enucleation

Key steps

1. A circumferential conjunctival incision is made at the limbus to preserve as much conjunctiva as possible.
2. The rectus muscles are isolated, sutures are placed for reattachment; the muscles are cut at the global attachment point.
3. The optic nerve is located with the enucleation scissors and either clamped with a right-angled clamp or cut with the enucleation scissors.
4. Pressure needs to be applied to the central retinal artery for 5 minutes. The enucleated globe and optic nerve need to be examined to be sure they are intact. If the enucleation is being done for a tumor, the globe must be inspected to be sure the tumor has not infiltrated the orbit.
5. After bleeding is controlled, a prosthesis is fitted into the socket.

In the past 100 years, there has been continued improvement in the surgical technique of enucleation and in the method of rehabilitating the anophthalmic socket. Orbital implants for sockets of enucleated eyes were introduced in 1886 by Frost and since then, there have been numerous modifications of orbital implants to provide continually improved cosmesis and motility of the overlying prosthesis (Shields et al., 1992).

A large number of globe prosthetics are on the market. They are made of glass, silicone, plastic, tantalum mesh, and hydroxyapatite. The major problem with most orbital prosthetics is migration, extrusion, and coupling of the implant to the prosthesis. Hydroxyapatite is the implant of choice because of fibrovascular ingrowth into the implant holding it in place.

6. The hydroxyapatite is covered with donor sclera, which is adjusted to the size of the implant, and the edges are sutured together.
7. The superior surface of the implant is scraped flat with a new knife blade for later insertion of an artificial eye.
8. Four small holes are cut into the sclera at the 12, 3, 6, and 9 o'clock positions for attachment of the rectus muscles.
9. Tenon's capsule is closed in two layers over the implant.
10. The conjunctiva is closed with absorbable suture.
11. A conformer is placed under the eyelids to maintain the space until the swelling goes down and an artificial eye is created. In 6 months a technetium-99 scan is done to see if the hydroxyapatite is vascularized.
12. If it is vascularized, a hole is drilled into the hydroxyapatite for the placement of the artificial eye where the visual axis should be.

13. A temporary peg is placed for 3 to 4 weeks to permit healing.
14. The peg is exchanged for a permanent pin, and the prosthesis is placed. Hydroxyapatite is the material of choice for extruded implant replacement.

The complications of the use of the hydroxyapatite implant are few. The implant allows motility of the artificial eye with few postoperative problems. It seems to be a well-tolerated integrated implant and is a base for future advancements in the rehabilitation of the socket of an enucleated eye. This implant provides the patient with satisfactory cosmesis and personal adjustment to living with an artificial eye (Shields et al., 1992).

STRABISMUS CORRECTION

Perioperative Nursing Considerations

The full definition of normal vision includes 20/20 visual acuity and the ability to use both eyes together, called binocular vision. Binocular vision sends the brain two slightly different views of any object on which the eyes focus. The brain then fuses the information transmitted by both eyes into a single image. This fusion makes normal three-dimensional vision possible. At birth an infant's eyes do not fix simultaneously on a single object. During the first year, most children develop the ability to focus on objects, hold both eyes parallel, and see the world in three dimensions. However, in some children, during early childhood, the eyes stop working together. This lack of coordination of the extraocular muscles prevents the eyes from looking at the same object at the same time. This problem is called strabismus. Amblyopia, a condition in which normal vision fails to develop in an eye despite the absence of disease or refractive error, often accompanies strabismus. For unknown reasons, the amblyopic eye sends a poor image to the brain. To protect the normal eye's clear image, the brain suppresses signals from the amblyopic eye. Double vision or diplopia results when the amblyopic eye turns inward or outward and focuses on an object different than the eye aimed straight ahead. The brain does not tolerate double vision so the image of the strabismus eye is often suppressed. As a result the eye does not "learn to see." Corrective surgery is performed to change the relative strength of individual muscles, therefore improving coordination.

Treatment should begin as soon as the diagnosis is made in order to ensure the development of the best possible visual acuity with good cosmetic result and to increase the chance for normal binocular visual function. The action of the extraocular muscles is influenced by the location of their insertion on the globe. The muscles do not act independently but must be coordinated with the opposing muscle. When one muscle contracts, the opposite, or antagonist, muscle must relax in order to produce smooth eye movement. A thorough understanding of these anatomical relationships forms the basis for a logical approach to extraocular muscle surgery.

The lateral rectus muscle abducts the eye and the medial rectus muscle adducts the eye. The other ocular muscles have both primary and secondary functions regarding elevation, depression, intorsion, and extorsion according to the position of the eye. Corrective extraocular muscle surgery for strabismus falls into three main categories:

1. Strengthening of a muscle by resecting the muscle or tendon
2. Weakening of the muscle by recessing the muscle on the globe
3. Transplanting a muscle to improve the rotation of a paralyzed muscle

Resection/recession of eye muscle

Key steps

1. Two bridle sutures are placed through the sclera at the level of the limbus. The sutures are used to expose the operative site.
2. The conjunctiva is incised with a toothed forceps and Westcott scissors over the muscle to be corrected.
3. The muscle is grasped with a large muscle hook.
4. A cotton-tipped applicator is used to clean and strip the muscle.
5. A Jameson muscle hook is inserted to hold the muscle while sutures are placed or the muscle is cut.

Resection

1. A caliper is used to measure the amount of muscle to be resected.
2. A Jameson muscle clamp is placed on the inside edge of the caliper.
3. The muscle is cut at its insertion point on the sclera, leaving a small stump.
4. Bleeding is stopped with cautery.
5. Two double-armed absorbable sutures are placed through the muscle behind the clamp.
6. The clamp is removed and the muscle superior to the suture is crushed with a hemostat and trimmed with Westcott scissors.
7. The muscle is stretched and reattached to the muscle stump on the sclera with the double-armed suture placed earlier.
8. The conjunctiva is closed with absorbable suture.

Recession

1. Two single-armed sutures are placed at the upper edge of the muscle.
2. The suture and the muscle clamp are held in one hand and the muscle is cut with Westcott scissors.
3. A caliper is used to measure the amount of recession on the globe.
4. The suture is placed through the superficial sclera at the recess point, and the muscle is reattached.
5. The conjunctiva is closed with absorbable suture.

The amount of adjustment is determined by tables developed over time and an examination used to determine the line of sight for the strabismus patient.

This surgery is normally done on children up to the age of 6 years when the neural pathways and receptors for sight become permanently established. After the age of 6 years the surgery is done mostly for cosmetic reasons. Extraocular muscle procedures are done in adults for the following reasons: diseases such as exophthalmos, Bell's palsy, muscular dystrophy, trauma to the eye with muscle injury, untreated childhood strabismus or unsatisfactory treatment in childhood, and muscular paralysis from a stroke. If the disorder is not corrected in early childhood, the nondominant eye, although fully functional, will essentially be blind.

The manipulation of the rectus muscle will usually cause transient bradycardia, which can be countered with atropine given intramuscularly early, or intravenously at the time of the attack. If the bradycardia is severe, the surgeon may need to stop manipulating the muscle until the heart rate returns to normal. The bradycardia is thought to be caused by the innervation of a branch of the vagus nerve.

CORNEAL PROCEDURES

Perioperative Nursing Considerations

The cornea's endothelium has an active sodium-pumping mechanism that draws water from the stroma of the cornea. If the endothelium is damaged, the sodium pump is damaged and edema results, creating a swollen, clouded cornea. The cornea has no blood supply, which prevents an immunologic response to foreign tissue. This phenomenon permitted the first successful human tissue transplantation in 1905 (Casey & Mayer, 1984). The first transplants in the United States were square and rarely sutured in place or were kept in place with suture bolsters attached to the sclera but not to the cornea. With the advent of better microsurgical instrumentation and microscopic suture in the 1950s, successful corneal transplantation became common. According to Casey, disorders that can lead to a corneal transplant are:

1. Keratoconus, a conical protrusion of the center of the cornea causing a thinning of the cornea and astigmatism
2. Fuchs' dystrophy, a gradual opacification of the stroma and a thickening and wart-like surface of Descemet's membrane
3. Corneal dystrophies, localized deposits of abnormal material disrupting the normal stroma arrangement
4. Herpetic keratitis, a viral infection of the cornea causing stromal scarring
5. Congenital endothelial dystrophy, a milky appearance of the corneal stroma with two to three times the normal thickness
6. Posterior polymorphous dystrophy, the formation of blister-like lesions in Descemet's membrane

7. Interstitial keratitis, bacterial, fungal, or yeast infections
8. Trauma
9. Aphakic bullous keratopathy, damage to the endothelium following cataract surgery

Corneal transplants

Before a corneal transplant can be done, cadaver corneal tissue must be obtained, tested, and preserved (Casey & Mayer, 1984). An eye bank that effectively screens the donor and its eye tissue for conditions that would prohibit its use is needed. Some of the indicators that would eliminate the donor tissue from being used are bacterial and fungal infections, any viral infection such as Creutzfeldt-Jakob's disease or AIDS, rabies, syphilis, hepatitis, diabetes, intrinsic eye diseases, death from unknown causes, some forms of leukemia, and Hodgkin's disease. After the death of the donor, the eye bank has 6 hours to procure the cornea before necrosis begins. The cornea is trephined at the level of the limbus with a 2.5- to 3-mm rim of scleral tissue. The donor eyes and cornea should be kept as cool as possible after death to slow metabolism and prevent necrosis between the time of death and the procuring of the cornea. The cornea is taken under sterile conditions and placed in a sterile glass or plastic container containing storage medium. The endothelial side of the cornea is never touched and is placed facing up in the bottle to prevent damage. The bottle is capped and placed in a cooler with ice. The eye bank will need to evaluate the corneal tissue in the lab and grade the tissue for transplantation. Each layer of the cornea is evaluated and graded separately. Short-term storage in the storage medium will preserve the cornea for up to seven days. If a suitable recipient has not been found during this period, the cornea can be cryopreserved. Before cryopreservation of the cornea, it should be run through special solutions before being submerged in liquid nitrogen at −197°C. When a suitable recipient is found, surgery is scheduled as early as possible.

There are two major techniques for transplanting corneal tissue, full-thickness penetrating keratoplasty and partial-thickness lamellar keratoplasty. The full-thickness penetrating keratoplasty is the most common form of transplant. Figure 2-9 shows specialized instruments used in keratoplasties.

Penetrating keratoplasty

Key steps

1. The scrub person sets up an independent table for cutting the donor corneal button. This table should be draped using sterile technique and have a toothed forceps, the trephine requested by the surgeon, 6 micro eye spears, a 3-ml syringe, and an individual container of balanced salt solution available.
2. The recipient eye is prepped and draped in the normal manner.
3. A ring is sutured to the sclera just inferior to the corneal scleral junction to prevent the sclera from collapsing during surgery.

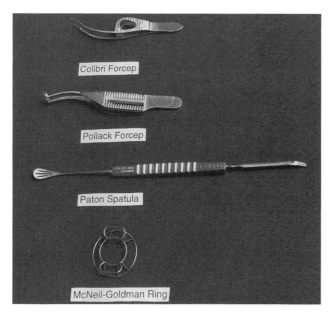

FIGURE 2-9 Keratoplasty instruments.

4. A McNeil-Goldman ring has the ability to hold the lids back as well as support the sclera. Care must be taken not to place tension on the cornea with the ring because it will alter the graft results.
5. The size of the corneal button is determined by a caliper; the appropriate trephines are requested. The donor button is cut 0.5 mm larger than the recipient cornea. The most frequently requested trephines are 7.7 mm for the donor and 7.5 mm for the recipient. After the trephine size has been determined, the recipient's eye is covered by a moist 4×4 gauze sponge while the donor button is cut. The cut of the donor button should be made as perpendicular as possible because any tilt will cause astigmatism. For example, a 10-degree tilt will cause 0.1 mm shift in circumference, causing a 4 diopter shift in astigmatism. There are a number of devices on the market to assist the surgeon in making a perpendicular cut. The Lieberman punch has single-use blades. The trephine and circular blades must always be cleaned with a balanced salt solution; micro eye spears are used to remove any metal fragments and metal polish used to make the blade. The blade should be inspected for any defects and should be discarded if any are found. Once the trephine has been mounted on its holder and cleaned, it should be protected from coming into contact with anything; even glove powder can lead to complications.

   When these steps have been taken, the surgeon will call for the donor tissue. The circulating nurse will open the container containing the donor cornea over a corner of the sterile table set up earlier by the scrub person to cut the donor button. This should be done in a slow, deliberate manner so as not to drop the tissue. The surgeon will use the 3-ml syringe to draw off some of the preservative solution and flush the cutting platform and the trephine with the solution. The surgeon will then place a drop of the solu-

tion on the cutting platform in preparation for receiving the tissue. The tissue is grasped along the scleral rim with a toothed forceps and placed on the cutting platform. The tissue is inspected and adjusted on the cutting platform so that the cut is made centrally. The trephine is lowered, and the cut is made as perpendicular as possible. The button should come off the trephine cleanly while the remaining rim will be left on the blade. The rim is removed and inspected for central placement of the cut. It is returned to the container it came from and returned to the eye bank for continued testing. The button should be covered with the preservative and moved to the Mayo stand, where it is covered, to prevent accidental damage by the surgical team. If the cut to obtain the button is not complete, the cut must be completed with curved Vannas scissors or curved corneal scissors.
6. The patient's eye is uncovered and dried with micro eye spears so it can be marked with the trephine for proper placement. The trephine is adjusted to the depth of cut needed. An indentation is made with the trephine to be sure the cut is central and the defect of the patient's eye is encompassed.
7. The cut is made as perpendicular as possible and only until penetration is achieved, so that the anterior chamber can be maintained and the underlying structures left undamaged. If the cut is too deep, a viscoelastic is used to maintain the anterior chamber and keep the iris and other structures back. Penetration is determined by aqueous fluid entering the field.
8. The remainder of the cut must be made with a knife blade and tightly curved Katzen corneal scissors, right and left. The patient's cornea is placed in a medicine cup filled with a balanced salt solution and placed on the back table. It should not be passed off the field until the donor cornea is sutured in place.
9. The wound edge is inspected for any defects or shelving from a nonperpendicular cut. If observed, curved Vannas or similar scissors are used to trim this tissue. The internal contents of the eye are now "open to the sky" and it is especially important that the patient not move or do anything that will increase intraocular pressure such as coughing, talking, or straining. Normally the intraocular contents of the eye are maintained under 20 mm Hg of pressure. When the cornea is removed, the contents can easily be expressed through the opening. To help prevent this, an ocular pressure–reducing device is frequently placed prior to surgery. If a viscoelastic such as Healon, Occucoat, Viscoat, or Provisc is available, it is spread around the edge and over the iris and lens.
10. The next sequence of steps should be done without the surgeon having to ask for the instruments. The donor cornea is scooped off the cutting block by a Paton spatula and delivered onto the viscoelastic. The stroma is grasped by a two-pronged Pollack forceps, being careful not to touch the endothelium. The Paton spatula is replaced with 10–0 monofilament nonabsorbable suture on a locking needle holder.
11. The first cardinal suture is placed between the prongs of the Pollack forceps to the level of Descemet's mem-

brane on the donor cornea. The Pollack forceps is replaced with a Colibri or similar forceps, and the suture is placed at the same level on the recipient's corneal rim at the 12 o'clock position.

12. The suture is tied loosely, and the second cardinal suture is placed at the 6 o'clock position with the Colibri forceps, a nonlocking needle holder, and the same suture. The other two cardinal sutures are placed at the 3 o'clock and the 9 o'clock positions. The surgeon will then see a triangle-shaped image, which he will evaluate for symmetry.
13. Four additional sutures are placed between the original four to help flatten the graft.
14. Finally, a continuous 11–0 monofilament nonabsorbable suture is used around the entire graft. Occasionally, 16 interrupted, evenly spaced 10–0 sutures will be used. Interrupted sutures are used for areas of necrosis or sectors of vascularization in the patient's cornea.
15. The suture knots are rotated into the corneal tissue to reduce discomfort, prevent the knots from coming undone from the friction of the lids, and reduce the chances of postoperative infection. The knots will cause visual distortion until they are removed.
16. A fluorescein strip is used to check the wound edges for leaks. This procedure is known as the Sydell test. If leaks are found, the suture may need to be replaced (the 10–0 suture is taken out usually at 6 months and the 11–0 suture is usually removed at 1 year but can remain indefinitely).

Cataract extraction with intraocular lens placement

An additional procedure that is frequently done with the "open sky" corneal transplant is a cataract extraction with an intraocular lens (IOL) placement.

Key steps

1. After the cornea is removed, the superior portion of the capsule of the lens is cut and removed with a small knife blade.
2. The nucleus is expressed with a lens loop, and the cortex material is removed with an irrigation-aspiration device (see Cataract Extraction for description).
3. An IOL is implanted into the capsule, and the corneal graft is sutured in place.

A frequent complication during this procedure, with aphakic patients, is the herniation of vitreous through the opening. An anterior vitrectomy will then need to be performed, and the necessary equipment should be on hand during these procedures. There are a number of cutting-suctioning mechanisms available with varying amounts of automation. Care must be taken not to place the vitreous under tension, which can lead to retinal detachment. The chances of vitreous herniation can be reduced by the preoperative placement of pressure on the eye, which reduces intraocular pressure by reducing the amount of fluid in the tissues of the eye. The pressure can be applied by several devices such as a Honan balloon. These devices squeeze the water out of the vitreous for 1 to 2 hours,

thereby reducing intraocular pressure. Another method of reducing intraocular pressure is the intravenous administration of 20% solution of osmolyte. A minor complication following full-thickness corneal grafting is the loss of full sensitivity. The cornea is innervated by the ophthalmic division of the fifth cranial nerve, which is cut during grafting. This reduces the cornea's ability to sense a foreign object, which could lead to damage of the corneal graft.

Lamellar keratoplasty

The lamellar keratoplasty procedure is technically more difficult and more time consuming than a penetrating keratoplasty but has a higher success rate (Casey & Mayer, 1984). The first successful keratoplasty was performed in 1886 between a rabbit and a human. The lamellar keratoplasty remained the most popular transplant until the mid 1950s when the results of full-thickness grafts improved. The success of the partial-thickness graft is due to the layered cellular arrangement of the corneal tissue and its avascularity.

The donor cornea is cut the same way as for a full-thickness graft (see previous section). However, older corneal tissue or cryopreserved tissue can be used because the endothelial layer does not have to be viable. Because cryopreserved tissue can be used, the tissue can be lathed, which affects its refractive abilities.

Key steps

1. The patient's eye is prepped and draped in the usual manner.
2. A wire lid speculum is used to retract the eyelids.
3. A trephine is used to mark the cornea and begin the partial-thickness cut.
4. The cornea is dried and kept dry by micro eye spears in order to better see the stromal layers.
5. Diamond and ruby knives are used to peel the tissue in a direction parallel to the bed of the stroma lamellae. An angled beveled knife is frequently used to keep the dissection in a parallel plane.
6. Once the cornea has been dissected, the lip of the recipient cornea is undermined to provide a fitted suturing plane.
7. The patient's cornea is washed with a balanced salt solution, and the donor tissue is delivered to the area with a Paton spatula.
8. A Pollack forceps is used to hold the donor cornea for the placement of the first cardinal suture.
9. The Paton spatula is exchanged with a locking needle holder and 10–0 monofilament nylon suture. The Pollack forceps is exchanged with a Colibri forceps.
10. The first suture is placed at the 12 o'clock position, the second suture is placed at the 6 o'clock position, the third suture is placed at the 3 o'clock position, and the fourth suture is placed at the 9 o'clock position.
11. The remaining 12 sutures are placed equidistant from each other and in opposition to the last suture placed.

12. The knots are buried into the corneal tissue. A continuous suture is frequently not used. As in full-thickness grafts, the donor cornea is 0.5 mm larger than the recipient wound. If Descemet's membrane is penetrated during the peeling process, a 10–0 monofilament nylon is used to close the wound. Due to the delicate, thin nature of Descemet's membrane, this suturing can be very difficult. If the endothelium is healthy and Descemet's membrane is intact, the lamellar disc will become repopulated with the host keratocytes and the epithelium will also be replaced in time (Casey & Mayer, 1984).

Refractive Procedures

The precepts of the surgical correction of astigmatism were delineated almost 100 years ago, and numerous techniques have been enthusiastically espoused only to be abandoned because of their poor reliability, unpredictability, and associated operative and postoperative hazards (Ibrahim et al., 1991). The optical qualities of the cornea can be altered by three related and similar procedures. The epikeratoplasty is a lamellar keratoplasty in which the donor cornea is altered on a computer-controlled lathe similar to one used to create contact lenses. This procedure is not popular because of all the problems related to it. These problems include: the lathe tissue may not be placed in the right orientation, which will lead to severe astigmatism; healing problems; the shape of the donor tissue is not right; or the correction is at fault.

The corneal wedge resection is used to correct severe astigmatism, especially after a corneal transplant. The wedge is taken out circumferentially, and the edges are sutured together. This procedure is usually done following a transplant to relieve severe astigmatism caused by the surgery. A keratometer is used to obtain an accurate corneal surface curvature measurement, which helps the surgeon estimate how much and where to resect.

A radial keratoplasty (RK) is used to reduce myopia. Radial incisions are made through most of the stromal tissue with a diamond knife, leaving a small circular optical center clear over the opening of the pupil. The incisions will heal, and the scar tissue that forms pulls and flattens the curvature of the cornea, correcting the refractive error. This procedure is frequently done in a clinic under topical anesthesia. Studies are currently under way to determine the long-term effectiveness of this corrective surgery.

RK is only done on a healthy eye, and the potential complications must be emphasized to the patient. Potential complications can be: glaring from the scars, permanent scarring, infection that could lead to possible loss of vision, cataract formation from an injury to the lens, and long-term variations in the level of correction. The amount of correction and the method used to do the correction are inaccurate, so results are frequently imperfect. The eye continues to go through vision changes with aging, and this may result in a return to glasses or contact lenses later. These patients may also develop astigmatism.

A new procedure that holds greater promise is the use of a 193-nm excimer laser to ablate the top of the cornea, causing the same flattening effect as the RK surgery without some of the problems. In contrast to radial keratotomy, there are minimal glare sensitivity problems and virtually no chance of perforation. Eyes that undergo photorefractive keratectomy have no recurrent erosion or structural weakening, both of which have been seen with RK (Sher et al., 1991).

Excimer ablation can be performed safely with topical anesthesia. The laser uses an argon-fluorine gas mixture to produce a 193-nm wavelength. The entire laser system is computer controlled. A head-restraint system is used, and a three-axis alignment is necessary to get a centralized abatement (Sher et al., 1991). Following the ablation, tobramycin dexamethasone suspension drops and 5% homatropine hydrobromide are instilled and the eye has a disposable soft contact lens placed. The contact lens is continued for the first 3 weeks to promote epithelial growth. The major complications of this procedure are overcorrection or undercorrection and corneal hazing (Sher et al., 1992).

Pterygium Excision

A special problem thought to be created by the constant irritation of wind, dust, and ultraviolet light is a pterygium. It is a frequent problem among farmers. Pterygium is a fibrovascular connective tissue overgrowth of the conjunctiva onto the cornea (Casey & Mayer, 1984). The growth is dissected off the cornea and conjunctiva down to the sclera. A dose of low-level radiation from technetium-99 may be used to prevent regrowth on the surgical wound before closing. The conjunctiva is undermined and closed over the top of the wound. Pterygiums have a regrowth rate of 20% to 40% (Casey & Mayer, 1984).

UVEAL TRACT PROCEDURES

Glaucoma

The major disease associated with the uveal tract is glaucoma. Glaucoma is an abnormal increase in intraocular pressure that can lead to a blind, painful, and hard eye. Intraocular pressure is measured by the amount of forces needed to indent a specific area of the cornea. Normal pressure readings are from 10 to 20 mm Hg. If intraocular pressure rises above 20 mm Hg, the patient may be diagnosed with glaucoma. The pressure increase causes devascularization and atrophy of the retina and degeneration of the optic nerve, which leads to a slow, painless, insidious loss of sight. Usually when problems of loss of sight are noticed, irreparable damage has already been done. Glaucoma is caused by a malfunction of the "plumbing" of the eye. Aqueous fluid, produced by the ciliary body, flows between the iris and the lens into the anterior chamber, where it nourishes the structures before passing through the trabecular meshwork into the canal of Schlemm, at the lateral edge of the iris (Fig. 2-10).

Glaucoma is classified as primary, secondary, congenital, or absolute. Primary glaucoma can be further divided into open angle and closed angle (Fig. 2-11). About 90% of all cases of glaucoma are open angle. The term *open angle* refers to the angle between the iris and Schwalbe's line at the edge of the cornea (Fig. 2-2). Schwalbe's line is at the beginning of the trabecular meshwork. Primary open-angle glaucoma is thought to be caused by degenerative changes of the trabeculum of the canal of Schlemm. The treatment program is aimed primarily at lowering production of aqueous fluid or improving its absorption. The trabeculum and the anterior chamber angle can be directly observed with a gonioprism (Fig. 2-12,*A* and *B*). A gonioscope-prism permits a clear view of the anterior chamber angle. Medical treatment is the treatment of choice.

The drugs used to treat glaucoma are:

1. Miotics such as pilocarpine 1% to 4%, to increase the efficiency of the outflow channels
2. Epinephrine hydrochloride, to decrease the production of aqueous fluid
3. Carbonic anhydrase inhibitors, such as acetazolamide, to decrease aqueous fluid production

Visual field tests are done to determine the degree of peripheral vision lost owing to high intraocular pressure. If the medical treatment is ineffective in controlling glaucoma, filtering surgery becomes necessary. There are two basic filtering procedures, but the intended result is to form a bleb or cyst to collect the excessive aqueous fluid and to create a channel from the anterior chamber to the bleb. Specialized glaucoma surgery instruments are shown in Figure 2-13.

Glaucoma filtering procedure

Key steps

1. The conjunctiva is opened and balanced salt solution is injected into the subconjunctiva to produce the bleb.
2. The conjunctiva is then dissected up to the level of the limbus and held out of the way with a smooth Chandler forceps.
3. The sclera is incised with a knife blade in an V or U shape, having the upper part of the shape at the level of the limbus.
4. A flap is dissected up and held in place with a fine toothed Pierse-Hoskin forceps.
5. An incision is made into the anterior chamber at the level of the trabeculum, and a Kelly punch is used to take out a small portion of the trabeculum and Schlemm's canal and sclera.
6. A small peripheral iridectomy is done with a #5 jeweler's forceps and small curved scissors.
7. The dissected scleral flap is sutured at the pointed bottom of the incision with a 10–0 monofilament nylon suture.

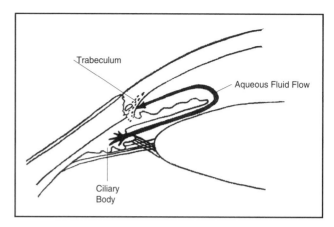

FIGURE 2-10 Aqueous fluid flows from the ciliary body for filtration and absorption in the trabeculum.

8. Before the conjunctiva is closed, the scleral incision is checked with micro eye spears to be sure it will leak.

The aqueous fluid will leak out of the wound into the bleb, to be absorbed by the sclera. Because of the protein and glucose content of the aqueous fluid, the conjunctiva and sclera will eventually wall off the bleb and form a closed cyst. Failure of the filtering bleb is a serious problem that occurs at various times after glaucoma filtering surgery. As the external aqueous drainage declines, the intraocular pressure may return to a level sufficient to produce optic nerve damage (Ewing & Stamper, 1990). To treat this problem, a bleb needling or a bleb revision may become necessary. Revision of a preexisting filtering site has several theoretical benefits: it preserves conjunctiva, is essentially an extraocular procedure, does not require the implantation of foreign materials, and does not damage the ciliary body (Ewing & Stamper, 1990). To prevent the bleb from closing, a neoplastic agent, 5-fluorouracil (5-FU) or mitomycin C, is applied to the sclera before the closure of the conjunctiva.

The use of postoperative subconjunctival 5-FU has been shown to increase the surgical success rate for eyes that have had previous surgery and undergone subsequent trabeculectomy (Ewing & Stamper, 1990). Currently, 5-FU is repeatedly administered by subconjunctival injections, which has many disadvantages, including the need for frequent dosing, discomfort associated with the injection, and ocular surface problems such as corneal epithelial defects and conjunctival wound leaks (Kitazawa et al., 1991). The advantage of this technique is the precise control over the amount of agent used to obtain the desired results.

A single application of mitomycin C at the time of surgery can have the same effect as the multiple applications of 5-FU without the complications. However, due to the toxic nature of the neoplastic agent, the wound must be irrigated with at least 90 ml of balanced salt solution and special precautions must be taken to dispose of the remaining neoplastic agent.

If the patient is unable to maintain a bleb, an artificial reservoir or valve can be implanted to keep it open. The procedure is similar to the trabeculectomy except the

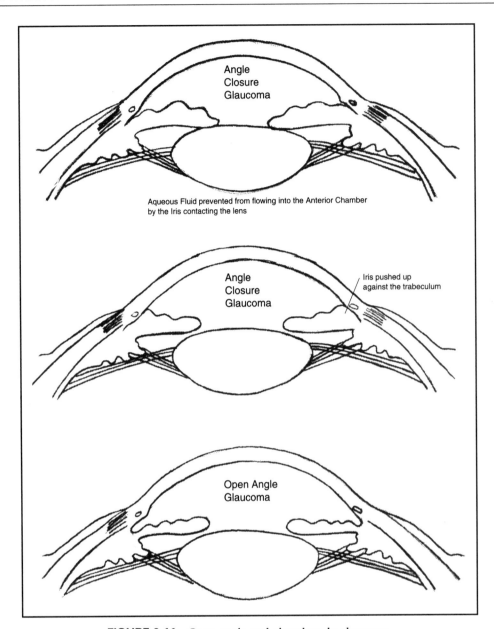

Aqueous Fluid prevented from flowing into the Anterior Chamber
by the Iris contacting the lens

FIGURE 2-11 Open-angle and closed-angle glaucoma.

conjunctival sac is enlarged to accommodate the reservoir and a silicone tube is passed into the anterior chamber. A large number of different types of valves are on the market but generally are an unrestricted tube about 0.3 mm in length connected to a reservoir.

Closed-angle glaucoma is usually acute and is caused by a sudden increase in intraocular pressure that causes the iris to block the outflow channels (see Fig. 2-11). The onset is usually rapid vision loss and pain. Subacute or chronic closed-angle glaucoma can be caused by the same factors that cause an acute attack but at a slower rate. Treatment is medical, but surgery is often indicated. The surgical procedure of choice for both an acute and a chronic closed-angle glaucoma is an iridectomy. The iridectomy is usually performed by an optical argon laser that creates a hole in the iris. Secondary glaucoma is caused by a dislocated lens that forces the iris up against the cornea and results in an obstruction,

changes in the uveal tract such as infection or bleeding that obstructs the drainage tracts of the trabeculum meshwork, and trauma that changes the anatomy and alters its normal function. Treatment entails correcting the underlying problem and treating the glaucoma with medications until it resolves.

Because of the ocular pressures involved and the potential for infection, a watertight closure is imperative. The watertight closure can be more difficult than normal because the constant pressure causes the tissue involved to become thin and delicate or, in a revision, to be thicker than normal.

Congenital glaucoma occurs in newborns and small children, usually as a result of a recessive genetic trait. Incomplete development of the outflow channels or a growth of tissue over the trabeculum prevents the outflow of aqueous fluid. Surgery is the treatment of choice. Cryotherapy is used to destroy the aqueus pro-

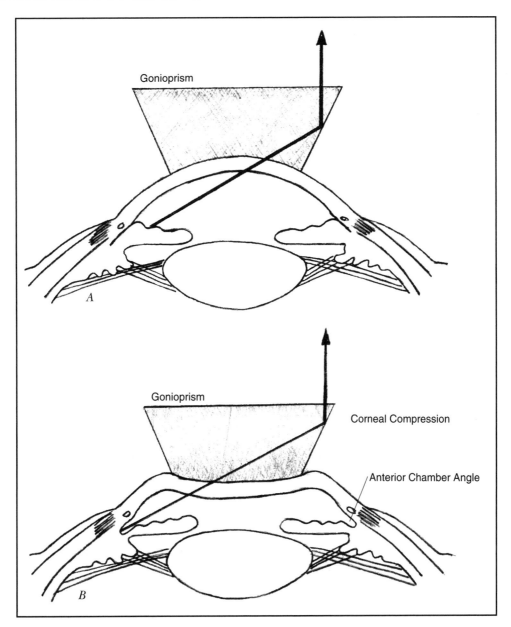

FIGURE 2-12   *A,* Observation for trabeculum and anterior chamber angle with a gonioprism. Unable to see anterior angle and trabeculum due to iris obstruction. *B,* Gonioprism used to compress the cornea opening the anterior chamber angle and permitting visualization of the trabeculum.

duction by freezing the ciliary body and destroying the tissue, thereby decreasing production of aqueous fluid. The cryoprobe is applied to the conjunctiva over the ciliary bodies, 4 to 5 mm posterior to the limbus, and an ice ball is generated (Fig. 2-14,*A, B,* and *C*). If there is tissue growth over the trabeculum, a goniotomy is performed. A gonioknife is inserted through the limbus, across the anterior chamber, and the tissue is incised through one quadrant under direct vision of a gonioscope (Fig. 2-15,*A* and *B*). This procedure can be done four times on each eye. Congenital glaucoma is easily recognizable by the large infant eyes that appear filled with iris, and eyes sensitive to light.

Absolute glaucoma is the end result of a failed treat-ment program or the lack of treatment. When this occurs, the blind, painful, hard eye frequently has to be enucle-ated.

CATARACT PROCEDURES

Perioperative Nursing Considerations

Opacification of the lens (cataract) can be caused by a number of factors and can occur at any time depending on the following factors.

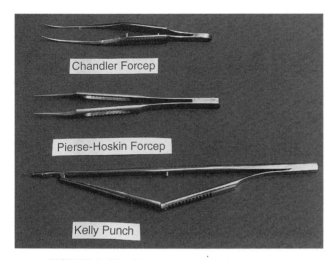

FIGURE 2-13 Glaucoma surgery instruments.

In infants, the etiology of cataract formation may be:

1. Infection
2. Developmental abnormalities
3. Heredity
4. Traumatic eye injury
5. Chemical imbalances like galactosemia and diabetes

In adults, all of the above can cause cataracts, along with:

1. Prolonged exposure to ultraviolet light
2. Some medications (e.g., those used to treat glaucoma)
3. Part of the normal aging process

The only disorders of the lens are opacification and dislocation. In either, removal of the lens is the only treatment.

Until the 1980s, intracapsular cataract extraction (ICCE) was the procedure of choice for the removal of cataracts. According to Wertenbaker (1981), the first ICCE was performed in 1753 by Samuel Sharp of London, but the procedure did not become common practice until the 1940s. The procedure remains relatively the same today. An 18-mm incision is made at the level of the limbus, and the cornea is retracted while the entire lens is grasped and removed. The method of grasping the lens has changed over the years with the advent of new technologies.

The lens can be removed with mechanical forceps, various suction devices, and a cryoextractor. The cryoextractor has been the instrument of choice because the tissue is firmly attached to the probe and reduces the chance that the capsule will rupture. If the cryoextractor is used, a bottle of balanced salt solution must be available to warm any tissue inadvertently frozen. Multiple peripheral iridectomies are occasionally done to prevent iris prolapse during extraction if dilation fails. Occasionally, alpha-chymotrypsin is injected to the area around the lens to help dissolve the zonules. The incision is closed tightly with 10–0 nylon. Because the capsule has been extracted, an intraocular lens (IOL) cannot easily be placed. (IOL placement will be discussed at the end of this section.) Another complication of this procedure is the herniation of vitreous from the posterior chamber. For these reasons, extracapsular cataract extraction (ECCE) has supplanted ICCE as the method of choice.

Extracapsular cataract extraction (ECCE)

Key steps

1. A conjunctival incision is made in the region of the limbus, and a small 3-mm incision is made at the level of the limbus.
2. A cystotome (Fig. 2-16), a bent 25-gauge needle, or a right-angled miniature knife is used to incise the anterior capsule of the lens.
3. Anterior capsulectomy is one of the most critical steps in extracapsular cataract extraction. Secure long-term capsular fixation and centralization of the posterior chamber intraocular lens can best be achieved if integrity of the central opening is maintained. Radial tears that extend toward the equator from the margin of the capsulectomy are associated with a high incidence of extrusion of at least one loop out of the capsular bag. Figure 2-17 shows four representative types of anterior capsulectomies. The circular continuous capsularhexis is the procedure of choice (Assia et al., 1991).
4. The complete circumferential incision can be made with the cystotome or with Utrata forceps (Fig. 2-18, *A* and *B*). If the circumferential incision is made with the cystotome, the edge is ragged and torn. If Utrata forceps are used, the circumferential incision is smooth.
5. Prior to the capsulotomy, a viscoelastic is injected into the anterior chamber to maintain the chamber and protect the corneal endothelium.
6. After the capsulotomy, a 27-gauge blunt needle, on a 3-ml syringe filled with balanced salt solution, is inserted into the cortex, and the balanced salt solution is injected. The hydrodissection loosens the nucleus, permitting easier extraction.
7. After the hydrodissection, the limbal incision is enlarged to permit the expression of the nucleus with a blunt instrument, which gently massages the area on the opposite side of the eye.
8. Sutures are generally placed prior to expression so that the eye can be closed quickly if complications occur.
9. After the lens is extracted, the limbal incision is temporarily closed and an irrigation–aspiration needle is inserted to extract the remaining cortex. The preferred irrigation solution is balanced salt solution plus (BSS Plus), which has trace amounts of chemical ions, making it totally isotonic to intraocular tissue. The BSS Plus should be used for all intraocular procedures. The aspiration part of the needle is usually attached to an automated suction device but may be just a syringe. An effort is made to leave the posterior capsule intact to prevent vitreous herniation into the anterior chamber and to provide a bag for the placement of the IOL.

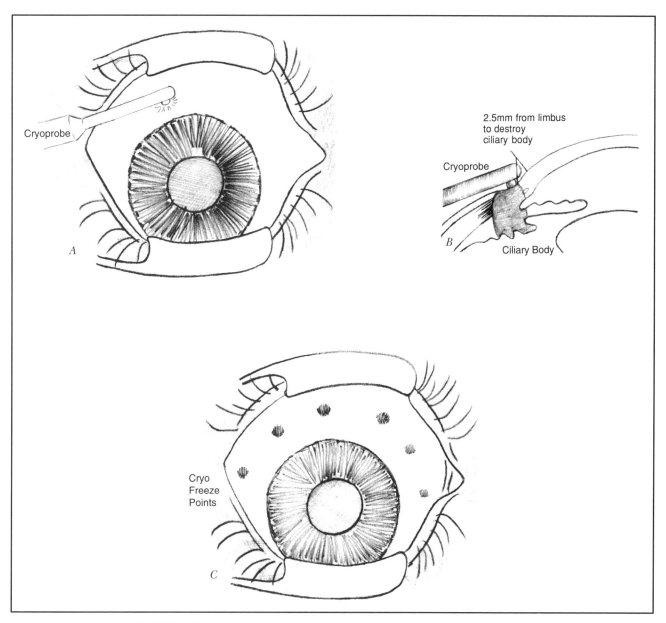

FIGURE 2-14 *A, B, C,* Cryotherapy used to destroy the aqueous production in congenital glaucoma.

10. If a primary IOL placed at the time of surgery is used, the sutures are loosened or cut and the IOL is eased into the capsular bag. Prior to the IOL placement, a viscoelastic may be used to keep the chamber and bag inflated and to help the IOL slide into place.
11. Once the IOL is placed, the limbal incision is closed with a 10–0 nylon suture and the viscoelastic is extracted with the irrigation–aspiration unit.
12. The incisional site is checked for leaks, using micro eye spears.
13. If no leaks are found, the conjunctiva is closed.

Phacoemulsification

Phacoemulsification has been available for cataract surgery in the United States for approximately 20 years. There have been major developments in equipment, instrumentation, and pharmaceutical agents intended to improve the outcome and ease of performance of this procedure. Currently, phacoemulsification is the procedure of choice in 25% to 30% of the ophthalmic surgeries in the United States. With cataract surgery the most frequently performed operation in the United States, this represents a large group of patients (Hattenhauer, 1991).

The phacoemulsifier uses a hollow titanium needle to fragment the hard nucleus of the lens while simultaneously flushing and aspirating the fragmented debris into the machine. Because of the size of the tip, the entire ECCE can take place through a 3-mm incision with minimal trauma to the eye. However, with the advent of the machine, strict preoperative safety checks must be performed on the irrigation and aspiration system, and the ultrasonic tip must

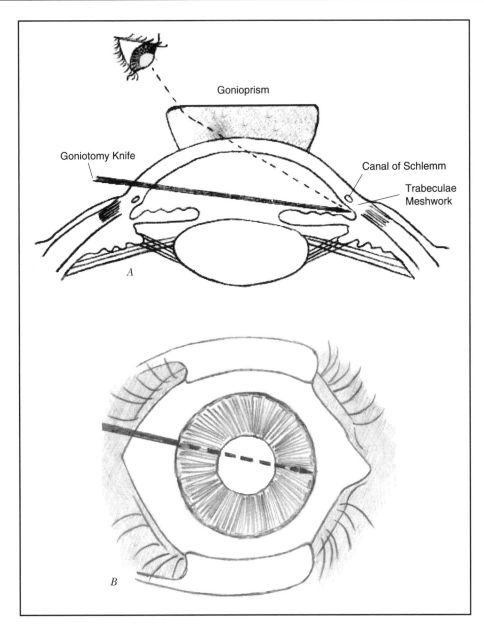

Gonioprism

Goniotomy Knife

Canal of Schlemm

Trabeculae Meshwork

A

B

FIGURE 2-15 *A,* Goniotomy. A gonioknife is inserted through the limbus, crossing the anterior chamber and incising the tissue over the trabeculum. *B,* Goniotomy. Goniotomy sweep with the goniotomy knife.

be tuned to function precisely. The ultrasound used to emulsify the lens is electrical energy that is converted to linear (back-and-forth) motion, which strikes the lens material 40,000 times a second. The ultrasonic tip is surrounded by a silicone sleeve that permits a constant flow of irrigation to keep the anterior chamber inflated and assists in keeping the tip cool. With the advent of flexible IOLs, the use of phacoemulsification continues to evolve. Flexible IOLs permit the entire procedure and the placement of the IOL through the same 3-mm incision. This development has led to a no-stitch phacoemulsification technique with IOL placement.

In the procedure, the conjunctival incision is made and a 3-mm limbal incision is made on a beveled plane, which permits the incision to close naturally from the top flap when the eye is soft and from the lower flap when the

eye is firm. The conjunctiva is reapproximated using electrocautery at the end of the procedure.

Although phacoemulsification is currently the procedure of choice in 25% to 30% of the ophthalmic surgeries in the United States, it is not indicated for every patient. It is contraindicated for dislocated lens, soft infantile lens, dense cataracts, and patients with shallow anterior chambers or difficult-to-dilate pupils as in glaucoma.

Cataracts in children are the main cause of deprivation amblyopia. Unlike the adult eye, the infant's eye will lose its potential for normal sight if a dense cataract is present. The current preferred treatment for congenital cataracts is surgical removal as soon as possible. Pediatric cataracts have a soft nucleus and can usually be taken out with just irrigation and aspiration. Two small incisions are made in the periphery of the cornea, one for the irrigation needle

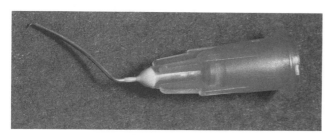

FIGURE 2-16 Cystotome, used to incise the anterior capsule of the lens in cataract extraction.

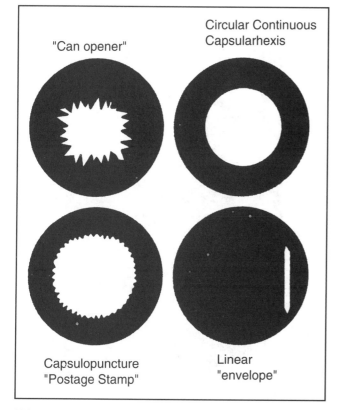

"Can opener"

Circular Continuous Capsularhexis

Capsulopuncture "Postage Stamp"

Linear "envelope"

FIGURE 2-17 Four methods of anterior capsulectomy. Circular capsularhexis is preferred.

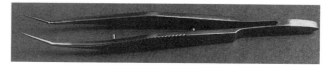

A

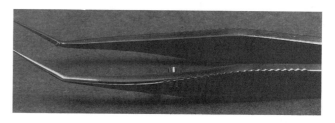

B

FIGURE 2-18 *A, B* Utrata forceps used for anterior capsulectomy.

and the other for the cutting aspirating tip of an ocutome (see the section on retinal procedures for further understanding of the ocutome).

Convalescence for cataract surgery is usually very short, with few restrictions after the second day. "After-cataracts" are caused by a failure to remove all of the cortex and epithelial cells during the initial extraction. The "after-cataract" causes a clouding of the capsule, which restricts vision. A posterior capsulotomy with laser therapy is usually done. The six most frequent complications subsequent to phacoemulsification are permanent corneal edema, disruption of the anterior hyaloid, late opacification of an intact posterior capsule, cystoid macular edema, retinal detachment, and posterior dislocation of the nucleus (Fastenberg et al., 1991). The treatment of these complications ranges from a corneal transplant to a posterior vitrectomy.

The most frequent complication is the dislocation of the lens during cataract surgery, which often leads to severe uveitis, glaucoma, and vitreous condensation. If untreated, vision may be permanently lost. Treatment of dislocated lenses and lens fragments has improved with the advances in vitrectomy techniques. Soft to moderately hard lenses are safely treated with the vitrectomy probe, microfragmentation probe, and microvitrectomy forceps. Nonetheless, removal of hard lenses remains hazardous (Spapiro et al., 1991).

Implantation of intraocular lens

When the lens is removed during cataract surgery, the eye loses its focusing ability and correction is needed to regain clear sight. The aphakic (without lens) patient sees objects larger than normal, but the objects are blurred and without detail. This problem can be corrected by glasses, contact lenses, or the placement of an IOL. Glasses are the poorest substitute because they are located in front of the eye and need to magnify the image by 35% to get clear vision. Because of this magnification, considerable adjustment must be made by the patient in judging distances and object sizes. Since only one cataract can be removed at a time, one eye will see a magnified image while the other eye sees the blurred world of the cataract patient. This causes severe visual impairment for the 6 months the patient must wait before the other eye can be operated on; if only one eye needs to be corrected, this may be a long-term problem. Contact lenses, because of placement directly on the cornea, have only a 7% magnification problem. It is much easier for the patient to adapt to these images. Also, the patient has a complete field of vision with contact lenses, whereas with glasses, the patient gets a clear image only in the direct center of the glasses. The contact lenses have the added advantage of being ultra-lightweight whereas the glasses are very heavy.

The best visual results are achieved by the placement of an IOL. The IOL was developed in 1944 by a British air force surgeon who noticed a lack of ocular reaction from plastic canopy fragments in the eyes of pilots whose planes were shot down. Dr. Harold Ridley made IOLs from the canopy plastic and inserted them into the anterior chamber after removing a cataract.

The IOL is now made of plexiglass or polymethyl methacrylate (PMMA) cut and polished to microscopic perfection (Fig. 2-19,A to C). The IOL has a center of clear plastic that can be either biconvex or convexoplano and two haptics (spring-hook appendages). The IOL can be made of a single piece or have two polypropylene haptics swaged on. The polypropylene haptics will break down over time and should not be used on young patients. Since the IOL cannot adjust its anterior-to-posterior dimensions, it provides only myopic, near-sighted, or hyperopic, farsighted, vision. The patient must decide whether there is a need for reading or driving glasses.

The power of the IOL is determined by a computer program that must consider the patient's corneal curvature, the anterior chamber depth, and the globe's axial length (Atkinson & Kohn, 1986). The anterior chamber IOL is placed on top of the iris with its edges wedged against the anterior chamber angle. The anterior chamber IOLs were found to have a high degree of serious complications, which include corneal damage, glaucoma, uveal inflammation, extrusion, and infections. Because of these complications, IOLs fell out of use until the 1980s, when posterior chamber IOLs were developed and tested. The posterior IOL is placed in the capsular bag after the lens is extracted, providing a natural placement for the IOL. If the capsule is missing or ruptured, the IOL haptics can be wedged between the ciliary body and the iris (ciliary sulcus) or the IOL can be trans-sclerally sutured in

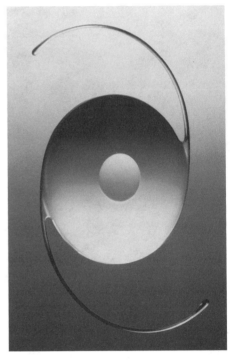

B

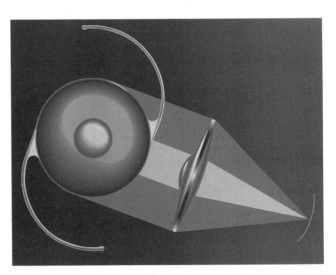

A

FIGURE 2-19 Examples of intraocular lens: *A,* Slimfit™ one-piece, modified "C" loop, posterior chamber, biconvex lens. *B,* Nuvue bifocal one-piece, modified "C" loop, posterior chamber, biconvex lens, 7.0 optic. *C,* Depiction of near (central portion) and distant (outer portion) simultaneous vision through a multifocal lens. (Courtesy of IOLAB, Inc., Claremont, California.)

C

place. Most IOLs placed today have ultraviolet protection impregnated into the plastic.

Two relatively new IOLs are now being used. The flexible or foldable IOL was developed to be placed through the 3-mm incision made to do phacoemulsifications. The other IOL has a suturing opening in the haptics so the IOL can be sutured into place. These IOLs are placed when no posterior capsule exists. A 10–0 polypropylene suture is used to secure this IOL in its position through two sclerotomies placed 180 degrees apart (Maguire, 1991).

RETINAL PROCEDURES

Perioperative Nursing Considerations

Defects in the continuity of the retina can be caused by a number of reasons, such as a blow to the side of the head, severe myopia, inflammation, noninflammatory degenerative diseases of the retina, diabetes, surgical trauma, and hereditary disorders. The patient will exhibit a loss of vision without pain or will see a slow decrease in the visual field as though someone was lowering a curtain over the eye. If there is bleeding into the posterior segment, as in diabetic retinopathy, the patient's vision will become progressively blurred. If the bleeding stops on its own and clears up after several weeks, the vitreous collagen fibrils may become stained, creating floaters. The most frequent disorders that require surgery are retinal detachment, endophthalmitis, and diabetic retinopathy. In retinal detachment, the retina becomes separated from the choroid. This can be caused by:

1. Severe myopia
2. A blow to the side of the head or to the eye
3. As a result of the normal aging process
4. Congenitally
5. Through adhesion formation from an inflammatory process

Retinal detachments are classified as primary detachments if there is a hole in the retina that permits fluid to enter the space between the retina and the choroid. In secondary retinal detachment, fluid or tissue is built up between the choroid and the retina without an opening (hole) in the retina. The location of the detachment and the cause determine the method of draining the fluid and reattaching the retina to the choroid.

Endophthalmitis is an inflammation of the eye that can be caused by bacteria, fungi, or viruses. In the natural growth media of the eye, endophthalmitis progresses rapidly. In a matter of days it can progress from a minor infection to one that is life-threatening. It needs to be treated aggressively with antibiotics, and if it is unresponsive to this treatment, a posterior vitrectomy with intraocular antibiotics is done or the eye is enucleated. If endophthalmitis is left untreated, the infection will travel by way of the optic nerve, infecting the brain and causing death.

Diabetic retinopathy is caused by the vascular changes that occur because of diabetes (Garcia & Ruiz, 1992). It is classified as nonproliferative or proliferative. Nonproliferative retinopathy is the early vascular changes that may lead to microbleeds or leakage that is frequently reabsorbed. Changes in the capillary wall lead to a rupture and eventual blockage of the blood supply to a small area of the retina, leading to retina ischemia. Proliferative retinopathy is caused by this ischemia and the retina's effort to relieve the anoxia. New blood vessels are formed in the area and in the surrounding tissue. This neovascularization is much weaker tissue and frequently ruptures, causing hemorrhage into the vitreous, leading to complete blindness. If left untreated, the blindness becomes permanent. If the hemorrhage is found early, laser therapy may be the only treatment needed. The laser light is absorbed by hemoglobin, melanin, and xanthophyll.

Xenon lasers were used originally, but they emitted a white light that contains all visible wavelengths, thereby destroying larger areas than desired and causing a decrease in visual acuity and a loss in peripheral visual fields. The argon laser has taken its place as the laser of choice. The argon beam contains both blue light (488 μm) and green light (514 μm), which are well absorbed by the xanthophyll in the retina. Anywhere from 400 to 1600 "burns" are done, depending on the area of the neovascularization. The peripheral retinal tissue is destroyed and its need for oxygen is reduced, thereby preventing neovascularization.

Lasers

Retinal detachment can be corrected only surgically. There are several techniques used to accomplish the reattachment. Diathermy, photocoagulation, and retinocryopexy have been effective prophylaxes against retinal detachment for retinal tears (Smiddy et al., 1991). The traditional therapy consists of insertion of microneedles into the sclera or use of a needle tip on a probe with shortwave radiofrequency (diathermy) energy being delivered to the needles. This causes thermal changes in the tissue, with scar formation, resulting in retinal reattachment at the adhesion points. This procedure is not done very frequently anymore.

A more popular method is the application of a −80°C cryoprobe (see Fig. 2-14,A to C) to the scleral area of detachment, producing a sterile inflammation that forms an adhesion, thus reattaching the retina. These two procedures produce the same type of adhesion, but because of the less invasive nature of the cryotherapy, it has fewer complications and has replaced diathermy.

Pneumoretinopexy, the injection of air or expansile gases into the vitreous cavity, is another method of retinal reattachment. Various gases are used, depending on the length of time the gas is needed to keep the retina reattached. Gases used and their expandability are the following:

Pure Gas Used	Amount Injected	Days It Will Last	Expandability
SF6	1.5 cc	7–10 days	2.5 times
CF4	2.0 cc	5 days	3 times
C2F6	0.8 cc	10 days	4 times
C3F8	1.0 cc	35 days	2 times
C4F10	0.6 cc	45 days	2 times

Pneumoretinopexy is usually done in the physician's office, with the use of cryotherapy to close and seal the hole before the gas is injected. If gas is injected, the gas bubble must be kept in the area of the detachment, so the patient is instructed to hold the head a certain way until the retina can reattach, usually in 2 weeks.

Laser therapy is used to "spot weld" the retina where it is detached. This procedure can be done in the physician's office with an indirect ophthalmoscope laser or in the operating room during the vitrectomy procedure. Indirect ophthalmoscope laser therapy will sometimes be needed in the operating room during a vitrectomy if the detachment or retinal hole is high anteriorly and there is the possibility of hitting the lens of the eye with the laser probe. For a sclerotomy 4.0 mm posterior to the limbus, there is about 1.0 mm separating the lens and the instrument shaft when approaching the ora serrata 90 degrees from the sclerotomy. For sclerotomies 3.0 mm posterior to the limbus, there is usually contact with the lens at the arc distance (Smiddy et al., 1991).

Two extensive surgical procedures that correct retinal detachments are scleral buckling and the posterior vitrectomy.

Scleral buckling

The scleral buckling procedure was developed by Dr. Schepens in the late 1950s. It consists of opening the conjunctiva circumferentially, isolating the rectus muscles with silk strands, dissecting a circumferential scleral flap, applying diathermy, placing a silicone band circumferentially in the scleral flap, closing the flap over the silicone band, and holding it in place. The band deforms the sclera, decreasing the circumference of the globe and thereby reducing vitreous traction circumferentially. Later modification of this technique eliminated the need to dissect a scleral flap and permitted the securing of the scleral buckle component to the outside of the sclera with nylon suture, along with the use of cryotherapy instead of diathermy (Fig. 2-20).

There are a large number of scleral buckle components on the market, and the surgeon will decide which component to use depending on the size and area of the detachment. This procedure was the method of choice for retinal detachments too large for other effective treatments or if the above-mentioned treatment programs were unsuccessful, until 1966, when Dr. Kasner performed the first planned vitrectomy.

Posterior vitrectomy

Indications for doing a vitrectomy instead of one of the above-mentioned procedures are:

1. Large retinal detachments
2. Diabetes
3. Trauma
4. Macular hole
5. Vitreoretinal traction
6. Vitreous media opacities
7. Diagnoses such as posterior malignancies, uveitis, and viral retinopathies
8. Complications of anterior segment surgeries, such as dislocated lens, expulsive hemorrhage, retained cortex, and epithelial downgrowth

The purpose of a posterior vitrectomy is to remove the vitreous humor without pulling on the retina or detaching the retina, thereby permitting the surgeon to work on the retina directly (Fig. 2-21). In order to accomplish this, the surgeon must rely on an ocutome, which cuts and aspirates the vitreous jelly.

According to Charles (1976), suction on the ocutome should be set at 60 to 80 mm of Hg and the cutting rate should be set as high as possible, usually 400 to 600 cycles per minute. These settings will reduce the amount of vitreous drawn into the probe before the vitreous is cut, thereby reducing the tension on the vitreous that is attached to the retina. Since the probe aspirates material out of the eye, there is a need to replace this material with fluid and to maintain normal eye pressure, which is 20 mm Hg. If the eye pressure is not maintained, the eye will become soft and will collapse, causing a massive detachment and expulsive choroidal hemorrhage. An infusion of BSS Plus, which is isotonic to the eye tissue, is used at an initial infusion pressure of 30 to 35 mm Hg. The higher pressure is needed to compensate for the probe's aspiration and the leaking that takes place around the instruments placed in the eye. The height of the infusion bottle may need to be changed at the surgeon's request if there is a need to control bleeding, to tamponade the bleeders, or to reattach the retina.

The posterior vitrectomy surgical procedure is as follows:

Key steps

1. Two U-shaped incisions are made in the conjunctiva at the 3 o'clock and the 9 o'clock positions 6 to 7 mm posterior to the limbus.
2. A diathermy is used to control bleeding.
3. A 20-gauge micro vitreoretinal (MVR) knife blade is used to puncture the globe 3 to 4 mm posterior to the limbus, 4 mm in phakic patients and 3 mm in aphakic patients (see explanation above).
4. A 5–0 nylon suture is placed on both sides of the puncture wound to secure the infusion cannula. The 20-gauge infusion cannula is flushed with BSS Plus before placement in the puncture wound and secured with the suture.

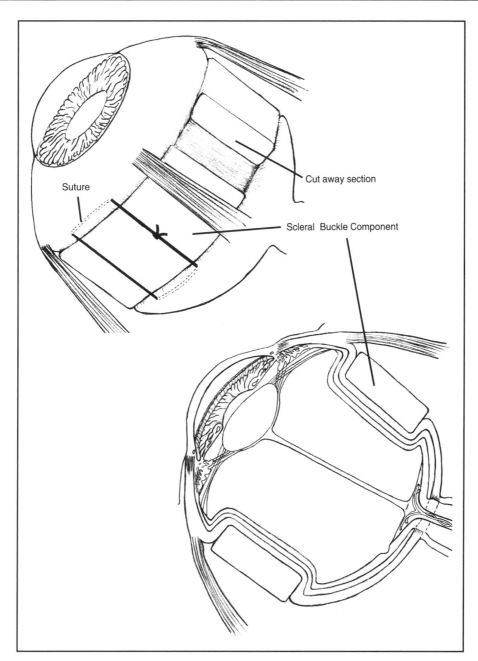

Suture

Cut away section

Scleral Buckle Component

FIGURE 2-20   Scleral buckling technique.

5. The infusion is not turned on until after the surgeon has checked the tip of the infusion cannula to be sure it is free of retinal tissue. The infusion is turned on or off only at the direct request of the surgeon.

6. Two other 20-gauge puncture wounds are made, one next to the infusion cannula and the other 180 degrees opposite to it, 3 to 4 mm from the limbus, in the pars plana. These two puncture wounds are used for an illumination probe (light pipe) and the ocutome vitreous cutting probe.

7. The light pipe and the ocutome probe are inserted, the infusion is turned on, and the vitreous is removed (see Fig. 2-21). The light pipe is used to help manipulate the eye and vitreous, as well as to illuminate the posterior segment. A large variety of 20-gauge instruments are used to cut membranes or vitreous bands or to manipulate retinal tissue.

8. An assistant is required to hold an irrigating handheld contact lens that focuses the operating microscope on the retina.

9. The assistant may also be called upon to depress the sclera, bringing the anterior portions of the retina into view. The surgeon must be cautious when working in this area not to jar the lens or it may need to be removed. Once the vitreous is removed, a number of techniques may be used to reattach the retina.

10. Filtered air can be infused instead of BSS Plus to reattach the retina. Then, argon laser therapy is used to

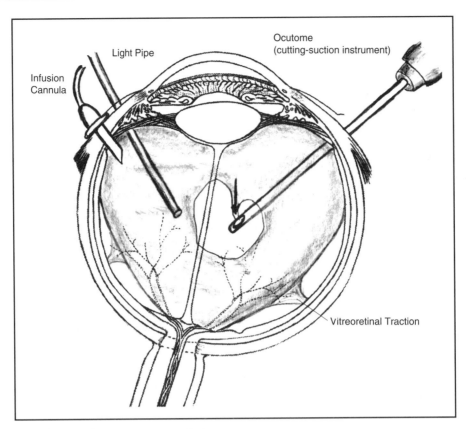

FIGURE 2-21 Vitrectomy technique.

"spot weld" the retina in place. If there is a retinal hole with fluid buildup behind the retina, the fluid must be drained so the retina will lie next to the choroid.

11. If there is no hole, a retinotomy is performed as posterior as possible, with an intraocular diathermy. A soft-tipped needle is inserted behind the retina, with application of a surgeon-controlled linear suction, to remove the fluid.

12. According to Echardt, et al., (1991), liquid perfluorocarbons are useful tools during vitreous surgery for complicated retinal detachments; their high specific gravity considerably facilitates reattachment of the retina.

In the case of giant tears where the entire retina has become detached, perfluorocarbon, which is two to three times heavier than water, is needed to flatten the retina so it can be "spot welded" with the argon laser. In these patients, 1000 centistoke silicone oil is usually infused at the end of the procedure to keep the retinal flap against the choroid. Since its introduction by Cibis et al. in 1962, vitreous replacement by silicone oil has become an increasingly accepted treatment for severe and complicated retinal detachments. Silicone oil is optically clear and possesses physical properties that promote retinal tamponade. The tolerance of various eye tissue to the oil is, however, a matter of ongoing controversy. This issue is further complicated by the fact that intraocular silicone oil can exist in two forms: large cohesive bubbles or minute dispersed droplets. Oil dispersion takes place over weeks to months in a process that has been called "emulsification."

Eyes that have been treated with silicone oil sometimes lose vision due to corneal decompensation, cataract, glaucoma, low-grade uveitis, or oil-induced retinopathy. Some of these complications have been associated with silicone oil emulsification. The cause of emulsification is unclear, but several investigators have attributed it to increased concentrations of protein and/or phospholipid that reduce the interfacial surface tension between oil and water (Ohira et al., 1991). The oil is left in for 3 to 4 months before it is removed, and it is for the complications associated with emulsification that it must be removed. Other vitreous substitutes are being investigated, such as the heavy liquid perfluorocarbon ($C10F18$), new inert gases, and continued refining of the silicone oil. The advantages of silicone oil therapy over other vitreal substitutes are:

1. Postoperative positioning of the eye is less of a problem than with the gases. A patient who is incapable of maintaining a face-down position (e.g., a child, a mentally incapacitated patient, or a patient with a spinal or neck problem) may fare better.

2. If the patient requires ambulatory vision in the only sighted eye

3. If the patient must travel by airplane after surgery, because intraocular pressure from expandable intraocular gases will increase during air travel

4. Some disease processes such as cytomegalovirus retinitis, in which silicone oil has been indicated
5. Patients who may fare better with silicone oil (e.g., those who have a large inferior retinotomy)
6. Previously vitrectomized eyes
(Adapted from Haller & Campochiaro, 1992)

The properties that make perfluorocarbon (new inert gas) useful in the treatment of retinal detachments are their ability to expand and their intraocular persistence. Both of these useful properties are attributable to the low solubility of perfluorocarbon gases in blood, with the expansion phase resulting from the entry of serum nitrogen and oxygen into the gas bubble and persistence resulting from the slow reabsorption of the gas. While the gas bubble is in the eye, its buoyant force holds the retina against the retinal pigment epithelium until the chorioretinal adhesions can become maximal. The buoyant force is directly proportional to the bubble volume and to the difference in specific gravities between the gas and saline solution. Thus, gases provide a markedly higher buoyant force than the force obtainable with silicone oil. The high surface tension and buoyant force of gases result in better internal tamponade properties (Lopez & Chang, 1992).

Posterior vitrectomies can be performed with any or all of the techniques for reattaching the retina, including the placement of a scleral buckle. The prognosis for these patients depends on the extent of the detachment and the length of time the retina is detached. Recovery can be complete or the patient may recover only light perception. It usually takes 6 weeks to get some of the vision back and up to 2 years for the final results to be known. More than 80% of the patients operated on will have improved vision.

There are a number of complications that can arise during a vitrectomy. In diabetic patients, all of the eye tissue is affected by the diabetes. The cornea may cloud up during the procedure, limiting the surgeon's ability to see the retina. The corneal epithelium can be scraped off with a knife blade, but this will give the surgeon only about an hour of clear vision.

The lens may become clouded because of jarring or osmotic pressure differences. In diabetics the lens is accustomed to higher concentrations of glucose, so 3 ml of dextrose is added to the BSS Plus infusion fluid to prevent osmotic shift. If the lens is bumped or becomes cloudy, it is removed by a pars plana fragmentation. A fragmatome is inserted posterior to the lens, and with increased fluid flow and suction the lens is cored by the fragmatome. The cortex and zonules are removed with the ocutome. Other complications that can occur include the collapse of the eye because the infusion fluid runs dry, the intravenous tubing becomes disconnected, or the stopcocks are not positioned properly. Vitreoretinal surgery is in its infancy, with new and better equipment coming on the market daily. A new avenue under investigation is mini-instrumentation, 25 gauge, adding possible additional puncture wounds in the eye to support additional instrumentation, essentially giving the surgeon an extra pair of hands.

The new frontiers of vitreoretinal surgery are:

1. Removal of subretinal hemorrhages and choroidal neovascular membranes
2. Evacuation of large pigment epithelial detachments
3. The treatment of diabetic macular edema that is nonresponsive to laser photocoagulation
4. Rotational retinal flaps, moving the fovea to healthy retinal pigmented epithelium
5. Implantation of transplanted retinal pigmented epithelium cells

TRAUMA TO THE EYE

Perioperative Nursing Considerations

Trauma to the eye can be classified as nonpenetrating or penetrating injuries. Nonpenetrating injuries include burns, both thermal and chemical, and blunt contusions to the globe, which can lead to retinal detachments and/or bleeding and increased intraocular pressure, leading to damage to the optic nerve. Chemical burns are particularly hazardous and should be treated immediately by flooding the cornea with water and neutralizing chemicals. Penetrating injuries can be either with or without a foreign body. Penetrating injuries without a foreign body are debrided and closed. Penetrating injuries with a foreign body require an extensive examination to accurately determine where the foreign body is located. Localization should include, but not be restricted to, direct ophthalmoscopic or indirect ophthalmoscopic examination, CT scan, ultrasound, and X-ray. Once the object has been localized, it should be removed. If it is metallic, an electromagnet can be used to remove it. A nonmagnetic object must be retrieved by instruments.

Four goals should be met during the repair of any injured tissue: the restoration of normal anatomical relationships, the restoration of functional architecture, the prevention of late complications, and preparation for any anticipated secondary procedure (Hamill & Thompson, 1990). The majority of the injuries occur to the cornea first, then to the eyelid, conjunctiva, anterior chamber, orbit, retina, and sclera, and finally to the lens.

Repair of Traumatic Eye Injuries

When intraocular contents are protruding through the wound, identification of the tissue should be attempted. Vitreous material should be excised, flush with the wound edge. Lens fragments should be cleared from the wound with irrigation. If necessary, an anterior vitrectomy and/or removal of the lens through a separate incision should follow corneal closure. Prolapsed iris, except for obviously necrotic or suppurative tissue, should be repositioned. Prolapsed retina or uvea should also be repositioned.

Concurrent with management of prolapsed intraocular tissue is the identification of landmarks. Landmarks of the cornea include the limbus, the interlocking edges of stellate lacerations, loose tissue, or pigmentation lines. These should be sought and reapproximated to restore proper anatomical relationships. The landmarks should be closed first, proceeding from periphery to center, using 9–0 black silk on the limbus and 10–0 nylon on the cornea. The anterior chamber should be reformed as soon as possible with air, saline, or a viscoelastic material to minimize the risk of inadvertent damage to intraocular structures and to facilitate subsequent suture placement (Hamill & Thompson, 1990). Postoperative infection and inflammation must be effectively prevented.

Complex orbital fracture with dislocation of the orbital rim and/or orbital walls should be repaired as soon as possible. The procedure consists of the accurate reconstruction of the dislocated bones with wire and/or plating. Early reconstruction is necessary to avoid contour deformities and the aesthetic deformities of enophthalmos and dystropia of the globe (Denny & Gonnering, 1990).

The goal of ocular trauma surgery is no longer just the ability to save the eye but to reconstruct it to a functioning level. The developments and refinements of the surgical procedures defined in this chapter make this possible.

SUMMARY

This chapter has examined the most commonly performed ophthalmic surgical procedures, perioperative considerations, and patient care. Using the nursing process, the nurse assesses the patient for visual disturbances, establishes nursing diagnoses, implements a plan of perioperative care, and assists with intraoperative therapies.

REFERENCES

Albiar, E., & Holds, J. B. (1992). Hydroxyapatite orbital implants: Indications for use and nursing considerations. *Journal of Ophthalmic Nursing and Technology, 11*(2), 71–75.

Assia, E. I., Apple, D. J., Barden, A., Tsai, J. C., Castaneda, V. E., & Hoggatt, J. S. (1991). An experimental study comparing various anterior capsulectomy techniques. *Archives of Ophthalmology, 109*, 642–647.

Atkinson, L. J., & Kohn, M. L. (1986). *Berry & Kohn's Introduction to operating room technique*, ed. 6, New York: McGraw-Hill.

Casey, T. A., & Mayer, D. J. (1984). *Corneal grafting*. Philadelphia: W. B. Saunders.

Christenbury, J. D. (1992). Translacrimal laser dacryocystorhinostomy. *Archives of Ophthalmology, 110*, 170–171.

Denny, A. D., & Gonnering, R. S. (1990). Early repair of complex orbital fractures. *Retina: The Journal of Retinal and Vitreous Disease, 10* (Suppl 1), S8–S19.

Echardt, C., Nicolai, U., Winter, M., & Knop, E. (1991). Experimental intraocular tolerance to liquid perfluorooctane and perfluoropolyether. *Retina: The Journal of Retinal and Vitreous Disease 11*, 375–384.

Ewing, R. H., & Stamper, R. L. (1990). Needle revision with and without 5-fluorouracil for the treatment of failed filtering blebs. *American Journal of Ophthalmology, 110*, 254–259.

Fastenberg, D. M., Schwartz, P. L., Shakin, J. L., & Golub, B. M. (1991). Management of dislocated nuclear fragments after phacoemulsification. *American Journal of Ophthalmology, 112*, 112–539.

Garcia, C. A., & Ruiz, R. S. (1992). Ocular complication of diabetes. *Clinical Symposia*, 6–26.

Garrity, J. A., Saggau, D. D., Gorman, C. A., Bartley, G. B., Fatourechi, V., Dardwig, P. W., & Dyer, J. A. (1992). Torsional diplopia after transantral orbital decompression and extraocular muscle surgery associated with Graves' orbitopathy. *American Journal of Ophthalmology, 113*, 363–373.

Gordon, D. M. (1962). *Diseases of the eye*, Summit, NJ: Ciba.

Haller, J. A., & Campochiaro, P. A. (1992). Oil and gas on troubled water. *Archives of Ophthalmology, 110*, 768–769.

Hamed, L. M., Tse, D. T., Glaser, J. S., Byrne, S. F., Schatz, S., & Norman, J. (1992). Neuroimaging of the optic nerve after fenestration for management of pseudotumor cerebri. *Archives of Ophthalmology, 110*, 636–639.

Hamill, M. B., & Thompson, W. S. (1990). The evaluation and management of corneal lacerations. *Retina: The Journal of Retinal and Vitreous Disease, 10* (Suppl 1), S1–S7.

Hattenhauer, J. M. (1991). To "Phaco" or not? *Archives of Ophthalmology, 109*, 315.

Ibrahim, O., Hussein, H. A., El-Sahn, M. F., El-Nawawy, S., Kassem, A., & Waring, G. O. III. (1991). Trapezoidal keratotomy for the correction of naturally occurring astigmatism. *Archives of Ophthalmology, 109*, 1374–1380.

Jones, L. T., & Wobig, J. L. (1976). *Surgery of the eyelids and lacrimal system*. Birmingham, AL: Aesculapius.

Kelman, S. E., & Elman, M. J. (1991). Optic nerve sheath decompression for nonarteritic ischemic optic neuropathy improves multiple visual function measurements. *Archives of Ophthalmology, 109*, 667–671.

Kitazawa, Y., Kawase, K., Matsushita, H., & Minobe, M. (1991). Trabeculectomy with mitomycin. *Archives of Ophthalmology, 109*, 1693–1698.

Krupin, T. (1992). Implanted aqueous shunt devices for glaucoma surgery. *Journal of Ophthalmic Nursing and Technology, 11*(1), 23–25.

Kwitko, S., Gritz, D. C., Garbus, J. J., Gaunderman, W. J., & McDonnell, P. J. (1992). Diurnal variation of corneal topography after radial keratotomy. *Archives of Ophthalmology, 110*, 351–356.

Lopez, R., & Chang, S. (1992). Long-term results of vitrectomy and perfluorocarbon gas for the treatment of severe proliferative vitreoretinopathy. *American Journal of Ophthalmology, 113*, 424–428.

Maguire, A. M., Blumenkranz, M. S., Ward, T. G., & Winkelman, J. Z. (1991). Scleral loop fixation for posteriorly dislocated intraocular lenses, *Archives of Ophthalmology*, 109: 1754–1758.

McDonnell, P. J., Moreira, H., Garbus, J., Clapham, T. N., D'Arcy, J., & Munnerlyn, C. R. (1991). Photorefractive keratectomy to create toric ablations for correction of astigmatism. *Archives of Ophthalmology, 109*, 710–713.

Murphy, W., and the Editors of Time-Life Books (1982). Remedies for eye complaints, foiling the thieves of sight, surgery under the microscope. *Touch, Smell, Taste, Sight and Hearing*, 62–136.

Ohira, A., Wilson, C. A., DeJuan, E., Murata, Y., Soji, T., & Oshima, K. (1991). Experimental retinal tolerance to emulsified silicone oil. *Retina: The Journal of Retinal and Vitreous Diseases, 11*, 259–265.

Opening your eyes to intraocular–drug administration (1994). *Nursing '94*, 24:44–45.

Patipa, M. (1992). Visual field loss in primary gaze and reading gaze due to acquired blepharoptosis and visual field improvement following ptosis surgery. *Archives of Ophthalmology, 110*, 63–67.

Paton, D. (1974). Cataracts, development, diagnosis, management. *Clinical Symposia, 26*(3), 22–25.

Sher, N. A., Barak, M., Daya, S., DeMarchi, J., Tucci, A., Hardten, D. R., Frantz, J. M., Eiferman, R. A., Parker, P., Telfair, W. B., Lane, S. S., & Lindstrom, R. L. (1992). Excimer laser photorefractive keratectomy in high myopia. *Archives of Ophthalmology, 110*, 935–941.

Sher, N. A., Chen, V., Bowers, R. A., Frantz, J. M., Brown, D. C., Eiferman, R., Lane, S. S., Parker, P., Ostroy, C., Doughman, D., Carpel, E., Zabel, R., Gothard, T., & Lindstrom, R. L. (1991). The use of the 193-nm excimer laser for myopic photorefractive keratectomy in sighted eyes. *Archives of Ophthalmology, 109*, 1525–1530.

Shields, C. L., Shields, J. A., & DePotter, P. (1992). Hydroxyapatite orbital implant after enucleation. *Archives of Ophthalmology, 110*, 333–338.

Smiddy, W., Michels, R. G., & Green, W. R. (1991). Lens and peripheral retinal relationships during vitrectomy. *Retina: The Journal of Retinal and Vitreous Disease, 11*, 199–203.

Smiddy, W. E., Flynn, H. W., Nicholson, D. H., Clarkson, J. G., Gass, D. M., Olsen, K. R., & Feuer, W. (1991). Results and complications in treating retinal breaks. *American Journal of Ophthalmology, 112*, 623–631.

Spapiro, M. J., Resnick, K. I., Kim, S. H., & Weinberg, A. (1991). Management of the dislocated crystalline lens with a perfluorocarbon liquid. *American Journal of Ophthalmology, 112*, 401–405.

Spires, R. (1991). Enucleation and the hydroxyapatite orbital implant. *Journal of Ophthalmic Nursing and Technology, 10*(5), 204–206.

Spires, R. (1992). Optic nerve sheath decompression in the treatment of progressive nonarteritic ischemic optic neuropathy. *Journal of Ophthalmic Nursing and Technology, 11*(2), 58–59.

Vaughan, D., Asbury, T., & Cook, R. (1971). *General Ophthalmology*, Norwalk, CT: Appleton & Lange.

Wertenbaker, L. and the Editors of U.S. News Books (1981). The imperfect eye, the mechanics of vision. *The Eye*, 27–37, 101–123.

Chapter 3

Otologic Surgery

Key Concepts

- Patients with sensory and perceptual (auditory) disorders have special communications needs. Hearing deficits usually result in increased patient anxiety.
- The perioperative nurse must assess the best way to communicate with the patient and validate that communications were understood.
- The operating room environment must be quiet and free of loud noises that could startle the otologic patient.
- Patient comfort during the procedure is essential so that movement is minimal. Positioning aids and a good assessment ensure comfort of the patient.
- Functionality of microsurgery instruments is critical to successful patient outcomes.
- Hearing-disabled patients are legally entitled to an interpreter.

INTRODUCTION

This chapter describes common otologic surgical procedures, preparation of the patient who may be hearing-impaired, and preparation of the room, instruments, and special equipment. A thorough patient plan of care includes effective modes of communicating, special patient concerns, and discussion of expected outcomes of the procedure.

ANATOMY

The ear serves two primary purposes, hearing and maintenance of equilibrium. It is divided into three anatomical divisions: external, middle, and inner (Fig. 3-1).

External Ear

The external ear consists of the auricle or pinna and the external auditory canal, which terminates at the tympanic membrane or eardrum. The tympanic membrane divides the external ear from the tympanic cavity and consists of three areas: the *pars flaccida*, the small upper portion; the *pars tensa*, the larger, vibrating portion; and the *annulus*, anchoring the tympanic membrane to the external canal.

Middle Ear

The middle ear, located in the temporal bone, contains the ossicles: the malleus, incus, and stapes. The facial nerve and the *chorda tympani nerve*, a branch of the facial nerve, are also in this space. Sensation within the middle ear is provided by the *glossopharyngeal* nerve (cranial nerve IV). The ossicles conduct vibrations to the oval window, an opening to the inner ear. The malleus (hammer) connects the eardrum to the incus; the incus (anvil) is in contact with the stapes (stirrup). The footplate of the stapes fits into the oval window. The middle ear and mastoid are supplied with blood from branches of the internal and external carotid arteries. The tympanic cavity communicates with the nasopharynx through the eustachian tube.

Inner Ear

The inner ear, located in the petrous portion of the temporal bone, contains the cochlea and the vestibular labyrinth. These small channels or structures contain the perilymph and the endolymph. The perilymph surrounds the inner ear and serves as a protective cushion to the end-organ receptors. The perilymph is continuous with the subarachnoid space and the cerebrospinal fluid through the aqueduct of the cochlea. The endolymph is contained in the endolymphatic system and bathes and nourishes the sensory cells.

Cochlea

The cochlea is divided into three compartments, the scala vestibuli, the scala tympani, and the cochlear duct. The scala vestibuli is associated with the round window, and the scala tympani is associated with the oval window. The scala tympani and vestibuli contain perilymph, and the cochlear duct contains endolymph.

The organ of Corti, the neural end-organ for hearing, is contained on the vestibular surface of the basilar membrane of the cochlea. The cochlea converts the mechanical wave movement energy from vibrations in the perilymph into electrochemical impulses by means of the hair cells of the organ of Corti.

The acoustic nerve (cranial nerve VIII) connects the inner ear to the brain.

Vestibular labyrinth

The vestibular labyrinth is composed of the utricle, saccule, and the semicircular canals. The semicircular canals are identified as the lateral, superior, and posterior. In each ear the canals are arranged at right angles to one another, so that any movement of the head excites at least one of the semicircular canals. The blood supply of the inner ear is provided by the internal auditory branches of the basilar artery.

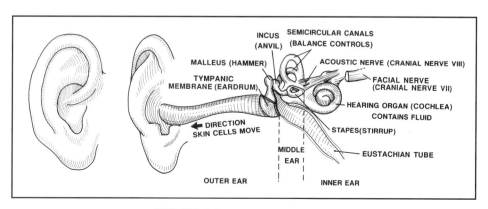

FIGURE 3-1 Anatomy of the ear.

Mastoid

The mastoid bone is a portion of the temporal bone. The cortex covers a system of interconnecting air cells, which are continuous with the middle ear cavity. The mastoid antrum is the largest air-containing cavity and connects directly with the middle ear.

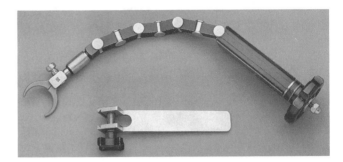

FIGURE 3-2 Universal otologic speculum holder.

NURSING CONSIDERATIONS

In planning perioperative care for the patient undergoing ear surgery, it is important to assess the hearing limitations of the patient. Hearing deficits may result in increased anxiety. A goal of preoperative care should be to decrease anxiety for the patient. To communicate effectively with the patient, the perioperative nurse should speak clearly to the patient and confirm that the patient heard and understood the communication.

The environment in the operating room should be kept quiet and free of loud noises that could startle the patient. If the procedure is being performed under local anesthesia, it is essential to stress to the patient the importance of remaining still and not moving during the surgery. It is important to identify any conditions, such as back pain or arthritis, that would prevent the patient's remaining in the prescribed position. Positioning aids may be useful for keeping the patient comfortable.

Hospitals, by law, must provide hearing-impaired services to patients requiring this assistance. Interpreters certified or qualified at the national or state level should be used for language interpretation. Financial arrangements should be made with local agencies to provide qualified interpreters for the hearing-impaired. A list of interpreters and their telephone numbers should be available in the operating room. Telecommunications Device for the Deaf (TDD) hearing-impaired telephone modems should be provided within the institution and portable units should be available for use in patient rooms.

Positioning

Most patients are in a dorsal recumbent position with the affected ear up. A foam cushion may be placed under the patient's head for comfort and to prevent pressure on the dependent auricle. If the procedure is being performed under local anesthesia, the head may be secured in position by a 2-inch piece of tape placed across the patient's forehead and attached to the operating room bed. A Mayo stand is placed over the patient's head, and drapes are placed to allow the patient to see and to allow the nurse to visualize the patient and reassure the patient during the procedure. A speculum holder (Fig. 3-2) may be attached to the operating room bed to allow the surgeon's hands to remain free, particularly should mastoid surgery be performed. The operative side should be placed as close to the edge of the bed as practical. The patient may be placed on the operating room bed in a reverse position

with the head at the foot of the operating room bed. This allows proper positioning of the microscope.

Prepping

For endomeatal incisions and stapedectomies, the surgeon may require that an area about 1 inch above and in front of the ear be clipped of hair to facilitate draping and postoperative dressing of the ear. For postaural and endaural incisions, a 2-inch wide area in front, above, and behind the ear should be clipped. Clipping is preferred to shaving, as shaving traumatizes the skin and increases the risk of infection. Males may prefer to have the entire head shaved to maintain symmetry. Females may be able to cover the shaved area with longer hair.

The ear is prepared by cleaning the meatus with cotton-tipped applicators. It may be desirable to place a plastic adherent drape around the ear prior to the surgical prep and to wipe the ear dry with a sterile towel after completion of the prep. The auricle is prepped with a topical antimicrobial solution for the prescribed period of time. Some surgeons may request that prep solution be instilled in the external canal with a syringe preoperatively.

A sterile plastic aperture drape is then applied with the auricle exposed through the opening. For procedures involving extensive irrigation, a drainage pouch may be attached to control the fluid.

Equipment

The operating microscope is required for otologic procedures. To be effective, a binocular eyepiece is essential and a teaching attachment may be required for educational purposes. Microscope lenses of different powers should be available in the room and should be carefully inspected preoperatively to be certain that they are clean and free of dust.

Power drills are essential for middle ear surgery. Several manufacturers and varieties of handpieces are available (Figs. 3-3 and 3-4). Drills may be pneumatic or electric. Electric drills may have the motor contained in the handpiece or separate from the handpiece. Pneumatic drills must be powerful, with high torque and speed, for example, more than 20,000 revolutions per minute (rpms). When using the drill, it is important to avoid overheating

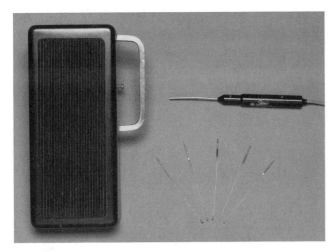

FIGURE 3-3 Otologic drill. *Left*, foot pedal control; *right top*, Skeeter ultra-lite Oto-tool. *Right bottom*, Oto-flex leur set.

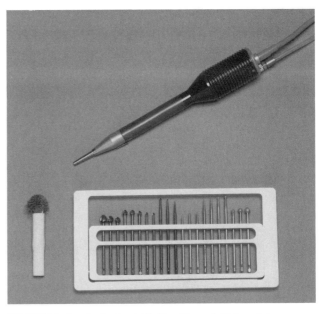

FIGURE 3-4 Otologic drill. *Top*, Shea drill handpiece. *Bottom left*, wire luer cleaner. *Bottom right*, Diamond Luer and burr set.

and localized desensitization of the bone through the use of continuous irrigation. It is also important to utilize intermittent rather than constant pressure with the drill bit. Overheating near the facial nerve may cause facial paralysis.

Diamond burrs cut more slowly but are not as likely to tear tissue; they tend to push soft tissue away. They may also assist in controlling bleeding from bone by pushing the vessel down into its channel and filling the channel with bone dust.

The teeth of each drill burr must be kept free of bone dust. Cutting burrs will require more attention because they tend to clog more easily than coarse-toothed burrs. Continuous flooding of the field with irrigation solution also helps to prevent clogging of burrs.

Bone dust has potent osteogenic properties; therefore, in procedures such as stapedectomies or tympanoplasties, or endolymphatic sac or fenestration procedures, it is most important to prevent bone dust from settling in areas where osteogenesis would create problems (Glasscock & Shambaugh, 1990). It is important to ascertain functionality of the appropriate burrs.

Suction irrigators are necessary to ensure adequate visibility of the surgical field. Copious irrigation washes away blood, bone dust, and bacteria from chronically infected ears.

Bone wax, while a valuable adjunct in controlling bleeding, especially bone marrow bleeding from the mastoid tip and the retrofacial nerve tract, is a foreign body and should be used judiciously.

Gelatinous sponge (e.g., Gelfoam) and oxidized cellulose (e.g., Surgicel) are useful for hemostasis in the mastoid process. Oxidized cellulose, however, must not be placed on the facial nerve or brain stem as its capacity to absorb fluid causes it to swell, causing compression in confined spaces. This may result in nerve deficit when the compression is over nerve tissue. A synthetic collagen sponge can be left in the wound, and when this is moistened with thrombin, stops venous bleeding (Glasscock & Shambaugh, 1990).

An effective mechanism for controlling bleeding is to place a moistened cottonoid against a piece of compressed Gelfoam over a bleeding point. After several minutes, the cottonoid can be removed, leaving the Gelfoam.

Instrumentation

Special instrumentation for otologic surgery includes alligator forceps, knives, curettes, periosteal elevators, rongeurs, and microsurgery instruments (Fig. 3-5, 3-6, 3-7, and 3-8). Sharp curettes are preferred over dull curettes as they cut with less pressure and are more effective. Large curettes present less risk of injury to the dura and facial nerve. Many of the instruments are extremely delicate and require special care and handling. It is essential that each instrument be inspected preoperatively to ensure that it is in perfect working order.

Incisions

Postauricular incision

The postauricular incision is used to expose the mastoid process and follows the curve of the postauricular fold, beginning at the upper attachment of the auricle and continuing to 1 cm behind the mastoid process. When making this incision, the surgeon and assistant may place digital pressure on either side of the incision to control bleeding, as the incision may cut across the posterior auricular artery.

Newborns do not have a mastoid process. Caution must be used when making this incision to avoid severing the facial nerve.

Following the incision and control of bleeding, the lateral surface of the mastoid process is exposed, using a periosteal elevator. A self-retaining mastoid retractor will

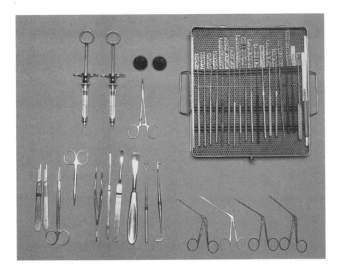

A

FIGURE 3-5 *(A)* Micro basic ear instrumentation: *Top, from left:* syringes, ear speculums, mosquito hemostat forceps. *Bottom, from left:* two #3 knife handles with #15 blades, pointed sharp scissors, baby Metzenbaum scissors, Adson-Brown tissue forceps (2), Shambrough elevator, Lempert elevator, wing-tip elevator, double skin hook, Miller-Senn retractors, alligator forceps (2), Bellucci scissors, large (2), *On tray, from left to right: (B)* #1 knife, #2 knife, weapon, (House-Rosen knife), gimmick (House elevator), Rosen needle, capsule knife. *(C)* Straight pick, mastoid searcher, fenestrometer, large right angle pick, fine right angle pick, Guilford canal knife, *(D)* Derlacki mobilizer, right and left Fisch microcurettes, right and left whirlybirds, Shambrough (duckbill) elevator, mirror (end covered).

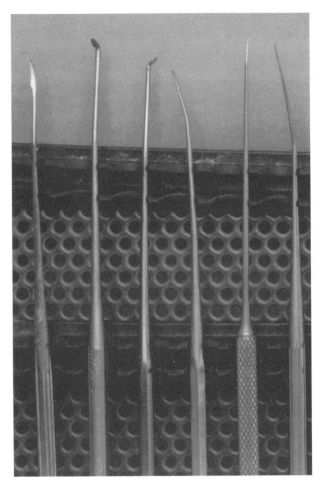

B

then be placed. The retractor should be spread carefully to avoid stripping the skin from the meatus.

Endaural incision

The endaural incision is made in two stages and may be made with a Lempert's triangular knife or a #15 blade. Assuming that the patient is in an upright position, the incision begins at the 12 o'clock position on the superior meatal wall about 1 cm from the outer edge of the meatus to nearly the 6 o'clock position. It is then taken outward 2.3 mm to the edge of the conchal cartilage. A second incision going upward about halfway between the meatus and the upper edge of the auricle allows for greater exposure.

Stapes incision

The stapes incision begins at the 6 o'clock position on the inferior meatal wall and slopes outward to 6 to 8 mm from the annulus, and extends forward to about 2 mm above the short process of the malleus. The periosteum and the meatal skin are elevated inward to the annulus and sulcus tympanicus with an angled lancet. Bleeding may be controlled by applying a suction to cotton balls soaked in lidocaine with epinephrine, the solution used for local injection, and/or electrocautery. The annulus tympanicus is then elevated and the posterior half of the

tympanic membrane is folded across the manubrium onto the anterior half, exposing the posterior portion of the tympanic cavity.

Dressings

Postoperatively, a cotton ball may be packed loosely in the patient's ear, 4 × 4 fluffs applied to maintain the auricle in an anatomical position, and a Kerlix-type dressing applied to maintain the dressing in place.

EXTERNAL EAR SURGICAL PROCEDURES

Bilateral myringotomy with tubes

Perioperative nursing considerations

Otitis media is a common occurrence in children. In the United States, one billion dollars is spent annually for the treatment of pediatric otitis media (Facione, 1990). The disease primarily affects children from 6 months to 3 years of age and results from a dysfunction of the eustachian tube. Negative pressure secondary to blockage of the

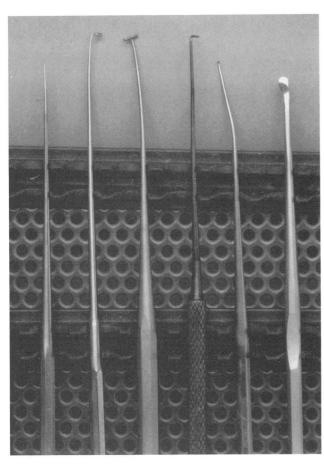

C

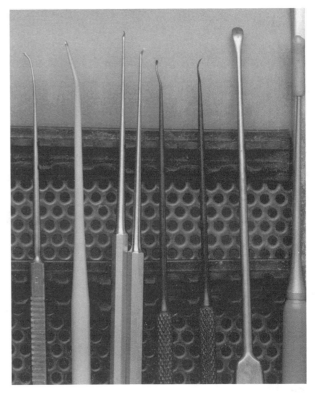

D

eustachian tube leads to a middle ear effusion. A bilateral middle ear effusion of longer than 90 days' duration puts a child at some risk of hearing loss, speech problems, and recurrent acute otitis media (AOM) (Schwartz, 1987).

The surgical procedure, bilateral myringotomy with tubes (BMT), is performed under general anesthesia with a small number of instruments (Fig. 3-9) and a microscope. An incision is made in the pars tensa of the tympanic membrane, and the effusion is aspirated, followed by placement of tiny, hollow tympanostomy tubes (Figs. 3-10 and 3-11).

The incision in the tympanic membrane can be made in the anteroinferior quadrant if the tube is to remain in place for a long period of time or in the posteroinferior quadrant if a short time is desired (Glasscock & Shambaugh, 1990).

Politzer first suggested the bypassing of the eustachian tubes with ventilation tubes 100 years ago (Facione, 1990). The benefits of adenoidectomy in conjunction with BMT remain unproven. The procedure is vigorously supported by some surgeons and not considered helpful by others.

Procedure

Key steps

1. No prep is necessary.
2. The head and microscope are positioned.
3. The external ear canal is cleaned with an ear curette.
4. The tympanic membrane is incised with a myringotomy knife.
5. Fluid is aspirated.
6. The tympanostomy tube is attached to alligator forceps for placement.
7. The tympanostomy tube is placed.
8. Suctioning is done.
9. Antibiotic ear drops are instilled.

Complications of tympanostomy tubes include acute and chronic otorrhea or cholesteatoma. *Pseudomonas* microorganisms often are the cause of chronic otorrhea.

Postoperatively, the child returns to normal activity soon after surgery, with the addition of earplugs for participation in water activities. About 20% of the children undergoing BMT will require the procedure two or more times (Schwartz, 1987).

MIDDLE EAR SURGICAL PROCEDURES

Stapedectomy/Stapedotomy

Perioperative nursing considerations

Otosclerosis, or otospongiosis, causes deafness through the formation of abnormal bone that locks the stapes in place and prevents it from vibrating and carrying the stimulus. In 1952, Rosen introduced stapes mobilization.

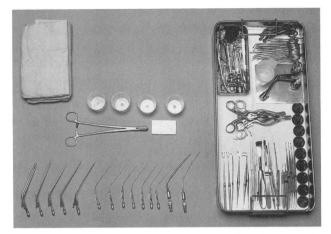

FIGURE 3-6 Basic ear tray. *Top, from left:* Towels, medicine glasses, fascia crusher with teflon block. *Bottom, from left:* suction irrigating tips (5), ear suction tips (9). *Tray contents:* short sponge stick, short Kelly hemostats (2), Crilewood needle holders (2), plastic needle holders (2), Providence hemostats (4), straight mosquito forceps (2), curved mosquito forceps (10), towel clips (small) (6), disposable towel clips (4), ear speculums (9), Miller-Senn retractors (2), wing-tip elevator (1), Lempert elevator (1), long skin hooks (2), short skin hooks (2), double skin hooks (2), bayonet forceps, long (1), bayonet forceps, short (1), short Adson-Brown tissue forceps (2), long Adson-Brown tissue forceps (2), Adson dura forceps (2), suture scissors, straight (1), baby Metzenbaum scissors (1), tubex syringes (2), teflon block (1), bone-holding forceps (1), Hoffman clamp (1), Beaver knife handle (1), irrigation spouts (2), endaural speculum (1), suction irrigating tips, Shambraugh elevator (1), I curettes (2), J curettes (2), small humpback Weitlaner retractors (2), large cupped forceps, Shea scissors, small; Shea alligator forceps, minimicro scissors, minimicro cupped forceps, mini alligator forceps, Derlacki mobilizer, wire crimper, malleus nipper, #3 knife handles (2), Metzenbaum scissors (2), 2-point sharp scissors (1), Bellucci scissors, mini House forceps, Shea cupped forceps.

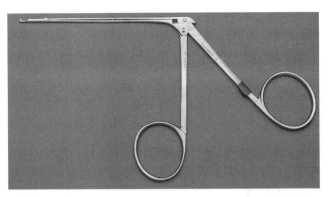

FIGURE 3-8 Malleus nipper.

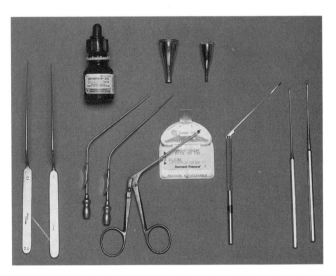

FIGURE 3-9 Myringotomy set. *Top, from left:* Cortisporin otic solution, ear speculums (2). *Bottom, from left:* Kas pick chisel, Kas pick, straight; #5 ear suction tip, #20 ear suction tip, alligator forceps with tympanostomy tube, myringotomy blade on Beaver handle, small curette, large curette.

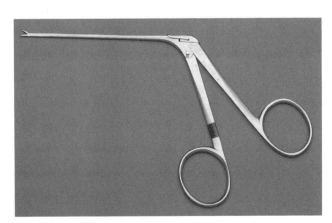

FIGURE 3-7 Wire crimper.

Shea introduced the stapedectomy operation in 1958 (Conrad, 1990). The volume of stapedectomies increased quickly in the 1960s, but the number of deaf patients with otosclerosis decreased to about 20% of its peak by the late 1970s (Conrad, 1990). Currently the diminishing pool of otosclerotic patients causes concern for resident training. Limited experience may compromise patient outcomes (Alford et al., 1988).

Stapes surgery has evolved from the original total stapedectomy, to partial stapedectomy, to small fenestra stapedectomy (SFS) or stapedotomy (Conrad, 1990). The procedure involves removal of the otosclerotic lesion at the footplate of the stapes and creation of an implant to maintain the conductive mechanism. Some otologists interpose a vein or connective tissue graft between the piston and the fenestra. Most otologists sever the stapedius tendon to avoid lenticular necrosis, which may allow the prosthesis to slip.

Carbon dioxide (CO_2) and potassium, titanyl, phosphate (KTP) crystal lasers may be used to create a hole in the footplate for insertion of the prosthesis. Lasers may be used to remove connective tissue and open the oval window for revisions (Smalley, 1990). The KTP laser provides precise focus and avoids the alignment concerns associated with the CO_2 laser. Caution is necessary to avoid the

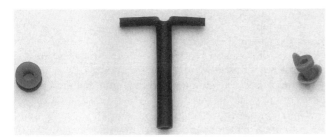

FIGURE 3-10 Examples of tympanostomy tubes: Sheehy collar button tube, Goode T-tube, Shea parasol tube.

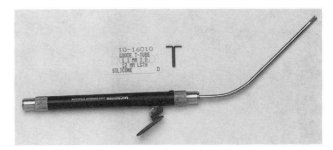

FIGURE 3-11 Goode T-tube for tympanostomy with inserter.

beam's penetrating to inner ear structures and causing sensorineural damage. When using the CO_2 laser, spot size must be reduced to less than 0.3 mm to prevent bone charring and ragged edges (Smalley, 1990). To be successful, the CO_2 laser must be coaxial and parfocal. Blood loss is minimal when using the laser. Patients may report an improvement in hearing while in the operating room.

As with any laser use, the field should be draped with wet towels, the laser placed in the standby mode when not in use, and a bowl of sterile water kept available on the back table to extinguish a possible ignition or fire. See Chapter 22, Vol. 1, for more information on lasers.

Documented outcomes include:

1. Vein and polyethylene procedures: 73% achieved lasting closure of the air–bone gap, and 5% had some residual improvement 6 to 11 years postoperatively.
2. Piston reconstruction through the posterior part of the footplate: 91% showed closure and 4% showed improvement 3 to 6 years postoperatively (Morrison, 1971).

About 90% of operated ears will have a permanent hearing gain, and 1% will be permanently worse (Conrad, 1990).

Stapedectomy

Key steps

1. Instruments (Figs. 3-12 and 3-13) are placed on the overhead Mayo stand.
2. A local anesthetic, usually lidocaine with epinephrine, is injected into four quadrants of the canal to control bleeding.
3. The canal is cleaned, the speculum is placed, and the microscope is positioned.
4. The tympanomeatal flap is lifted, using a Guilford or House knife.
5. The posterior bony ledge is removed with the "weapon."
6. The incustapedial joint is cut.
7. The stapedial tendon is cut with a Bellucci scissors.
8. The stapes superstructure is fractured with a Rosen needle and cups.
9. Stapedotomy is performed with a drill hole in the footplate, using the Skeeter drill.

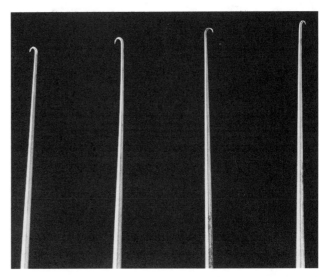

FIGURE 3-12 Stapedectomy footplate hooks: 3.0-mm anterior footplate hook, 6.0-mm anterior footplate hook, 6.0-mm posterior footplate hook, 3.0-mm posterior footplate hook.

10. The prosthesis is placed and the patient's hearing is tested verbally.
11. The prosthesis is secured with a graft (vein, fascia, gelatinous sponge).
12. The tympanomeatal flap is replaced, using a drum elevator and Rosen needle.
13. The external ear is packed and a dressing is applied.

Tympanoplasty

Perioperative nursing considerations

Perforations of the tympanic membrane that persist may require surgical closure. Chronic perforations may be relatively painless and have foul-smelling otorrhea. Central perforations (tubotympanic type) may be repaired with a simple surgical procedure. Marginal perforations more frequently require surgical reconstruction (tympanoplasty) of the tympanic membrane. Perforations in the posterior superior pars tensa and perforations in the pars flaccida (attic position) of the tympanic membrane have a high correlation with cholesteatoma forma-

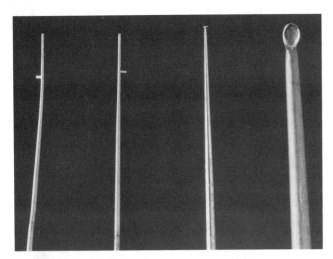

FIGURE 3-13 Stapedectomy instruments: 4.0-mm measuring rod, 4.5-mm measuring rod, Mushroom gauge, stapes curette.

tion (Falcione, 1990). Cholesteatomas are the result of skin cell migration from the external ear through a perforation in the tympanic membrane.

Five types of tympanoplasties have been employed:

I. Covering the perforation in the tympanic membrane with a graft, the same as myringoplasty
II. Closing the perforation with the graft, primarily contacting the body of the incus
III. Depressing the graft against the stapes when the malleus and incus are missing
IV. Invaginating the graft into the oval window when all the ossicles are missing except a mobile stapes footplate
V. Invaginating the graft into the oval window much as in IV but in the presence of an immobile stapes footplate

The approach may be through the ear canal, postauricularly, or through both areas. The surgeon removes the remnants of the tympanic membrane. The diseased portion of the middle ear is then removed with picks, curettes, or a drill. Irrigation is required to remove debris and maintain a clean operating field.

A temporalis fascial graft, which may be harvested prior to or following the ear procedure, will be allowed to dry on a flat surface or may be pressed to facilitate handling. The surgeon will trim the graft and position it with alligator forceps or picks. The graft may be held in place by a gelatinous sponge.

A word of caution about nitrous oxide anesthesia is in order here. Nitrous oxide, which is 34 times more soluble than nitrogen, enters air-filled cavities such as the middle ear more rapidly than air can leave, resulting in an elevation of middle ear pressures. Therefore, inhaled nitrous oxide concentrations should be limited to 50%, with discontinuance of the inhalations at least 5 minutes before placement of the graft (Stoelting & Miller, 1989).

Ossicular Chain Reconstruction

Ossicular chain interruption most frequently occurs as a result of otitis media but may result from a head injury. Repair may require two surgical procedures: first, the removal of infected/pathologic tissue, and second, reconstruction.

Ossicular chain reconstruction may be accompanied with a partial ossicular replacement prosthesis (PORP) or a total ossicular replacement prosthesis (TORP).

PORP involves replacement of a diseased or eroded malleus or incus. A TORP is used when all ossicles are diseased or eroded.

Ossicular chain reconstruction procedure

Steps 1, 2, 3, and 4 are the same as for stapedectomy, except that a larger flap may be turned.

Mastoidectomy

Perioperative nursing considerations

In 1873, Hermann Schwartz established the indications and technique of the simple mastoid operation (Glasscock & Shambaugh, 1990). Mastoidectomy is the surgical removal of the mastoid process to eradicate diseased bone. Mastoidectomy may include removal of some ossicles and the canal wall or, if radical removal is required, will include removal of the canal wall and the ossicles. Modified radical mastoidectomy is indicated for cholesteatoma removal and tympanic membrane repair. A second operation 6 months later is necessary to remove any residual cholesteatoma and perform the ossicular reconstruction.

General anesthesia is usually used, but local anesthesia can be used. Either endaural, postauricular, or both incisions may be used, but the postauricular incision offers better exposure and may be preferred. Diseased bone is removed with a drill. Caution must be used to avoid the facial nerve. Facial nerve damage results in immobility of the affected side, mouth droop, and inability to close the eye, drink water, or whistle.

Tympanamastoidectomy

Key steps

1. Four quadrants of the canal are injected with lidocaine with epinephrine.
2. The tympanomeatal flap is raised.
3. A postauricular incision is made to harvest the fascia graft.
4. The graft is smoothed and set aside to dry.
5. Diseased mastoid bone is removed with a drill.
6. Results are checked with a pick, Rosen needle, gimmick, and mastoid searcher.
7. Diseased ossicles are removed using Bellucci scissors, weapon, gimmick, or other microsurgical instruments.
8. All evidence of cholesteatoma is eradicated.

9. The fascial graft is placed.
10. The mastoid cavity and middle ear are packed with absorbable pledgets soaked in balanced salt solution or Cortisporin solution.
11. Incisions are closed, the external canal is packed, and dressings are applied.

INNER EAR SURGICAL PROCEDURES

Cochlear Implants

Perioperative nursing considerations

Cochlear implants are available for patients who are diagnosed as being profoundly deaf. The House 3M Cochlear Implant system was approved for use in adults by the Food and Drug Administration (FDA) in 1984. In 1990, the FDA approval was granted for its use in children 2 to 17 years of age. The device may be used in children who are born deaf. One in every thousand U.S. children is born deaf.

A platinum electrode is placed in the scali tympani of the cochlea (Fig. 3-14). A mastoidectomy and opening of the facial recess are required to provide access. At about 2 months postoperatively, the patient is fitted with the external device.

Key steps

1. An incision from above the pinna extending to the mastoid tip is made.
2. A recess in the mastoid cortex is created with a trephine and osteotome.
3. The tympanic membrane is elevated.
4. The posterior bony canal is grooved for electrode leads.

5. The promontory bone is drilled to allow visibility of the first cochlear turn.
6. The electrode wire tip is guided into the cochlea.

Endolymphatic Sac Shunt Procedure

Endolymphatic hydrops (Meniere's disease) is an inner ear condition, caused by labyrinthine dysfunction. Symptoms include vertigo with nausea and vomiting, tinnitus, and neurosensory hearing loss. Patients may respond to a salt-free diet and a diuretic.

Surgical procedures available to correct the condition are the endolymphatic sac shunt procedure and labyrinthectomy.

Key steps

1. The mastoid approach is used.
2. The endolymphatic sac is opened.
3. The fluid is drained.
4. A shunt is placed between the sac and the subarachnoid space or the mastoid.

Labyrinthectomy

The vestibular labyrinth can be removed to correct vertigo but results in loss of vestibular function and loss of hearing.

ACOUSTIC NEUROMA

An acoustic neuroma arises from Schwann cells of the vestibular portion of cranial nerve VIII (acoustic). Although the tumors are benign, their size may produce cerebellar or brain stem symptoms. Symptoms may in-

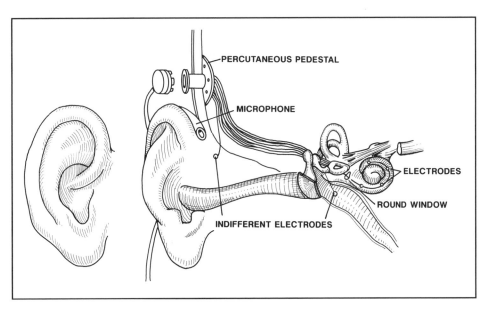

FIGURE 3-14 Cochlear implant.

clude unilateral hearing loss, tinnitus, vertigo, diplopia, and decreased lacrimation. The tumor may be diagnosed by a brain stem auditory evoked-response test. Confirmation of the diagnosis is made by magnetic resonance imaging of the brain and internal auditory canals. If the tumor extends into the cranium, its removal becomes a neurosurgical procedure.

Excision of Acoustic Neuroma

Key steps

1. A postauricular incision is made, similar to a mastoidectomy incision.
2. Ossicles and semicircular canals are exposed.
3. The incus is removed with alligator forceps.
4. The semicircular canals are excised with a drill.
5. The bone is removed.
6. The dura is opened with a #11 blade.
7. The tumor is dissected with a gimmick and other microinstruments.
8. The mastoid cavity is packed with fat, fascia, or muscle.
9. The incision is closed.

SUMMARY

Otologic surgery requires a calm atmosphere, devoid of noise, comfortable for the patient, and conducive to minute and precise surgical "moves." This chapter has described care and preparation that help ensure the environment described.

Common otologic procedures of the outer, middle, and inner ear were described, along with the required instrumentation, equipment, and care of the patient. The goal of most otologic surgery is to correct sensory deficits and disorders of the ear leading to optimal patient functioning.

REFERENCES

Alford, B. R., Cocker, N. J., Duncan, N. O. III, Jenkins, H. A., & Wright, G. L. (1988). Stapedectomy trends for the resident. *Annals of Otology, Rhinology and Laryngology, 97,* 109–113.

Coligado, E. J. et al. (1993). Multichannel cochlear implantation in the rehabilitation of post-traumatic sensorineural hearing loss. *Archives of Physical Medicine and Rehabilitation, 74,* 653–657.

Conrad, G. J. (1990). Collective stapedectomy (an approach to the numbers problem). *The Journal of Laryngology and Otology, 104,* 390–393.

Facione, N. (1990). Otitis media: An overview of acute and chronic disease. *Nurse Practitioner, 15* (10), 11–20.

Glasscock, M. E., & Shambaugh, G. E. Jr. (1990). *Surgery of the ear* (4th ed.). Philadelphia: W. B. Saunders

Goldenberg, R. A., Brown, M., and Cunningham S. (1992). Laser stapedectomy: A new method of correcting deafness. *AORN Journal, 55,* 759, 761–762, 764.

Graves, M. (1991). Otologic surgery, pp. 501–527, in M. H. Meeker and J. C. Rothrock (eds.). *Alexander's care of the patient in surgery* (9th ed.). St. Louis: Mosby–Year Book.

Kane, D. M. (1992). Practical points in the management of a postoperative acoustic neuroma patient. *Journal of Post Anesthesia Nursing, 7,* 262–266.

Morrison, A. W. (1971). *Diseases of the ear, nose and throat* (3rd ed., pp. 351–394). St. Louis: C. V. Mosby.

Saunders, S. H. (1989). Tonsils, adenoids, & grommets. *Midwife Health Visitor & Community Nurse, 25* (12), 516–517.

Schwartz, R. H. (1987). A practical approach to chronic otitis. *Patient Care,* July 15, 91–109.

Smalley, P. J. (1990). Lasers in otolaryngology. *Nursing Clinics of North America, 25* (3), 645–656.

Stoelting, R. K., & Miller, R. D. (1989). *Basics of anesthesia* (2nd ed., pp. 362–363). New York: Churchill Livingstone.

ADDITIONAL READINGS

Alberti, P. W. (1987). The future of cochlear implants: A summary of the national forum. *The Journal of Otolaryngology, 16* (5), 322–323.

Atkinson, L. J. (1992). *Berry & Kohn's operating room technique* (7th ed.) St. Louis: Mosby–Year Book.

Brunner, L. S., & Suddarth, D. S. (1988). Assessment and management of patients with hearing problems and ear disorders. In *Textbook of Medical-Surgical Nursing* (6th ed., pp. 1370–1392). Philadelphia: J. B. Lippincott.

Campbell, C. (1991). Acoustic neuroma: Nursing implications related to surgical management. *Journal of Neuroscience Nursing 23* (1), 50–56.

Flood, J. (1989). Glue ear. *Nursing Times 85* (36), 38–41.

Fuller, J. R. (1986). Eye, ear, nose, throat and mouth surgery—Part II. In *Surgical technology principles and practice* (2nd ed., pp. 511–525). Philadelphia: W. B. Saunders.

Hepworth, S. (1990). Communicating with a hearing impaired patient. *The Lamp,* July, 31–34.

Iadarola, G., & Kerrigan, M. B. (1986). Do you hear what I hear? *AORN Journal 43,* 478–481.

Jackson, P. D., & Rupp, R. R. (1986). Primary care for the hearing impaired: A changing picture. *Geriatrics, 41* (3), 75–80.

Mair, I. W. S. (1989). Occasional stapes surgery—a Norwegian experience. *The Journal of Laryngology and Otology, 103,* 259–262.

Mallett, J. (1989). Talking patients round. *Nursing Times, 85* (38), 37–39.

Maniglia, A. J. (1989). Implantable hearing devices. *Otology—Current Concepts and Technology, 22* (1), 175–200. Philadelphia: W. B. Saunders

News focus (1989). Extra-sensory aid. *Nursing Times 85* (50), 14–15.

Chapter 4

Nasal Surgery

Key Concepts

- With the increase in endoscopic procedures, a thorough understanding of equipment, its care, and sterilization is essential.
- Anticipated equipment (headlight, endoscopy equipment, suction, positioning aids) should be in the room preoperatively, especially if the procedure is done under local anesthesia.
- Patients are usually placed in supine or modified supine position.
- The nose is often injected/packed with vasoconstricting and/or localizing anesthetic agents prior to the procedure (lidocaine with epinephrine; oxymetazolone or phenylephrine; cocaine topical solution, 5% to 10% strength), which can result in cardiac arrhythmias.
- The skin preparation for nasal surgery is still done even though most of the procedures are considered to be clean procedures only. Because the surgeon needs access to the eyes on many procedures, a nonirritating solution should be used to prevent eye irritation.
- CT scans and X-ray films need to be available in the operating room for surgical reference.
- Blood loss must be carefully monitored. The potential for hemorrhage exists due to the extensive vascularity of the nose and face.
- Morbidity and bleeding are less if the patient is in the subacute phase of nasal disease at the time of surgery. Preoperative assessment should include time of last dose of antibiotic.
- Scrub persons should be alert for eye or eyelid movement while the surgeon is removing any tissue. Collected specimens that float in a saline-filled container should be brought to the immediate attention of the surgeon; this specimen/ tissue may be periorbital fat. Either occurrence could indicate that periorbital or optic damage (blindness) is in progress.
- Nasal packing is used to support internal structures and aid in hemostasis. Impregnating the packing (iodoform, plain, or petrolatum gauze) with an antibiotic ointment prior to insertion will prevent trauma upon removal and reduce the incidence of infection.
- Nasal packing can cause significant alterations in respiratory physiology and arterial blood gases in elderly patients, as well as increase anxiety levels in all patients.
- Dressings made of 2 × 2 sponges, called drip pads or moustache dressings, are taped under the nose postoperatively.

INTRODUCTION

Nasal surgery is varied and not without risks, since many of the procedures take place near vital structures of the head. Respiratory functioning is most affected by nasal surgery, as is the patient's body image and perceived appearance. This chapter discusses a number of nasal procedures, including those done endoscopically. The perioperative nurse has many opportunities to contribute to the outcomes of the surgery as well as to provide supportive care and information to the patient.

ANATOMY

The nose, being the most prominent feature of the face, has many functions: it is the organ of the sense of smell and it assists the sense of taste by discriminating food properties; it also helps regulate and control the temperature and humidity of inspired air, acts to remove particulate matter from inspired air, and assists in speech resonance and in flow regulation during inspiration. The nose is composed of an external, or outer, nose and an internal part, the nasal fossae. The outer nose is the pyramid-shaped structure positioned on the middle third of the face. It is constructed of bone, fibrous tissue, cartilage, and skin (Fig. 4-1). Ethmoid, sphenoid, maxillary, and frontal bones assist in the framework. The internal nose is situated between the roof of the mouth and the cranial base, and is anterior to the nasopharynx (Fig. 4-2). Air enters into the right and left nasal cavities through two nostrils (nares). The nasal septum, which separates the cavities into halves, is situated in the midline. The septum has both a cartilaginous and a bony framework. Cartilage forms the anterior part (columella), while the vomer and perpendicular plate of the ethmoid form the upper, lower, and posterior portions.

Just inside the nostril is the vestibule, lined with skin and stiff hairs, which serve to trap particulate matter before reaching the lungs. A mucous membrane lining is continuous from the interior of the nose past the vestibule to the lungs. Turbinate bones (or conchae) are found on the lateral walls of each cavity (Fig. 4-3). The primary function of these sagging projections (superior, middle, and inferior) is to humidify and regulate air temperature. Therefore they have the thickest and most vascular mucous membrane in the nose.

Located in facial bones surrounding the nasal cavities are the paranasal sinuses. These air (or bony) sinuses, which are lined with mucous membrane, drain into the nasal cavities through openings in grooves between the turbinates. There are four pairs of sinuses: the frontal, sphenoidal, ethmoidal, and maxillary (Fig. 4-4).

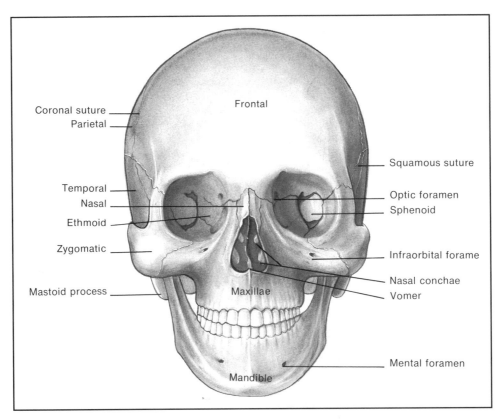

FIGURE 4-1 Frontal, lacrimal, zygomatic, maxillary, and nasal bones of the skull. (From Anderson, P.D. [1984]. *Basic Human Anatomy and Physiology.* Boston: Jones and Bartlett Publishers.)

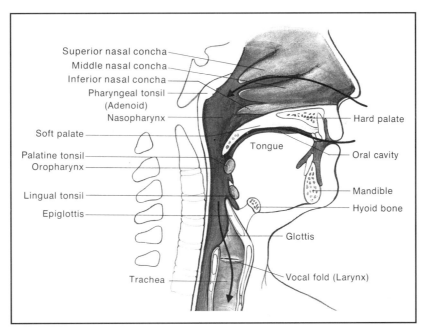

FIGURE 4-2   Sagittal section of the head and neck.   (From Anderson, P.D. [1984]. *Basic Human Anatomy and Physiology.* Boston: Jones and Bartlett Publishers.)

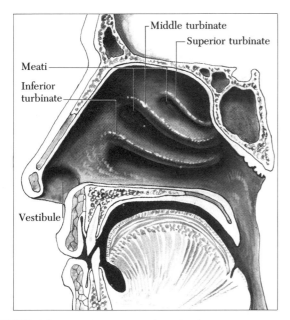

FIGURE 4-3   Nasal turbinates (conchae).   (From Grimes, J. and Burns, E. [1992]. *Health Assessment in Nursing Practice* [3rd ed.]. Boston: Jones and Bartlett Publishers.)

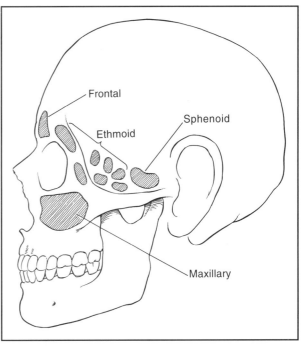

FIGURE 4-4   Lateral view of the head, showing sinuses.

A nasolacrimal duct opens into each nasal cavity below the inferior turbinate onto each side. Tears drain into the nose and serve as an added source of humidification. The sense of smell (olfactory) is located in the superior septum and turbinate of the mucous membrane. Blood supply for the external nose is from the facial, superior coronary, ophthalmic, and infraorbital arteries. The nerve supply for the muscles is from the facial nerve, and that of the skin is from the infraorbital, infratrochlear, and ophthalmic nerves. The fossae receives blood supply from the ophthalmic, the internal maxillary, and the superior facial arteries. Termination of blood supply is the ophthalmic and facial veins. The internal nose receives its nerve supply from the olfactory, vidian, sphenopalatine, ophthalmic, superior maxillary, and palatine nerves, and from Meckel's ganglion.

NURSING CONSIDERATIONS

Along with an extensive history, a complete physical examination of the nose is necessary to confirm or rule out abnormalities. The external nose is checked for symmetry, nostril shape, and anterior position of the septum. Endoscopic or gross physical examination is then done to look for obstructions caused by nasal septal deviations, polyps, fractures, spurs, hypertrophied tissues, or masses. Obstructions in airflow can be measured by using manometers, mirror tests, rhinomanometry, and flowmeters. Manageable epistaxis can be cauterized in the office with silver nitrate sticks. Cultures and smears from drainage can be done to detect bacterial sinusitis. Imaging may be done on those patients who have abnormalities without detectable symptoms, or for those who may need functional endoscopic sinus surgery. Computed tomography (CT) scanning is superior to plain X-ray studies because of better images and less radiation exposure; however, CT scans are expensive. CT scans show abnormalities that sinus X-ray series and nasal endoscopy may not show. Currently CT images provide the most preoperative information for patients undergoing endoscopic sinus surgery. Because bone is not visualized, magnetic resonance imaging (MRI) studies are primarily used to differentiate soft tissue abnormalities. Therefore, MRI images are better than CT scans for detecting nasal and sinus tumors. Benefits of using MRIs include no radiation exposure and the fact that the study can be done for patients who are unable to hyperextend their heads; the significant drawback is the cost of the study.

SURGICAL PROCEDURES

Submucosal Resection (SMR)

Nursing considerations

Deviations of the nasal septum in adults can result in the need for surgical correction. This type of obstruction can precipitate acute and chronic sinusitis and upper respiratory infection. Submucosal resection (SMR) involves removal of cartilage and bony septum causing the obstruction while preserving an adequate caudal and dorsal strut of quadrangular cartilage. However, there may be complications to this procedure: internally, these may be septal perforations and a potential for airway obstruction; externally, SMR may cause a sagging of the nose, loss of nasal tip support, and retraction of the columella (Beeson, 1987). Instrumentation will be from a nasal set (Figs. 4-5 and 4-6).

Desired outcomes are successful and calm anesthetic emergence with unobstructed mouth breathing and minimal blood loss during the procedure as well as postoperatively. The patient will be positioned in high Fowler's position postoperatively.

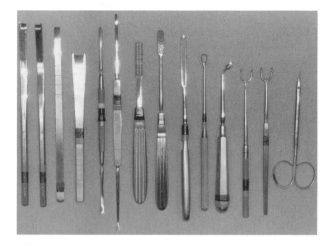

FIGURE 4-5   Nasal instrument set. *Left to right:* left and right guarded osteotomes, Cottle osteotome, bilateral guarded osteotome, Freer elevator, Cottle elevator, diamond rasp, Maltz rasp, Ballenger swivel knife, Coakley curette, Wellaminski antrum perforator, Joseph double-hooked retractor, Cottle guarded double-hooked retractor, iris scissors.

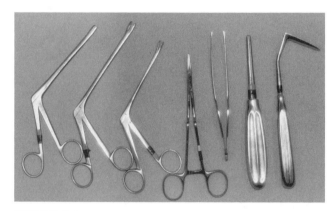

FIGURE 4-6   Nasal instrument set. *Left to right:* small Takahashi forceps, medium Takahashi forceps, duckbill forceps, bayonet needle holder, bayonet forceps, Cottle crusher, Aufricht retractor.

Procedure

Key steps

1. After nasal injections/vasoconstricting packing is removed, the nostril is exposed with a nasal speculum.
2. A mucoperichondrial-mucoperiosteal flap is created on one side of the septum by first incising the septal cartilage with a #15 blade and then using a Cottle or Freer elevator.
3. The bony septum is further freed up until the quadrangular cartilage is disarticulated from the perpendicular plate of the ethmoid and the vomer.
4. The remaining nostril is exposed and an opposing mucoperichondrial-mucoperiosteal flap is incised.
5. The bony septum is freed up as before, with care not to create any communication to the other side. Any spurs or deviations are removed at this time.

6. The septum may be manipulated to a more midline position at this time. Cartilage grafts placed in the flaps may also be used.
7. The mucoperichondrial flaps are repositioned and septal segments are stabilized for closure. Typically, a rapidly absorbing suture on a small cutting needle (plain or chromic catgut) is used on the incision.
8. Nasal packing is placed and a 2 × 2 gauze moustache dressing (drip pad) is taped in place. An external splint of rigid plastic may be applied prior to dressing.

Septoplasty (Nasal Septal Reconstruction, NSR)

Nursing considerations

Spurs and protrusions can be removed in a septoplasty by freeing the quadrangular or anterior septal cartilage. This procedure is preferred to an SMR because of access to other bony and cartilaginous structures while preserving septal support (Beeson, 1987). External nasal deformities caused by a deviated nasal septum and dislocation of the columella can be corrected with this procedure. A rhinoplasty may be done in addition if part of the deformity is due to displacement of the bony framework (Loré, 1988). Instrumentation is the same as for SMR.

Desired outcomes are as for the SMR procedure.

Procedure

Key steps

1. Using a #15 blade, an incision is made along the nasal tip (caudal) end of the deviated side.
2. If the deviation occurs at the base of the septum, bone and cartilage are involved. Because of this, blunt dissection cannot be achieved using the conventional Freer method. Sharp dissection and use of osteotomes will be necessary.
3. Once the mucoperichondrium is elevated medially and laterally on the affected side, a convex wedge is removed to allow straightening of the septum.
4. If proximal deviation is present, further elevation of the mucoperichondrium is required. Cuts or wedges of the offending deviation are done to remove buckling.
5. Because cartilage has memory, cartilage grafts or Teflon splints should be sutured strategically into place if the mucoperichondrium is not intact.
6. If a nasal deformity exists, an incision should be made between the lateral nasal cartilage and the septum. If this is not done, the deformity will most likely resume its original position.
7. Incisions are closed using an absorbable suture on a small cutting needle. Teflon splints may be sutured into place with nylon on a cutting needle.
8. If splints are not used, the nose may be packed; otherwise a moustache dressing may be applied (Loré, 1988).

Rhinoplasty

Nursing considerations

Rhinoplasty is the reconstruction of the external nose. It is done for patients desiring a tip elevation, a hump removal, or a smaller, straighter, or narrower nose (also see Chapter 16 in this volume). If there are existing obstructive symptoms, a septoplasty is done first. This is because the septoplasty in itself can change the external appearance of the nose. A rhinoplasty nasal set is used for instrumentation.

This procedure should not lead to any further deformities or cause any internal nasal obstructions.

Procedure

Key steps

1. Depending on which correction is done, a #11 or #15 blade is used to incise through the skin and cartilage. Adequate retraction may be obtained with a speculum or double-pronged skin hooks for good exposure.
2. Elevation of perichondrium and periosteum is accomplished with Freer elevators, scissors, and osteotomes.
3. A hump may be removed with chisels or cutting forceps; a small curved button-end knife may be used to sever the bony hump (Loré, 1988).
4. If the septum needs correction, it can be done with septal scissors; rough bony edges can be rasped.
5. If soft tissue needs correction, this can be accomplished with small scissors and bayonet forceps; grafting may be necessary at this time.
6. Suturing is done with nylon or chromic suture on cutting needles of different sizes, depending on the correction being done. Blood loss is checked. If nasal packing is used, it is gently placed at this time. A nasal splint made of rigid plastic, metal, or tape may be applied.

Nasal Polypectomy

Nursing considerations

Nasal polyps are hypertrophied nasal mucosa that can result from chronic edema. They are typically found in patients who suffer from allergic rhinitis. They are usually found in the middle meatus (turbinate) and may occur singly or in numbers (Fig. 4-7). Mature polyps have pedunculated bases, whereas the newer ones are attached at the base. If the polyp becomes obstructive, a nasal polypectomy is indicated.

A choanal polyp may stem from the maxillary sinus mucosa. The choana is the communicating passageway between the nasal fossae and the pharynx. If a choanal polyp grows large enough to obstruct the nasopharynx, a Caldwell-Luc procedure is indicated to prevent possible recurrence (Goldman, 1988). In severe or recurrent nasal polyposis, the KTP 532 laser is helpful in allowing the removal of the bulk of intranasal polyps without bleeding. The aim is to prevent bleeding rather than to attempt he-

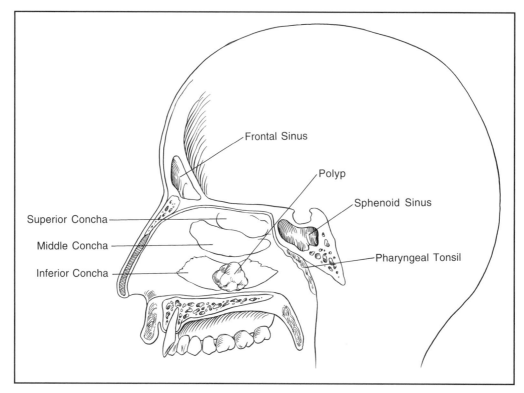

FIGURE 4-7 Nasal polyps.

mostasis once bleeding is present (Kennedy & Zinreich, 1988). Further explanation of this procedure will be found under Functional Endoscopic Sinus Surgery. A nasal set plus polyp snares (Fig. 4-8,*A* and *B*) is used.

Procedure

Key steps

1. After vasoconstricting agents have reached a therapeutic level, the offending nasal cavity is retracted using a nasal speculum.
2. The base of each polyp is located for positioning a wire around it. The polyp is then removed, using the loaded nasal polyp snare and forceps (Fig. 4-9). The surgeon will then identify if there are more polyps after removal of the first one (Goldman, 1988).
3. No suturing is required. Any blood loss is checked prior to nasal packing.

Ethmoidectomy

Nursing considerations

An ethmoidectomy is removal of the diseased portion of the middle turbinate, removal of ethmoidal cells, and removal of diseased tissue in the nasal fossa through a nasal or an external approach. This is done for patients who suffer from chronic ethmoid sinusitis and ethmoid polyps. Chronic ethmoid sinusitis easily spreads to the maxillary and frontal sinuses because the anterior ethmoid attaches to folds and fissures in the middle meatus. The mucus be-

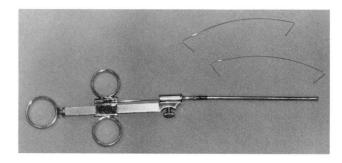

A
FIGURE 4-8 Nasal polyp snare. *A*, Unloaded; *B*, loaded.

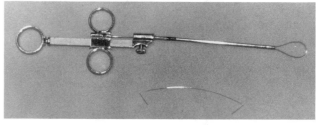

B

tween the contacting or inflamed mucosal areas is retained and provides ideal conditions for bacterial growth. Therefore, the health of the maxillary and frontal sinuses is dependent on the health of the ethmoid (Loré, 1988). Depending on the approach, a sinus endoscopy set (see Figs. 4-10 to 4-13) or nasal set of instruments is used.

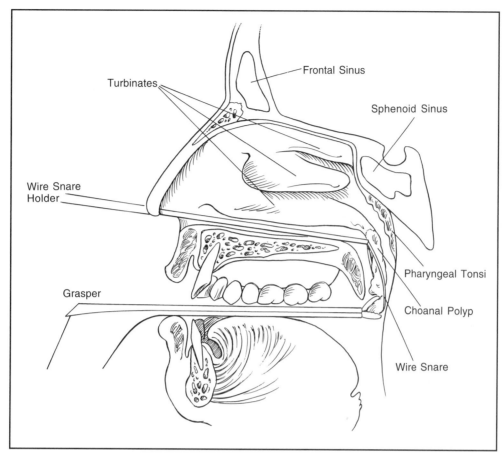

FIGURE 4-9 Removal of choanal polyp.

The patient should recover fully without evidence of any of the following complications: blindness, visual disturbances, bleeding, or neurological deficits. Unobstructed mouth breathing should be present.

Intranasal approach procedure

Key steps

1. The ethmoid sinus is reached laterally to the attachment of the middle meatus (turbinate). Care must be taken not to injure or remove any turbinate unless it is cystic.
2. Gentle use of forceps and curettes is done in the ethmoid sinus to remove diseased tissue. Orbital tissue can be inadvertently tugged on or removed at this time. If eyelid movement is observed, the surgeon must be informed immediately.

External approach procedure

Key steps

1. A brow incision is made using a #15 blade.
2. All tissues are very gently retracted and dissected to reach the lacrimal bone, the frontal process of the maxilla, and occasionally the nasal bone.
3. The anterior portion of the middle turbinate is removed to allow entrance to the ethmoid.

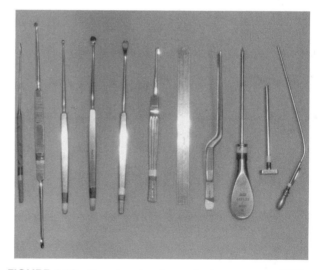

FIGURE 4-10 Functional endoscopic sinus surgery (FES) instrumentation. *Left to right:* sickle knife, Cottle elevator, small curette, large curette, Coakley curette, septal knife, ruler, bayonet forceps, trocar, trocar sheath, Frazier suction tip.

4. Diseased tissue is removed from the ethmoid sinus. Bleeding must be controlled to prevent ocular impingement resulting in blindness.

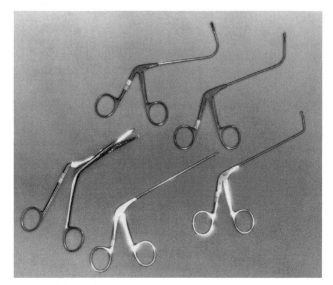

FIGURE 4-11 FES instrumentation. *Top row, left to right:* 100-degree horizontal spoon forceps, 70-degree horizontal spoon forceps. *Bottom row:* Knight septal scissors, straight nasal scissors, angled nasal scissors.

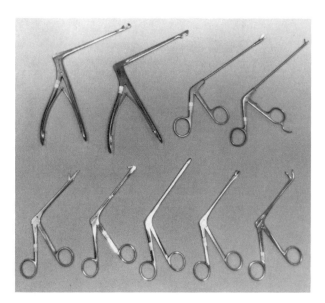

FIGURE 4-12 FES instrumentation. *Top row, left to right:* upbiting punch forceps, downbiting punch forceps, angled nasal scissors, biopsy scissors. *Bottom row:* Struyken forceps; back-biting nasal cutting forceps, straight Takahashi forceps, straight Blakesley forceps, angled Blakesley forceps.

5. The surgeon may need to do some reconstructive surgery with nonabsorbable suture on a small cutting needle on the nasofrontal duct and medial canthal ligament (Loré, 1988).
6. Packing may be placed gently in the operative site with the end out. If there is any question about postoperative bleeding, Loré (1988) prefers use of rubber band drains. (Sterilized rubber bands are cut to the desired length, placed unsutured in the incision upon closing, and removed postoperatively by gentle pulling.)

Intranasal endoscopic approach procedure

Key steps

1. A 0 or 30-degree telescope is used to landmark the middle turbinate or the anterior wall of the sphenoid.
2. If the middle turbinate obstructs the view or is cystic, its removal may be necessary.
3. Gentle grasping forceps are used to remove diseased tissue. The eyes of the patient must be observed at all times. If swelling occurs, an immediate external approach must be done to decompress the orbit (Bumsted & Corey, 1989).

Turbinectomy

Nursing considerations

An anterior inferior turbinectomy is removal of the anterior end of the inferior turbinate. Inferior turbinectomy is removal of the greater part of the lower border of the hypertrophied inferior turbinate. Anterior middle turbinectomy is removal of the anterior end of the middle turbinate body. Any polyps are removed at this time.

Turbinectomy relieves obstructive symptoms and promotes drainage (McNeely, 1991). A nasal set of instruments is used.

Expected patient outcomes should be similar to those of ethmoidectomy.

Procedure

Key steps

1. After the preferred vasoconstricting agents are instilled, the nostril is retracted with a nasal speculum to expose the offending turbinate.
2. A #15 blade is used to made an incision over the turbinate.
3. All or part of the turbinate is removed, along with any polyps.
4. In some cases, a sharp, two-pronged electrocoagulation instrument may be used for several seconds to desiccate the tissue.
5. Nasal packing may be used, followed by a drip pad.

Sphenoidectomy

Nursing considerations

Patients with recurrent sinusitis may require evacuation of the diseased tissue. This opening may be for one or both of the sphenoid sinuses by the intranasal or external ethmoidectomy approach. Instrumentation commonly used is a nasal set.

Expected patient outcomes are the same as those for ethmoidectomy.

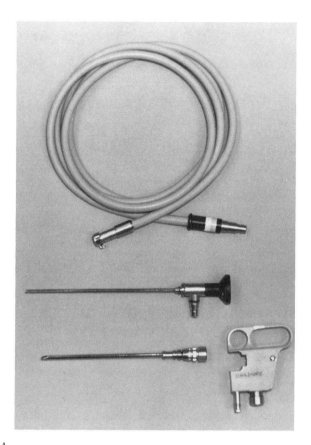

A

FIGURE 4-13   FES instrumentation. *A, Top to bottom*: fiberoptic cord, telescope, scope sheath, suction irrigator handpiece. *B*, Assembled nasal endoscopy lens.

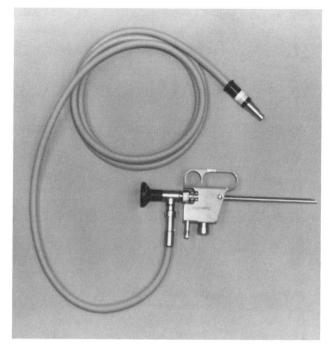

B

an opening in the lateral wall of the nose under the middle turbinate and the removal of the anterior end of the inferior turbinate. A nasal set is used for instrumentation.

Desired patient outcomes are for unobstructed breathing. Because of the close proximity of the procedure site to the orbital floor, the patient should be watched for any visual disturbances. Any neurological deficits may suggest an air embolism.

Procedure

Key steps

1. Entry to the sphenoid sinus must be made carefully between the middle and superior turbinates. The more superior the position will be, the less dense the bone. The surgeon must remain close to the midline to avoid the carotid artery branches.
2. Downward deflecting bone-cutting instruments are used to break through the anterior wall of the sphenoid. If necessary, an X-ray film may be done to check placement.
3. The opening is carefully enlarged until the surgeon is able to remove the diseased tissue.
4. If the surgeon encounters any obstructions from deviations in the septum or polyps, these may first need to be corrected.
5. If an external ethmoid approach is used, packing may be placed gently.

Procedure

Key steps

1. The inferior turbinate is located and incised with a #15 blade.
2. The tissue is elevated by periosteals and elevators.
3. If the antral window is made for gravity drainage, a trocar or chisel is used to puncture into the antral wall of the maxillary sinus.
4. Enlarging the antral window can be done with a curved rasp or cutting forceps and punches (Loré, 1988).
5. Diseased tissue is removed, as are polyps, using a nasal polyp snare.
6. The sinus can be irrigated and suctioned. Packing may be used afterward.
7. A moustache dressing is applied.

Intranasal Antrostomy (Antral Window)

Nursing considerations

Patients suffering from recurrent maxillary sinus infections may benefit from this procedure. It involves making

Radical Antrostomy (Caldwell-Luc)

Nursing considerations

Patients who have recurrent maxillary sinus infections may require a radical antrum or Caldwell-Luc procedure.

This procedure is done through an intraoral incision to create an opening between the nostril and maxillary sinus to permit gravity drainage. Because the surgeon has open visualization of the sinus, any diseased tissue may be removed. A nasal set of instruments, with primary emphasis placed on bone-cutting instruments, is used.

Any postoperative nausea and vomiting can be curtailed with an antiemetic. The patient should be warned of a foul taste in the mouth if iodoform packing is used.

Procedure

Key steps

1. The upper lip is retracted on the affected side. A #15 blade is used to make a horizontal incision over the canine fossae down to the bone.
2. A periosteal elevator is used to free up fascia and muscles over the anterior wall of the antrum (maxillary sinus).
3. The antrum is entered well above the teeth, using chisels, burrs, or osteotomes. A rongeur or bone-cutting forceps may be used to enlarge the opening.
4. Diseased tissue may now be removed with soft tissue–grasping forceps.
5. A nasoantral opening may be made beneath the inferior turbinate (meatus) to facilitate gravity drainage (Loré, 1988).
6. Nasal packing may be done and the intraoral incision closed with absorbable (chromic) suture on a cutting needle.

Functional Endoscopic Sinus Surgery (FES)

Nursing considerations

Endoscopic sinus surgery is purported to increase visualization, which leads to better and safer surgery. This is based on the premise that chronic, recurrent sinusitis of bacterial origin stems from diseased ethmoids. Because of this disease process, maxillary sinuses are frequently involved. This type of procedure allows access to all sinuses and is done for the following conditions: polyps, mucoceles, periorbital cellulitis, and sinusitis that is acute or chronically untreatable with antibiotics. Disadvantages of using this approach include expense and time in training, initial cost of instrumentation and equipment, subsequent upkeep of instruments and equipment, poor visualization due to bleeding, monocular vision, poor depth field, and difficulties with revisions or large polyps (Gibson, 1991). Currently, two FES techniques are used: the Messerklinger and the Wigand. The Wigand technique approaches all the sinuses on the affected side and works best for those with extensive disease or when the Messerklinger technique has failed (Rice, 1989). FES instrumentation is shown in Figures 4-10 through 4-13.

Procedure

Key steps

1. According to Kennedy and Zinreich (1988), a 0-degree telescope that has been defogged is carefully introduced into the nostril of the affected side.
2. An incision is made with a #15 blade around the anterior and inferior attachment of the uncinate process. This bony structure is removed to gain access to the ethmoidal infundibulum, a tube-shaped passage.
3. Diseased ethmoid cells are then opened and removed, using delicate forceps.
4. Dissection is completed in an anterior to posterior fashion when all disease visualized on the CT scan has been removed.
5. In the event a KTP laser is being used to remove intranasal polyps, endoscopic equipment should be set up, with an attached laser fiber.
6. After carefully introducing the scope, the polyp is grasped with suction forceps and cut along the base by bringing the fiber in contact with the tissue. It is advanced slowly through the polyp mass.
7. Smoke is aspirated, using either a separate suction or suction forceps.
8. No suturing is required and usually no packing is placed.

Frontal Sinusotomy (Trephination)

Nursing considerations

Patients who have acute frontal sinusitis that creates pressure on the orbit need a hole made in the frontal sinus to allow drainage of pus or fluid accumulation. This is done when conventional measures are unsuccessful. A nasal set is used for instrumentation.

Care must be taken to prevent orbital or intracranial injury during the procedure. Neurological status is checked. Drainage tubes will remain in place under the dressing. Blood loss should be minimal. Postoperatively the drainage tubes should function to prevent dehiscence.

Procedure

Key steps

1. Using a #15 blade, an incision is made just below the medial curve of the eyebrow down to the bone.
2. The periosteum is elevated and placement of the burr hole is confirmed by X-ray (Loré, 1988).
3. The hole is made with a small burr or curette. The drainage is cultured.
4. Gentle saline irrigation may be done at the surgeon's discretion (Loré, 1988).
5. Drainage tubes are placed before any suturing is done. Wound closure material is according to the surgeon's preference. Dressings are applied.

Frontal Sinus Surgery

Nursing considerations

Frontal sinus surgery approaches the frontal sinus in an effort to obliterate the sinus, cleanse it, and drain it. Patients presenting for this type of surgery have chronic recurrent sinus infections unresponsive to antibiotics. They may already have had a trephination done. A cosmetic incision is made coronally or across the brow (do not shave), depending on the surgeon's and the patient's choices. Fat harvested from the abdomen may be used in obliterating the sinus. The circulating nurse should receive a sterilized or high-level disinfected X-ray template from the surgeon for use on the field. A nasal set and Stryker power saw are used for this procedure.

The patient's neurologic signs should remain normal throughout the procedure. Blood loss should be minimal. According to Loré (1988), the following complications are possible: fracture of the inner wall or table, leading to a possible cerebrospinal fluid leak; fracture to the orbital roof; air embolus; recurrent disease; osteomyelitis; and other infectious processes.

Procedure

Key steps

1. If the coronal approach is used, the incision is made in the scalp skin from ear to ear. This incision should not be used on balding persons. Raney clips may be applied for hemostasis of the scalp. If the brow approach is used, the incision is made above the eyebrow line and may extend bilaterally (McNeely, 1991).
2. The periosteum is left attached to the bone. The flap is retracted away so the template can be placed over the sinus. Once the template is in position, an incision is made through the periosteum along the superior, medial, and lateral edges. The inferior edge is left so the blood supply to this created flap is not compromised (Loré, 1988).
3. A sagittal or oscillating saw is used to cut through the bone overlying the sinus. An elevator or osteotome may be used to facilitate elevation of the bony flap.
4. The diseased mucosal tissue is removed with burrs. Harvested fat is placed in the cavity.
5. The bony flap is positioned back in place after any rough edges are smoothed. Absorbable suture is used on the flap. The skin flap is closed with noncolored suture.
6. Dressings are applied.

Repair of Nasal Fracture

Nursing considerations

Fractures of the nasal bones or nasal septum are more common than generally thought. In children they often occur from accidents. In adults they are associated with automobile accidents or physical assaults. Many times there is no obvious external deformity or internal ob-

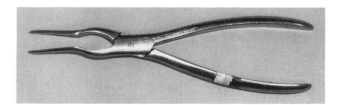

FIGURE 4-14 Asch septal straightening forceps.

struction so the patient does not realize there is a fracture. Fractures should be manipulated within 10 days because thereafter the nasal bones will have started to unite and reduction will be difficult (Saunders et al., 1979).

Procedure

Key steps

1. The patient should be placed in a dorsal recumbent or supine position if manipulation under local anesthesia is to be done.
2. Fractures with displacement to the side may require external manipulation using an inserted elevator to check for midline placement.
3. Fractures with depression of nasal bones may require elevation internally with an elevator or Asch forceps (Fig. 4-14). External manipulation is used to shape bones as elevation is done.
4. Nasal packing may be used at the surgeon's discretion. An external nasal splint and tape are applied.

Control of Epistaxis

Nursing considerations

Patients presenting in the surgical suite for epistaxis must not be taken lightly. These persons most likely have been treated in a physician's office with silver nitrate sticks, balloon catheters, packing, and ice therapy with pressure point control. Unmanageable in the office, the bleeding tends to be more diffuse and oozes more than from a single site. If the origin is from an anterior site, it is most commonly from the ethmoid artery. If bleeding arises posterior in the nose, it is from the sphenopalatine artery. Both of these arteries branch off of the internal maxillary artery, which in turn stems from the carotid. This should be kept in mind because blood not remaining in the carotid artery tree means blood may not be getting to the brain. To further complicate this situation, preoperative nasal packing in the elderly can decrease both oxygen and carbon dioxide levels. With this contributing to a decreased level of consciousness, carbon dioxide retention/hypoxia can lead to lethal arrhythmias. Preoperative nursing care should include the skin integrity of the nose if packing is in place, hematocrit level, and visual acuity (Lee, 1989).

Prevention of shock and respiratory embarrassment must be priorities throughout the procedure. Appropriate antibiotic therapy should be started to prevent infection or toxic shock syndrome from preoperative nasal packing.

Procedure

Key steps

1. Depending on the possible origin of the bleed and surgeon preference, entry may be intranasally or through a Caldwell-Luc approach. See previous procedures for each of these.
2. Preparation should be made to include sterile microscopic examination with appropriate instrumentation.
3. Once the offending artery is located, a small hemoclip is securely placed.
4. Further inspection must be done to ensure there are no other bleeding branches.
5. Closing suture is done according to the surgeon's preference after the bleeding is stopped. A rubber band drain may be used. Nasogastric suctioning may be indicated.
6. Dressings are applied if appropriate.

SUMMARY

This chapter has presented the most common nasal procedures, indications for these procedures, nursing considerations, and key steps in the surgeries. The perioperative nurse plays a significant role in assessing patient risks and preventing complications.

REFERENCES

Beeson, W. H. (1987). The nasal septum. *The Otolaryngologic Clinics of North America, 20,* 743–767.

Bumsted, R., & Corey, J. (1989). Revision endoscopic ethmoidectomy for chronic rhinosinusitis. *The Otolaryngologic Clinics of North America, 22,* 801–807.

Dedo, D. (1984). *The atlas of aesthetic facial surgery.* Orlando: Grune & Stratton.

Gibson, B. (1991). Great debates in otolaryngology: Intranasal vs endoscopic ethmoidectomy. *Archives of Otolaryngology—Head and Neck Surgery, 117,* 19.

Goldman, M. (1988). *Pocket guide to the operating room.* Philadelphia: F. A. Davis.

Kennedy, D., & Zinreich, S. (1988). The functional endoscopic approach to inflammatory sinus disease: Current perspectives and technique modification. *American Journal of Rhinology, 2,* 89–96.

Lee, K. (1989). *The textbook of otolaryngology and head and neck surgery.* New York: Elsevier Science Publishing.

Loré, J. Jr. (1988). *An atlas of head and neck surgery* (3rd ed.). Philadelphia: W. B. Saunders.

McNeely, K. S. (1991). Rhinologic and sinus surgery, pp. 528–544 in Meeker, M., & Rothrock, J. *Alexander's care of the patient in surgery* (9th ed.). St. Louis: C. V. Mosby Co.

Rice, D. (1989). Techniques and variations of endoscopic sinus surgery. *The Otolaryngologic Clinics of North America, 22,* 713–726.

Saunders, W., Havener, W., & Keith, C. (1979). *Nursing care in eye, ear, nose, and throat disorders* (4th ed.). St. Louis: C. V. Mosby.

Chapter 5

Laryngologic and Head and Neck Surgery

Key Concepts

- Most head and neck procedures can be done with a single surgical team; however, several complex operations require more than one surgical team (e.g., resection of advanced head and neck tumors with immediate reconstruction).

- Wound closures in head and neck procedures include direct closure, skin grafting, and tissue transfer.

- Various specialties may be involved: general surgery, otorhinolaryngology, radiology, plastic surgery, dentistry, oral surgery, ophthalmology, and neurosurgery.

- Extensive disease may be present even with a short-time history of symptoms.

- Procedures may be performed under local anesthesia, local anesthesia with intravenous conscious sedation, or under general anesthesia.

- Patients may require extensive preoperative preparation, as some procedures will have major psychological and physical impact, including cosmetic deformity and loss of function (e.g., voice).

- Resuscitative equipment, including suction and oxygen, must always be readily available.

INTRODUCTION

Laryngologic and head and neck surgery consists of minimally invasive procedures, such as a laryngoscopy performed under local anesthesia in a same-day surgery setting, and radical procedures, such as a laryngectomy, which requires extensive surgery and rehabilitation. Many of the procedures performed on adults are for malignancies (Dougherty, 1990). It also includes removal of the tonsils and adenoids, a procedure once very common but now performed very judiciously. This chapter describes the intricate anatomy involved in this type of surgery, the technology used, and the many anxieties and concerns of patients and families.

ANATOMY

The head and neck region is one in which a large number of important structures are compressed into a relatively small area.

The oral cavity and oropharynx have a functional role in the ingestion, deglutition, and digestion of food, in speech articulation, and in respiration. The oral cavity extends from the lips anteriorly to the faucial arch posteriorly (Fig. 5-1). Included in this cavity are the lips, teeth, floor of the mouth, oral tongue, gingiva, retromolar trigone, buccal mucosa, and hard palate. The oropharynx includes the soft palate, palatine tonsils, base of the tongue, and the posterior pharyngeal wall (Fig. 5-2). It extends inferiorly to the level of the hyoid bone and epiglottis.

The salivary glands consist of the paired major glands—the parotid, submandibular, and sublingual—in addition to hundreds of minor salivary glands throughout the mouth and oropharynx. The major salivary glands are intimately associated with the regional cranial nerves, including the facial nerve, lingual nerve, and hypoglossal nerve. The hypopharynx (laryngopharynx) is continuous with the oropharynx and extends inferiorly to the inlet of the esophagus. It includes the piriform sinuses and the thyrohyoid membrane.

The larynx and pharynx have major roles in respiration, deglutition, and speech production. The pharyngeal musculature guards the entry to both the alimentary and respiratory tracts. At the lower border of the cricoid, the hypopharynx joins the esophagus, and the larynx continues the airway through the trachea. The primary role of the larynx is in respiration. It protects the airway and controls airflow. Exhalation of air through the larynx is controlled by voluntary muscles, enabling the larynx to become the organ of voice. During swallowing, the larynx is pulled upward and forward, closing the air passageway and thus shunting food into the esophagus. When any foreign material enters the larynx, a cough reflex occurs in an attempt to expel the material. Anteriorly the larynx is covered by the sternohyoid, sternothyroid, thyrohyoid, and omohyoid muscles and posteriorly by the inferior constrictor muscle. The larynx is continuous with the trachea from below and opens into the pharynx above. It is composed of nine cartilages that are joined together by ligaments and controlled by skeletal muscles (Fig. 5-3). There are three single cartilages (cricoid, thyroid, and epiglottis) and three paired cartilages (arytenoid, corniculate, and cuneiform). Except for the vocal cords, the larynx is lined with ciliated mucous membrane. The

Two pairs of mucous membrane folds project into the laryngeal cavity. The upper paired folds are called the ventricular folds, or false vocal cords. The lower paired folds are called the vocal cords, or true vocal cords. Each fold plays an important part in sound production. The

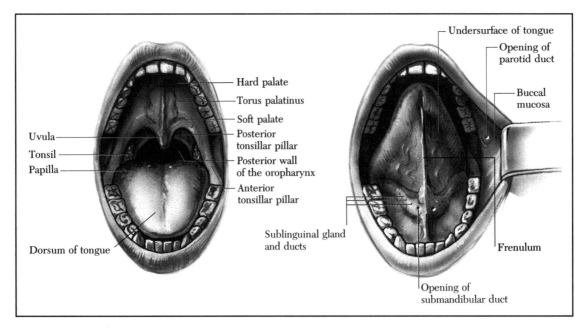

FIGURE 5-1 Anatomy of the oral cavity. (From Grimes, J. and Burns, E. [1992]. *Health Assessment in Nursing* Practice (3rd ed.). Boston: Jones and Bartlett Publishers.)

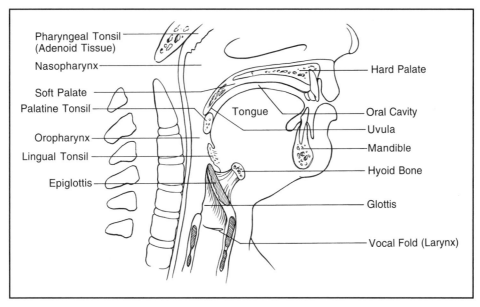

FIGURE 5-2 Anatomy of the oropharynx.

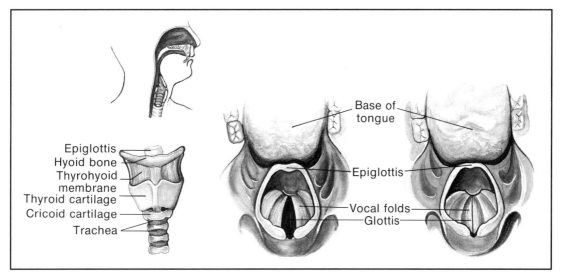

FIGURE 5-3 Larynx—posterior view. (From Anderson, P. D. [1984]. *Basic Human Anatomy and Physiology*. Boston: Jones and Bartlett Publishers.)

opening between the vocal cords is called the glottis. The trachea, or windpipe, is a flexible, tubular structure that extends from the larynx downward, lying in front of the esophagus, through the midline of the neck and into the thorax. The walls of the trachea are comprised of approximately 16 to 20 U-shaped cartilages, placed one above the other at close intervals. The open end of the U is at the back, facing the esophagus. Connective tissue and muscle bridge this gap. The cartilage rings keep the trachea open at all times for the passage of air to and from the lungs (Meyerhoff & Rice, 1992).

Metastases in the head and neck area spread principally through the lymphatics (Fig. 5-4). There are three main groups of lymphatic tissue in the head and neck. The first contains the palatine tonsils, lingual tonsils, adenoids, and adjacent submucosal lymphatics. This area is known as Waldeyer's ring. The second contains the transitional lymphatics, and the third contains the cervical lymph nodes. Lymph nodes are also categorized by level within the neck. Lymphatic flow is predictable unless it has been distorted by tumor, previous surgery, or irradiation (Way, 1991).

NURSING CONSIDERATIONS

General Information

Although lesions and malignancies are often readily visible in the head and neck area, extensive disease may be present even with a short-time history of symptoms. The

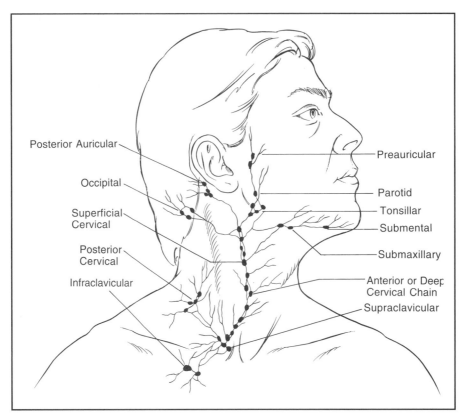

FIGURE 5-4 Lymph nodes of the head and neck area.

four most common presenting symptoms are pain, bleeding, obstruction, and a mass. A careful history is taken, including noting social habits such as the use of tobacco products and excessive alcohol consumption. A physical examination, visual and by palpation, is conducted of the entire head and neck area, including the oropharyngeal cavity. The examination of the intraoral cavity may include probing of the ducts and needle biopsy. Further testing such as by computed tomography (CT scan), magnetic resonance imaging (MRI), X-rays, and bone scans may be used to confirm what was found on the physical examination as well as to detail the extent of the disease process. Clinical staging of head and neck cancers permits a method of classification, estimation of prognosis, and basis for a treatment plan. Included in the staging are: size and location of primary tumor; existence, size, number, and location of neck nodes involved; and the presence or absence of distal metastases.

Nursing Diagnoses

Altered nutrition: less than body requirements may be present if the patient has been unable to eat owing to difficulty in swallowing or nausea and vomiting related to preoperative radiation or chemotherapy.

High risk for infection is present for all surgical patients but especially when the lymphatic system may be compromised or when tissue has been compromised by preoperative radiation.

Impaired gas exchange: due to obstruction of the airway may be seen in patients who have obstructing tumors. It may

also be seen in patients with severe swelling of the oropharynx due to an upper airway infection.

Impaired tissue integrity may be seen in patients who have diseased mucous membranes or skin damaged by preoperative radiation.

Altered mucous membrane may be seen in patients who have oral pain or discomfort, stomatitis, oral lesions or ulcers, lack of or decreased salivation, or edema.

Impaired verbal communication may be seen in patients who have hoarseness due to disease or treatment and in those with a tracheostomy or laryngectomy. Preoperative plans should be made, when possible, for methods to communicate postoperatively when patients are undergoing a tracheostomy or laryngectomy.

Impaired swallowing due to mechanical obstruction or facial paralysis: patients with this diagnosis may not be able to swallow their saliva and also are at risk for aspiration.

Body image disturbance may be seen especially in patients undergoing a radical neck procedure or in those scheduled for a laryngectomy, which will change forever the sound of their voice.

Anxiety is seen in all surgical patients but may be seen especially in children having surgery or in patients undergoing diagnostic procedures.

Intraoperative preparation

Routine positioning for laryngologic and head and neck procedures is the supine position with a small shoulder roll for hyperextension of the neck. Pressure points and major nerve areas should be well padded and supported. A safety belt should always be applied. The surgeon's preference and the procedure will determine what body hair, if any, is to be removed and whether this is to be done on the ward or in the operating room. An electrosurgical grounding pad is applied for most procedures. Skin prepping may range from none in certain laryngeal procedures to extensive in head and neck procedures; therefore, the surgeon's preference is followed. Draping of the patient may also range from minimal to extensive and varies according to the individual surgeon (Silcox, 1991).

SURGICAL PROCEDURES

Endolaryngeal Procedures

Endolaryngeal procedures are done for diagnoses and treatment with the use of a rigid or flexible scope and a light source.

Indirect laryngoscopy

The development of the technique of indirect mirror examination of the larynx in 1854 was the forerunner of airway endoscopy. For the first time physicians had a technique with which they could examine the larynx (Meyerhoff & Rice, 1992). Another 40 years passed before the development of methods for obtaining direct access to the airway.

Indications for indirect laryngoscopy include performing a visual inspection of the oral cavity as part of a complete ear, nose, and throat examination; to examine the larynx for specific symptoms such as hoarseness or stridor; and for taking biopsy specimens and possible removal of small benign tumors from the larynx. Visual functioning of the cranial nerves can be observed during this examination, including the functioning of cranial nerve X (symmetrical elevation of the soft palate) and cranial nerve XII (movement and protrusion of the tongue).

Perioperative nursing considerations Cooperation of the patient throughout the examination is required, and therefore this procedure may not be suitable for young children. The patient requires constant reassurance during the procedure and should be provided with explanations of techniques as they are being performed. All equipment should be ready prior to the commencement of the procedure. Any artificial dentition needs to be removed prior to the procedure (i.e., dentures, bridges). Any loose teeth should be noted. Suction equipment, oxygen, and resuscitative equipment must be immediately available. If intravenous sedation is used during the procedure, institution policy should be followed for monitoring the patient and the required documentation. The patient should maintain an NPO status until return of gag reflex if a topical anesthetic spray is used. The patient should remain in an ambulatory care recovery room or lounge until reflexes return.

Instruments and supplies include the following: coaxial light source, wooden tongue blades, gloves, gauze sponges, laryngeal mirrors of various sizes, defogger or warming solution, specimen container, suction apparatus, selection of fine curved punches, forceps and double-cupped forceps for biopsy and specimen removal, syringe and needle if an aspiration is to be done, epiglottic retractor, and emesis basin (the gag reflex is easily triggered).

Key steps

1. The patient will be instructed to breathe normally and will be told that a laryngeal mirror will be introduced into the oral cavity without initially touching anything. To bring the epiglottis forward, the patient will be requested to say "e-e-e" when asked. To evaluate the function of the larynx, the patient may be requested to cough during the examination.
2. The tongue is grasped and gently held with a gauze sponge by the examiner as a prewarmed (to avoid condensation) laryngeal mirror is introduced into the oral cavity. The gag reflex may be incited if the dorsum of the tongue is touched. With the mirror positioned gently against the uvula and soft palate, visual inspection of the following structures is completed: base of the tongue, vallecula, epiglottis, posterior portions of the larynx and pharyngeal wall, and the pyriform fossae (Fig.5-5).
3. The patient should be reassured and asked to continue mouth breathing, and as the patient relaxes, the ventricular and vocal cords (false and true cords) can be visualized. When the patient makes the requested "e-e-e" sound the entire larynx can be viewed, including the anterior commissure.
4. If during phonation the epiglottis does not come forward enough, an epiglottic retractor may be used (Freund, 1979).
5. With an active gag reflex or when biopsy and specimen removal is needed, a topical anesthetic spray may be used.

Flexible fiberoptic examination

Indications for the use of the flexible fiberscope are as stated for indirect laryngoscopy, except for the taking of biopsies, but in addition include the following: for patients with hypersensitive gag reflexes, immobilized patients, small children, patients with cervical spine abnormalities or with limited jaw opening, and as a guide for inserting endotracheal tubes transnasally.

Perioperative nursing considerations Suction equipment, oxygen and resuscitative equipment must be immediately available. If the procedure is being performed in young children, restraint can be applied by wrapping the child in a sheet. The patient requires constant reassurance and adequate explanations during the procedure. All equipment should be ready prior to the commencement of the procedure.

Equipment and supplies include the following: fiberoptic instrument, light source and cables, lubricant, topical anesthetic, defogger or warming solution, cotton

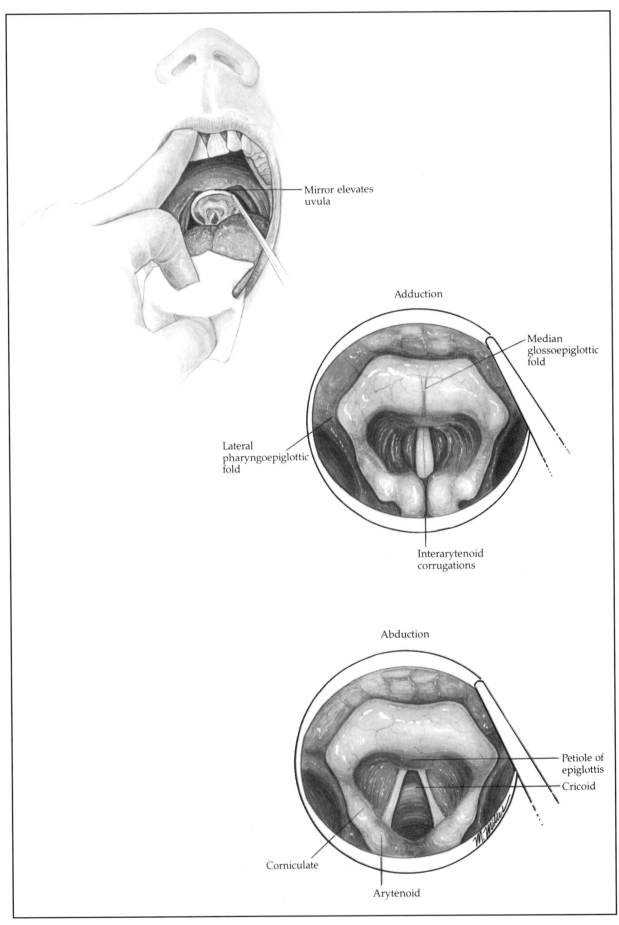

Mirror elevates uvula

Adduction

Median glossoepiglottic fold

Lateral pharyngoepiglottic fold

Interarytenoid corrugations

Abduction

Petiole of epiglottis

Cricoid

Corniculate

Arytenoid

FIGURE 5-5 Indirect laryngoscopy. (From Johns, M. E., Price, J. C., & Mattox, D. E. [1990]. *Atlas of head and neck surgery* (vol. 1). Philadelphia: B. C. Decker. Reprinted by permission of Mosby-Year Book, Inc.)

pledgets, and suction apparatus; videoscopic equipment may be required (Fig. 5-6).

Key steps

1. A cotton pledget thoroughly soaked with the selected topical anesthetic is inserted into one naris. Some of the anesthetic will flow through the post choana area into the pharynx and larynx (Meyerhoff & Rice, 1992).
2. The end of the fiberscope is lubricated to facilitate its insertion, and the tip is introduced into the nasal passage. When the nasopharynx is reached, the tip of the scope is angulated downward and the hypopharynx can be visualized (Fig. 5-7).
3. As the scope is advanced further, the following structures are observed: vallecula, epiglottis, supraglottic larynx, cords, and pyriform fossae.
4. The patient may be requested to cough, breathe deeply, or phonate in order to assess vocal fold motion.

Direct laryngoscopy

Indications for direct laryngoscopy include assessment of laryngeal malignancy and biopsy, foreign body removal, removal of benign lesions with forceps or laser, dilation or laser excision of laryngeal stenosis, evaluation of laryngeal injuries, and drainage of abscesses and cysts (Meyerhoff & Rice, 1992).

Perioperative nursing considerations Direct laryngoscopy may be performed under local or general anesthesia. If performed under local anesthesia, the patient

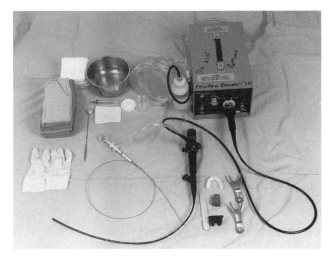

FIGURE 5-6 Flexible fiberoptic examination table set-up.

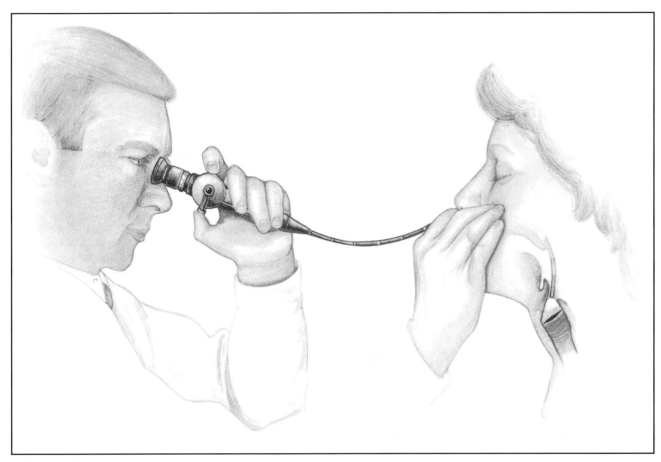

FIGURE 5-7 Flexible fiberoptic examination of larynx. (From Johns, M. E., Price, J. C., & Mattox, D. E. [1990]. *Atlas of head and neck surgery* (vol. 1). Philadelphia: B. C. Decker. Reprinted by permission of Mosby-Year Book, Inc.)

needs to receive adequate preoperative explanations as well as constant reassurance during the procedure. If intravenous sedation is used during the procedure, institution policy for patient monitoring and required documentation must be followed. All equipment should be ready prior to the commencement of the procedure. Proper positioning of the head by the examiner is vital. A contraindication to direct laryngoscopy is disease of the cervical spine, wherein marked extension of the cervical spine is impossible or dangerous. Artificial dentition should be removed prior to the procedure, and any loose teeth should be noted. Suction equipment, oxygen, and resuscitative equipment must be immediately available.

Severe bradycardia may occur in newborns and young infants examined without any anesthesia. Some examiners prefer to use a laryngeal nerve block. If microscopic examinations are required, a 400-mm lens should be used. Patients who have foreign bodies lodged in the larynx may present with pain, laryngospasm, dyspnea, and inspiratory stridor proportionate to the degree of upper airway obstruction. In conscious patients with adequate air exchange, indirect laryngoscopy and X-rays of the neck will confirm the position of the foreign body (Way, 1991). Removal may be accomplished with direct laryngoscopy using alligator forceps, with the patient under general anesthesia. When direct laryngoscopy is performed under general anesthesia, visual time is limited if no endotracheal tube is used.

Equipment and supplies include laryngoscopes sized to the patient, light source and cord, topical anesthetics, suction apparatus, gauze pads or mouth guard, laryngeal biopsy forceps, specimen jar, gloves, defogger or warming solution, emesis basin, syringe and fine needles for aspiration, and a self-retaining laryngoscope holder for suspension laryngoscopy and microlaryngoscopy (Fig. 5-8). For microlaryngoscopy, a basic laryngoscopy setup, a microscope with a 400-mm objective lens, and the following microlaryngeal instruments are needed: grasping forceps; straight, upbiting, and cup forceps; knives (curved and straight); suction tube; mirror; laryngeal probe; and laryngeal caliper.

Key steps

1. With the patient in a supine position, moderate flexion of the neck with an upward motion of the head is accomplished. The surgeon may request a head drape and full sheet to cover the patient.
2. The end of the laryngoscope is introduced into the right side of the patient's mouth (Fig. 5-9). Examination of the hypopharynx, vallecula, epiglottis, supraglottic larynx, and glottis is conducted (Freund, 1979).
3. Direct laryngoscopy also permits visualization of the postcricoid area. The glottis may be spasmodically closed. This spasm may not be present with very thorough topical anesthesia or with deep general anesthesia. When the larynx opens widely, the cords may be seen.
4. The lifting motion and elevation of the patient's head are increased as the examination continues. The laryngoscope may be passed through the cords to examine the subglottic region and upper trachea.

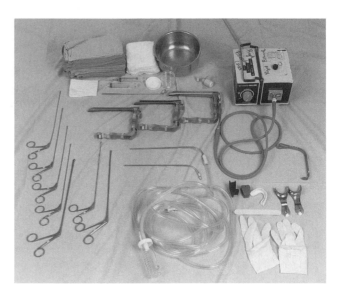

FIGURE 5-8 Direct larynogoscopy table set-up.

Esophagoscopy

Indications for the direct visualization of the esophagus and cardia of the stomach include the following: for removal of a foreign body, injection of esophageal varices, dilation of stenoses, dysphagia, hematemesis, examination of lesions, and removal of tissue and secretions.

Perioperative nursing considerations Flexible or rigid endoscopes may be used. A rigid esophagoscope is contraindicated in patients with limited jaw mobility and cervical spine deformities. Artificial dentition should be removed prior to the procedure, and any loose teeth should be noted. Usually a general anesthetic is given; however, with the use of a flexible endoscope, local anesthesia and sedation may be used. If the procedure is performed under local anesthesia, the patient needs to receive adequate preoperative explanations as well as constant reassurance during the procedure. If intravenous sedation is used during the procedure, institution policy for patient monitoring and required documentation is to be followed. All equipment should be ready prior to the commencement of the procedure. Suction equipment, oxygen, and resuscitative equipment must be immediately available. With the use of a rigid endoscope, the patient is supine, and with the use of a flexible endoscope, the patient is placed in a lateral position.

Instruments and supplies include the following: esophagoscope of surgeon's preference, suction apparatus and tubes, coaxial light source and cords, a selection of forceps, specimen containers, lubricant, gauze sponges, mouth guard, and sterile saline (Fig. 5-10).

Key steps

1. The esophagoscope is usually introduced on the right side of the mouth and is advanced forward until the uvula and posterior wall are visible.
2. As the head is extended further, the scope is passed between the two arytenoid cartilages.

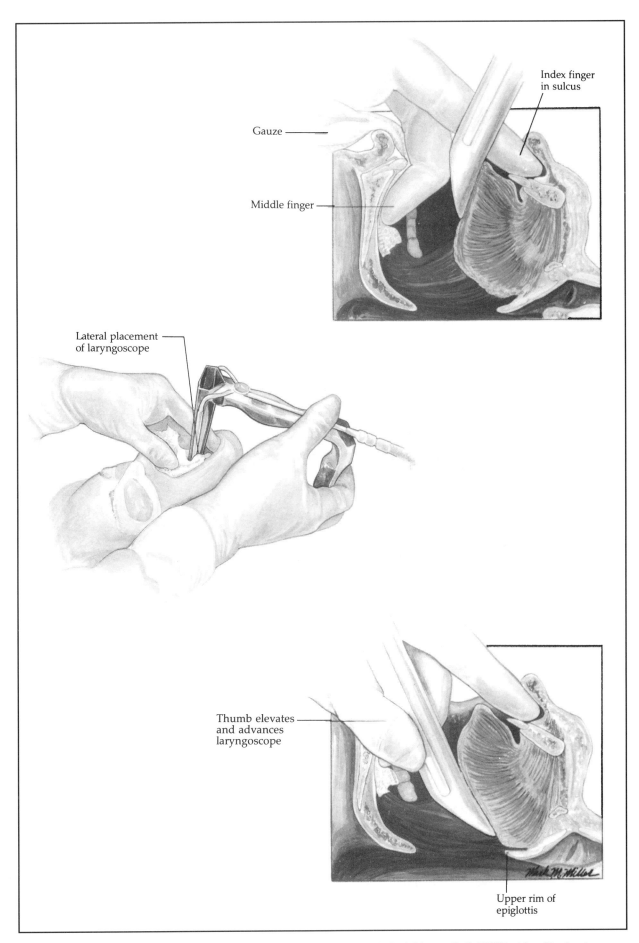

Gauze

Index finger
in sulcus

Middle finger

Lateral placement
of laryngoscope

Thumb elevates
and advances
laryngoscope

Upper rim of
epiglottis

FIGURE 5-9 Operative laryngoscopy. (From Johns, M. E., Price, J. C., & Mattox, D. E. [1990]. *Atlas of head and neck surgery* (vol. 1). Philadelphia: B. C. Decker. Reprinted by permission of Mosby-Year Book, Inc.)

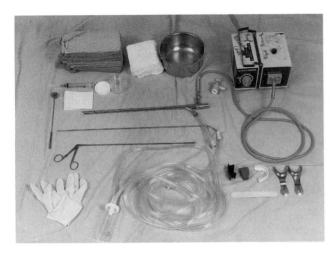

FIGURE 5-10 Rigid endoscopy table set-up.

3. As the cricoid cartilage is elevated slightly, the scope is passed as far as the beginning of the esophagus, with continuous careful pressure and slight turning movements.

4. The scope is advanced further until the cardia is exposed. The head of the patient must be maximally extended (Fig. 5-11).

5. During the examination and dependent on the indication for the procedure, secretion and biopsy specimens are taken.

Carbon dioxide laser surgery with laryngoscopy

Indications for laser surgery of the larynx include removal of webs, vocal cord papillomas, and carcinoma in situ.

Perioperative nursing considerations The method of operation and the power and safety requirements of the carbon dioxide laser as well as all lasers are discussed in Chapter 22 of Volume 1. While the laser is in operation, all personnel must wear safety glasses that have side shields. Regular personal prescription glasses or contact lenses are not sufficient protection. The surgeon will test the laser to ensure alignment of the beams. Signs indicating that a laser is in use should be placed on the outside door of the operating room. The use of laser equipment requires thorough education of surgical, nursing, and anesthesia staff. The patient is positioned and draped as for laryngoscopy.

Instruments for the procedure include the basic set-up for laryngoscopy and microlaryngoscopy. An emergency tracheostomy set and a variety of tracheostomy tubes, a ventilating bronchoscope, and grasping forceps should be immediately available.

Key steps

1. The patient's eyelids should be closed with tape and protected with wet saline gauze pads.

2. Wet gauze pads or cottonoid patties may also be placed in the oral cavity and peritracheal area.

3. If the patient is intubated, a laser-resistant endotracheal tube must be used.

4. Proper laser smoke evacuation should be employed.

5. The laser energy vaporizes tissue, producing minimal damage to surrounding tissue and excellent hemostasis for small blood vessels that are transected.

Surgery of the Oral Cavity

Indications for surgery include chronic inflammation of glands, congenital anomalies, and the removal of benign and malignant lesions. Small, superficial lesions may be excised under local anesthesia and sedation. Frequently, lesions of the oral cavity require more extensive dissection than planned and may even require a radical neck dissection and resection of the mandible and the tongue. Extensive preoperative preparation of the patient is vital, including any plans for immediate reconstruction. This includes possible flaps to reconstruct large defects and bone reconstruction with plates or grafts. For excision of oral tumors, a tracheostomy may be performed to ensure an adequate airway postoperatively. This may be done under local anesthesia. For some procedures, a pharyngeal pack of moist gauze may be used.

Tonsillectomy and adenoidectomy

Indications for surgical removal include lymphoid hypertrophy causing respiratory obstruction, dysphagia for solid food, speech distortion, tonsillar hemorrhage, cor pulmonale (secondary to tonsillar hypertrophy), peritonsillar abscess (quinsy), recurrent tonsillitis, recurrent adenoiditis, recurrent otitis media, orthodontic complications, and suspicion of malignancy.

Perioperative nursing considerations History of aspirin use should be determined and aspirin use should be stopped at least 1 week prior to surgery. Patients with anemia and bleeding disorders require further work-up prior to surgery. A modified adenoidectomy may be performed in patients with palate abnormalities (including repaired cleft palate) to prevent hypernasal speech postoperatively. Tonsillectomy and adenoidectomy are frequently performed on children. Chapter 18 in Volume 2 provides general information regarding pediatric surgery.

Postoperative airway management may present difficulties in patients with altered neurologic tone and physical abnormalities of airways, including patients with cerebral palsy, Down syndrome, Treacher Collins syndrome, or Crouzon's disease. Extremely young children, owing to their small airway size and the edema following surgery, are also at greater risk. These patients may require special monitoring in an intensive care setting postoperatively.

Recording of blood loss during the operative procedure should follow institution policy.

After ensuring that a safety belt is secured over the patient, a sandbag or roll is placed under the patient's shoulders to hyperextend the neck. The patient is in

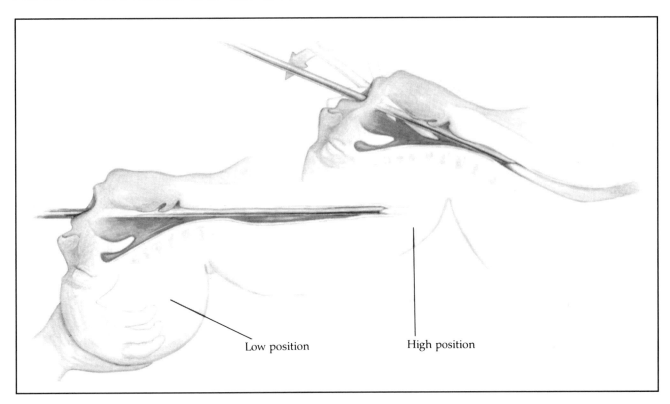

FIGURE 5-11   Rigid esophagoscopy. (From Johns, M. E., Price, J. C., & Mattox, D. E. [1990]. *Atlas of head and neck surgery* (vol. 1). Philadelphia: B. C. Decker. Reprinted by permission of Mosby-Year Book, Inc.)

slight Trendelenburg's position. An electrocautery pad is applied to the patient, and the surgeon may request an antimicrobial solution to cleanse the patient's face prior to the placement of a head drape and full sheet.

Instruments and supplies include the following: tonsillectomy and adenoidectomy (T&A) set and, dependent upon the indication for the surgery, additional instrumentation such as biopsy forceps (Fig. 5-12).

Key steps

1. A self-retaining mouth retractor is inserted and may be secured to the Mayo stand. A tongue depressor may also be used for visualization of the operative area. Efficient suction must be available throughout the procedure.
2. There are two basic surgical techniques for performing tonsillectomy and adenoidectomy. In one technique, the electrocautery is used to dissect the tonsil from its fossa. Better hemostasis is achieved with this technique, but postoperative complications such as increased pain and delayed healing may occur.
3. In the alternative technique, the mucosa of the anterior pillar is incised with a knife, followed by blunt dissection with scissors along the posterior pillar. The tonsil is then removed with a snare.
4. Electrocautery or a tonsil sponge placed in the fossa is used to obtain hemostasis.

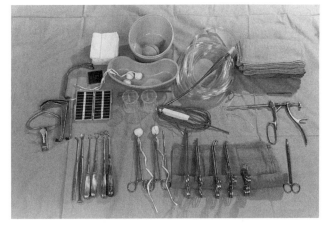

FIGURE 5-12   Tonsillectomy and adenoidectomy instrument table.

5. Occasionally, a ligature is required to control a bleeding vessel. Electrocautery may be used, but if a biopsy procedure is being done, this technique will not be used.
6. The adenoids are then removed using curettes or an adenotome, followed by pressure applied with tonsil sponges.
7. After careful visual inspection of the fossa to determine complete hemostasis, the mouth retractor is removed.

8. Once the endotracheal tube has been removed, the patient should be placed on his or her side or in a semirecumbent (Fowler's) position to prevent aspiration.

Submandibular gland excision

Indications for this procedure include a mass in the gland, chronic or recurrent acute sialoadenitis (*sialo* = of the salivary gland), glandular dysfunction, abscesses, and sialolithiasis.

Perioperative nursing considerations A preoperative work-up may have included a fine needle biopsy, computed tomography (CT scan), and magnetic resonance imaging (MRI) in order to assess the extent of the submandibular disease. These studies have mostly replaced the sialogram, wherein the duct system was infused with a contrast medium. Preoperative preparation of the patient is important and should include discussion of potential damage to the facial nerve as well as to the lingual and hypoglossal nerves. In patients with possible malignancy, more extensive preoperative preparation is required, including the possible need for neck dissection and resection of nerves, mandibular segment, and floor of the mouth. The patient is placed in the supine position with the affected side uppermost. The skin prep and draping are done as for thyroid surgery.

Instruments and supplies include the following: minor neck dissection set, lacrimal probes, and nerve stimulator. A major neck dissection set-up and tracheostomy set with tubes should be readily available.

Key steps

1. A small skin incision is made below the lower edge of the horizontal portion of the mandible and then is continued through the platysma muscle and cervical fascia, developing the skin flaps.
2. The mandibular branch of the facial nerve is located and gently retracted.
3. The external maxillary artery and anterior facial vein are clamped and ligated. (The external maxillary artery is double clamped, doubly ligated, and transected.) The gland is freed by blunt dissection.
4. Wharton's duct is ligated and divided.
5. The submandibular gland is removed (Loré, 1988).
6. A small drain is inserted, and the wound is closed with fine sutures. A light gauze dressing may be applied.

Parotidectomy

Indications for partial or total parotidectomy include the following: removal of benign and some malignant tumors, inflammatory lesions, vascular anomalies, and for metastatic cancer involving lymph nodes overlying the gland (Fig. 5-13).

Perioperative nursing considerations Preoperative preparation of the patient is extremely important, as the surgery may be the first part of much more extensive surgery in the head and neck area. Special care will be taken to locate and dissect the facial nerve and its branches. The patient must be aware of the possible complication of facial nerve weakness or paralysis. When a total parotidectomy is being done for malignant tumor, a free nerve graft to reestablish continuity of the facial nerve may be done. Following parotidectomy, many patients experience gustatory sweating (Frey's syndrome). The smell and taste of food can produce sweating and redness of the skin overlying the parotid region.

The patient is positioned supine, with a shoulder roll in place, and the affected side of the face is uppermost. Skin preparation includes the entire side of the face, neck, and forehead. Draping is as for thyroid surgery.

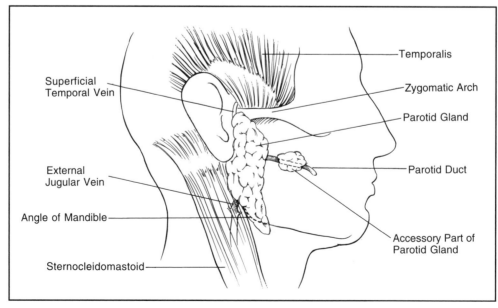

FIGURE 5-13 Parotid gland and surrounding structures.

Instruments and supplies include a major neck dissection set, nerve stimulator, lacrimal probes, and optical loupes.

Key steps

1. A preauricular and postauricular incision is made, with a curved extension following the skin crease below the angle of the jaw.
2. Skin flaps are elevated and retracted. Using blunt dissection, the gland is separated from the mastoid process and the cartilage of the external auditory canal.
3. The main nerve trunk of the facial nerve is located, and using sharp dissection, the nerve branches are followed through the gland. The superficial portion of the gland is removed. Stensen's duct (parotid gland duct) may be transected and ligated.
4. If the deep portion of the parotid gland needs to be removed, the facial nerve is retracted to provide exposure.
5. Hemostasis is obtained by ligature and electrocautery.
6. The wound is closed in layers, and a small drain may be inserted. A pressure dressing is applied.

Uvulopalatopharyngoplasty

Uvulopalatopharyngoplasty (UPPP) is performed to relieve oropharyngeal obstruction by excising redundant soft tissue of the soft palate, uvula, and posterior pharyngeal wall.

Perioperative nursing considerations Although there is improvement with this surgery, many patients still meet the criterion for a diagnosis of obstructive sleep apnea postoperatively (i.e., five or more apneas per hour of sleep). In nearly all cases, snoring is eliminated (Lee, 1989). Most patients with obstructive sleep apnea are overweight and may have special positioning needs in the operating room. Medications with sedative effects worsen sleep apnea and should not be given to these patients. A tracheostomy may be performed prior to the UPPP because of possible airway obstruction due to postoperative edema. An emergency bronchoscopy or tracheostomy may be required if obstruction occurs following anesthesia induction. Extensive resection may result in nasal air leak during speech and nasal regurgitation during swallowing. Postoperative recovery from UPPP is very painful for the patient. Positioning and draping are done as for tonsillectomy.

Instruments and supplies include the following: tonsillectomy instrument set, bronchoscopy equipment, tracheostomy instruments, and a variety of tracheostomy tubes.

Key steps

1. After placement of a self-retaining mouth gag, the surgeon may inject the area to be excised with small amounts of epinephrine, 1:100,000 solution.
2. The mucosa on either side of the uvula is clamped with hemostats and incised.
3. A box-shaped incision using a knife blade or electrocautery is made through the mucosa at the tongue base, ascending in the sulcus between the anterior pillar and mandible, and turning medially to cross the soft palate about midway between the edges of the soft and hard palates. Suture ligation may be necessary to control bleeding.
4. Using dissection, mucosa, glands, fat, and fibrous tissue are removed down to the muscular layers.
5. The uvula is amputated at the edge of the soft palatal muscle fibers. If tonsils are present, they are excised. Dense fibrous scar tissue may be encountered if a previous tonsillectomy has been done.
6. The posterior tonsillar pillar is trimmed and fixated to the corner of the palatopharyngeal incision.
7. Suturing is continued downward to the base of the tongue. This procedure of dissection and closure is repeated on the opposite side.
8. The palatal closure is completed by suturing the nasal surface of the mucosa to the incised edge of the oral surface (Meyerhoff & Rice, 1992).

Head and Neck Procedures

The earliest attempts at head and neck surgery were confined to easily accessible lesions of the lips and tongue. With the advent of modern anesthesia and the availability of blood for transfusion, antibiotics, radiation therapy, improved diagnostic techniques, and instrumentation, the ability to safely manage patients has greatly improved and more radical and complex procedures are evolving.

Laryngofissure repair

Indications for laryngotomy include bilateral abductor cord paralysis, malignancy, excision of laryngeal webs, and correction of strictures, benign lesions, and impacted foreign bodies.

Perioperative nursing considerations Tracheostomy is usually done as part of the procedure. A feeding tube is inserted prior to the start of the procedure.

The patient is supine, with a shoulder roll in place and the head slightly extended. The entire neck, shoulders, and upper anterior chest are prepped and draped as for thyroidectomy. The procedure may be performed under local anesthesia with conscious sedation or with general anesthesia. Suction equipment, oxygen, and resuscitative equipment must be immediately available. If intravenous conscious sedation is used during the procedure, institution policy should be followed for monitoring the patient and the required documentation.

Instruments and supplies include a head and neck set, oscillating power saw, and a variety of tracheostomy tubes.

Key steps

1. For the laryngofissure, a midline anterior incision is made with dissection proceeding down to the external perichondrium of the thyroid cartilage.

2. The thyroid cartilage is divided in the midline, using an oscillating saw. The internal soft tissues are divided as the two halves of the thyroid cartilage are retracted.

3. The true vocal cords are visualized through an incision into the cricothyroid membrane.

4. The interior of the larynx is exposed as the true vocal cords are divided in the midline (anterior commissure). Depending on the indication for the laryngofissure, further surgery is performed.

5. For closure, the thyroid cartilages are approximated and fixed, the muscles are closed in layers, a drain is inserted, and the soft tissues are closed.

6. If a tracheostomy was performed, a tracheostomy tube is inserted and a split gauze dressing is applied around the tube.

7. A pressure dressing of soft gauze is applied over the skin incision and fixed with a circular gauze bandage.

Teflon injection (for adductor vocal cord paralysis)

Indications for this procedure include the following: damage to cranial nerve X and paralysis secondary to traumatic, degenerative, and congenital disorders and surgery. The normal vocal cord is unable to approximate the fixed adducted vocal cord, resulting in vocal dysfunction. As there is increased air escaping during phonation, the vocal quality is whispery, and there may be limited phrase length. Spontaneous recovery occurs within 6 to 12 months of injury in most cases of unilateral vocal cord paralysis (Meyerhoff & Rice, 1992).

Perioperative nursing considerations Cooperation of the patient throughout the examination is required. The patient needs reassurance during the procedure and should be provided with explanations of the procedure as it is being performed. All equipment should be ready prior to the commencement of the procedure. Any artificial dentition needs to be removed prior to the procedure, and any loose teeth should be noted. Suction equipment, oxygen, and resuscitative equipment must be immediately available. The patient should maintain an NPO status until the gag reflex returns, as a topical spray or gargle will be used.

Instruments and supplies include the following: coaxial light source, gauze sponges, wooden tongue blades, laryngeal mirrors of various sizes, defogger or warming solution, suction apparatus, topical anesthetic, Teflon paste and gun (Fig. 5-14), #18 and #19 reusable laryngeal needles, and emesis basin.

Key steps

1. After the use of a topical gargle or spray, the tongue is grasped and gently held with a gauze sponge as a prewarmed laryngeal mirror is introduced into the oral cavity.

2. As the Teflon paste gun is positioned, the patient is asked to speak during injection in order to determine if a sufficient amount of the paste has been introduced.

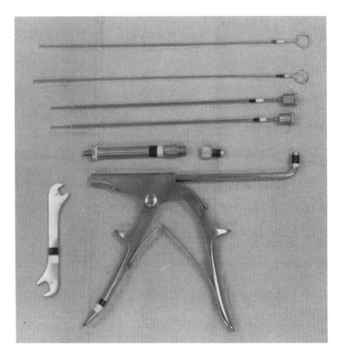

FIGURE 5-14 Teflon paste gun with #18 and 19 laryngeal needles and stylets, barrel and hub, and wrench.

Tracheostomy

Indications for tracheostomy include acute respiratory obstruction, stenosis of the larynx and trachea, trauma to the larynx or trachea, for long-term respiratory treatment, and as a preliminary procedure for more extensive surgery.

Perioperative nursing considerations The procedure can be done under local or general anesthesia, depending on the indication for the surgery. The tracheostomy may be temporary or permanent. The procedure can be performed over an endotracheal tube or a bronchoscope.

Extensive preoperative preparation of the patient is vital and should include postoperative tracheostomy care and discussion of how the patient can continue to communicate in the immediate postoperative period (e.g., with a writing board). Suction equipment, oxygen, and resuscitative equipment must be immediately available. An extra tracheotomy tube of the same size that the patient receives is to be kept with the patient at all times. All equipment should be ready prior to the commencement of the procedure. The patient is positioned supine on the operating room bed, with the neck extended and shoulders elevated with a roll or sandbag. The entire neck, shoulders, and upper anterior chest are prepped and draped as for thyroidectomy.

Instruments include a minor neck dissection set with the following instruments: tracheal dilator, Jackson tracheal hook, and Cushing nerve hook (Fig. 5-15). A variety of sizes of tracheostomy and endotracheal tubes are required, along with a local anesthetic set-up. Figure 5-16 shows a tracheostomy tube with obturator.

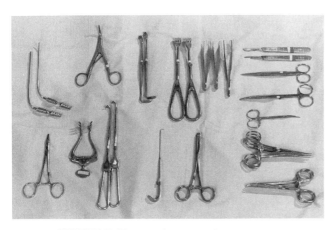

FIGURE 5-15 Tracheostomy instruments.

Key steps

1. Two types of incisions can be made: horizontal or vertical. A midline skin incision is made from the center of the thyroid cartilage to the sternal notch. After the initial skin incision, the remainder of the procedure can be almost totally done with electrocautery or by blunt dissection through subcutaneous fatty tissue, cervical fascia, and sternohyoid muscles.
2. The isthmus of the thyroid gland is retracted to expose the underlying second, third, and fourth tracheal rings. In some cases, it may be necessary to transect the isthmus.
3. Using a hypodermic needle, a few drops of topical anesthetic may be injected into the lumen of the trachea to reduce the coughing reflex.
4. A knife blade is then used to cut a window the same size as the diameter of the tracheostomy tube directly above the tracheal ring of choice. The opening into the trachea is usually made at or below the second tracheal ring; otherwise subglottic stenosis may result.
5. The tracheostomy tube is inserted, the obturator is removed, and the airway is verified prior to the removal of any endotracheal tube or bronchoscope that was in place.
6. Wound edges are lightly approximated. The tube is sutured to the skin; tapes are tied with a square knot and secured behind the neck.
7. The inner tube is then inserted. A split gauze dressing is applied around the tracheostomy tube.

Laryngectomy

Indications for laryngectomy are primarily for removal of tumors and as an extension of a planned surgical procedure where the disease process has invaded the larynx. A vertical (hemi) laryngectomy, removing one true vocal cord, one false cord, arytenoid, and one-half of the thyroid cartilage, is performed for superficial neoplasms confined to one vocal cord or for tumors extending a short distance below the cord. Postoperatively the patient has a hoarse voice with normal airway and no problem swallowing.

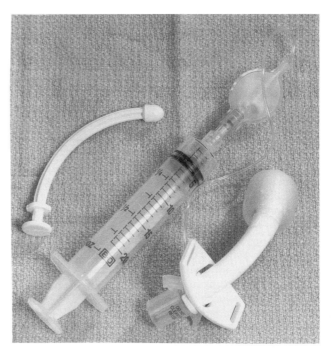

FIGURE 5-16 Tracheostomy tube with obturator.

A supraglottic (horizontal) laryngectomy removing the false cords, epiglottis, and hyoid bone is performed for tumors of the epiglottis and false vocal cords. Postoperatively, the patient retains a normal voice and airway but may aspirate occasionally, particularly liquids.

A total laryngectomy includes the removal of the hyoid bone, entire larynx, cricoid cartilage, and two or three rings of the trachea. Postoperatively the patient loses his voice and breathes through a tracheostomy stoma, but should have no problem swallowing.

Perioperative nursing considerations In most cases where total laryngectomy is required, radical neck dissection is also a necessary part of the procedure. Extensive preoperative preparation of the patient is vital, including discussion of how the patient can continue to communicate in the immediate postoperative period (e.g., with a writing board). The patient is positioned supine on the operating room bed, with the neck extended and shoulders elevated with a roll or sandbag. The entire neck, shoulders, and upper anterior chest are prepped and then draped as for thyroidectomy. A tracheostomy may be performed for airway control. An extra tracheostomy tube of the same size that the patient receives should be kept with the patient at all times.

Instruments and supplies include the following: a major neck dissection set, oscillating saw, and tracheostomy tubes.

Key steps

1. A single midline incision from the suprasternal notch to just above the hyoid bone is made, developing lat-

eral skin flaps. Palpation of lymph nodes is done to ascertain the presence of any lymphadenopathy.

2. The sternohyoid, sternothyroid, and omohyoid muscles (strap muscles) are transected.

3. Using sharp and blunt dissection, the thyroid gland is separated from the cricoid cartilage and the upper rings of the trachea.

4. The inferior laryngeal vessels and laryngeal nerve are transected, as are the superior laryngeal vessels and nerves.

5. With the hyoid bone exposed, the attached muscles are transected.

6. The trachea is transected over a small curved clamp, which has been inserted in the plane between the trachea and esophagus.

7. A Lahey clamp is used to retract the upper resected portion of the trachea and cricoid cartilage.

8. Sharp dissection is used to further separate the esophagus from the cricoid cartilage. The inferior pharyngeal constrictor muscles are transected. If the endotracheal tube was removed to perform this step, it is reinserted.

9. To prevent leakage of blood into the trachea, a moist gauze is placed around the endotracheal tube.

10. Depending on the extent of the laryngeal tumor, further resection may include a portion of the esophagus.

11. The hypopharynx is entered and the lateral hypopharyngeal wall is incised to the level of the hyoid bone, with dissection continuing along the remaining sides of the esophagus.

12. With the larynx retracted, the final attachments are cut; this may include a portion of the base of the tongue. The specimen is removed en masse.

13. After a nasal feeding tube is inserted through one naris into the esophagus, the pharyngeal and esophageal defect is closed, with the neck being placed in slight flexion.

14. The edges of the inferior pharyngeal constrictor muscle as well as the suprahyoid muscles are approximated.

15. The skin edges or the walls of the trachea may need further excision in order to approximate the margins, thus avoiding stenosis of the tracheostomy.

16. One or two suction drains are inserted through separate stab sounds and secured.

17. Final closure approximates the cervical fascia and platysmal muscles (Loré, 1988).

18. A light pressure dressing of soft gauze is applied over the skin incision and fixed with a circular gauze bandage.

19. The endotracheal tube may be exchanged for a metal tracheostomy tube, or a cuffed endotracheal tube may be used until postoperative edema subsides.

20. Tracheostomy tapes are tied with a square knot behind the neck, and a split gauze dressing is applied around the tracheostomy tube.

Radical neck dissection

The basic objective of this procedure is the complete removal of the tumor and surrounding structures, including the lymphatic system on one or both sides of the neck in an en bloc resection. This includes the removal of the sternocleidomastoid muscle, jugular vein, and spinal accessory nerve. The modified neck dissection is a variation of the radical neck dissection in which the spinal accessory nerve and the jugular vein are preserved either separately or together. The functional neck dissection is a complete cervical lymphadenectomy, preserving the spinal accessory nerve, sternocleidomastoid muscle, and jugular vein (Johns & Price, 1990).

Perioperative nursing considerations Extensive patient preoperative preparation is required, addressing the psychosocial and physical impact of the procedure on the patient. Prior radiotherapy may produce increased bleeding and difficult dissection, with possible rupture of vessels. Adequate amounts of blood should be available. Depending on the surgeon's preference, the patient may require removal of body hair prior to the procedure. Areas for hair removal include the face, neck, chest, and shoulders. Special care to protect the carotid artery may be achieved by using dermal grafts or rotation or muscular flaps. If the external jugular vein is accidentally opened before ligation, bleeding must be stopped immediately in order to prevent air embolism. Control of bleeding during and at the end of the procedure is essential.

Once the neck dissection has been completed, immediate reconstruction may be planned, requiring a second surgical set-up and team (e.g., plastic surgeons). Depending on the type of reconstruction involved, the patient may need to be reprepped and redraped in order to complete the procedure. Positioning and draping are done in a way that allows the surgeon the ability to turn and adjust the patient's head during the procedure. The anesthesia apparatus is not fixed to the table. The patient is placed in a supine position, and a Mayfield headrest may be used. A safety belt is placed, and if possible, a foot rest should be secured to the operating room bed. This will prevent the patient from sliding when the operating room bed is tilted at a 30- to 45-degree angle (Fowler's position). This position assists in the control of bleeding by preventing engorgement of veins. The head is draped, and sheets are applied as directed to mark out the operative field. Sutures may be used to secure towels in place. Wing sheets to cover the area immediately adjacent to the operative field are applied (i.e., anesthesia area).

The preoperative skin prep is extensive, involving the face, neck, shoulders, and chest. As the eyes are usually part of the operative field, care is taken to avoid corneal abrasion by the use of ointment and tape, suturing the eyelid closed or using a corneal protector.

Instruments and supplies include a major neck dissection set (Fig. 5-17) and tracheostomy tubes. For immediate reconstruction, an additional set-up and a second team may be required.

Key steps

1. A tracheostomy may be performed. The incisions for the neck dissection are made through the skin and

platysma muscle, depending on the site of the primary tumor. Examples of incisions are shown in Figure 5-18.

2. Skin flaps are developed and retracted to expose the lateral aspect of the neck. Bleeding vessels are controlled by ligatures or electrocautery. The flaps may be covered with moist laparotomy sponges.

3. Branches of the jugular veins are clamped, ligated, and divided. Attachments of the sternocleidomastoid muscle are transected, the deep fascia is incised, and the omohyoid muscle is divided at its scapular attachments.

4. Using blunt dissection, the internal jugular vein is isolated, double clamped, suture ligated, and transected.

5. As the internal carotid artery and vagus nerve are retracted, the internal jugular vein and associated nodes are removed.

6. Dissection continues upward along the anterior edge of the superior belly of the omohyoid muscle. The inferior belly is transected, and the dissection posteriorly follows the edge of the trapezius muscle, transecting cervical vessels.

7. The omohyoid muscle is severed from the hyoid bone. The cervical plexus and spinal accessory nerve are transected.

8. At the mandibular edge, the external maxillary artery and the anterior facial vein are divided. The mandibular branch of the facial nerve is preserved if feasible.

9. The submental triangle is dissected, reflecting the nodes, fat, and fascia downward as the transection continues along the trapezius muscle, removing all the contents of the posterior triangle.

10. The spinal accessory nerve and the internal jugular vein are dissected.

11. The submaxillary space is then dissected with transection of Wharton's duct and branches of the lingual vein.

12. With the muscle and lymph node mass reflected upward, the upper end of the internal jugular vein is clamped, suture-ligated, and divided. The dissection continues upward, transecting the external maxillary artery.

13. The posterior facial vein is doubly ligated as the tail of the parotid and the attachment of the sternocleido-

mastoid muscle are transected (Loré, 1988). The surgical specimen is removed.

14. The entire field is inspected for bleeding and is irrigated with warm saline solution.

15. If any immediate reconstruction is planned, it will begin at this point.

16. If the wound is to be closed without further reconstruction, suction drains are placed in the wound, and approximation of platysma muscle, subcutaneous tissue, and skin is completed.

17. If Penrose drains are used, a bulky pressure dressing is applied, and if suction drainage is used, the surgeon may prefer only a light gauze dressing or no external dressing.

18. If a tracheostomy is present, the dressing should be done as discussed for the tracheostomy procedure.

Reconstruction Following Head and Neck Surgery

The aims of surgery are to eradicate the disease while maintaining or improving function and appearance. Reconstructive procedures are tailored to the patient and the site and extent of the defect or disease.

Large defects in the oral cavity and oropharynx may be closed with skin grafts. New tissue used to close surgical defects may include local rotation or transposition skin flaps for the skin of the face and neck. For small defects in the oral cavity, local flaps of buccal or tongue mucosa may be used. To close larger defects, tissue can be transferred from more distant sites using skin flaps (deltopectoral flap and forehead flap), myocutaneous flaps (pectoralis major flap and latissimus dorsi flap), and vascularized free tissue transfers, also called free flaps (radial forearm flap). When a segmental resection of the mandible is required, the resulting deformity can affect eating, speech, and appearance, so reconstruction should be done if at all possible (Way, 1991). Plastic and reconstructive procedures are covered in Chapter 16 in this volume.

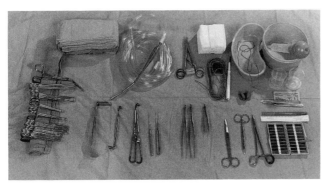

FIGURE 5-17 Neck dissection instruments.

SUMMARY

This chapter has described laryngologic and head and neck procedures, the equipment and supplies involved, and the role of the perioperative nurse in caring for patients undergoing this type of surgery. The nurse caring for these patients will be especially aware of the many concerns and anxieties seen in patients having laryngologic or head and neck surgery. Since a high percentage of head and neck procedures in adults are done because of malignancies, it is suggested that the nurse review Chapter 20, Oncologic Surgery, in this volume.

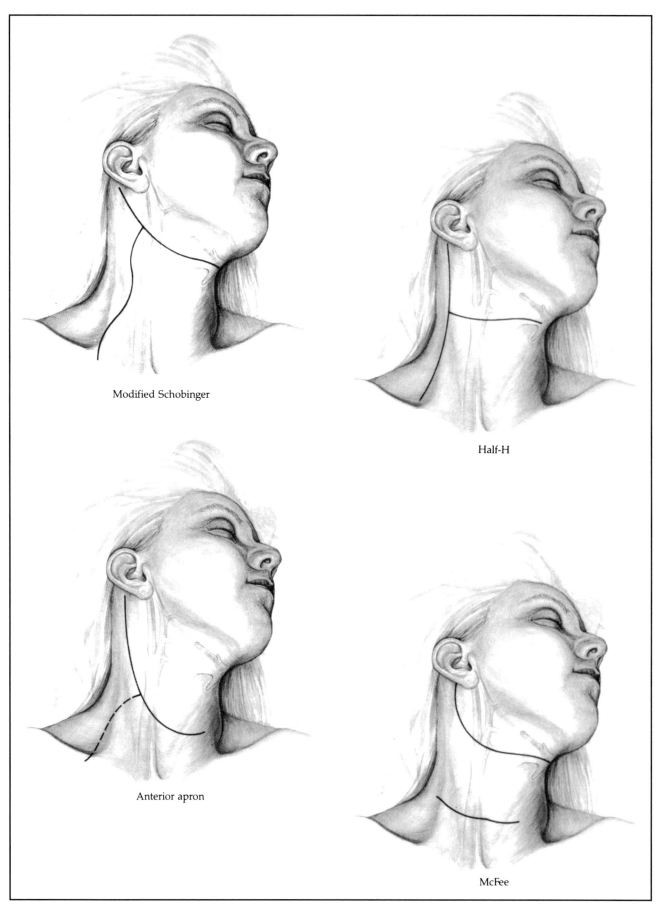

Modified Schobinger

Half-H

Anterior apron

McFee

FIGURE 5-18 Incisions for radical neck dissection. (From Johns, M. E., Price, J. C., & Mattox, D. E. [1990]. *Atlas of head and neck surgery* (vol. 1). Philadelphia: B. C. Decker. Reprinted by permission of Mosby-Year Book, Inc.)

REFERENCES

Cummings, C. W. (1989). *Otolaryngology—Head and neck surgery* (Update I). St. Louis: C. V. Mosby.

Cummings, C. W. (1990). *Otolaryngology—Head and neck surgery* (Update II). St. Louis: C. V. Mosby.

Dougherty, K. D. (1990). Otolaryngologic surgery. In J. C. Rothrock. *Perioperative nursing care planning,* St. Louis: C. V. Mosby.

Freund, H. R. (1979). *Principles of head and neck surgery* (2nd ed.). New York: Appleton-Century-Crofts.

Johns, M. E., Price, J. C., & Mattox, D. E. (1990). *Atlas of head and neck surgery,* Volume I. Philadelphia: B. C. Decker.

Lee, K. J. (1989). *Textbook of otolaryngology and head and neck surgery.* New York: Elsevier.

Loré, J. (1988). *An atlas of head and neck surgery* (3rd ed.). Philadelphia: W. B. Saunders.

Meyerhoff, W. L., & Rice, D. H. (1992). *Otolaryngology—Head and neck surgery.* Philadelphia: W. B. Saunders.

Naumann, H. H. (1984). *Head and neck surgery* (Vol. 4, Neck). Philadelphia: W. B. Saunders.

Silcox, S. (1991). Laryngologic and head and neck surgery, pp. 545–573 in Meeker, M. H. & Rothrock, J. C. *Alexander's care of the patient in surgery* (9th ed.) St. Louis: Mosby-Year Book.

Silver, C. E. (1986). *Atlas of head and neck surgery.* New York: Churchill Livingstone.

Snell, R. S. (1986). The head and neck. In *Clinical anatomy for medical students* (3rd ed.). Boston: Little, Brown, & Co.

Way, L. W. (1991). Head and neck tumors. In *Current Surgical Diagnosis and Treatment* (9th ed.). New York: Appleton and Lange.

Chapter 6

Thyroid/Parathyroid Surgery

Key Concepts

- The thyroid gland regulates the body's metabolism. Although removal of the gland will affect metabolism, the disease within the gland may create even more of a metabolic imbalance.

- Thyroid glands produce and synthesize the thyroid hormones triiodothyronine (T_3) and thyroxine (T_4). Their function is to maintain the metabolic rate of the body, stimulate the nervous system, and regulate growth and development in children.

- People who are at a higher risk for thyroid carcinoma include those exposed to radiation in the head and neck area and those with a family history of medullary thyroid cancer.

- Due to the proximity of the recurrent laryngeal nerve and the superior laryngeal nerve to the thyroid gland, they are at risk of damage during the operative procedure.

- Hemostasis is important in thyroid procedures. The superior thyroid artery, which originates at the carotid artery, and the two inferior thyroid arteries, which originate at the subclavian arteries, provide the majority of the blood supply to the thyroid gland.

- Patients undergoing thyroid surgery may exhibit anxiety concerning their self-image.

- The four pea-sized parathyroid glands are found lateral and posterior to the thyroid gland.

- Several specimens may be sent to the pathologist for identification of parathyroid tissue during the surgical procedure involving parathyroid glands. Multiple specimen jars should be readily available and labeled.

- The parathyroid glands produce parathormone, the primary regulator of calcium and phosphorus metabolism.

- Hypoparathyroidism is the most common serious complication of surgery on the thyroid gland.

INTRODUCTION

This chapter includes care of the surgical patient with thyroid or parathyroid disorders, perioperative nursing considerations, and key steps of the most common procedures. Indications for surgery and the importance of these endocrine glands for human body functioning are also discussed.

ANATOMY

Thyroid Gland

Historical perspective

Because of the shape of the thyroid itself or the shape of the thyroid cartilage, in 1646 Wharton renamed the "laryngeal" gland the thyroid gland (*thyreos* = shield).

By 1875, experiments with dogs showed that death from excision of the thyroid gland could be averted by a previous graft of the gland. Murray and Howitz successfully treated hypothyroidism in 1890 by using a thyroid extract. Most of the early studies on the thyroid gland were done in Switzerland, where, due to a lack of iodine, there were numerous people with enlarged thyroid, or "goiters." The primary problem was that the people suffocated from pressure on the trachea caused by the goiters (Haeger, 1988). In 1909, Theodore Kocher was awarded a Nobel Prize for his work in the field of thyroid surgery. During the 1800s he performed over 2,000 surgeries on the thyroid, with only a 4.5% mortality (Kaplan, 1989).

Anatomy

The thyroid is positioned at the base of the neck and on both sides of the larynx and the upper rings of the trachea (Fig. 6-1). This vascular gland is composed of two lateral lobes that are connected by an isthmus that crosses in front of the trachea. It is surrounded by a fibrous capsule. The weight of a normal thyroid gland is approximately 15 to 20 g.

The major blood supply to the thyroid gland consists of two superior thyroid arteries that come from the external carotids and descend to the upper poles of the thyroid. The two inferior thyroid arteries originate at the subclavian arteries and enter the lower part of each thyroid lobe. In some cases there is another artery that comes from the aortic arch to the midline of the gland, called the thyroidea ima. Both the superior and middle thyroid veins empty into the internal jugular vein. The inferior thyroid veins drain into the innominate vein (Kaplan, 1989).

Innervation of the thyroid gland is from the sympathetic and parasympathetic divisions of the autonomic nervous system. The anatomical position of the recurrent laryngeal nerve frequently varies. Generally, it lies lateral to the tracheoesophageal groove and medial to the carotid artery. A nerve stimulator can be used during the surgical procedure to confirm the identification of this nerve. Because of the proximity of the recurrent laryngeal nerve and superior laryngeal nerve to the thyroid gland, there is a risk of nerve injury during surgery (Kaplan, 1989). The nonrecurrent laryngeal nerves are usually found in close proximity to the inferior thyroid artery and close behind the carotid, only on the right side.

The functions of the laryngeal nerves are the following:

- The external superior laryngeal nerve innervates the cricothyroid muscle, which affects the vocal pitch.
- The recurrent laryngeal nerve innervates the vocal cords.

Endocrine glands produce an internal secretion that is released into the blood and lymph system and is circu-

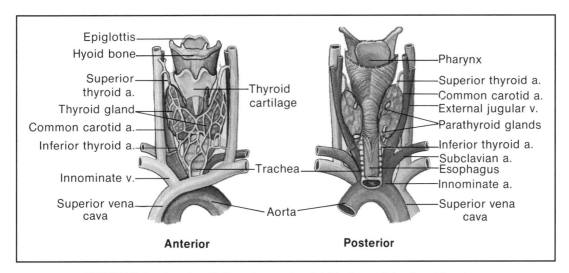

FIGURE 6-1   Anterior (*left*) and posterior (*right*) views of the thyroid and parathyroid glands.   (From Anderson, P. D. [1984]. *Basic Human Anatomy and Physiology.* Boston: Jones and Bartlett Publishers.)

lated throughout the body. The thyroid gland consists of follicle cells that produce and synthesize thyroid hormones and calcitonin. Release of these hormones is controlled by the hypothalamus and pituitary glands. Two of the thyroid hormones that are secreted are thyroxine (T_4) and triiodothyronine (T_3). These hormones function to increase the rate at which energy is released from carbohydrates and the rate at which protein is synthesized. They also regulate the rate of growth and development in children and stimulate the nervous system.

The primary function of the thyroid gland is to maintain an appropriate metabolic rate. The calcitonin produced by the thyroid gland is important in the metabolism of calcium and acts to reduce the blood plasma calcium concentration. This prevents the formation of new osteoclasts (Martinelli & Fontana, 1990). An imbalance may lead to a weakening of the bones.

The functions of the thyroid gland are as follows:

- Increases blood volume
- Increases cardiac output
- Increases the need for vitamins
- Regulates the metabolic rate
- Regulates growth and development
- Metabolizes iodine
- Stimulates protein synthesis
- Increases oxygen consumption

The entire thyroid gland and isthmus can be removed without compromising the life of the patient. The metabolic rate of a person whose thyroid has been removed can be regulated with supplemental drug therapy.

Parathyroid Glands

The parathyroid glands were first described in medical literature in 1889. In 1891 and 1900, animal research demonstrated that tetany and death resulted when the parathyroids were removed. By 1908 the connection between the parathyroid and blood calcium level regulation was determined (Kaplan, 1989).

These four very small pea-sized endocrine glands are located lateral and posterior to the thyroid gland. The inferior parathyroid is located near the terminal branch of the inferior thyroid artery near the back of the thyroid gland. The superior parathyroid is generally located near the upper terminal branch of the inferior thyroid artery and from the middle to upper third of the lobe. Occasionally, the parathyroids can be found in the thyroid tissue. A fifth supernumerary gland may be found in 5% of the population (de Francisco et al., 1991). Blood supply to the superior parathyroid gland is from the inferior thyroid artery. The lower gland receives its blood supply from a branch of the descending inferior thyroid artery.

The parathyroid glands secrete parathormone. This hormone is the primary regulator of calcium and phosphorus metabolism. It stimulates the kidneys to activate vitamin D, which enables the intestines to absorb more calcium and increases the reabsorption of calcium by the kidneys and decreases calcium loss. A disruption in this metabolism will result in diseases of the bone, renal calculi, or tetany.

NURSING CONSIDERATIONS

It is important for the perioperative nurse to understand the etiology of thyroid and parathyroid disorders in order to plan appropriate care for the patient.

Indications for Surgery

Thyroid carcinoma

Tumors of the endocrine system are rare. However, of those tumors, thyroid cancer is the most commonly diagnosed. These tumors vary from inactive or slow-growing tumors to malignant, fast-growing carcinomas. Thyroid cancer accounts for about 0.2% of cancer deaths per year (Donehower, 1991). The slow-growing tumors are most likely to be confined locally and they respond successfully to surgical intervention (Table 6-1).

According to the American Cancer Society approximately 12,500 new cases of thyroid cancer will be diagnosed in the United States in 1992. Of that number, 9,100 patients will be females and 3,400 patients will be males. It is estimated 1,000 people will die of this disease (American Cancer Society, 1992). Most of these cancers will occur in people between the ages of 25 and 65. Tumors of the endocrine system are rarely seen in children (Donehower, 1990).

Between 1920 and 1950, thousands of children were given low doses of radiotherapy for the treatment of en-

TABLE 6-1 Recommended Surgical Therapy for Thyroid Carcinomas

Type of Tumor	Tumor Size	Recommended Treatment
Papillary without node involvement	< 1.5 cm	Thyroid lobectomy, total thyroidectomy, postoperative scan,[131]I
Follicular without node involvement	1.5–4 cm	Thyroid lobectomy, total thyroidectomy, postoperative scan,[131]I
Papillary and follicular with node involvement	All patients	Total thyroidectomy and neck dissection, postoperative scan,[131]I
Medullary	All patients	Total thyroidectomy, modified or radical neck dissection
Anaplastic	All patients	Biopsy, palliative surgery only

larged tonsils or adenoids and other conditions of the head and neck such as acne and ringworm. There is a direct correlation between these childhood treatments and an increase in thyroid neoplasms. The majority of these tumors are benign. These patients have an increased risk for developing thyroid cancer from 5 years to 35 years following the radiation.

Assessment of a patient presenting with a thyroid mass includes a complete history; a history of any previous exposure to radiation; a thorough head and neck examination; definition of the size, location, and texture of the mass; a thyroid function test; and blood calcium, calcitonin, phosphorus, and thyroglobulin tests. The first sign of a thyroid tumor may be a small lump in the neck. As the mass grows on the thyroid gland, it can cause compression on the larynx, trachea, and esophagus. Compression of these structures can result in symptoms that include:

• Dysphonia
• Dyspnea
• Dysphagia

The four primary thyroid carcinomas are papillary, follicular, anaplastic, and medullary. Of these, the papillary and follicular carcinomas are well-differentiated. The cells are histologically comparable to the original tissue (Donehower, 1990).

Papillary carcinoma Papillary carcinoma composes 50% of thyroid cancer, and 90% of radiation-induced thyroid cancer is papillary. This cancer usually manifests before the age of 40, but the age range is from the early teens to 80 years or older. Women are more likely to have this disease, but they have a better prognosis than men. Of patients diagnosed with differentiated carcinoma of the thyroid, 70% to 90% present with a thyroid nodule or enlargement of a lymph node (Block et al., 1990). Treatment for patients with well-differentiated carcinoma of the thyroid includes appropriate preoperative evaluation, surgical intervention, and operative management with continued medical follow-up. Papillary cancer is the least aggressive of the thyroid tumors, and its overall mortality rate is low. Growth of the tumor is usually confined within the thyroid gland and to the pericapsular tissues and lateral neck lymph nodes. The cancer may exist in the gland for several years and not spread. If it does metastasize, the lungs and bones are the most common sites. The disease seems to be more aggressive and have a higher mortality rate in patients over the age of 50.

Follicular carcinoma Follicular carcinoma is potentially more invasive than papillary carcinoma. It is seen in an older group of patients. The thyroid gland is more likely to continue to produce thyroid hormones (T_3 and T_4) and in some cases this may cause hyperthyroidism. There is seldom enlargement of the lymph nodes in follicular carcinoma. The patient may have a history of a goiter that has changed in size or characteristics. The treatment modality for follicular carcinoma is total thyroidectomy followed by treatment with iodine-131 (^{131}I). If there is cervical node involvement, a modified radical neck dissection is recommended (Block et al., 1990).

Medullary carcinoma This disease accounts for only 5% to 10% of thyroid cancers. It appears spontaneously in 80% of the cases. Medullary carcinoma of the thyroid (MCT) is genetically transmitted by an autosomal dominant trait in 20% of cases. The age range for this disease is from 2 to 80 years old, with the median age being in the twenties. Patients may present with hoarseness, dysphagia, or flushing. More than 30% of the patients develop diarrhea.

There is usually node involvement when MCT is diagnosed. This disease metastasizes to the superior mediastinum and then to the lungs, bones, and liver. The survival rate of these patients is dependent on their age, sex, and stage of the disease when found. Because this type of tumor does not concentrate radioactive iodine, it does not respond to treatment with ^{131}I or external radiation. The surgical intervention in these cases is a total thyroidectomy, and if the lymph nodes are involved, a modified or radical neck dissection (Kaplan, 1989).

Anaplastic carcinoma Anaplastic carcinoma often appears outside of the thyroid capsule, rapidly invading the surrounding tissues. The patients often have a history of a rapidly growing hard mass in the neck. Metastases are usually to the mediastinum and the lungs.

This is the most lethal of the thyroid cancers. It is diagnosed more often in the 70- to 80-year-old age group. The patients present with a painful enlarged thyroid gland and lymph nodes. A long-standing history of goiter is present in 80% of these patients (Donehower, 1990). A needle biopsy is done to confirm the diagnosis. If the lesion is not resectable, surgical intervention is palliative. The goal of the surgery is to minimize the size of the tumor and relieve tracheal or esophageal compression. Treatment depends on the extent of the disease. Selected patients may be treated with Adriamycin or radiotherapy.

The prognosis for these patients is poor regardless of what therapy is done. These patients usually die within months of being diagnosed (Donehower, 1990).

Thyrotoxicosis/hyperthyroidism

The symptoms of hyperthyroidism are caused by an overproduction of thyroid hormones. This is reflected in several diseases, including Graves' disease, toxic multinodular goiter, and toxic adenoma.

Symptoms of hyperthyroidism

• Increased appetite
• Weight loss
• Muscle weakness
• Intolerance to heat
• Tachycardia
• Fine tremors

Graves' disease Ninety percent of the patients with hyperthyroidism have Graves' disease. It is six times more common in women than in men. The primary characteristics of the disease are manifested in the symptoms of hyperthyroidism and exophthalmos. A patient may have one or all of the symptoms. The treatment modalities include antithyroid drugs, ^{131}I, and subtotal thyroidectomy. The incidence of recurrent hyperthyroidism after one year of medical therapy has been reported at 43% during the first year after the medication is withdrawn (Falk, 1990). Considerations for treatment include the underlying pathologic process and the patient's age, sex, personal philosophies, and ability to comply with the therapy.

The major risk with surgery to the thyroid gland is damage to the recurrent laryngeal nerve, which could result in temporary or permanent vocal cord paralysis. This damage has been reported to occur in less than 0.4% of cases. Hypothyroidism resulting from surgery can be treated with medication.

Several weeks before surgery is scheduled, therapy with antithyroid drugs may be started to produce a euthyroid state. Iodine may be added to the therapy 8 to 10 days before the surgery. This will reduce the vascularity of the gland.

Thyroxine is sometimes added to the therapy regimen. It helps to prevent hypothyroidism and to decrease the size of the gland (Kaplan, 1989).

Propranolol administration has given an added safety margin to the patient with Graves' disease who is facing surgery. This beta blocker works to block the peripheral effects of T_3 and T_4. It decreases the pulse rate and tremor associated with thyrotoxicosis (Kaplan, 1989).

Toxic multinodular goiter These goiters contain several nodules. They may cause esophageal and/or tracheal obstruction. Treatment is with antithyroid drugs, ^{131}I, or surgical excision.

Toxic adenoma Toxic adenoma is usually a slow-growing single tumor. Treatment is the same as for toxic nodular goiter. Occasionally the adenoma will spontaneously necrose and hemorrhage and spontaneously go into remission (Kaplan, 1989).

Hypothyroidism

Hypothyroidism is caused by the failure of the thyroid gland to produce an adequate supply of hormones. It can be caused by surgically removing the thyroid gland or by ablation of the gland by radiotherapy. It may also be the result of the failure of the gland to develop properly. This disease can also be attributed to a goiter, tumors, or thyroiditis.

Medical treatment using L-thyroxine to restore the normal metabolic state is very effective. Approximately 80% of the patients presenting with symptoms of hypothyroidism are female (Kaplan, 1989).

Symptoms of hypothyroidism

- Weight gain
- Headaches
- Tiredness

- Speech impairment
- Hoarseness
- Dry skin

Hashimoto's thyroiditis

This autoimmune disease is associated with goiters and is seen more often in females over the age of 50. These patients may present with a neck mass that is tender and painful. The treatment is with suppressive drugs and/or surgery. Indications for a subtotal thyroidectomy are for cosmetic reasons and to relieve pressure and obstruction from the trachea or esophagus. Surgery may be done if the mass does not respond to medical treatment.

Hyperparathyroidism

This disease is usually the result of a parathyroid adenoma, hyperplasia, or carcinoma. Malignancy of the parathyroid is very rare and is seen in only 1% to 3% of parathyroid tumors (Kaplan, 1989). Hyperparathyroidism is seen primarily in postmenopausal female patients. Patients may exhibit signs of renal stone disease, hypertension, ulcers, bone disease, or joint pain. They may also complain of depression, confusion, irritability, or fatigue. A parathyroidectomy is done to remove the diseased gland or glands.

Hypoparathyroidism

The most common serious complication of surgery on the thyroid gland is hypoparathyroidism. It is usually a temporary condition that occurs in approximately 6.9% to 29% of total thyroidectomies (Netterville et al., 1990). Temporary hypoparathyroidism is common. The perioperative nurse should observe the patient for signs of tetany. If this is a permanent condition, administration of calcium and vitamin D replacement will be necessary. Permanent hypoparathyroidism is rare.

SURGICAL PROCEDURES

Perioperative Nursing Considerations

A thorough preoperative assessment of the patient's respiratory, cardiovascular, and renal function and central nervous system is vital for evaluating significant factors that could increase perioperative surgical risks. The patient with thyroid dysfunction should be closely monitored for any signs of altered metabolic rate. This would include hyperthermia, tachycardia, irritability, and exaggerated emotions. The perioperative nurse should be prepared to assist the anesthesia provider by labeling and sending tubes of blood for arterial blood gas studies, recording urine output, and initiating cooling of the patient if necessary. Results of thyroid function tests (T_3 and T_4) and current medication should be reviewed in the patient's chart. The severity of the disease process and the patient's age are also considered. In general, older patients are at a higher surgical risk than are younger patients. These patients may exhibit symptoms of congestive heart failure or atrial fibrillation.

Patients undergoing thyroid surgery are not only facing a possible diagnosis of cancer and that disease process but may also exhibit anxiety concerning their self-image. This assessment is important in the patient's plan of care done by the perioperative nurse. The incision line for thyroid surgery is in a highly visible area of the neck, and many patients are concerned about the cosmetic outcome of the surgery. Reassurance should be given that the placement of the incision for a thyroidectomy will be in a natural crease line of the neck. If the tumor is large there may be significant cosmetic and functional disability, but this can be minimized with appropriate reconstruction techniques.

Instrumentation (Fig. 6-2)

- Head and neck instruments and retractors
- Gelpi, spring, and rake retractors
- Lahey clamps
- Fine-tip right-angle forceps
- Greene retractors
- Tracheostomy tray available

The Mayo stand will be set up with the following items:

- #15 blades on #3 knife handles
- Sharp and blunt small right-angle forceps
- Mosquito clamps, curved hemostats
- Small Metzenbaum and suture scissors
- Tissue forceps and Adson forceps with teeth
- Miller-Senn and spring retractors
- Gelpi, Greene, and small Richardson retractors

Equipment

- Padded footboard
- Electrosurgical unit
- Suction

Supplies

- Minor set-up pack, which includes gowns, basins, towels, and needle container
- #15 blades; clips and staples if needed
- Kittner dissectors
- $1/4$-inch Penrose drain or small, soft Silastic suction drain
- 3-0 and 4-0 silk ties and 3-0 and 4-0 silk sutures
- Nonabsorbable suture on small cutting needle
- Asepto syringe
- Suction tubing
- Electrosurgical handpiece

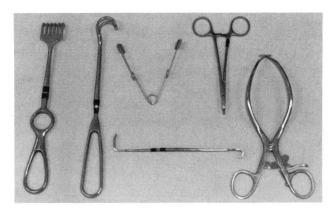

FIGURE 6-2 Instruments used in thyroid/parathyroid surgery. *From left:* Six-pronged rake retractor, Greene retractor, spring retractor, baby right-angle forceps, Miller-Senn retractor (at bottom), and Gelpi retractor.

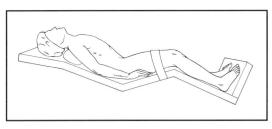

FIGURE 6-3 Positioning for thyroid and neck surgery (reverse Trendelenburg's position modified for thyroid and parathyroid procedures).

Positioning

Patients with hypothyroidism may have lower extremity edema and fragile skin. To ensure skin integrity, a foam pad may be placed on the operating room bed.

The patient is positioned supine with a folded sheet under the neck and scapulae (Fig. 6-3). This will extend the neck and allow the surgeon better access to the operative site. After properly padding the elbows, the arms can be positioned at the patient's side or extended on armboards. A padded footboard is attached to the operating room bed before positioning the patient in reverse Trendelenburg's position. This position will decrease the venous pressure, reducing the blood flow to the thyroid gland and facilitate the surgeon's access to the operative site.

Draping and prepping

The antimicrobial prep solution used for surgery will depend on the patient's skin sensitivity and the surgeon's preference.

Surgical prepping of the patient will include the area from the anterior neck and cheek and below the lower lip to above the ear on the affected side. The outer surfaces of the shoulders and chest are prepped to the table on both sides. The dispersive pad for the electrosurgical unit is connected.

The surgical field is draped with sterile towels, followed by a drape with a small fenestration.

Thyroidectomy

Thyroidectomy involves the removal of all or a portion of the thyroid gland. When a subtotal thyroidectomy is performed for Graves' disease, one lobe and a portion of the other lobe are removed. From 3 to 5 g of tissue with its blood supply is left intact on one side. A thyroid lobectomy involves removing the affected lobe and part of the isthmus. The surgical approach is the same as for a total thyroidectomy.

Key steps

1. The transverse incision line, approximately 2 cm above the sternal notch, is marked. A skin marker or a piece of silk suture pressed into a natural neck crease can also be used. The skin incision is made with a #15 blade.
2. The fascia and platysma are divided. The flap is elevated with small rakes or skin hooks. Stay sutures may be used for retraction. Hemostats or mosquito clamps in combination with a nonabsorbable suture or electrocoagulation are used to control the bleeding vessels.
3. The strap muscles are divided and retracted laterally. The superior flap is raised to the level of the thyroid cartilage, approximately 3 inches above the sternal notch. The inferior flap is undermined to the suprasternal notch. A sharp #15 blade or electrosurgical handpiece is used to undermine the flaps. The flaps are retracted with Greene thyroid retractors or Gelpi or spring retractors.
4. To rule out any undetected anomaly, the normal side of the gland is examined first.
5. The middle thyroid vein is dissected and ligated with a nonabsorbable suture. If the thyroid internal mammary artery is present, it is ligated. Dissection is done with a mosquito clamp to free the thyroid from the fascia. The superior pole is dissected free and the vessels ligated. The inferior pole is dissected and the vessels identified.
6. The parathyroids and recurrent laryngeal nerve are identified and preserved, followed by ligation of the inferior thyroid vessels.
7. Using hemostats and Metzenbaum scissors, the tissue is dissected away from the back of the gland, turning the gland medially. Lahey clamps may be used to elevate the lobe.
8. The isthmus is carefully dissected. The tissue attached to the trachea and cricoid cartilage is divided.
9. In a thyroid lobectomy the remaining thyroid tissue is sutured to the trachea after hemostasis has been obtained. When subtotal or total thyroidectomy is done, the remaining lobe is excised using the same method. It is imperative that hemostasis be maintained throughout the procedure. The field must remain dry to enable the surgeon to visualize the parathyroid glands and the recurrent laryngeal nerves. Excessive postoperative bleeding could cause edema, resulting in pressure on the trachea and esophagus and leading to respiratory distress.

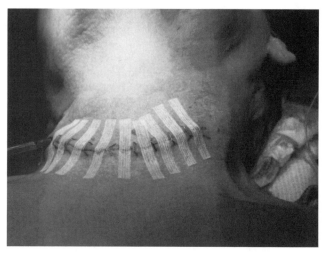

FIGURE 6-4 The thyroidectomy incision is closed with skin staples and sterile adhesive strips.

10. A small Penrose drain or small, soft Silastic suction catheter is generally used to drain the thyroid bed. Placing it laterally through the sternohyoid muscle results in better healing and cosmetic effects.
11. The fascia is closed, and the transected muscles are reapproximated with nonabsorbable suture.
12. An absorbable suture on a small cutting needle is used to reapproximate the dermis. Small sterile adhesive strips or skin staples are used to reapproximate the skin (Fig. 6-4).
13. Sterile gauze and tape are used for the dressing. A "Queen Anne's collar," made with a tri-folded towel placed around the patient's neck, crossed in the front, and secured with tape, can be used to secure the gauze dressing. A modified "Queen Anne's collar," made using 3-inch or 4-inch adhesive or elastic tape and padded with gauze, may also be used.

Substernal intrathoracic thyroidectomy

Intrathoracic goiters are seen in approximately 1% of thyroidectomy patients. The enlarged goiter extends into the intrathoracic region, receiving its blood supply from the inferior thyroid artery. A trans-sternal incision may be necessary if the tumor:

- Is too large to remove through the cervical incision
- Extends into the mediastinum with an extensive blood supply
- Has superior vena cava involvement
- Has evidence of superior mediastinal lesions

Key steps

1. The cervical incision is expanded vertically from the suprasternal notch to a horizontal incision at the level of the third interspace. This provides visualization of the vascular supply as well as the recurrent laryngeal nerve (Kaplan, 1989). Longer instruments should be available.

Thyroglossal duct cystectomy (Sistrunk procedure)

The thyroglossal duct is an embryologic remnant. It extends from the base of the tongue through the hyoid bone to the thyroid gland. It usually disappears in infants, but sometimes remains as an anomaly in adults. It is often seen in children and adolescents.

Key steps

1. The incision is made between the hyoid bone and the thyroid cartilage. The sternohyoid muscles are separated and divided at the midline, and lateral flaps are raised.
2. Sharp and blunt dissection is used to mobilize the cyst and duct. A complete excision of the thyroglossal duct and cyst is performed.
3. The mid portion of the hyoid bone containing the tract is removed as this prevents recurrence.
4. The closure is similar to that following a thyroidectomy.

In addition to a routine thyroid set-up, some small orthopedic instruments such as rongeurs, periosteal elevators, and a bone cutter should be available.

Radical neck dissection

When cervical node involvement is present with differentiated thyroid cancer the recommended surgical treatment is a total thyroidectomy and radical neck dissection (see Chapter 5, this volume). This involves excision of the cervical lymph nodes, sternocleidomastoid muscle, internal jugular vein, and spinal accessory nerve on the affected side. A second head and neck instrument set-up is used to decrease the possibility of spreading the cancer cells to an unaffected area.

The perioperative nursing team will plan for the additional skin preparation, instrumentation, and drapes needed. This may include a dermatome and mesher, tracheostomy tray, and basic major instrument set for gastrostomy.

Postoperative nursing care

In the postoperative period, thyroidectomy patients have the potential for:

- Airway obstruction
- Thyroid storm
- Recurrent laryngeal nerve damage
- Hypothyroidism
- Hypoparathyroidism

Postoperative edema and hemorrhage in the thyroid bed may cause an obstruction of the trachea. If left untreated, it could lead to respiratory complications and death. A suture removal set should be available in the patient's room. Some hospitals require a tracheostomy tray be available in case an emergency tracheostomy is necessary. However, if the wound is opened, the obstruction is usually relieved.

Thyroid storm is the result of a release of an excessive amount of thyroid hormones into the blood stream. It may be triggered by stress, surgery, or infection, but the primary cause is surgical. The symptoms may appear from 6 to 18 hours postoperatively (Martinelli & Fontana, 1990). Occasionally a thyroid storm will manifest during the intraoperative period. The symptoms to be aware of are a sudden onset of tachycardia, hyperpyrexia, diaphoresis, shock, vomiting and diarrhea, and deteriorating mental status. The treatment for thyroid storm includes the use of steroids, acetaminophen, and propranolol. If a hypo/hyperthermia blanket is being used, it is turned to cooling. Cool iced saline applied to the patient's skin and cool saline infused intravenously can be used to lower the temperature.

Intraoperative damage to the laryngeal nerve may be temporary or permanent and bilateral or unilateral. The incidence of recurrent laryngeal nerve damage reported by Gould et al. was 0.2% (Kaplan, 1989). The patient may exhibit symptoms from hoarseness, stridor, and airway obstruction to a change of vocal quality. If both recurrent laryngeal nerves are damaged, the patient will be aphonic and unable to breathe as the cords come to the midline.

Parathyroidectomy

Parathyroidectomy involves the excision of one or more of the parathyroid glands. Removal of all four glands will cause tetany and death if not treated. Most, but not all, of the parathyroid tissue can, however, be safely removed.

Key steps

1. The surgical approach is the same as for a thyroidectomy. Mosquito clamps, electrocautery, and 3-0 or 4-0 silk sutures are used to maintain hemostasis.
2. The thyroid gland is exposed and rotated medially.
3. The recurrent laryngeal nerve is identified. The inferior parathyroid is usually located near the intersection of the laryngeal nerve and the inferior thyroid artery. The superior parathyroid is usually located 1 or 2 cm above that area and on the posterior surface of the thyroid (Kaplan, 1989). All four glands are carefully examined before excision begins (Fig. 6-5). This will protect against excising three parathyroid glands only to find that the patient does not have a fourth gland.
4. Dissection is accomplished using Metzenbaum scissors, mosquito clamps, and Kittner sponges.
5. Closure is done as in a thyroidectomy.

Autotransplant of parathyroid tissue

When a total parathyroidectomy is performed for removal of an adenoma it may be desirable to autotransplant a piece of the parathyroid tissue. The remaining parathyroid tissue can be marked with a nonabsorbable suture and reimplanted in the sternocleidomastoid muscle or into the brachioradialis muscle. The advantage of an autotransplant is that it is placed in a location that is more easily accessible than the neck. If the patient needs

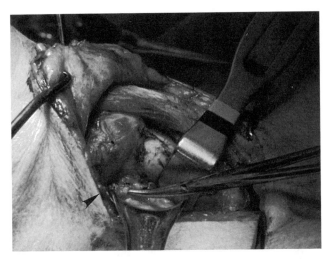

FIGURE 6-5 Identification of parathyroid gland (*arrow*) after right thyroid lobectomy.

further surgery to remove additional parathyroid tissue, it may not necessitate additional general anesthesia. Risks associated with surgery on the parathyroid are similar to the risks of thyroidectomy.

SUMMARY

This chapter has discussed surgical procedures on the thyroid and parathyroid glands. Responsibilities of the perioperative nurse include a detailed understanding of anatomical structures and relationships, disorders necessitating surgery, diagnoses through testing, the patient's physiological and emotional reactions to the surgery, and the patient's understanding of the expected outcomes of surgical intervention.

REFERENCES

American Cancer Society (1992). *Cancer facts and figures.* Atlanta: American Cancer Society.

Block, B. L., Spiegel, J., & Chami, R. (1990). The treatment of papillary and follicular carcinoma of the thyroid. *Otolaryngologic Clinics of North America, 7,* 403–412.

de Francisco, A. L. M., Amado, J. A., Casanova, C., Britz, E., Riancho, J., Cotorruelo, J., de Bonis, E., Canga, E., & Arias, M. (1991). Recurrence of hyperparathyroidism after total parathyroidectomy with autotransplantation: A new technique to localize the source of hormone excess. *Nephron, 58,* 306–309.

Donehower, M. G. (1990). Endocrine cancers. In *Cancer Nursing: A Comprehensive Textbook.* Philadelphia: W. B. Saunders.

Falk, S. A. (1990). The management of hyperthyroidism: A surgeon's perspective. *Otolaryngologic Clinics of North America, 23,* 361–380.

Goldman, M. (1988). *Pocket guide to the operating room.* Philadelphia: F. A. Davis.

Haeger, K. (1988). *The illustrated history of surgery.* New York: Bell Publishing.

Kaplan, E. (1989). Thyroid and parathyroid. In S. I. Schwartz (Ed.), *Principles of Surgery* (5th ed., p. 1626). New York: McGraw-Hill.

Martinelli, A. M., & Fontana, J. L. (1990). Thyroid storm, potential perioperative crisis. *AORN Journal, 52,* 305–313.

Netterville, J. L., Aly, A., & Ossoff, R. H. (1990). Evaluation and treatment of complications of thyroid and parathyroid surgery. *Otolaryngologic Clinics of North America, 23,* 529–551.

Chapter 7

Surgery of the Abdominal Wall, Gastrointestinal Tract, and Accessory Organs

Key Concepts

- The patient undergoing gastrointestinal (GI) surgery is at risk for fluid and electrolyte imbalance related to (a) preoperative bowel preparation, (b) water evaporation from abdominal cavity exposure, and (c) preoperative symptoms such as vomiting, diarrhea, or sequestration of fluid related to obstruction.
- The patient is at increased risk for hypothermia related to loss of body heat through exposure of the abdominal cavity.
- The risk for infection is increased because of the unsterile nature of the GI tract.
- GI tract dysfunction is associated with malnutrition. When disturbances in metabolism occur, problems with wound healing and fluid balance develop.
- Alteration in nutrition makes surgery more difficult and often creates a risk for infection related to poorly vascularized subcutaneous tissue.
- Frequently, abdominal surgery is performed for conditions that are associated with pain. This may make preoperative assessment difficult.
- The potential for blood loss in intraabdominal surgery is great, owing to the presence of highly vascular intraabdominal organs and large blood vessels.
- Manipulation of the intestine during surgery results in temporary postoperative paralytic ileus.
- Postoperative abdominal wound infections often lead to ventral hernias.
- When a combined abdominal and perineal approach is used during surgery, two surgical teams may be required.

INTRODUCTION

Surgery of the abdominal wall, gastrointestinal (GI) tract, and accessory organs involves multiple body systems. Included in surgery of the GI tract are the accessory organs—such as the spleen, pancreas, liver, gallbladder, and ducts—and supportive structures of the abdomen.

This chapter contains an extensive review of structural anatomy of the "abdominal" organs, a discussion of nursing considerations in patient care, and key steps of surgical procedures. Both conventional and laparoscopic approaches to surgery are covered. Expected outcomes for the patient are discussed at the end of the chapter.

ANATOMY

Abdominal Wall

The many layers of the abdominal wall (Fig. 7-1) protect the intraabdominal organs. Under the skin lies the subcutaneous fat. A concentration of connective tissue lies above the muscle layer. The linea alba, a tendinous structure, divides the abdominal wall into two parts. The transversalis fascia, considered the strongest layer of the abdominal wall, lies under the muscle layer, just above the peritoneum. The principal structures that make up the anterior abdominal wall (Fig. 7-2) are the rectus (vertical muscle enveloped between anterior and posterior rectus sheaths), the transverse abdominis, and the external and internal oblique muscles (Morton, 1989).

The blood supply to the abdominal wall is furnished by the superior and inferior epigastric, lower intercostal, lumbar, and iliac circumflex arteries. The venous drainage corresponds to the arterial supply (Guyton, 1986).

In addition to protecting the intraabdominal organs, the abdominal muscles function as an accessory respiratory apparatus. They aid in defecation by increasing intraabdominal muscle pressure with contraction (Guyton, 1986).

The inguinal canal (Fig. 7-3) passes obliquely downward and medially as a tunnel from the internal ring. The inguinal ligament is the curved inner free edge of the external oblique muscle between its origin on the iliac crest and its insertion at the pubis. The spermatic cord passes downward through the inguinal canal from the internal ring. The cord lies superior to the inguinal ligament and anterior to the floor of the inguinal canal. It emerges through the external inguinal ring to pass into the scrotum (Morton, 1989).

Gastrointestinal Tract and Accessory Organs

The GI tract is a series of hollow viscera that begins at the mouth and ends at the anus (Fig. 7-4). The intraabdomi-

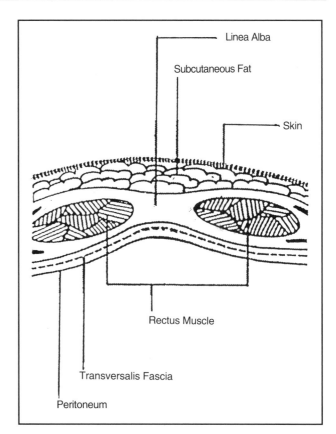

FIGURE 7-1 Layers of the abdominal wall. (Courtesy of Ethicon Inc.)

nal portion includes the distal esophagus, stomach, small intestine, colon, and proximal rectum. The distal rectum and anal canal lie below the peritoneum, outside of the abdominal cavity.

The GI tract consists of layers of tissue that have various purposes. The innermost layer, the mucosa, contains cells that are secretive. The submucosa is composed of connective tissue, whereas the muscularis contains both longitudinal and circular muscle. These layers facilitate movement of food and waste through the tract. The outer layer, the serosa, is fibrous and protects the intraabdominal organs (Fig. 7-5). The largest serous membrane of the body is the peritoneum, which covers the walls of the abdominal cavity. It also drapes most of the abdominal organs and covers the upper surface of the pelvic organs. The distal rectum and anal canal do not have a serosal layer (Guyton, 1986).

The intraabdominal accessory organs include the liver, gallbladder, pancreas, and spleen (see Fig. 7-4). These organs have unique anatomical construction that does not correspond to the layers of the GI tract. They contribute to digestion through secretive functions, and their surfaces are covered with peritoneum.

The primary function of the GI tract is to provide the body with a continual supply of water, electrolytes, and nutrients. Food must be moved along the tract at an appropriate rate for the digestive and absorptive functions to take place.

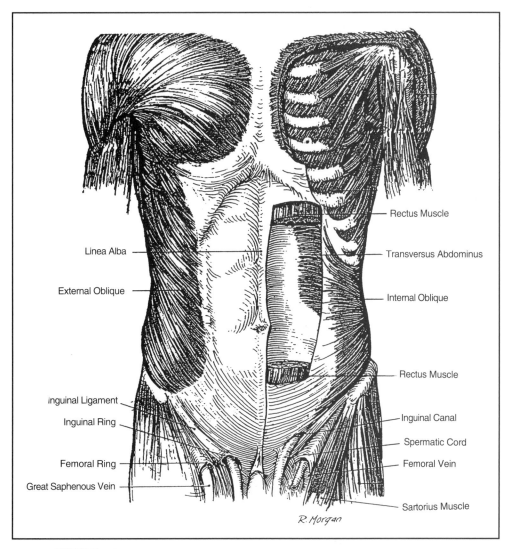

FIGURE 7-2 Muscles of the anterior abdominal wall. (*Stedman's medical dictionary* [1990]. Baltimore: Williams & Wilkins.)

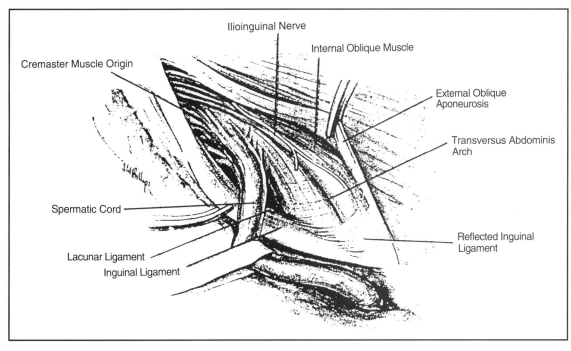

FIGURE 7-3 Inguinal canal. (Condon, R. E. [1989]. In L. M. Nyhus & R. E. Condon [Eds.]. *Hernia* [3rd ed.]. Philadelphia: J. B. Lippincott.)

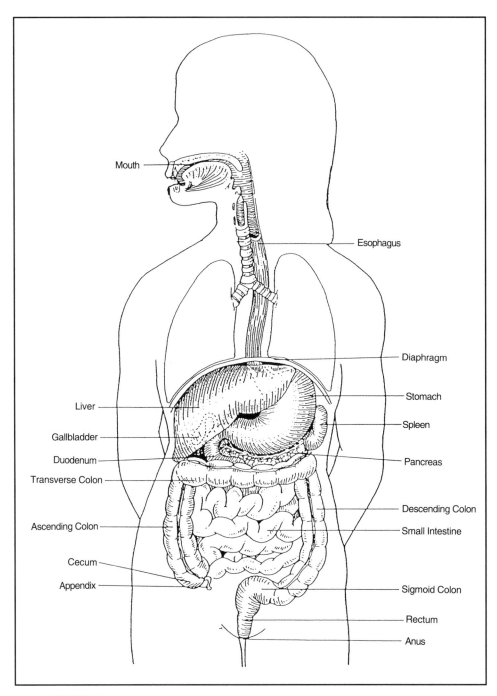

FIGURE 7-4 Gastrointestinal tract with accessory organs. (Broadwell, D. B., & Jackson, B. S. [1982]. *Principles of ostomy care.* St. Louis: C. V. Mosby.)

Esophagus

The esophagus is a muscular tube that passes through the diaphragm to join the stomach at the gastroesophageal junction (Fig. 7-6). The esophageal submucosa is thick and fatty, to permit considerable mobility, which is an advantage when constructing anastomoses. The muscular layer conducts food along the esophagus to the stomach through peristaltic waves stimulated by the vagus nerve, while lubrication is provided by the mucus-secreting mucosa. At the lower end of the esophagus, the circular muscle functions as a sphincter, which remains constricted unless swallowing has occurred. This prevents reflux of stomach contents into the esophagus (Guyton, 1986).

The blood supply of the abdominal esophagus is provided by supplemental arteries on the abdominal side of the diaphragm as well as the left gastric artery. Venous drainage takes place through azygos and left gastric veins (Murray & Keagy, 1987).

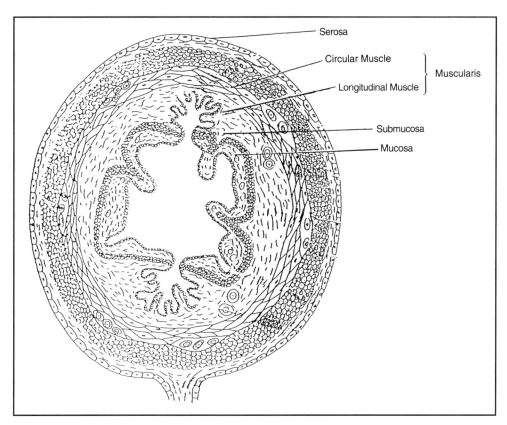

FIGURE 7-5 Cross-section of the gastrointestinal tract. (Guyton, A. C. [1986]. *Textbook of medical physiology.* Philadelphia: W. B. Saunders.)

Stomach

The stomach lies in the upper left portion of the abdomen just below the diaphragm (Fig. 7-7). The upper portion of the stomach, the fundus, accepts food from the esophagus through the gastroesophageal junction. The food then passes into the thicker, more muscular portion, the antrum, where it is ground and mixed with gastric secretions. The distal portion of the stomach, the pylorus, is delineated by a thick band of circular muscle that effects gastric emptying at a rate suitable for proper digestion and absorption by the small intestine (Guyton, 1986).

The gastric blood supply comes from the celiac artery and its three branches, the gastric, splenic, and hepatic arteries. The venous drainage correlates with the arterial supply and drains almost entirely into the portal system (Guyton, 1986).

The functions of the stomach are controlled predominantly by the vagus nerves (see Fig. 7-7). Vagal stimulation results in secretion of hydrochloric acid, pepsinogen, and instrinsic factor by the gastric glands in the fundus and body of the stomach as well as secretion of mucus, some pepsinogen, and gastrin by the pyloric glands in the antrum (Guyton, 1986).

Spleen

The spleen is a soft, oblong organ, dark purple in color, that lies below the diaphragm, posterior and lateral to the stomach. It is held in position in the left upper quadrant by suspensory ligaments. Peritoneum surrounds the spleen except for its hilus, where arteries and nerves enter and veins and lymphatics emerge. A capsule encloses the pulp of the spleen (Quinlan, 1991).

The splenic artery runs along the upper border of the pancreas and enters the spleen at the hilus (Fig. 7-8). The venous drainage occurs through the splenic vein, which joins the superior mesenteric vein to form the portal vein (Quinlan, 1991). Dilatation of these vessels causes the spleen to store several hundred milliliters of blood in the venous sinuses and in the pulp (Guyton, 1986).

The spleen is the site of phagocytosis, proliferation of plasma cells and lymphocytes, and filtration of particulate matter from red blood cells. It is a harbor for platelets and influences immunity through antigen production (Quinlan, 1991).

Liver

The liver lies in the right upper quadrant of the abdomen above the right kidney, colon, stomach, pancreas, and intestines and immediately below the diaphragm. It is divided into right and left lobes, which start anteriorly at the gallbladder bed and extend posteriorly to the vena cava (Fig. 7-9). A network of connective tissue covers the entire organ and extends into the parenchyma along blood vessels and bile ducts. The most exterior layer of this connective tissue covers the liver and is referred to as Glisson's capsule (Guyton, 1986).

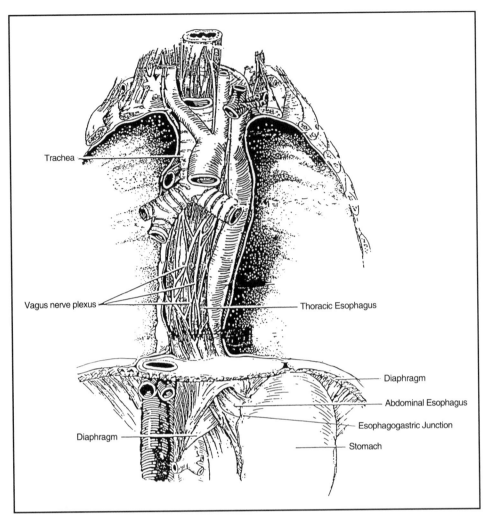

FIGURE 7-6 Anatomy of the esophagus. (Pelligrini, C. A., & Way, L. W. [1991]. In L. W. Way [Ed.]. *Current surgical diagnosis & treatment.* Norwalk, CT: Appleton & Lange.)

The liver's basic functional unit is the liver lobule, which is constructed around a small vein that empties into the hepatic veins and then into the vena cava. The lobule is composed of hepatic plates one or two cells thick. Between these cells lie small bile canaliculi that empty into terminal bile ducts. Through this system, the liver converts bilirubin, a breakdown product of hemoglobin, into bile. The terminal bile ducts merge into the hepatic duct to leave the liver (Guyton, 1986).

Arterial blood flows into the liver from the hepatic artery and venous blood through the portal system (Fig. 7-10). Venous sinusoids, offshoots of both vessels, are lined by endothelial and Kupffer cells, which phagocytose bacteria and other foreign matter in the blood. The liver drains by the hepatic vein into the inferior vena cava (Guyton, 1986).

Gallbladder and common bile duct

The gallbladder is a saclike organ that lies on the underside of the liver and is attached by connective tissue, the peritoneum, and blood vessels (Fig. 7-11). As the sac narrows, it continues as the cystic duct to join the common bile duct. The gallbladder provides a passageway for bile from the liver to the intestine and regulates its flow. Bile is concentrated in the gallbladder by mucosal absorption of water, sodium, chlorides, and other electrolytes and is stored there until the presence of fat causes its release. This in turn causes the contraction of the gallbladder muscle to empty and bile to flow through the common duct into the duodenum (Guyton, 1986).

Pancreas

The pancreas is a thin, elliptical organ that lies within the retroperitoneum in the upper portion of the abdomen. It can be divided into three portions—head, body, and tail. The head of the pancreas is intimately adherent to the middle portion of the duodenum and lies in front of the inferior vena cava. Anteriorly, the stomach and first portion of the duodenum lie partly in front of the pancreas. The tail of the pancreas lies in the hilum of the spleen. The main pancreatic duct (the duct of Wirsung)

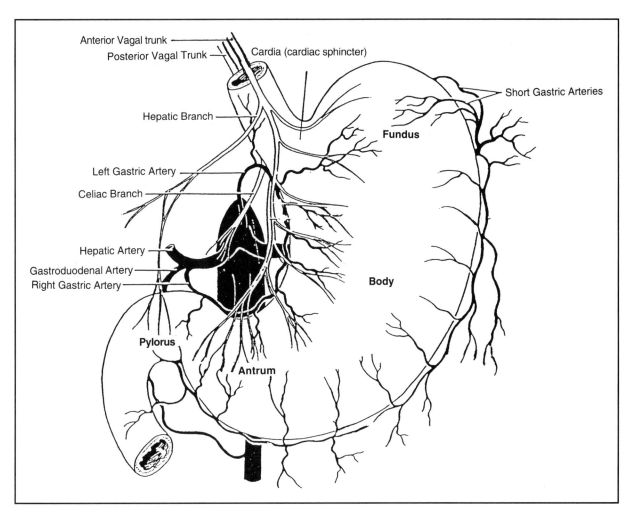

FIGURE 7-7 Anatomy of stomach with vagus nerves. (Way, L. W. [1991]. *Current surgical diagnosis and treatment.* Norwalk, CT: Appleton & Lange.)

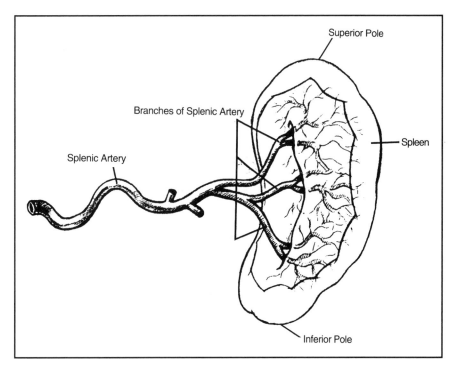

FIGURE 7-8 Anatomy of spleen. (Gray, S. W., & Skandalakis, J. E. [1985]. *Atlas of surgical anatomy.* Baltimore: Williams & Wilkins.)

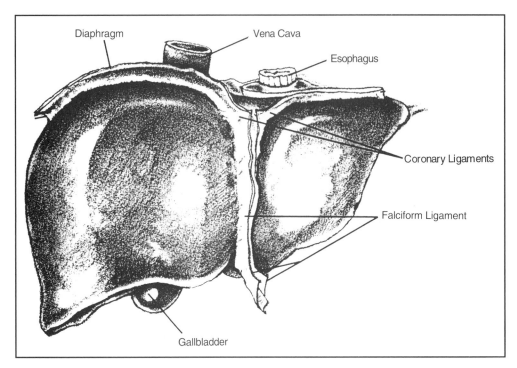

FIGURE 7-9 Anatomy of liver. (Modified from Gray, S. W., & Skandalakis, J. E. [1985]. *Atlas of surgical anatomy*. Baltimore: Williams & Wilkins.)

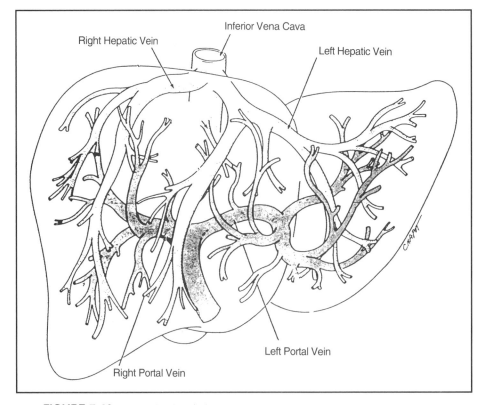

FIGURE 7-10 Hepatic circulation. (Campra, J. L., & Reynolds, T. B. [1988]. In I. M. Arias, W. B. Jakoby, H. Popper, D. Schacter, & D. A. Shafritz [Eds.]. *The liver: Biology and pathobiology* [2nd ed.] New York: Raven.)

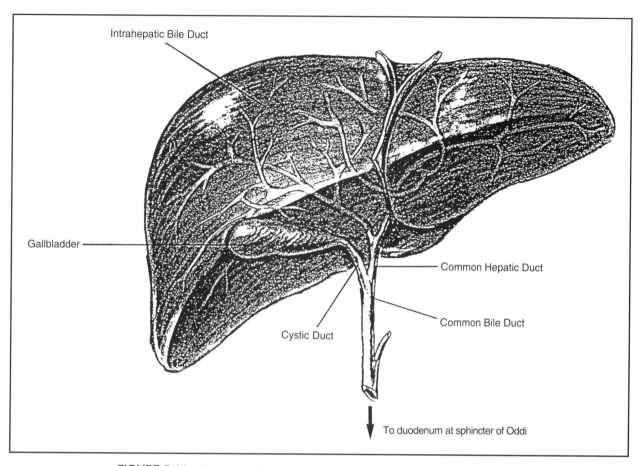

FIGURE 7-11 Anatomy of the gallbladder. (Hermann, R. E., & Vogt, D. P. [1987]. In J. H. Davis [Ed.]. *Clinical surgery.* St. Louis: C.V. Mosby.)

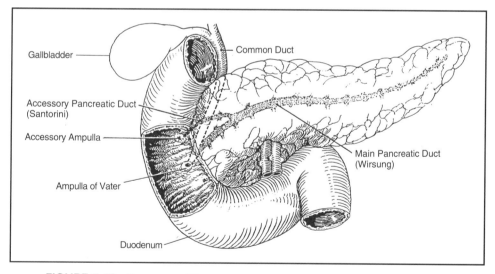

FIGURE 7-12 Pancreas. (Silen, W. [1964]. Anatomic configuration of the intrapancreatic duct. *Surgical Clinics of North America, 44*[5], 1253–1262.)

runs along the pancreas from the tail to the head and joins the common bile duct before entering the duodenum at the ampulla of Vater. The accessory pancreatic duct (the duct of Santorini) enters the duodenum proximal to the ampulla of Vater (Fig. 7-12) (Silen & Steer, 1989).

The blood supply of the pancreas is derived from branches of the celiac and superior mesenteric arteries. The spenic artery provides tributaries that supply the body and tail of the pancreas. The venous supply of the gland parallels the arterial supply (Guyton, 1986).

The function of the pancreas is to facilitate storage of foodstuffs by release of insulin after a meal and to provide

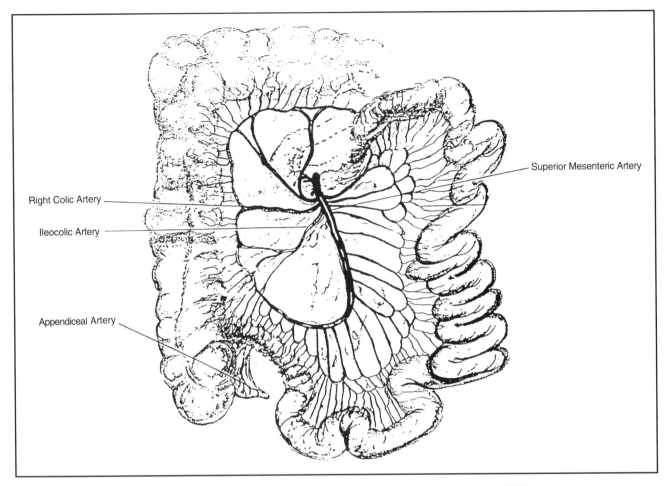

FIGURE 7-13 Small intestine. (Adapted from Morrow, M., & Jaffe, B. M. [1987]. In J. H. Davis [Ed.]. *Clinical surgery.* St. Louis: C. V. Mosby.)

a mechanism for their mobilization by release of glucagon during periods of fasting. Insulin and glucagon, as well as pancreatic polypeptide and somatostatin, are produced by the islets of Langerhans. These hormones are released through the blood while the digestive enzymes travel through the pancreatic duct to reach the duodenum (Guyton, 1986).

Small intestine

The small intestine extends from the pylorus of the stomach to the cecum and can be divided into three parts: the duodenum, the jejunum, and the ileum. The length of the small intestine is estimated to be 12 to 22 feet. The jejunum and the ileum are suspended on the mesentery, which contains fat, blood vessels, lymphatics, and lymph nodes. The mesentery fans out, to account for the small intestine's relative mobility within the abdominal cavity (Fig. 7-13).

The blood supply of the small intestine arises from the superior mesenteric artery and its branches. The venous drainage is through the superior mesenteric vein to the portal circulation (Guyton, 1986).

The small intestine secretes mucus and gastrointestinal hormones to aid digestion. It also facilitates absorption of water, sodium, chloride, calcium, iron, carbohydrates,

protein, and fat. The muscular layer of the small intestine is responsible in part for intestinal movement through segmental contraction (Guyton, 1986).

Appendix

The appendix is an extension of the cecum that averages 10 cm in length (Fig. 7-14). The tip of the appendix may be found in a variety of locations, most commonly behind the cecum. The appendiceal artery provides the blood supply and is a branch of the ileocolic artery (Sabiston, 1987). It is thought that the appendix participates in the secretory immune system in the GI tract; however, removal of the appendix produces no detectable defect in the functioning of this system (Schwartz, 1989a).

Colon and rectum

The colon, approximately 3 to 5 feet long, extends from the ileum to the rectum. The first portion of the colon, the cecum, is the widest portion. The colon progresses from the cecum up the ascending or right colon, traverses the upper abdomen at the transverse colon, and descends in the left colon to the sigmoid, which is the narrowest portion. The sigmoid empties into the rectum (Fig. 7-15).

The superior mesenteric artery supplies the cecum, as-

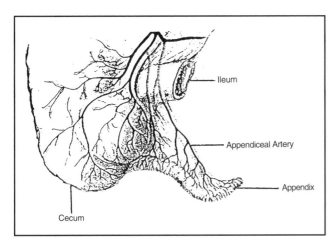

FIGURE 7-14   Anatomy of appendix.   (Courtesy of Ethicon Inc.)

cending colon, and transverse colon through its ileocolic, right colic, and middle colic branches. The inferior mesenteric artery supplies the descending colon, sigmoid colon, and upper rectum through its left colic, sigmoidal, and superior rectal branches. The veins draining the colon follow the same course as the corresponding arteries, except for the inferior mesenteric vein, which drains the descending colon, sigmoid colon, and proximal rectum and enters the splenic vein (Kodner et al., 1993).

The colon absorbs water, sodium, and chloride, and secretes potassium, bicarbonate, and mucus. The site of digestion of certain carbohydrates and proteins, it provides the environment for the bacterial production of vitamin K (Guyton, 1986). The colon contains a dense microbial population that suppresses the emergence of pathogenic microorganisms. Because of this microbial population it is necessary to have complete preoperative bowel preparation to help prevent postoperative infections. Bowel cleansing is necessary also to prevent explo-

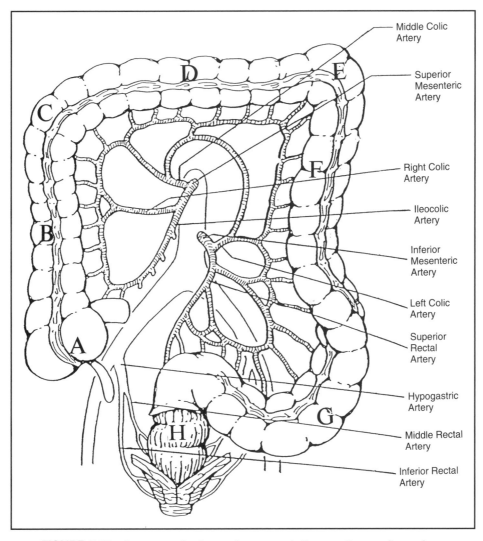

FIGURE 7-15   Anatomy of colon and rectum. *A*, Cecum; *B*, ascending colon (right); *C*, hepatic flexure; *D*, transverse colon; *E*, splenic flexure; *F*, descending colon (left); *G*, sigmoid colon; and *H*, rectum. (Kodner, I. J., Fry, R. D., Fleshman, J. W., and Birnbaum, E. H. In S. I. Schwartz [Ed.]. *Principles of surgery.* New York: McGraw-Hill. Reprinted with permission of McGraw-Hill.)

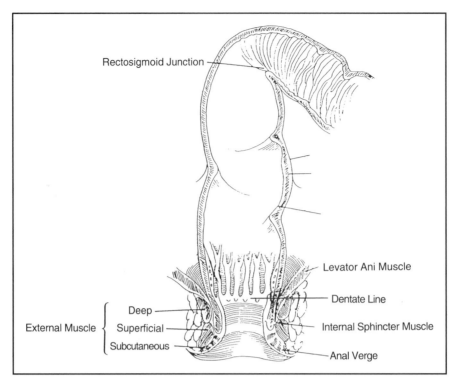

FIGURE 7-16 Rectum and anus. (Pemberton, J. B. [1991]. In G. D. Zuidema [Ed.]. *Shackelford's surgery of the alimentary canal* [3rd ed.]. Philadelphia: W. B. Saunders.)

sions when intracolonic electrocautery is used. This may occur because of the presence of hydrogen and methane gas in the colon. These gases occur normally from swallowed air, diffusion from the blood, and intraluminal production (Kodner et al., 1993).

The rectal wall consists of mucosa, submucosa, and two complete muscular layers, the inner circular and outer longitudinal.

The rectum is approximately 12 to 15 cm long and extends from the sigmoid colon to the anal canal following the curve of the sacrum (Fig. 7-16). The upper third of the rectum is covered by peritoneum on its anterior and lateral surfaces. The middle third of the rectum is covered by peritoneum only on its anterior surface, and the lower third of the rectum is below the peritoneal reflection (Pemberton, 1991).

The left and right branches of the superior rectal artery supply the upper and middle rectum. The middle and inferior rectal arteries supply the lower two thirds of the rectum. The venous drainage of the rectum parallels the arterial supply and empties into both the portal system and the inferior vena cava (Kodner et al., 1993).

Anal canal

The anal canal starts at the dentate line and ends at the anal verge (see Fig. 7-16). It is approximately 4 cm long and normally exists as a collapsed anteroposterior slit. The anal canal is surrounded by an internal and an external sphincter, which together make up the anal sphincter mechanism (Kodner et al., 1993).

NURSING CONSIDERATIONS

General Information

Surgery of the abdominal wall, gastrointestinal tract, and accessory organs is performed for diagnosis or treatment of pathology or defects in the abdominal wall, esophagus, stomach, spleen, liver, gallbladder, bile duct, pancreas, small intestine, colon and rectum, and anal canal.

The perioperative nurse who cares for patients having these surgeries will plan for possible problems related to fluid and electrolyte balance, hypothermia, nutrition, and bowel elimination patterns. Nursing diagnoses will reflect these alterations and will help the team plan appropriate interventions.

Surgery of the abdominal wall, gastrointestinal tract, and accessory organs includes many diverse procedures and variations in instrumentation, positioning, and equipment, and also distinct variations in patient responses and preparations. These aspects of patient care are covered in each of the categories of surgical procedures.

ABDOMINAL WALL SURGERY

Perioperative Nursing Considerations

Surgery of the abdominal wall most frequently involves repair of a hernia (a sac of peritoneum). A hernia can push through a defect or weakness in the layers of the abdominal wall. Along with the peritoneal sac, intraabdominal tissue can protrude through the defect and result in strangulation of this tissue. When this occurs, surgery is performed urgently.

The majority of hernias occur in the inguinal canal; 50% are indirect and 25% direct. Ventral hernias account for 10% of all hernias; 5% are femoral and 3% umbilical. The remainder are types of rare hernias (Kortz & Sabiston, 1987).

The essential steps to consider in the repair of a hernia are (1) management of the peritoneal sac and its contents and (2) repair of the fascial defect. When the defect is very large or the hernia is recurrent, a polypropylene, Dacron, or other mesh graft may be incorporated in the repair. Mesh is less likely to be rejected because the surrounding tissue grows into the graft (Morton, 1989).

Herniorrhaphies

Direct inguinal herniorrhaphy (Fig. 7-17)

A direct inguinal hernia protrudes through the floor of the inguinal canal and results from a weakening in the floor. It occurs medial to the epigastric artery (Morton, 1989).

Key steps

1. The bulge in the floor of the inguinal canal is exposed by retracting the spermatic cord, usually with a Penrose drain (Fig. 7-17,A).

2. Muscle fibers are excised to free the hernia (Fig. 7-17,B).
3. The fascia is sutured to the ligament while the hernia sac is depressed (Fig. 7-17,C).
4. The fascial flap is sutured over the transversalis fascia using nonabsorbable suture (Fig. 7-17,D).
5. A new external ring is created by placing a purse-string suture in the fascia (Fig. 7-17,E).

Indirect inguinal herniorrhaphy (Fig. 7-18)

An indirect inguinal hernia leaves the abdominal cavity at the internal ring and passes with the structures of the spermatic cord along the inguinal canal (Morton, 1989).

Key steps

1. The connective tissue of the external oblique muscle is incised, and the muscle fibers are pushed back to expose the hernia sac (Fig. 7-18,A).
2. The internal spermatic fibers are separated from the internal ring by blunt dissection (Fig. 7-18,B).
3. The hernia sac is freed and a ligature is placed at its base. The hernia sac is excised (Fig. 7-18,C).
4. The fascia is sutured to ligament as the internal oblique muscle is retracted (Fig. 7-18,D).
5. The floor of the inguinal canal is repaired by suturing fascia to fascia (Fig. 7-18,E).

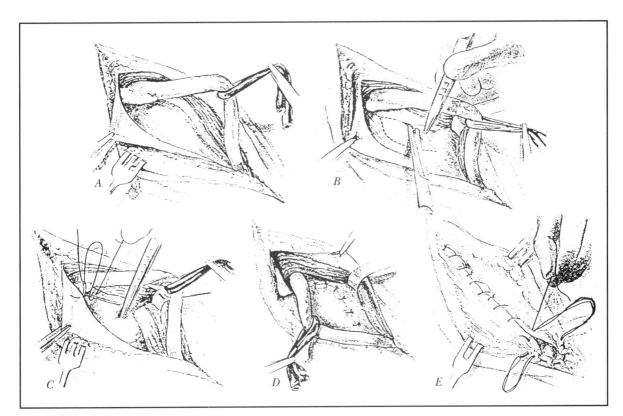

FIGURE 7-17 Direct inguinal herniorrhaphy. (Courtesy Ethicon Inc.)

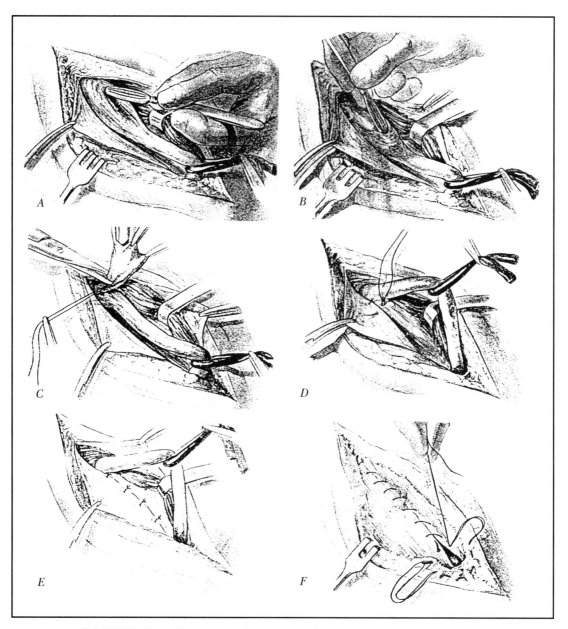

FIGURE 7-18 Indirect inguinal herniorrhaphy. (Courtesy Ethicon Inc.)

6. The external oblique muscle is sutured, and a new external ring is created with a purse-string suture in the fascia (Fig. 7-18,*F*).

Femoral herniorrhaphy

A femoral hernia is visible below the inguinal ligament as the peritoneal sac passes under the ligament into the femoral canal (rather than following the course of the direct hernia anteriorly into the inguinal canal) (Nyhus et al., 1990). The hernia may be repaired using a technique similar to the inguinal herniorrhaphy, or a preperitoneal approach can be used.

A preperitoneal approach through a low midline or Pfannenstiel's incision provides exposure that ensures a strong, secure repair that is less likely to allow recurrence of the hernia. This approach facilitates bowel resection, should it be necessary (Jackson, 1987).

Key steps

1. The skin and subcutaneous tissues, the anterior abdominal wall, the rectus sheath, and the external oblique aponeurosis are incised to reveal the internal oblique muscle.
2. The internal oblique, the transversus muscle, and the transversalis fascia are then divided. This exposes the preperitoneal fat and the peritoneum. When opened, the hernia sac can be seen extending into the femoral canal.
3. The sac is dissected free.

4. The hernia repair is accomplished by suturing a fold of transversalis fascia and aponeurosis of the transversus muscle to ligament with nonabsorbable sutures.

Laparoscopic herniorrhaphy

Laparoscopic herniorrhaphy represents an extension of current technology. Based on the principles of preperitoneal herniorrhaphy, this procedure is accomplished by internal incision of the peritoneum and identification and repair of the fascial defect through a laparoscope (Schultz et al., 1990). To protect the urinary bladder, a Foley catheter is inserted. The skin prep includes the genitalia and upper thigh. Laparotomy instrumentation is available, should it be necessary to make an abdominal incision.

Key steps

1. Pneumoperitoneum is established.
2. Additional port sites are established under direct visualization on either side of the midline.
3. The hernia sac is grasped and incised.
4. Downward traction is placed on the sac, so that the defect is visualized.
5. Rolls of polypropylene mesh secured with suture are passed through the trocar and placed into the hernia until it is filled.
6. Mesh is then placed over the defect, and the peritoneal edges are brought together and secured with clips.
7. Gas in a male patient's scrotum is gently evacuated into the abdominal cavity.
8. The trocar sites are then closed with clips or suture (Schultz et al., 1990).

Umbilical herniorrhaphy (Fig. 7-19)

An umbilical hernia occurs when a defect at the umbilicus is covered only by a peritoneal sac. This hernia can represent a congenital defect, or it may develop during adult life (Morton, 1989).

Key steps

1. A curved incision is made below the umbilicus, and the tissue is dissected to expose the rectus muscle (Fig. 7-19,*A*).
2. The peritoneal sac is freed and incised (Fig. 7-19,*B*).
3. The peritoneum and fascia are brought together with interrupted nonabsorbable sutures (Fig. 7-19,*C*).
4. The dead space between the fascia and the undersurface of the umbilical skin is obliterated with absorbable sutures (Fig. 7-19,*D*).
5. The skin is closed with subcuticular absorbable sutures (Fig. 7-19,*E*).

Ventral herniorrhaphy

A ventral hernia occurs in the area of a previous incision where the fascial layer is interrupted. Frequently, this defect is the result of postoperative wound infection. The surgery involves opening the incision to approximate the fascia. When the tissue will not approximate, mesh may be used to create a fascial layer.

Key steps

1. The old incisional scar is excised or a new incision is made perpendicular to the old one.
2. Dissection is completed down to normal fascia.
3. The peritoneal sac is dissected and opened to reduce the contents.
4. The excess peritoneum is excised and the peritoneum is closed.
5. The fascia is brought together and sutured with nonabsorbable suture.
6. Closure of the remaining layers of the abdominal wall is accomplished (Morton, 1989).

GASTROINTESTINAL TRACT AND ACCESSORY ORGAN SURGERY

Perioperative Nursing Considerations

Nutrition

The GI tract prepares food for cellular absorption by altering its physical and chemical composition. Digestion of food is accomplished through the secretion of various digestive enzymes and juices and the presence of bacteria and other flora, which aid in digestion. Because of this process, the GI tract is considered an unsterile system.

A malfunction along the GI tract can produce far-reaching metabolic disturbances that eventually can threaten life. The nutritionally depleted patient has diminished ability to form antibodies; superficial atrophy of mucous membranes, which increases susceptibility to infection; and diminished supplies of protein and vitamin C, which retard wound healing and increase susceptibility to shock from hemorrhage. The lowered albumin level causes increased fluid collection in the third space, rendering the malnourished patient more susceptible to alteration in skin integrity. Because of the high caloric requirements imposed by the physiologic stress of surgery and recovery, many debilitated patients receive a nutritional boost through hyperalimentation (Eisenberg, 1987).

Fluid and electrolyte balance

Many factors contribute to fluid deficit in patients undergoing abdominal surgery. Preoperatively, fluids can be depleted by bowel preparation and by withholding oral fluids. Symptoms related to GI diseases, such as diarrhea, vomiting, or sequestration of fluid because of obstruction, also contribute to this deficit. Intraoperatively, the abdominal cavity is exposed and evaporation of water occurs. Blood loss can be rapid and voluminous because of the large intraabdominal vessels and the vascular nature of intraabdominal organs. Postoperatively, the patient may

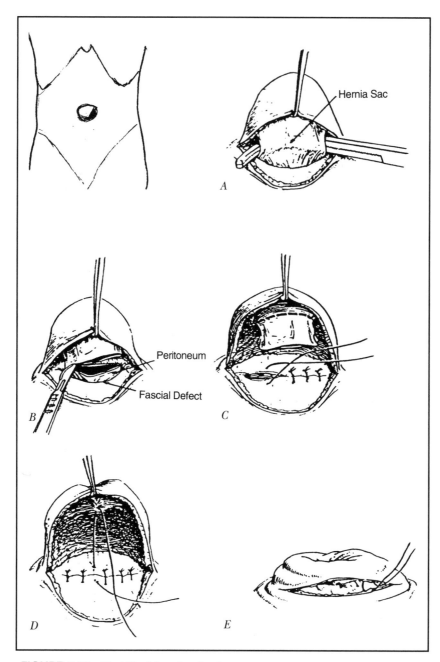

FIGURE 7-19 Umbilical herniorrhaphy. (Harmel, R. P. [1989]. In L. M. Nyhus & R. E. Condon [Eds.]. *Hernia* [3rd ed.]. Philadelphia: J. B. Lippincott.)

continue to experience fluid loss because of drains and tubes used for decompression.

Hypokalemia, hyponatremia, and *hypocalcemia* are associated with fluid loss from the GI tract, medication (i.e., diuretics, steroids), or underlying illness (i.e., renal disease, anemia). Muscle contractility, nerve conduction, and dispersement of body fluids depend on appropriate proportions of electrolytes (Sabiston, 1991).

The perioperative nurse must be alert for patient conditions that contribute to fluid and electrolyte imbalance. Appropriate measures to maintain this balance perioperatively include monitoring the use of irrigation fluids, weighing sponges, monitoring vital signs, and having knowledge of invasive hemodynamic monitoring devices.

Hypothermia

Hypothermia occurs when heat lost to the environment exceeds metabolic heat production. Measures should be taken to ensure that patients undergoing abdominal surgery are protected from loss of body heat. In addition to keeping the patient's immediate environment warm, intraabdominal irrigation fluids should be warmed to normal body temperature to minimize heat loss (Sessler, 1990).

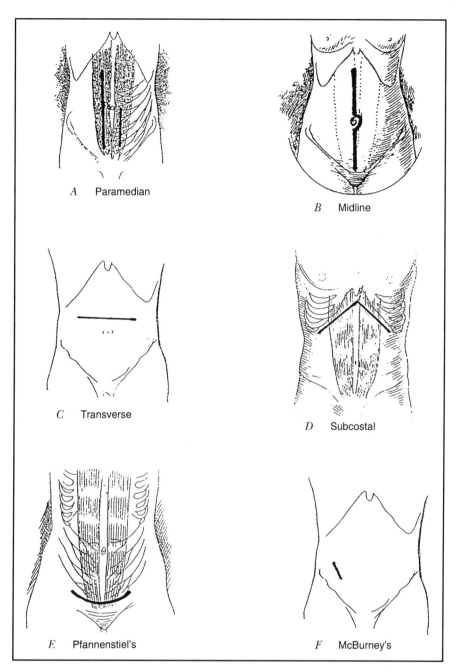

FIGURE 7-20 Abdominal incisions. (Courtesy of Ethicon Inc.)

Abdominal incisions

The considerations for making an abdominal incision include adequate exposure to the abdominal organ involved, the type of surgery proposed, the body habitus (or size) of the patient, and the presence of previous abdominal incisions (Ellis, 1989). Other concerns include avoiding undue physiologic stress and ensuring the best cosmetic result (Rout, 1991). The most frequently used incisions are identified by location (Fig. 7-20).

Paramedian A paramedian incision is made on either side of the midline, in the upper or lower portion of the abdomen. The anterior sheath of the rectus muscle is di-vided lateral to the midline, and the rectus muscle is separated in the midline to expose the posterior rectus sheath and peritoneum. These incisions are thought to heal more rapidly because of the abundant blood supply, and they are believed to provide stronger healing because an intact rectus muscle overlies and supports the suture line (Rout, 1991).

Midline A midline incision is made through the skin and subcutaneous tissue from a point just below or above the umbilicus to just below the xiphoid process or just above the symphysis pubis. The right and left rectus sheaths, with their contained rectus muscles, are retracted

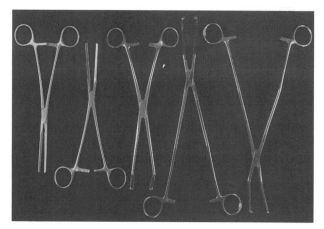

FIGURE 7-21 Intestinal instruments. Noncrushing clamps for use on the gastrointestinal tract.

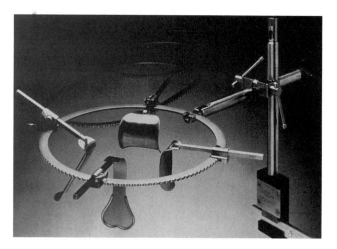

FIGURE 7-23 Bookwalter self-retaining retractor for abdominal wall. (Courtesy of Johnson & Johnson Professional, Raynham, MA)

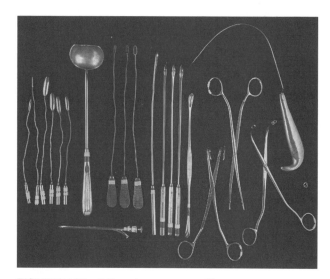

FIGURE 7-22 Biliary instruments: dilators, scoops, stone forceps, retractor, and trocar.

laterally, exposing the underlying transversalis fascia and peritoneum (Rout, 1991).

Transverse A transverse incision is made through the skin and subcutaneous tissue from one lateral border of the rectus muscle to the other at the desired level on the abdominal wall. Both anterior rectus sheaths are exposed and incised transversely from the lateral margin of one to the lateral margin of the other. The posterior rectus sheaths, transversalis fascia, linea alba, and peritoneum are carefully incised (Rout, 1991).

Subcostal A subcostal incision is made on either the right or the left side. The skin incision begins exactly in the midline at a point about one third of the distance from the tip of the xiphoid process to the umbilicus. The surface of the anterior sheath of the rectus muscle and

the surface of the external oblique muscle are cleared of subcutaneous tissue for the width and length of the incision. The anterior sheath of the rectus muscle can be incised transversely or obliquely in the line of the skin incision. The posterior rectus sheath, transversalis fascia, and peritoneum are then carefully incised in a transverse direction. The internal oblique and transverse abdominal muscles are divided in the direction of their fibers; unnecessary injury to the intercostal nerves is avoided (Rout, 1991).

Pfannenstiel's Pfannenstiel's incision is usually used for pelvic operations. It is designed to produce the maximum cosmetic effect: the scar will be within the area covered by the pubic hair. The anterior rectus sheath is incised transversely and the muscle is separated. The posterior rectus sheath and peritoneum are incised by a vertical incision. Care is taken with the urinary bladder, as it lies just below this incision (Rout, 1991).

McBurney's The McBurney's incision is a very short incision made in the right lower quadrant of the abdomen and provides limited exposure. It was devised for appendectomy.

Closure

Closure of abdominal incisions involves bringing the layers of the abdominal wall together in correct anatomic position. Absorbable sutures may secure the peritoneal layer. Slowly absorbable or nonabsorbable sutures are used to close the fascial layer, in an interrupted or running technique. Muscles are allowed to fall into normal position unless they have been incised. Incised muscles may be brought together and sutured. When the subcutaneous layer is closed, absorbable suture is used. The skin may be closed with staples, clips, or monofilament nonabsorbable suture.

Instrumentation

In addition to a basic instrument set, abdominal surgery may require long instruments, vascular instruments (see Chapter 15 in this volume), intestinal instruments (Fig. 7-21), biliary instruments (Fig. 7-22), and deep or specialized retractors. Since many abdominal operations require large incisions, self-retaining retractors are used to enable the surgical team to operate without continuously retracting the abdominal wall by hand (Fig. 7-23).

Hemostasis may be obtained with clamps and ligating sutures, monopolar and bipolar electrocautery (see Chapter 23 in Volume 1), lasers (see Chapter 22 in Volume 1), and surgical clips (see Chapter 31 in Volume 1). In certain abdominal surgeries a "cell-saver" may be used to recycle blood for transfusion.

Supplies such as catheters and tubes are used to provide decompression of specific organs or as monitoring devices during abdominal surgery. Closed wound drains, Penrose drains, or sump drains are used, depending on

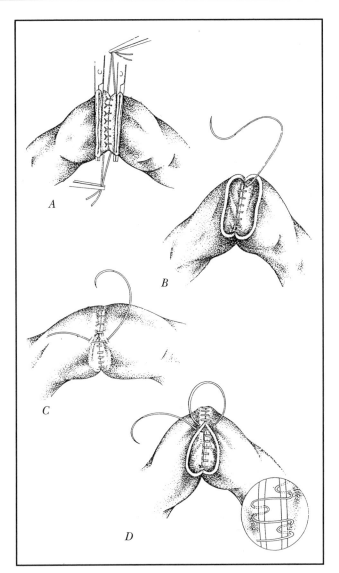

FIGURE 7-25 Double-layer sutured anastomosis. (*A*) Stay sutures approximate the transected bowel and the outer seromuscular layers of the bowel are joined by interrupted nonabsorbable sutures. (*B*) The inner posterior layers are joined with a continuous absorbable suture. (*C*) Absorbable suture is used on the posterior inner layer to close the inner anterior layers. (*D*) The anastomosis is completed by closing the anterior seromuscular layer with inverting nonabsorbable sutures. (Courtesy of Ethicon Endo-Surgery, Cincinnati, OH.)

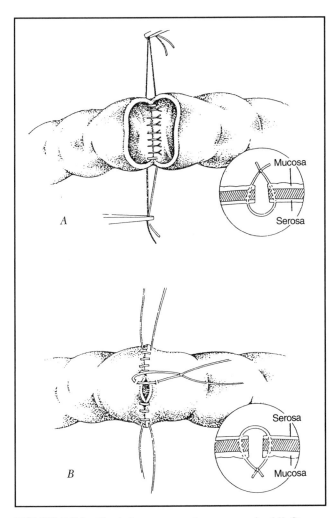

FIGURE 7-24 Single-layer sutured anastomosis. (*A*) Stay sutures are placed to approximate the transected bowel, and the posterior walls of bowel are joined by interrupted absorbable or nonabsorbable sutures. (*B*) The anterior bowel walls are also joined with interrupted sutures. (Courtesy of Ethicon Endo-Surgery, Cincinnati, OH.)

type of surgery and surgeon's preference. When these catheters, tubes, or drains are not removed at the end of the operation they should be clearly labeled to avoid confusion during postoperative care.

Anastomosis techniques

When a portion of the GI tract is removed, continuity is provided by creating an anastomosis of the remaining ends of the tract. To accomplish this, the surgeon may use absorbable and nonabsorbable sutures to complete the anastomosis in a single (Fig. 7-24) or a double layer (Fig. 7-25).

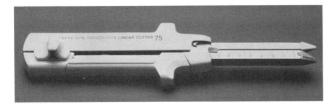

FIGURE 7-26 Linear cutter, a stapling instrument that places a double row of staggered staples and cuts between the staples. Available in 55- and 75-mm lengths. (Courtesy of Ethicon Endo-Surgery, Cincinnati, OH.)

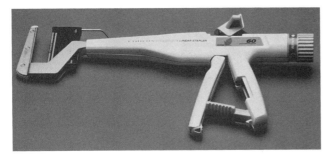

FIGURE 7-27 A linear stapling instrument places a double row of staggered staples. (Courtesy of Ethicon Endo-Surgery, Cincinnati, OH.)

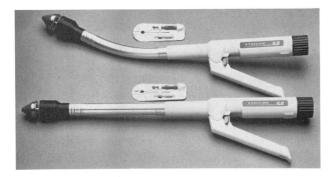

FIGURE 7-28 A circular stapler places a staggered row of staples in a circle formation and cuts out the tissue within the circle to create an end-to-end anastomosis. (Courtesy of Ethicon Endo-Surgery, Cincinnati, OH.)

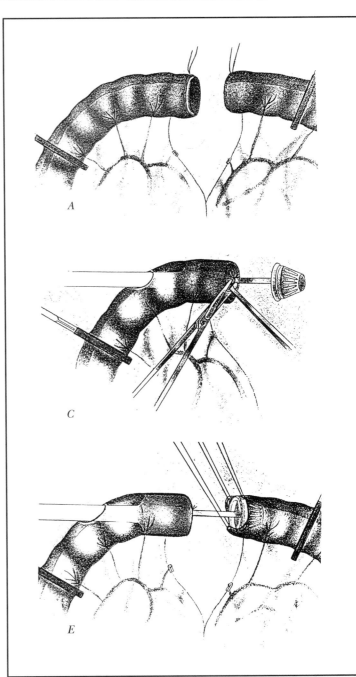

FIGURE 7-29 End-to-end stapled anastomosis: (*A*) Purse-string sutures are placed on each end of transected bowel. (*B*) Circular stapler is introduced through the enterotomy and purse-string suture is tied. (*C*) Stapler anvil is advanced into bowel lumen and the purse-string suture tied over anvil. (*D*) Ends of stapler are brought together and fired. (*E*) Enterotomy is closed with linear stapler. (*F*) Completed end-to-end anastomosis. (Courtesy Ethicon Endo-Surgery, Cincinnati, OH.)

More often, stapling instruments (Figs. 7-26 through 7-28) are used to complete the anastomosis. Techniques for using stapling instruments vary with surgeons' preference and the location of the anastomosis. These techniques include end-to-end (Fig. 7-29), functional end-to-end (Fig. 7-30), and end-to-side (Fig. 7-31) anastomoses.

Bowel technique

The presence of normal bacteria and flora makes the GI tract an unsterile system, so efforts are taken to protect the abdominal cavity from intraluminal contents. Instru-ments or supplies that come into contact with the lumen are discarded or isolated from the sterile field. The technique for accomplishing this is determined by institutional policy or surgeon's preference.

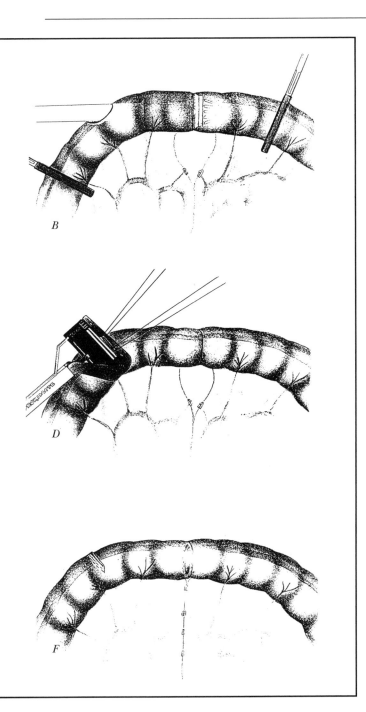

B

D

F

Esophageal Procedures

Most frequently, esophageal procedures are performed transthoracically (see Chapter 14 in this volume). However, when the distal esophagus is involved, some operations can be performed through an abdominal approach. Because of its integral function, the stomach is usually involved in esophageal surgery.

Antireflux procedures are performed to prevent reflux of the stomach contents into the lower esophagus. This reflux frequently occurs because of a hiatal hernia at the esophagogastric junction that permits the stomach to slide into the thoracic cavity (sliding hiatal hernia) or to

protrude into the thoracic cavity in a peritoneal sac (paraesophageal hiatal hernia) (Fig. 7-32). When symptoms cannot be controlled with medication and alteration of diet, surgical correction is required (Skinner, 1991).

Nissen fundoplication

A fundoplication is an approach to repairing a hiatal hernia by wrapping the fundus of the stomach around the esophagus (Fig. 7-33). This procedures secures the distal esophagus in the abdomen. With the patient in a supine position, an upper midline or left subcostal incision is performed. A nasogastric tube is used to provide gastric decompression (Zinner, 1992).

Key steps

1. The esophagogastric junction is freed by incising the ligaments of the left lateral lobe of the liver and the peritoneal attachments of the stomach.
2. A portion of the stomach is mobilized by ligating and dividing the short gastric arteries and mobilizing the esophagus at the hiatus. Care is taken to protect the vagus nerve (Fig. 7-33,*A*).
3. The peritoneal surface of the esophagus is divided. A large rubber dilator is used as an intraesophageal stent to protect the inside surface of the esophagus (Fig. 7-33,*B*).
4. Nonabsorbable sutures are placed posterior to the esophagus when the distal esophagus is retracted into the abdomen (Fig. 7-33,*C*).
5. The dissected portion of the stomach is passed posteriorly to wrap the distal esophagus in a 360-degree manner. This wrap is secured with nonabsorbable sutures placed through the seromuscular wall of the stomach, the anterior wall of the esophagus, and the seromuscular portion of the other side of the stomach (Fig. 7-33,*D*).

Laparoscopic fundoplication

Esophageal procedures can be accomplished laparoscopically, and the operative portion of the procedure is nearly identical to that of the conventional approach. The patient is in lithotomy position utilizing reverse Trendelenburg's to cause the abdominal contents to fall away from the diaphragm (Bagnato, 1992).

Key steps

1. Pneumoperitoneum is established using a closed or open technique.
2. The umbilicus is used to provide access for the laparoscope and camera, while additional sites provide access for instrumentation.
3. The left lobe of the liver is retracted using a blunt probe while the peritoneum over the gastroesophageal area is excised using an electrocautery hook dissector.
4. The distal esophagus is mobilized by blunt and sharp dissection, taking care not to enter the chest cavity when operating close to the diaphragm.

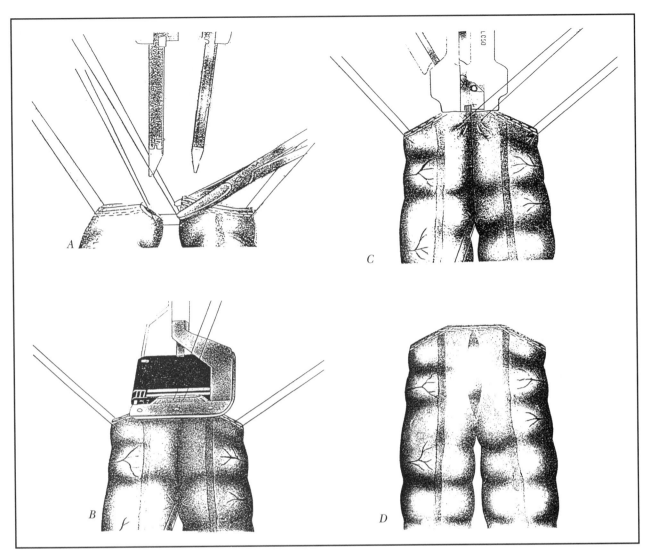

FIGURE 7-30 Functional end-to-end stapled anastomosis. (*A*) Corners of previously stapled bowel ends are excised to allow introduction of each limb of linear cutter. (*B*) Linear cutter is locked and fired. (*C*) The common opening of the bowel is closed with a linear stapler. (*D*) Completed functional end-to-end anastomosis. (Courtesy Ethicon Endo-Surgery, Cincinnati, OH.)

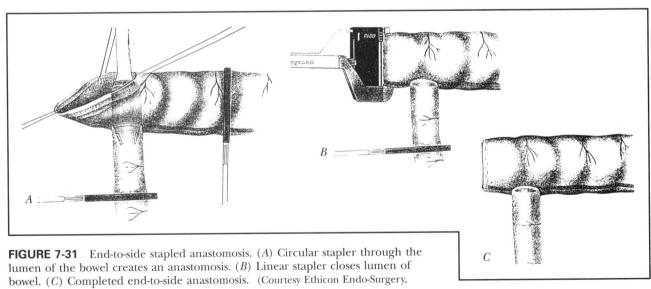

FIGURE 7-31 End-to-side stapled anastomosis. (*A*) Circular stapler through the lumen of the bowel creates an anastomosis. (*B*) Linear stapler closes lumen of bowel. (*C*) Completed end-to-side anastomosis. (Courtesy Ethicon Endo-Surgery, Cincinnati, OH.)

FIGURE 7-32 Types of hiatal hernias. (Skinner, D. B. [1991]. In D. C. Sabiston, Jr. [Ed.]. *Textbook of surgery.* Philadelphia: W. B. Saunders.)

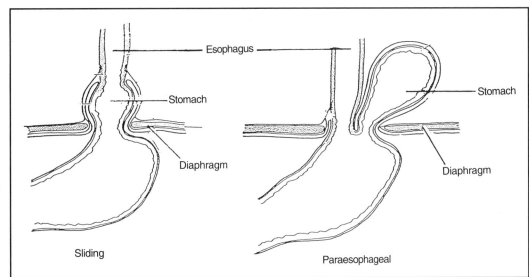

FIGURE 7-33 Nissen fundoplication. (Zinner, M. J. *Atlas of gastric surgery.* New York: Churchill Livingstone. [1992].)

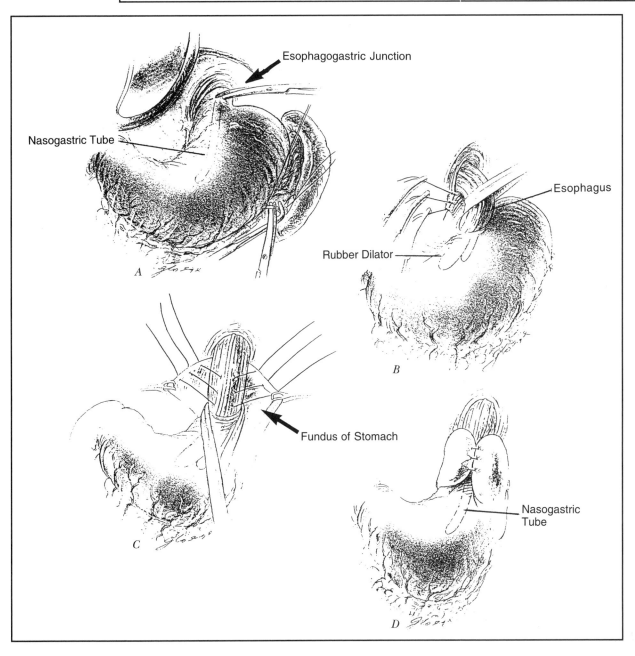

5. The anterior and posterior vagus nerves may be identified before completing the esophageal dissection.
6. A large rubber dilator is placed transesophageally to maintain the patency of the esophagus.
7. The stomach is mobilized by ligating the short gastric veins.
8. The distal esophagus is lifted anteriorly and the posterior fundus of the stomach is passed behind the esophagus. The stomach is then wrapped around the distal esophagus and secured with interrupted nonabsorbable sutures. These may be tied intra- or extracorporeally.
9. Teflon pledgets may be used to secure the repair. (Bagnato, 1992; Hinder & Filipi, 1992)

Gastropexy

A gastropexy can be performed to narrow the opening of the diaphragm at the gastroesophageal junction. This secures the position of the esophagus.

Key steps

1. The gastroesophageal junction is mobilized.
2. Posteriorly, sutures are placed in the diaphragm to narrow the opening at the area through which the esophagus passes into the abdominal cavity.
3. The gastropexy is performed by placing nonabsorbable sutures to anchor the gastroesophageal junction as well as the curvature of the stomach to the ligament of the diaphragm (Zinner, 1992).

Transhiatal esophagectomy

The operation to remove an esophageal tumor or diverticulum varies according to the portion of the esophagus to be resected and extent of disease (Fig. 7-34). Surgical resection with reestablishment of GI continuity by means of esophagogastric anastomosis is the most widely used surgical procedure for attempted cure. A "blind esophagectomy" through separate abdominal and cervical incisions is a means of removing the affected portion of the esophagus. Because the vagus nerves are resected, some form of gastric outlet procedure, such as pyloroplasty (see Stomach), is performed in conjunction with the resection (Murray & Keagy, 1991).

The esophagectomy is performed with the patient supine with a small roll placed transversely across the shoulders to hyperextend the neck. The entire neck, chest, and abdomen are prepped for the combined midline abdominal and cervical incisions. Self-retaining retractors are used to retract the liver and the left costal margin (Zinner, 1992).

Key steps

1. The stomach is mobilized by transecting the ligaments and short gastric arteries, and prepared for transposition into the chest. The right gastroepiploic artery is preserved to maintain a blood supply (Fig. 7-34,A).
2. Pyloroplasty is performed (see Gastric Procedures).

3. Once the stomach is mobilized, the resection begins at the esophageal hiatus. The entire esophagus is mobilized bluntly (Fig. 7-34,B).
4. The neck incision is made and dissection between the trachea and the esophagus is completed. The esophagus is retracted with a Penrose drain and dissected free of the trachea (Fig. 7-34,C).
5. When the esophageal dissection is complete, a Penrose drain is stapled to the distal esophagus and pulled down through the tunnel. The esophagus is divided from the drain, which is left as a guide. The tumor is then resected (Fig. 7-34,D).
6. The tube of stomach is attached to the drain and pushed up to the cervical incision (Fig. 7-34,E). The esophagogastric anastomosis is completed through the cervical incision (Fig. 7-34,F). A large rubber dilator may be used as an intraesophageal stent during the anastomosis.
7. A tube jejunostomy (Fig. 7-34,G) is placed at the end of the operation, to provide a means of maintaining nutrition until oral intake is resumed.

Gastric Procedures

Gastric operations are performed for peptic ulcer disease when complications such as hemorrhage, obstruction from scarring or edema, or perforation occur. It is also indicated when nonoperative management fails. These surgeries attempt to create a balance between the rate of secretion of gastric juice and the degree of protection of the mucosal layer of the stomach (Carrico & Stevenson, 1987).

Vagotomy

Vagotomy, or division of the vagus nerve, causes a reduction in gastric secretion (Fig. 7-35) and is frequently used in combination with other procedures for the treatment of ulcer disease. *Truncal vagotomy* (total abdominal vagotomy) consists of resection of a 1- to 2-cm segment of each vagal trunk as it enters the abdomen on the distal esophagus. *Selective vagotomy* is transection of each abdominal vagus nerve at a point just beyond its division. Some branches of the posterior vagus are maintained. *Parietal cell vagotomy* may be referred to as a highly selective, superselective, or proximal gastric vagotomy. It involves dividing all vagal branches on the proximal two thirds of the stomach (Carrico & Stevenson, 1987).

Pyloroplasty

A pyloroplasty may be done in conjunction with vagotomy to aid in the emptying of the stomach or may be indicated to relieve scarring from chronic peptic ulcer disease (Kirk, 1989).

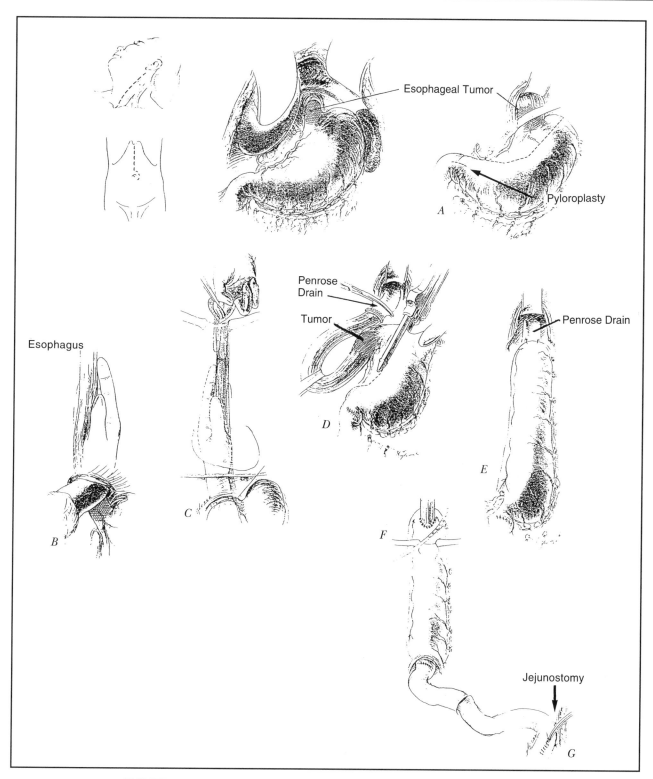

FIGURE 7-34   Transhiatal esophagectomy.   (Zinner, M. J. *Atlas of gastric surgery.* New York: Churchill Livingstone. [1992].)

Key steps

1. After the narrowest portion of the pyloroduodenal canal has been identified, a longitudinal incision (Fig. 7-36,*A*) is made across the pylorus.

2. A wider canal is produced by closing the incision transversely (Fig. 7-36,*B*).

3. The closure at the pylorus can be accomplished with single- or double-layer sutures or by stapling (Fig. 7-36,*C*).

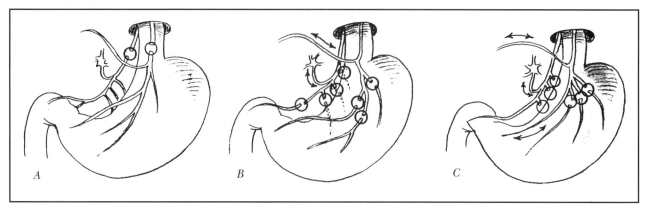

FIGURE 7-35 Types of vagotomy. (*A*) truncal, (*B*) selective, and (*C*) highly selective or parietal cell. (Carrico, C. J. & Stevenson, J. K. [1987]. In J. H. Davis [Ed.]. *Clinical surgery.* St. Louis: C. V. Mosby.)

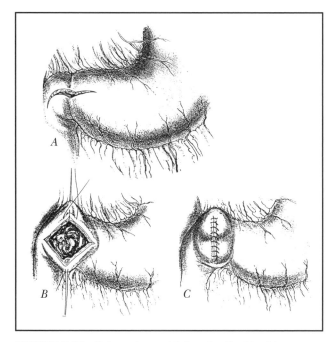

FIGURE 7-36 Pyloroplasty with longitudinal incision converted to transverse closure. (Kirk, R. M. [1989]. In Schwartz, S. D., & Ellis, H. [Ed.]. *Maingot's abdominal operations.* Norwalk, CT: Appleton & Lange.)

Gastric resection is performed for peptic ulcer disease or removal of gastric tumors. These surgeries often involve the first or second portion of the small intestine, the duodenum and jejunum, respectively.

Subtotal gastrectomy

Subtotal gastrectomy consists of resection of the distal two thirds to three quarters of the stomach with restoration of gastrointestinal continuity, either as a gastroduodenostomy (Billroth I) or gastrojejunostomy (Billroth II) (Zinner, 1992). Both operations are performed through an upper midline incision with the patient supine.

Gastroduodenostomy (Billroth I)
Key steps

1. The greater and lesser curvatures of the stomach are mobilized from the site of the duodenum to just beyond the level of gastric resection. The omental vessels are ligated.
2. After mobilization, a 90-mm stapling device is used to close the proximal stomach (Fig. 7-37,*A*).
3. The duodenum is divided just beyond the pylorus, between intestinal clamps.
4. An intestinal clamp is placed at the distal line of resection and a portion of the stomach is removed (Fig. 7-37,*B*).
5. The duodenum is then anastomosed to the remaining stomach using suture or stapling techniques (Fig. 7-37,*C*).
6. The completed anastomosis shows the gastroduodenostomy (Fig. 7-37,*D*).

Gastrojejunostomy (Billroth II)
Key steps

1. The greater and lesser curvatures of the stomach are mobilized from the site of the duodenum to just beyond the level of gastric resection. The omental vessels are ligated.
2. After mobilization, a 90-mm stapling device is used to close the proximal stomach. A stapling device that places two rows of staples and cuts between them is used since the duodenum is not involved in the anastomosis (Fig. 7-38,*A*).
3. The duodenal stump is inverted with nonabsorbable sutures. Intestinal clamps are placed across the distal stomach and the tip of the stomach is removed (Fig. 7-38,*B*).
4. A loop of jejunum is brought through a clear area of the mesentery of the transverse colon (Fig. 7-38,*C*).
5. The jejunum is anastomosed to the stomach (Fig. 7-38,*D*).
6. Once the anastomosis is completed, it is brought below the transverse colon and the stomach is sutured to the mesentery (Fig. 7-38,*E*).

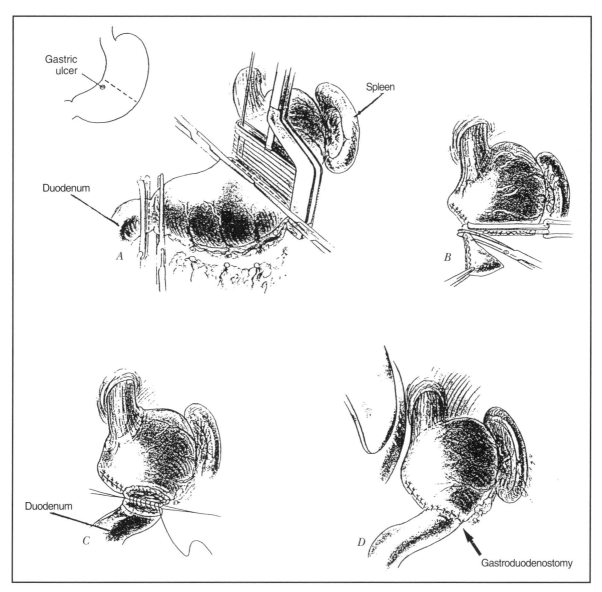

FIGURE 7-37   Gastroduodenostomy (Billroth I).   (Zinner, M. J. *Atlas of gastric surgery.* New York: Churchill Livingstone. [1992].)

Total gastrectomy

Total gastrectomy has come to mean the removal of the entire stomach with the cardia (cardiac sphincter), at least some esophageal tube, and a cuff of duodenum. When performed for cancer, the operation often incorporates removal of the spleen, the body and tail of the pancreas, the omentum, and the lymph nodes draining the stomach (Fig. 7-39,*A*) (Zinner, 1992).

Key steps

1. The greater and lesser curvatures of the stomach are mobilized by dividing the omentum, ligaments, branches of the left and right gastric vessels, and the gastroepiploic vessels.
2. The duodenum is divided just distal to the pylorus and

is closed. The esophagus is divided above the gastroesophageal junction (Fig. 7-39,*B*).
3. Reconstruction is begun by identifying a section of jejunum and dividing it with a stapling device (Fig. 7-39,*C*).
4. The jejunum is brought up to the esophagus. End-to-side jejunojejunostomy is performed (Fig. 7-39,*D*).
5. Gastrointestinal continuity is restored by anastomosing the esophagus to the jejunum (Fig. 7-39,*E*).

Gastrostomy

A gastrostomy is an opening in the stomach through which a catheter can be placed and then brought through the abdominal wall. This can provide gastric decompression as a temporary measure in conjunction with other GI surgery, or access to the GI tract for administration of nutrients or medication. Stamm's method is frequently used for creating a gastrostomy (Chassin, 1980).

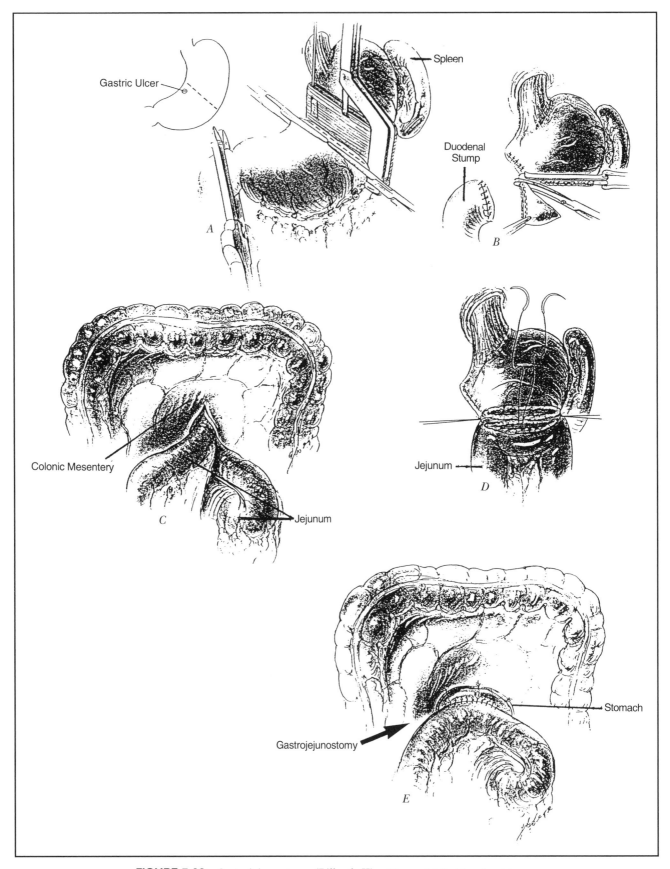

FIGURE 7-38 Gastrojejunostomy (Billroth II). (Zinner, M. J. *Atlas of gastric surgery.* New York: Churchill Livingstone. [1992].)

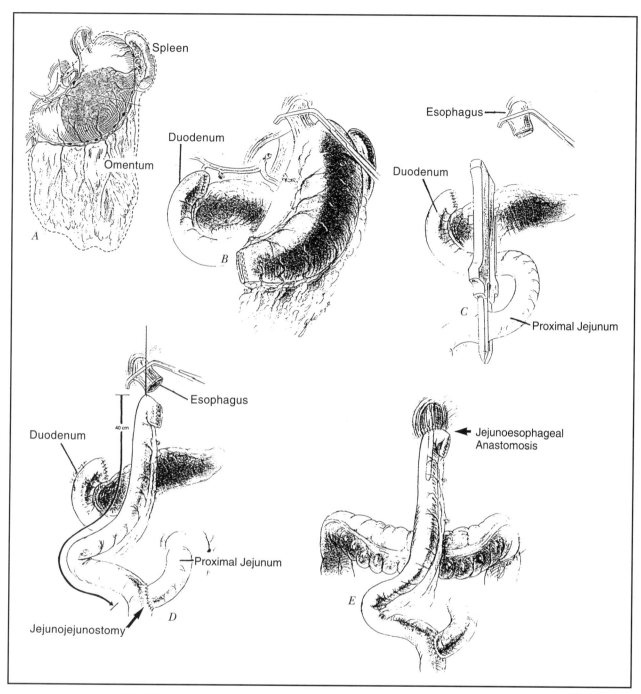

FIGURE 7-39 Total gastrectomy. (Zinner, M. J. *Atlas of gastric surgery.* New York: Churchill Livingstone. [1992].)

Key steps

1. An incision is made through the layers of the stomach, and the tube is inserted into the lumen. An absorbable suture is placed as a purse string around the tube (Fig. 7-40,*A*, *B*).
2. The open end of the tube is brought through the layers of the abdominal wall and secured with a nonabsorbable suture at the skin level.
3. The stomach is fixed to the abdominal wall by placing absorbable sutures through the layers of the stomach and the peritoneum (Fig. 7-40,*C*).

Splenic Procedures

The indications for splenic surgery include hypersplenism, certain hemolytic anemias, cysts, abscesses, tumors, and splenic artery aneurysm. Abdominal trauma may result in splenic lacerations that require repair or splenectomy. Inadvertent laceration may occur during abdominal surgeries because of the spleen's proximity to other organs (Quinlan, 1991).

Surgery of the spleen involves complete removal, partial resection, or repair. Blood loss is of most concern because of the large quantity of blood the organ con-

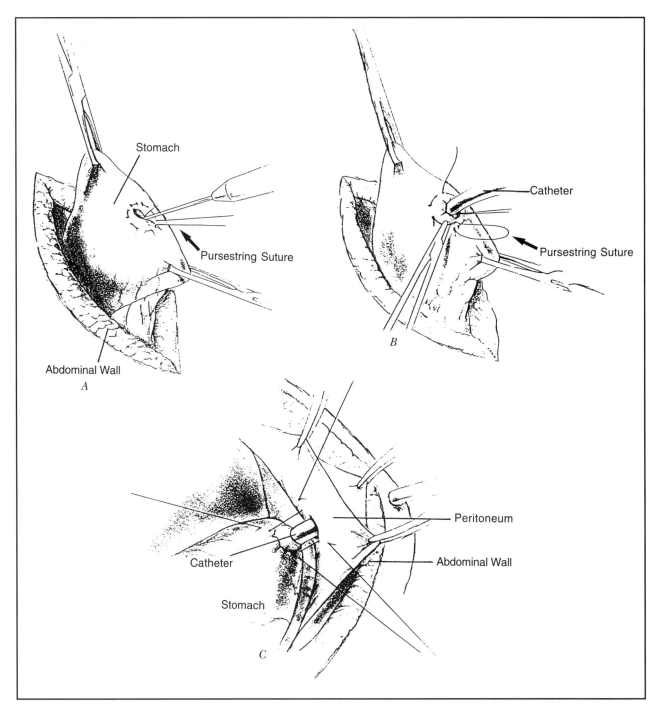

FIGURE 7-40 Gastrostomy (Stamm). (Chassin, J. L. [1980]. *Operative strategy in general surgery.* New York: Springer-Verlag.)

tains. Also, the patient's preoperative status may reflect existing anemia. When the spleen is removed, a sudden change may occur in the patient's hemodynamic status (Quinlan, 1991). Blood products and extenders must be available.

A midline, left subcostal, paramedian, or transverse incision is utilized to provide adequate exposure. In addition, the stomach is decompressed by a nasogastric tube to make exposure better and dissection easier. Long instruments, vascular instruments, and vessel clips should be available.

Splenectomy (Fig. 7-41)

Key steps

1. The spleen is mobilized to expose the pedicle of splenic artery and vein.
2. The ligamentous attachments are transected as well as the gastric veins that run from the spleen to the greater curvature of the stomach.
3. The splenic artery and vein are ligated using double or suture ligatures.
4. The spleen is removed.

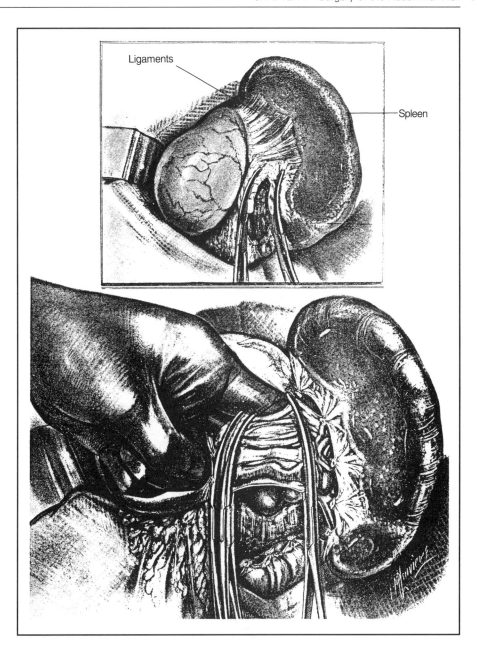

FIGURE 7-41 Splenectomy. (Schwartz, S. I. [1989]. In S. I. Schwartz & H. Ellis [Eds.]. *Maingot's abdominal operations.* Norwalk, CT: Appleton & Lange.)

Because loss of the immune functions of the spleen following splenectomy is thought to contribute to the incidence of serious postoperative infections, more efforts are being taken to repair lacerations of a healthy spleen that occur during trauma or by intraoperative injury (Hansen et al., 1991).

These splenic lacerations can be controlled with pressure and application of a synthetic coagulant, suturing the laceration (splenorrhaphy, Fig. 7-42), or applying an omental patch. A fractured spleen requires at least partial resection. In the hemodynamically unstable patient, splenectomy remains the treatment of choice (Hansen et al., 1991).

Hepatic Procedures

The multiple metabolic functions of the liver make it essential for survival, so extensive preoperative assessment must

determine the feasibility of surgery. The additional compromise of liver function caused by disease may increase the risk of performing hepatic surgery (Quinlan, 1991).

Hepatic resection

Liver resection is indicated for benign and malignant conditions and is an option after it is determined that at least 15% of healthy liver tissue will remain and that its vascular and biliary systems will function. Metastatic lesions may be resected when the inferior vena cava and portal veins are not involved and the primary tumor has been resected (Beckermann & Galloway, 1989).

Types of liver resections include right and left lobectomy, right trisegmentectomy (right lobe with the medial segment of the left lobe), and left lateral segmentectomy (Fig. 7-43). With the patient in the supine position, a subcostal, bilateral subcostal, or upper midline incision with

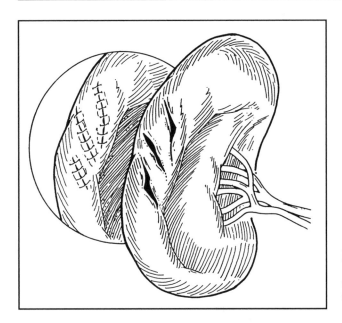

FIGURE 7-42 Direct suturing of splenic laceration. (Reprinted with permission, *AORN Journal,* 53, p 1526, June 1991. Copyright AORN Inc., 2170 South Parker Road, Suite 300, Denver, CO 80231.)

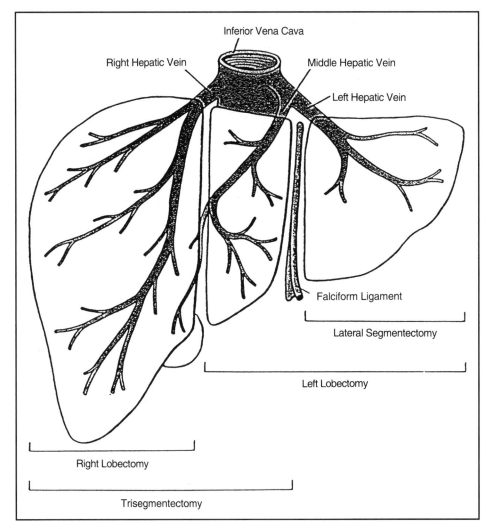

FIGURE 7-43 Hepatic resections. (Starzl, T. E., Bell, R. H., Beart, R. W., & Putnam, C. W. [1975]. *Surgery, Gynecology and Obstetrics, 41.* By permission of SURGERY, GYNECOLOGY & OBSTETRICS.)

extension to the chest may be utilized (Steuer, 1990). An ultrasonic aspirator may assist in dissection of the liver (Fig. 7-44). This instrument vibrates at an ultrasonic frequency to dissect the liver parenchyma while leaving vascular and biliary structures intact for ligation.

Left hepatic lobectomy

Key Steps

1. The hepatic ligaments are divided, and the left hepatic vein is identified and surrounded by a vessel loop.
2. The lesser omentum is sectioned and the hepatic artery is identified and the left branch is divided.
3. The cystic artery is ligated and divided and the cystic duct is dissected free. When the gallbladder is removed, the cystic duct is ligated, leaving a stump.
4. With the common duct exposed, the hilus of the liver is dissected to reveal the right and left hepatic ducts. A rubber catheter may be placed into the right hepatic duct and used to control bile leaks.
5. Following division of the left hepatic duct, the left branch of the portal vein is identified and ligated. A suture ligature is used to reinforce the ligation.
6. The inferior vena cava is controlled by tapes or tourniquets. When the left hepatic lobe is devascularized, the left hepatic vein is clamped and divided.
7. The parenchyma of the liver is incised and the left lobe removed. The caudate lobe may be excised or left in place.
8. Following the resection, the raw surfaces of the liver are inspected for hemostasis (Kittur & Smith, 1991).

Right hepatic lobectomy

Key steps

1. The hepatic and hepatocolic ligaments are divided and the colon is displaced downward. The liver is rotated to the left, and the right hepatic vein is identified and looped.
2. The gallbladder is removed, and the cystic duct stump is left long so it may be used to check for bile leaks.
3. The right hepatic artery is ligated and divided. The right branch of the portal vein is ligated and secured with a suture ligature.
4. Hilar dissection is accomplished to expose the right and left branches of the common bile duct. The right hepatic duct is divided and ligated. Inferior vena caval bleeding may be controlled with tapes or tourniquets.
5. The right hepatic vein is transected. The liver is retracted to the left and, beginning at the right hepatic vein, the liver parenchyma is dissected from the right lateral wall of the vena cava to expose the multiple small right hepatic veins. These are divided individually.
6. The liver capsule is transected from the level of the right hepatic vein and continued to the gallbladder bed.

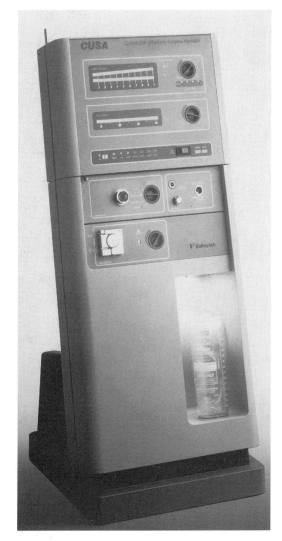

FIGURE 7-44 Cavitron ultrasonic aspirator. (Courtesy of Valleylab Inc.)

7. The middle hepatic vein is preserved, ligating only its branches.
8. The devascularized lobe of the liver is resected and the raw surfaces checked for hemostasis (Kittur & Smith, 1991).

Left lateral segmentectomy

Key steps

1. The round and falciform ligaments are divided. The left triangular and small left coronary ligaments are sectioned.
2. The left hepatic vein is identified at the base of the coronary ligament.
3. With the left lateral segment freed of its attachments and the left hepatic vein controlled, the liver capsule is incised to the left of the falciform ligament.
4. The left hepatic vein is clamped and divided.
5. The dissection of the parenchyma is completed, and the resected liver is removed (Kittur & Smith, 1991).

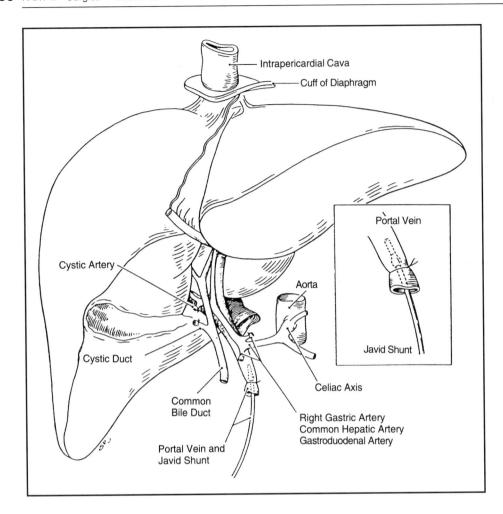

Portal Vein

Javid Shunt

Intrapericardial Cava
Cuff of Diaphragm

Cystic Artery

Aorta

Cystic Duct

Common
Bile Duct

Celiac Axis

Right Gastric Artery
Common Hepatic Artery
Gastroduodenal Artery

Portal Vein and
Javid Shunt

FIGURE 7-45 The donor liver. (Turcotte, J. G., et al. [1991]. In G. D. Zuidema [Ed.]. *Shackelford's surgery of the alimentary tract* [3rd ed.]. Philadelphia: W. B. Saunders.)

Right trisegmentectomy

Key steps

1. The hepatic ligaments are divided and the liver is rotated to the left. Branches of the right inferior phrenic vessels in the ligaments are ligated.
2. The right hepatic vein is isolated, and packs are placed to displace the liver inferiorly.
3. The gallbladder is removed with the specimen, so it is not necessary to perform a formal cholecystectomy. The cystic artery is divided, and the cystic duct is ligated and divided, leaving a long stump.
4. The right hepatic artery is traced to its origin and ligated. The portal vein is identified and the right branch is divided.
5. The common duct is traced to its bifurcation, and the right duct is transected.
6. Dissection of the vascular and ductal structures to the left lobe is carried out, making sure that no vessels and ducts to the lateral segment are injured.
7. The inferior vena cava is controlled and the liver is retracted to the left and inferiorly. The right hepatic vein is cross-clamped and divided. The caval end is closed with nonabsorbable suture and the hepatic end is suture ligated. The numerous right hepatic veins entering the vena cava are ligated individually.
8. The liver parenchyma is dissected, taking care to preserve the left hepatic vein. The liver is elevated anteriorly and the resected portion is removed.
9. The remaining small raw liver surface is inspected for hemostasis (Kittur & Smith, 1991).

Liver transplantation

Transplantation has become an option for patients with end-stage liver disease. The most common indications are primary biliary cirrhosis, posthepatitic cirrhosis, chronic active hepatitis, and sclerosing cholangitis. Transplantation is effective therapy for some hepatic tumors for which a low rate of recurrence has been documented (Turcotte et al., 1991).

Transplantation may be accomplished by replacement of the host liver with a donor liver (orthotopic) or by implantation of an extra liver (auxiliary). The most successful technique has been orthotopic transplantation. The most common explanation for transplantation failure is preexisting hepatic injury in the donor organ; so careful screening of donors is essential. In addition to adequate liver function, the donor is screened for circumstances of death, past history, associated diseases, cardiorespiratory stability, severe chemistry profile abnormalities, need for excessive pressor support, and length of time from brain death or organ procurement (Gordon et al., 1989).

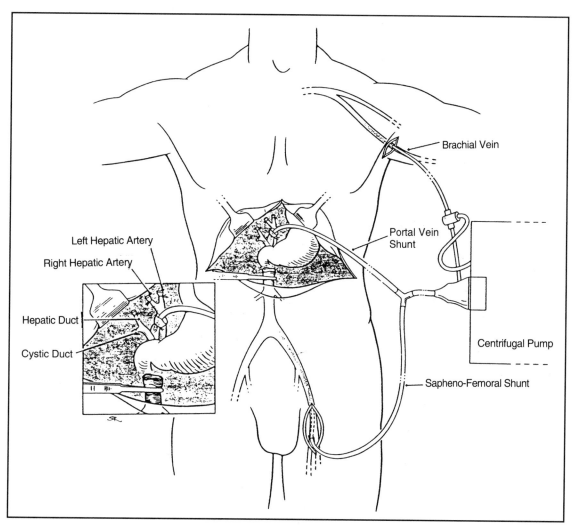

FIGURE 7-46 Venovenous bypass. (Turcotte, J. G., et al. [1991]. In G. D. Zuidema [Ed.]. *Shackelford's surgery of the alimentary tract* [3rd ed.]. Philadelphia: W. B. Saunders.)

Preservation of the donor liver is accomplished by immediate cooling and careful removal of a portion of aorta just below the diaphragm, a cuff of diaphragm, a segment of aorta, hepatic artery, right gastric artery, common duct, and portal vein. A Javid shunt can be tied into the portal vein to infuse cold lactated Ringer's solution during implantation of the liver (Fig. 7-45). The liver can be maintained by cold preservation as long as 24 hours (Turcotte et al., 1991).

Orthotopic liver transplantation The transplantation is performed through a bilateral subcostal incision with midline extension to the chest. Equipment needed for the surgery includes an extra setup for preparation of the donor liver, vascular instruments and supplies, chest instruments, and biliary instruments.

During the procedure, the portal vein and inferior vena cava are temporarily cross-clamped. Venovenous bypass (Fig. 7-46) is used by many surgeons during the vascular anastomoses, to avoid venous hypertension and resultant swelling of the colon, third space sequestration of fluid, and postoperative renal failure (Turcotte et al., 1991).

Key steps

1. Dissection of the donor hepatic hilum, division of the hepatic artery and bile duct, and skeletonization of the portal vein are accomplished. Venous bypass is begun.
2. The suspensory ligaments of the liver are taken down, and the vena cava is freed above and below the liver.
3. The vena cava is clamped and divided above and below, and cut up along the base of the liver, often leaving a portion of the back wall of the infrahepatic vena cava.
4. The liver is removed by dividing the common bile duct and the portal vein. The right and left hepatic arteries are ligated and divided while the proper hepatic artery is mobilized.
5. The adrenal vein orifice is identified and oversewn.
6. The graft is now implanted while cold lactated Ringer's solution drips continuously through the portal vein.
7. The suprahepatic caval, infrahepatic caval, and hepatic artery and portal vein anastomoses are per-

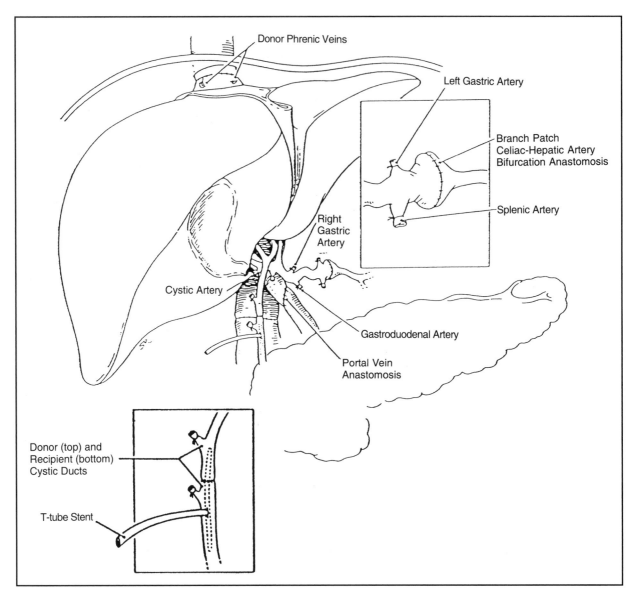

FIGURE 7-47 Orthotopic liver transplantation. (Turcotte, J. G. et al. [1991]. Hepatic transplantation. In G. D. Zuidema [Ed.]. *Shackelford's surgery of the alimentary tract* [3rd ed.]. Philadelphia: W. B. Saunders.)

formed (Fig. 7-47). The liver is flushed with warm blood by temporarily unclamping the portal vein before removing the suprahepatic clamp. The recipient is given calcium, bicarbonate, and extra blood at the time of declamping.

8. The portal vein cannula is removed just before reanastomosing the portal vein, and the other two limbs are removed after the liver has been revascularized. The portal anastomosis is completed, and the venous clamps are removed.

9. The arterial anastomosis is performed by anastomosing the celiac axis of the donor to the proximal hepatic artery. When the arterial supply cannot be used for anastomosis, a donor iliac artery graft may be anastomosed to the donor celiac artery and then passed to the aorta just below the left renal vein.

10. Biliary reconstruction is accomplished by direct duct-to-duct reconstruction over a T-tube stent. When the bile ducts are diseased, the donor duct is anastomosed to the recipient jejunum (Turcotte et al., 1991).

The transplanted liver must function immediately following the anastomosis. Postoperatively, maintenance immunosuppression is accomplished with cyclosporine. This drug has contributed to the increase in liver transplantations in Europe and the United States (Gordon et al., 1989).

Biliary Procedures

Surgery of the biliary system is performed for stones, tumor, stricture, drainage, and duct obstruction. It is

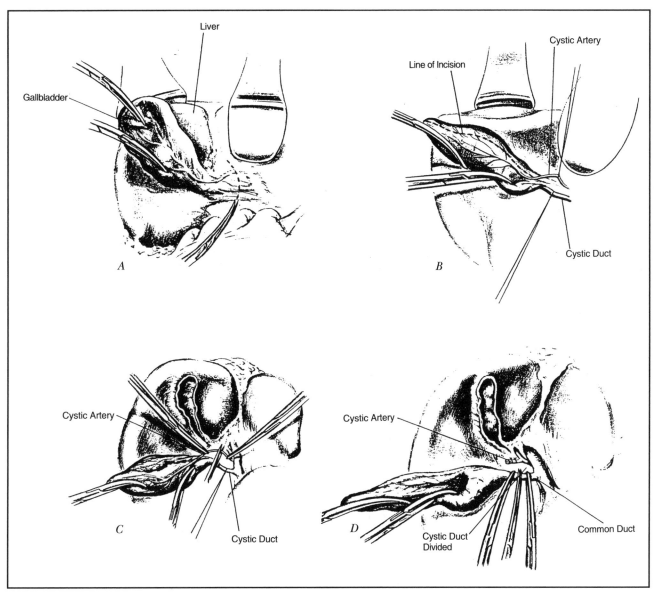

FIGURE 7-48 Cholecystectomy. (Hoerr, S. O., & Hermann, R. E. [1987]. In L. W. Way and C. A. Pellegrini [Eds.]. *Surgery of the gallbladder and bile ducts.* Philadelphia: W. B. Saunders.)

most often performed with the patient in the supine position. Some surgeons request that the patient's right upper quadrant be elevated by placing an inflatable pillow under the patient. The patient should also be positioned to accommodate a cassette for intraoperative radiographic visualization of the ductal system. Biliary instruments, T tubes, and closed-system drains should be available. A choledochoscope may be used to view the lumen of the common bile duct. Care should be taken to isolate the gallbladder contents from the sterile field.

Cholecystectomy

When stones form in the gallbladder they can migrate into the common bile duct or the cystic duct to produce biliary colic or acute cholecystitis. Cholecystectomy is of-

ten the treatment for this condition, especially when the symptoms are recurrent or persistent. The gallbladder may also be removed for tumor.

Key steps

1. The peritoneum overlying the gallbladder and ducts is opened (Fig. 7-48,*A*).
2. The cystic duct is isolated by placing a ligature around it (Fig. 7-48,*B*). The cystic artery is identified and divided (Fig. 7-48,*C*).
3. If an intraoperative cholangiogram is to be done, the cystic duct is cannulated with a cholangiogram catheter.
4. If no stones are identified in the common duct, the cystic duct is ligated with nonabsorbable ligatures and divided (Fig. 7-48,*D*).

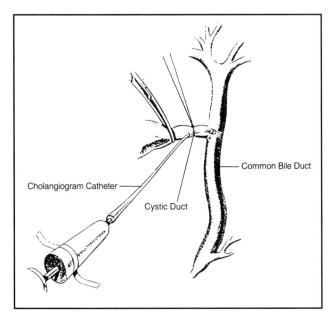

FIGURE 7-49 Cystic duct cholangiogram. (Hoerr, S. O., & Hermann, R. E. [1987]. In L. W. Way and C. A. Pellegrini. *Surgery of the gallbladder and bile ducts.* Philadelphia: W. B. Saunders.)

5. Next, the peritoneum along the gallbladder is incised, and the gallbladder is retracted toward the fundus. The gallbladder is dissected free and removed.
6. The gallbladder bed is inspected for bleeding and may be left open or closed with running absorbable suture.

Intraoperative cholangiogram (Fig. 7-49)

Operative cholangiograms are frequently taken during biliary surgery to locate ductal stones and ensure patency of ducts. Important aspects of technique include the following:

Key steps

1. Protective radiographic equipment is used.
2. The operating room bed must accommodate a radiographic cassette.
3. The patient must be positioned on the bed to facilitate taking intraoperative films. A scout film is often taken at the beginning of the procedure, following positioning, to ensure adequate exposure.
4. The cholangiogram catheter is filled with sterile saline with all air expelled, and held in a position with catheter tip down and syringe above, to ensure that no air is in the catheter.
5. The catheter is passed to the surgeon with saline in the syringe.
6. After the catheter is positioned in the duct, the saline-filled syringe is replaced with the dye-filled syringe.
7. X-rays are taken following injection of the dye.

Laparoscopic cholecystectomy

Preparation for laparoscopic cholecystectomy includes placing the patient in the supine position, with the arms extended at 90 degrees on armboards. A nasogastric tube and urinary catheter are inserted. An abdominal setup should be ready for possible laparotomy. The patient's position is secured, as the operating room bed will be put into reverse Trendelenburg's position with the right side slightly elevated to improve exposure (Partain, 1991).

Key steps

1. After pneumoperitoneum is achieved, the secondary trocars are placed under direct vision.
2. The gallbladder fundus is grasped, pushing it up and over the liver.
3. The gallbladder is dissected to the cystic artery or cystic duct. The cystic duct is separated from any surrounding structures.
4. An intraoperative cholangiogram may be used to detect stones in the common bile duct and to evaluate the length and course of the cystic duct.
5. The cystic duct is severed with microscissors and the gallbladder–cystic duct junction is grasped. A ligature is placed around the cystic duct.
6. The cystic duct is dissected down to the junction with the common bile duct. The cystic duct is ligated. A clip is placed on the cystic duct remnant distal to the ligature.
7. The cystic artery is dissected, clipped, and severed in a similar manner. Clips are placed proximally for control of the artery.
8. The gallbladder is dissected by laser or electrocautery as it approaches the liver and liver bed.
9. After the gallbladder has been removed from its bed, the gallbladder bed itself is inspected and irrigated, to make certain there is no active bleeding.
10. Under direct visualization, the gallbladder is brought up to the blunt-tipped trocar and is removed through the periumbilical incision.
11. Carbon dioxide is released from the abdomen, and the fascia in the umbilical incision is reapproximated with subcuticular absorbable sutures (Gadacz, 1991c).

Common bile duct exploration

The presence of common duct stones may be determined preoperatively or intraoperatively. Often, the stones can be palpated during the operation. Frequently, they can be removed by opening the duct and manipulating the stones with index finger and thumb. Other instruments that are helpful in removing stones are stone forceps, scoops (see Fig. 7-22), biliary catheters, choledochoscopes, and irrigation.

Following the exploration to remove stones from the common duct, a T tube may be placed to keep the duct patent. The tube is sized to fit the duct.

1. The common duct is exposed, and stay sutures are placed in the anterior wall and used for traction.
2. The lumen of the duct is opened and explored. Stones are removed as they are encountered.
3. Following removal of the stones, the duct is dilated and the sphincter of Oddi is calibrated.

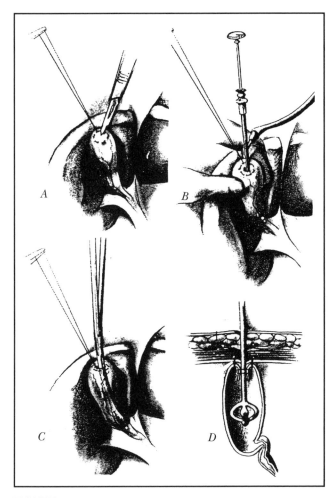

FIGURE 7-50 Cholecystotomy. (Schwartz, S. I. [1989]. *Principles of surgery* [5th ed.]. New York: McGraw-Hill. Reproduced with permission of McGraw-Hill.)

4. The ductal system is then irrigated with saline. The T tube is inserted and the duct is closed around the external limb of the tube with interrupted absorbable sutures. The T tube is brought through the abdominal wall and secured to the skin with nonabsorbable suture.

Cholecystotomy

When a person who is too debilitated to withstand a surgical procedure to remove the gallbladder is experiencing acute cholelithiasis with cholecystitis, the choice of treatment may be to open and drain the gallbladder. This is accomplished by inserting a drainage tube in the gallbladder and securing the tube with a purse-string suture.

Key steps

1. A purse-string suture is placed in the saclike portion of the gallbladder (Fig. 7-50,*A*).

2. Within the circle of the suture, a trocar is used to puncture the gallbladder and aspirate its contents (Fig. 7-50,*B*).
3. When stones are present, they may be removed by using stone forceps, scoops, or suction (Fig. 7-50,*C*).
4. A catheter is placed in the opening and secured with the purse-string suture. The catheter is brought through the abdominal wall and secured to the skin by a nonabsorbable suture (Fig. 7-50,*D*).

Choledochoduodenostomy (Fig. 7-51)

Obstruction of the common bile duct may be caused by calculi, tumor, or inflammatory lesions due to cholecystitis, pancreatitis, or sclerosing cholangitis (Braasch & Gasbarro, 1990). When bypass is necessary to correct this condition, the duodenum has frequently been used. A direct anastomosis can be made between the dilated, thick-walled portion of the common bile duct and the duodenum (Hoerr & Hermann, 1987).

Key steps

1. The obstructed common duct is located and dissected proximally.
2. A longitudinal opening is made in the common bile duct and the duodenum. The duct opening is pulled transversely to approximate to the longitudinal opening in the duodenum (Fig. 7-51,*A*).
3. The anastomosis is constructed as a single layer of through-and-through interrupted absorbable or nonabsorbable sutures. The posterior wall of the anastomosis is sutured (Fig. 7-51,*B*); then the anterior wall is sutured (Fig. 7-51,*C*).
4. When the completed anastomosis has a large diameter a stent is not necessary (Fig. 7-51,*D*). When it is small, the proximal duct may be stented with a T tube (Hoerr & Hermann, 1987).

Pancreatic Procedures

Pancreatic surgery is performed because of damage to the pancreas through inflammation and cyst formation, to remove tumors, or for indications that result in the destruction of pancreatic tissue, such as trauma.

Cysts or pseudocysts form when the pancreatic duct is disrupted and secretions leak into the surrounding tissue. This usually occurs as a result of chronic pancreatitis. To correct this situation, cysts may require a drainage procedure. When internal drainage is most desirable, the cyst may be anastomosed to an adjacent organ, either the stomach or the duodenum (Becker, 1992).

As chronic pancreatitis progresses, the pancreas becomes more hardened, smaller, and fibrotic. Once severe complications of chronic pancreatitis have developed, pancreaticojejunostomy may be considered (Silen & Steer, 1989). This procedure allows return of pancreatic juice to the intestine. With the patient in the supine position, an upper midline, paramedian, or subcostal incision is performed.

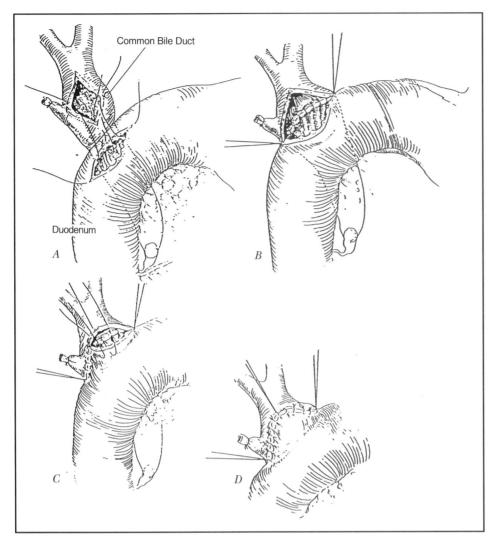

FIGURE 7-51 Choledocho-duodenostomy. (Gliedman, M. L., & Gold, M. S. [1989]. In S. I. Schwartz & H. Ellis [Eds.]. *Maingot's abdominal operations* [9th ed.]. Norwalk, CT: Appleton & Lange.)

Pancreaticojejunostomy (Fig. 7-52)

Key steps

1. A strip of pancreatic tissue is excised on the anterior surface of the pancreas. This groove extends from the head to the tail of the pancreas (Fig. 7-52,*A*).
2. Ductal stones are removed and strictures of the duct are released.
3. A limb of jejunum is brought to the anterior surface of the pancreas. Continuity of the intestine is established through jejunojejunostomy. A side-to-side anastomosis is completed between the limb of jejunum and the opened duct of the pancreas (Fig. 7-52,*B*).

Resections of the pancreas are performed for chronic pancreatitis in patients who have not benefited from a bypass procedure, or to remove tumor. Resections may include some or all of the pancreas, depending on the

FIGURE 7-52 Side-to-side pancreaticojejunostomy. (Braasch, J. W., & Rossi, R. L. [1982]. In O. H. Beahrs and R. W. Beart, Jr. [Eds.]. *General surgery: Therapy update service, Update 8.* New York: John Wiley & Sons.)

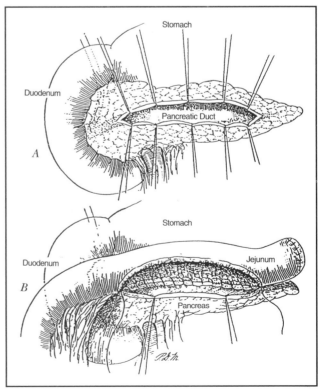

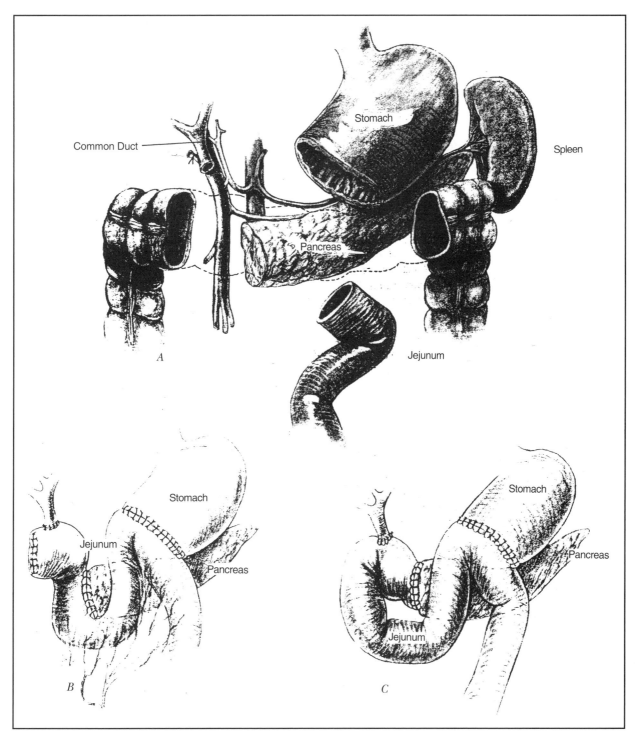

FIGURE 7-53   Pancreatoduodenectomy (Whipple procedure).   (Keith, R. [1987]. In J. H. Davis [Ed.]. *Clinical Surgery.* St. Louis: C. V. Mosby.)

extent of disease, status of the bile ducts, and previous pancreatic surgery. Surgery of the distal pancreas leaves a rim of pancreatic tissue attached to the duodenum and preserves the blood vessels and common duct. When the head of the pancreas is involved, the surgery becomes more complex (Keith, 1987). When tumor involves the head of the pancreas, the surgery also involves the biliary system, the duodenum, and both pancreatic ducts.

Pancreaticoduodenectomy

Removing the head of the pancreas for tumor is commonly referred to as the Whipple procedure. Because of the intricate ductal system and relationship to the duodenum, the surgery involves duodenectomy, partial gastrectomy, and partial removal of the jejunum and common duct (Fig. 7-53,*A*). Intestinal continuity and provision for drainage of the common bile duct must be established.

Key steps

1. The pancreatic head is exposed by dividing the gastrocolic ligament and mobilizing the transverse colon. The colon is deflected downward to provide exposure.
2. The peritoneum is incised along the pancreas, and the neck is freed from the superior mesenteric vessels and the portal vein. A Penrose drain may be placed around the neck of the pancreas to facilitate its manipulation.
3. The common bile duct is freed and encircled with a tape or Penrose drain. The duodenum is dissected free. The gastroduodenal artery is ligated and divided away from the hepatic artery.
4. The duodenum and head of the pancreas are mobilized, as is the first portion of the jejunum.
5. The stomach is mobilized by dissecting the gastrocolic ligaments. The stomach is divided by clamping or stapling. The proximal portion of the stomach is left intact.
6. After the stomach is divided, the distal portion is deflected. The duodenum and jejunum are divided.
7. The gallbladder is dissected and the junction of the cystic duct and the common bile duct is identified. The common duct is divided just above the junction of the cystic duct, leaving as much stump as possible for the anastomosis.
8. The pancreas is elevated away from underlying vessels. Sutures are placed on the superior and inferior margins of the pancreas on either side of the line of resection. The pancreas is transected, and sutures are placed on the pancreatic duct in preparation for pancreaticojejunostomy.
9. Gastrointestinal continuity is restored by creating an anastomosis of the common duct stump to the end of the jejunum. The remaining portion of pancreas and pancreatic duct are connected in side-to-side fashion. A more distal loop of jejunum is brought up to the level of the remaining portion of the stomach, and a gastrojejunostomy is created (Fig. 7-53,*B*).
10. An alternative approach is to connect the remaining pancreas to the end of the jejunum and an end-to-side anastomosis of the common duct to the jejunum. In this method, a loop of jejunum is used to create the gastrojejunostomy (Fig. 7-53,*C*).

Pancreatic transplantation

Pancreatic transplantation is performed as an attempt to achieve normal carbohydrate metabolism in patients with insulin-dependent diabetes mellitus (IDDM). Destruction of the pancreatic beta cells of the islets of Langerhans is thought to produce the characteristic decreased insulin production. Diabetes-related complications and insulin dependency result from hyperglycemia and other metabolic disturbances (Dafoe, 1991; Ball, 1986). The goal of transplantation is to provide functioning beta cells, thereby eliminating the need for insulin administration, and stopping or slowing the progression of diabetic complications (Brayman, Najarian, & Sutherland, 1992).

Transplantation of a functioning islet cell mass, either as a vascularized pancreas graft or as a particulate graft of islets, has been performed in an effort to restore normal glucose metabolism. Whole pancreatic transplants are preferred to segmental grafts (tail of pancreas) because of the higher success rate. They are preferred also to avoid placing related living donors at risk of surgery and of developing diabetes in the future. Because the transplant recipient often has developed end-stage renal failure, a kidney transplant may be performed in conjunction with the pancreatic procedure (Dafoe, 1991).

One of the problems associated with pancreatic transplantation has been the management of the pancreatic duct. Because the duct secretes digestive and proenzyme secretions, autodigestion of surrounding tissue can occur. The methods utilized to manage the duct include external drainage through a fistula to the skin, ligation of the duct, free intraperitoneal drainage, injection of polymer to occlude the duct, and drainage into the intestine (Mittal & Toledo-Pereyra, 1986). The method most preferred is use of donor duodenum as a conduit to drain the secretions into the urinary bladder. This technique appears to be the most successful, and it provides a method of determining graft dysfunction through urine amylase measurement (Brayman et al., 1992).

The criteria for selection of cadaver pancreas donors include the general considerations for any organ donation. In addition, the donor must have no history of glucose intolerance, infection, malignancy, or significant hyperamylasemia. The preferred technique is perfusion in situ with cold preservation solution and a maximum 24 hours' cold storage time (Dafoe, 1991).

The donor pancreas (Fig. 7-54) is dissected with the duodenum, the gastroduodenal artery, and the spleen intact. It is then prepared for grafting. Arterial grafts may be used to lengthen the arterial components of the allograft, for ease in reconstructing arterial supply at the time of transplantation (Brayman et al., 1992).

Whole pancreatic transplantation   The operation is performed through a midline incision. A separate back table is set up for preparation of the graft. Vascular instruments, vascular suture, intestinal instruments, sterile slush, culture tubes, heparinized saline, and antibiotics for intraoperative use are available.

Key steps

1. The right common, internal, and external iliac arteries and veins and the right ureter are mobilized. The cecum is mobilized as necessary for ureteral and vessel exposure. All posterior branches of the common and external iliac veins are ligated and divided, including the internal iliac vein.
2. The urinary bladder is mobilized.
3. Following systemic heparinization, the venous anastomosis is performed by end-to-side connection of the portal vein to the external iliac vein.
4. The arterial anastomosis involves connecting a patch of aorta containing the celiac axis and the superior mesenteric artery to the external iliac artery or by us-

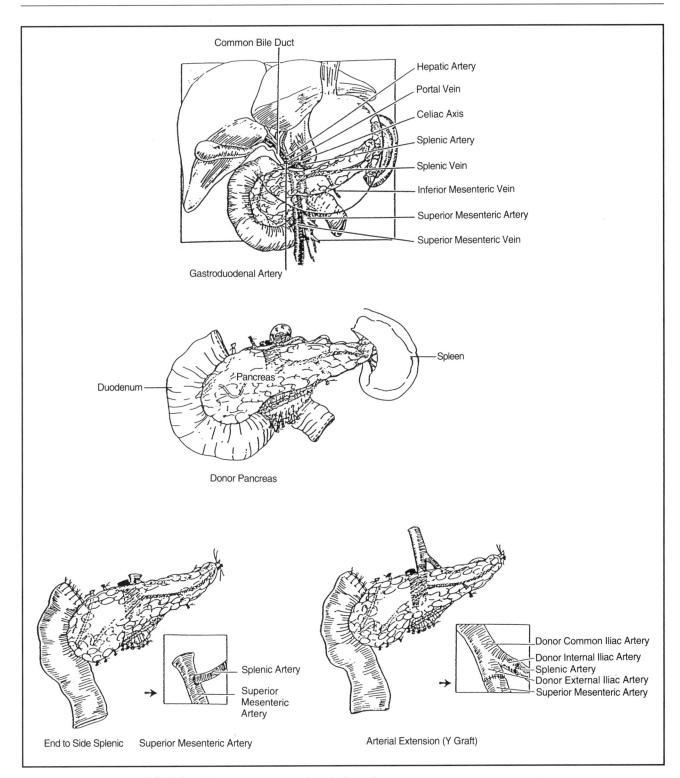

FIGURE 7-54   Pancreaticoduodenal allograft.   (Brayman, K. L., Najarian, J. S., &
Sutherland, D. E. R. [1992]. In J. L. Cameron [Ed.]. *Current surgical therapy.* St. Louis:
Mosby–Year Book.)

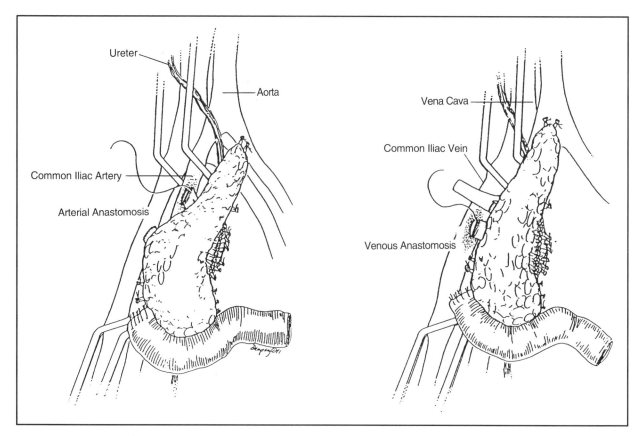

FIGURE 7-55 Revascularization of the pancreaticoduodenal allograft.
(Brayman, K. L., Najarian, J. S., & Sutherland, D. E. R. [1992]. In J. L. Cameron [Ed.].
Current surgical therapy. St. Louis: Mosby–Year Book.)

ing the common iliac artery of the vascular graft (Fig. 7-55).

5. The anastomosis between the duodenal segment and the urinary bladder can be hand sewn, or a circular stapler can be used (Fig. 7-56).
6. Following the completion of the anastomosis, the cystotomy is closed in layers with absorbable suture.
7. The operative area may be drained by a closed wound system.

When the pancreatic transplant functions well, the recipient no longer requires insulin. The patient may return to a liberal diet and realize control of diabetes complications. The patient may experience psychological as well as physiological benefits.

Small Intestine Procedures

Small intestine resection

Key steps

1. The extent of the resection is determined.
2. The mesentery is ligated with ties, suture ligature, clips, or staples and is divided.
3. The small intestine is transected, and the specimen is removed.
4. The ends of the small intestine are anastomosed end-to-end or side-to-side using sutures or staples.

Stricturoplasty

Inflammatory processes may cause scarring and resultant narrowing in the lumen of the intestine. When this occurs in the small intestine, care is taken to avoid unnecessary resection, lest the nutritional function of the small intestine be impaired. When narrowing occurs as a result of a benign process, stricturoplasty is an alternative to resection.

Key steps

1. The area of stricture is identified. A longitudinal incision is made over the stricture. This involves the layers of the anterior wall of the bowel (Fig. 7-57,*A*).
2. The layers of the anterior wall of the bowel are closed in a horizontal fashion by placing a single layer of absorbable or nonabsorbable suture (Fig. 7-57,*B*).

Ileostomy

An ileostomy is created to divert intestinal flow. An end ileostomy is constructed as a permanent measure for treatment of inflammatory bowel disease; a loop ileostomy may be a temporary measure to protect an anastomosis or to allow healing of distal disease.

The ideal stoma site must be determined preoperatively, as proper location is essential to rehabilitation of the patient. At the completion of the procedure, the skin

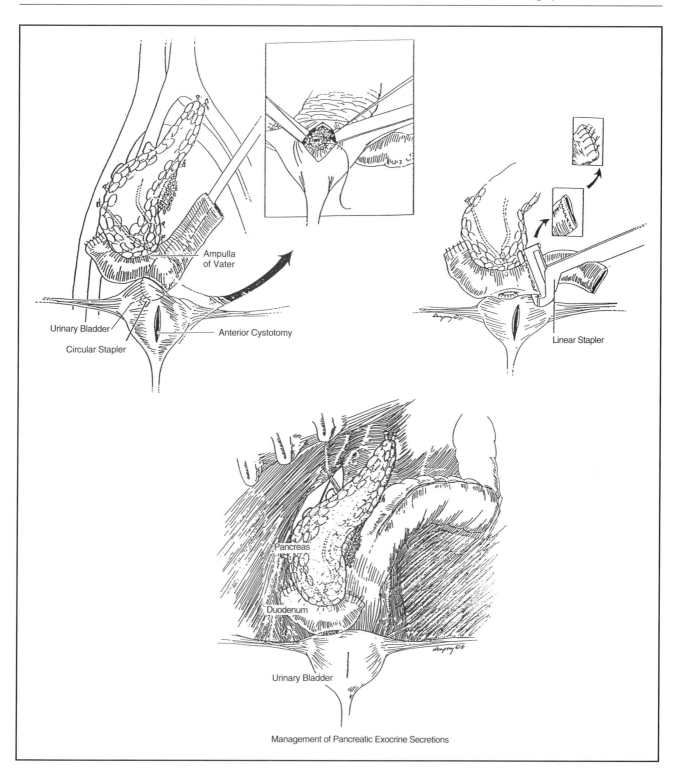

Ampulla
of Vater

Urinary Bladder

Circular Stapler

Anterior Cystotomy

Linear Stapler

Pancreas

Duodenum

Urinary Bladder

Management of Pancreatic Exocrine Secretions

FIGURE 7-56 Pancreaticoduodenocystostomy. (Brayman, K. L., Najarian, J. S., & Sutherland, D. E. R. [1992]. In J. L. Cameron [Ed.]. *Current surgical therapy.* St. Louis: Mosby–Year Book.)

is protected by a skin barrier and a simple, drainable pouch. The pouch should be held in position over the stoma by taping the edge of the pouch to the abdomen in picture-frame fashion using nonallergenic tape. The pouch should be directed to the side, as the patient will be in bed most of the time during the immediate postop-

erative period, and this arrangement is more comfortable and facilitates drainage of the pouch (Kodner, 1978).

End ileostomy (Fig. 7-58,A)
Key steps

1. A circular incision is made at the stoma site, and a disk of skin is excised.
2. The layers of the abdominal wall are incised down to the fascial layer. The peritoneum is incised to provide

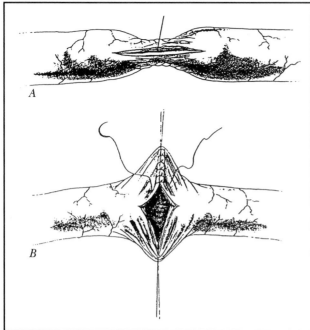

FIGURE 7-57 Stricturoplasty of the small intestine. (Corman, M. L. [1987]. *Colon and rectal surgery.* Philadelphia: J. B. Lippincott.)

access for the end of the ileum to be brought through the abdominal wall after the ileum has been divided.

3. The end of the ileum with its mesentery is delivered through the stoma site, and the mesentery is sutured to the peritoneum with running or interrupted sutures.

4. The mesentery is then transected flush with the abdominal wall by clamping, incising, and suturing.

5. A circumferential row of interrupted sutures is placed between the seromuscular layer of intestine and subcutaneous tissue, isolating the stoma from the abdominal cavity and fixing its position and length.

6. The stump of the intestine is resected, leaving a 6-cm length of bowel that can be nourished by the subserosal vessels.

7. Sutures are placed through full-thickness bowel and skin. The bowel is everted and the sutures are secured.

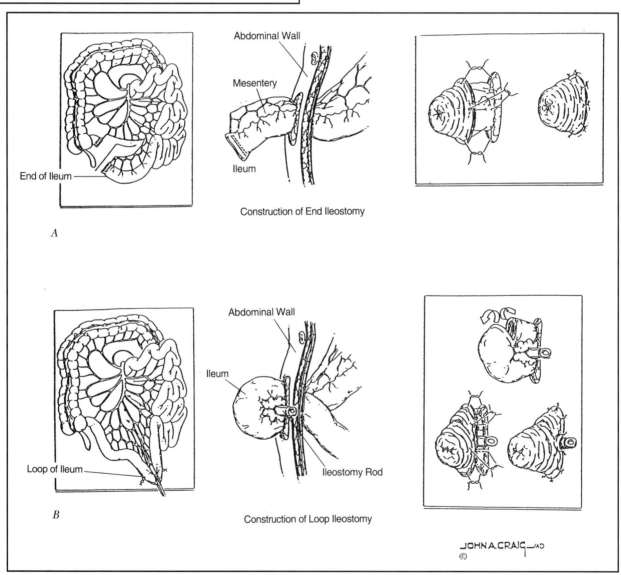

FIGURE 7-58 Construction of an ileostomy (end and loop). (Kodner, I. J., Fry, R. D., & Fleshman, J. W. [1989]. In S. I. Schwartz and H. Ellis [Eds.]. *Maingot's abdominal operations* [9th ed.]. Norwalk, CT: Appleton & Lange.)

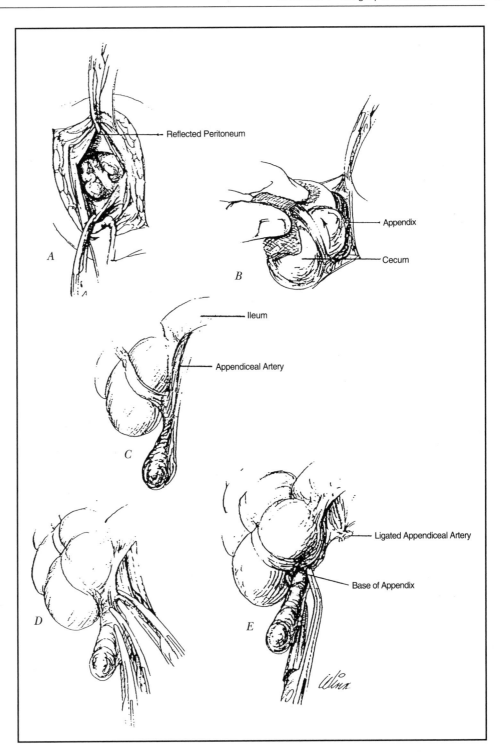

FIGURE 7-59 Appendectomy. (Lewis, F. [1987]. In J. H. Davis [Ed.]. *Clinical surgery*. St. Louis: C. V. Mosby.)

Loop ileostomy (Fig. 7-58,B)
Key steps

1. A loop of small intestine is brought through the stoma site.
2. The intestine is opened circumferentially, about 0.5 cm above the abdominal wall.
3. Sutures are placed between full-thickness bowel and dermis. The sutures are gently drawn taut, everting the bowel over a supporting rod.
4. A pouch may be fitted directly over the rod.

Appendiceal Procedures

Appendectomy (Fig. 7-59)

Appendicitis is the most common indication for removal of the appendix, though this surgery may be performed for tumors, such as carcinoid or adenocarcinoma. The appendix may be involved in inflammatory diseases of the cecum and ileum such as tuberculosis, typhoid fever, or Crohn's disease (Schwartz, 1989a).

Key steps

1. A transverse, midline, or McBurney's incision is made, and the peritoneum is reflected (Fig. 7-59,*A*).
2. Once the appendix is exposed (Fig. 7-59,*B, C*), the mesentery is transected beginning at its free border by taking small bits of tissue between pairs of hemostats.
3. When the appendix is freed, a crushing clamp is applied to the base of the appendix and then is moved distally, so that a ligature may be placed in the resulting groove (Fig. 7-59,*D*).
4. The appendix is transected, and the appendiceal stump may be ligated or inverted by placing a purse-string suture through the seromuscular layers of the cecum (Fig. 7-59,*E*).

Laparoscopic appendectomy

Key steps

1. Following establishment of pneumoperitoneum, a 10-mm trocar is placed through the midline adjacent to the umbilicus. In addition, an 11-mm trocar is placed in the right upper quadrant and the left lower quadrant.
2. The patient is placed in Trendelenburg's position, and the intestine is gently pushed out of the pelvis.
3. The appendix is grasped at its margin adjacent to the cecum.
4. A dissecting instrument is used to identify two open spaces in the immediate appendiceal mesentery.
5. Two reinforced clips are applied to the inflamed appendiceal stump.
6. The distal appendix is incised with the laser or electrocautery.
7. Once the appendix is freed, it is drawn through a 10-mm reducing sleeve or delivered through the 11-mm trocar in the left lower quadrant.
8. The fascial layer is closed, the carbon dioxide is evacuated, and all trocars are removed. The skin is approximated with suture, and puncture sites are covered with dressings (Schultz et al., 1991).

Colon and Rectal Procedures

Colon resection

A colon resection can be limited (wedge resection) or segmental (right, transverse, left), or it can involve the entire colon (subtotal or total). Indications for resection include tumors (benign or malignant), volvulus, ischemic processes, and inflammatory processes. The area of resection is determined by location of disease and the blood supply to the involved portion of the colon (Fig. 7-60). For resections not involving the left colon or upper rectum, a supine position is used. The surgery may be performed through paramedian, midline, or transverse incisions. Intestinal instruments are available as well as staplers or intestinal suture for anastomosis.

Key steps

1. The extent of resection is determined.
2. The main artery supplying the segment of colon to be removed is ligated and divided.
3. The mesentery is resected in continuity with the bowel.
4. The bowel is divided and the resected specimen is removed.
5. Intestinal continuity is reestablished by suturing or stapling the anastomosis.
6. The mesenteric defect is closed with running long-lasting absorbable sutures.

Laparoscopic colon resection

Colon resection is being performed more frequently with laparoscopic techniques. The surgical principles for colon resection apply to laparoscopic surgery. The variation of technique lies in choosing an intracorporeal or extracorporeal anastomosis.

Key steps

1. Following creation of pneumoperitoneum, three to four cannulas are inserted. This is determined by the site of resection and the patient's body habitus (body size). The camera is introduced through the infraumbilical site.
2. Dissection along the lateral avascular colon attachments is completed.
3. The ureter is identified.
4. Mobilization of the colon is completed. When the anastomosis is to be completed extracorporeally, a small abdominal incision is made. The mobilized colon is delivered through the incision, and the anastomosis is completed (Corbitt, 1992).
5. When the anastomosis is to be completed intracorporeally, the proximal portion of the bowel is divided first by an intraabdominal stapler. The distal portion is divided, and the specimen is placed immediately in a bag. When the anastomosis is completed below the peritoneal reflection, the specimen is removed through the anus. In other cases, the specimen is removed through the umbilical incision.
6. A transanal anastomosis can be accomplished by delivering the anvil of a circular stapler to the proximal limb of the anastomosis through the umbilical incision. Pneumoperitoneum is reestablished. The stapler is introduced through the anus and coupled with the anvil intraabdominally (Redwine & Sharpe, 1991).

Low anterior resection of rectum

When rectal disease requires a low resection, the anastomosis occurs deep in the pelvis (Fig. 7-61). The connection may even involve anastomosis of colon to anus. When coloanal anastomosis is established, a temporary colostomy is often constructed to protect this connection (Fig. 7-62).

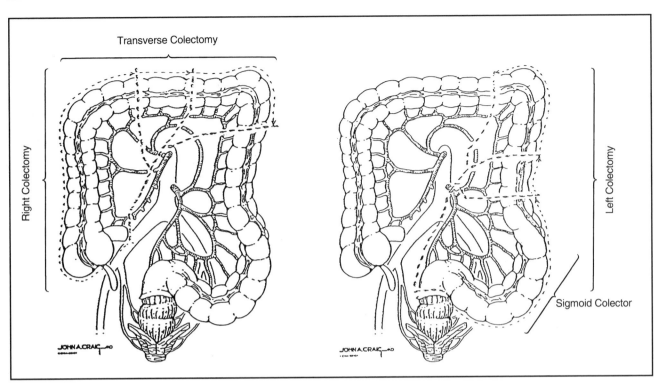

FIGURE 7-60 Resections of the colon. (Kodner, I. J., Fry, R. D., Fleshman, J. W., & Birnbaum, E. H. [1993]. In S. I. Schwartz [Ed.]. *Principles of surgery.* New York: McGraw-Hill. Reprinted with permission of McGraw-Hill.)

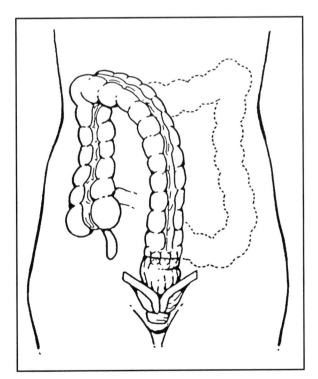

FIGURE 7-61 Low anterior resection. (Kodner, I. J., Fry, R. D., Fleshman, J. W., & Birnbaum, E. H. [1993]. In S. I. Schwartz [Ed.]. *Principles of surgery.* New York: McGraw-Hill. Reprinted with permission of McGraw-Hill.)

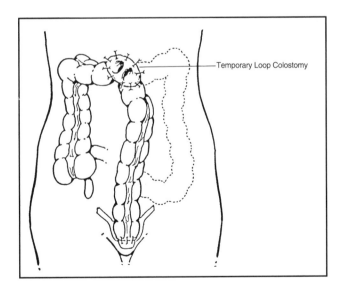

FIGURE 7-62 Coloanal anastomosis. (Kodner, I. J., Fry, R. D., Fleshman, J. W., & Birnbaum, E. H. [1993]. In S. I. Schwartz [Ed.]. *Principles of surgery.* New York: McGraw-Hill. Reprinted with permission of McGraw-Hill.)

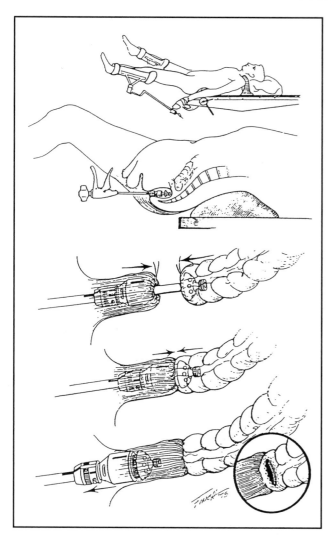

FIGURE 7-63 Transanal end-to-end anastomosis. (Goldberg, S. M., Gordon, P. H., & Nivatvongs, S. [1980]. *Essentials of anorectal surgery.* Philadelphia, PA: J. B. Lippincott. Reprinted with permission of S. M. Goldberg.)

These anastomoses are accomplished transanally. The patient is positioned in a "modified" lithotomy position, to provide access to the perineum. A circular stapler may be introduced transanally (Fig. 7-63).

Hartmann's resection

When an anastomosis cannot be constructed for reasons such as inflammation, debilitation, tumor fixation, or body habitus (size) of the patient, Hartmann's resection may be performed. This involves resection of the diseased portion of colon and construction of an end colostomy. This leaves the patient with a rectal stump that can be permanent or can be reconnected to the colon later (Fig. 7-64).

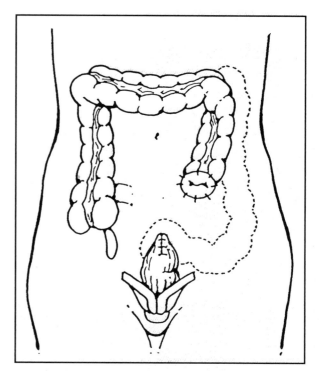

FIGURE 7-64 Hartmann's resection. (Kodner, I. J., Fry, R. D., Fleshman, J. W., & Birnbaum, E. H. [1993]. In S. I. Schwartz [Ed.]. *Principles of surgery.* New York: McGraw-Hill. Reprinted with permission of McGraw-Hill.)

Colostomy

A colostomy is constructed to treat malignant or benign disease of the colon or rectum. It can be a temporary measure to divert colonic flow or to decompress the colon. The temporary colostomy is usually a loop stoma constructed in the midtransverse colon. A permanent end colostomy is constructed of descending colon when the rectum must be removed (Kodner, 1978). The site of the colostomy is determined preoperatively. A pouching system should be available to apply over the stoma at the end of the operative procedure.

***End colostomy* (Fig. 7-65,A)**
Key steps

1. The left colon is mobilized to allow the stoma site to be brought to the anterior abdominal wall.
2. The colon is divided, and the proximal end is brought to the anterior abdominal wall through the site for the stoma.
3. The mesentery of the left colon may be fixed to the abdominal wall with a running nonabsorbable suture, thus closing the defect to the level of the stoma.
4. The colostomy is constructed by suturing the full thickness of bowel to the full thickness of skin with absorbable suture.
5. A pouch is applied over the stoma after the construction is complete.

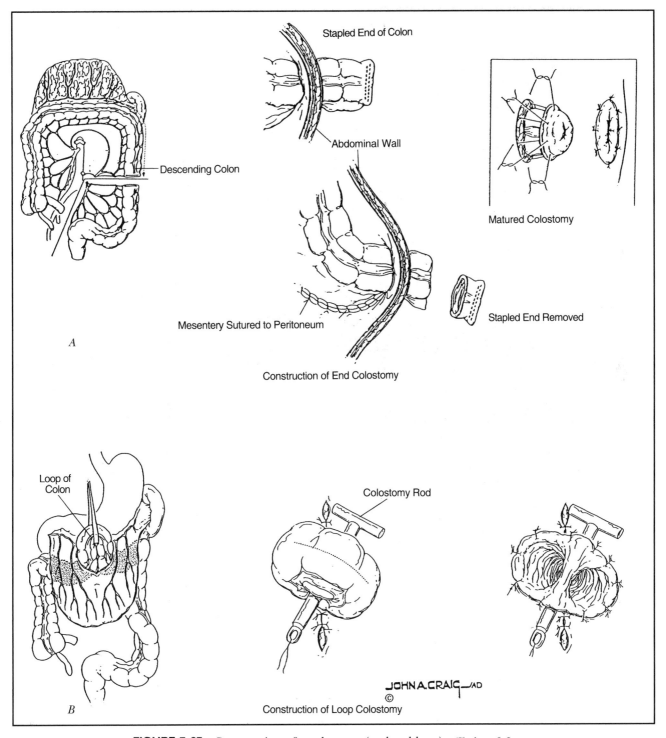

Stapled End of Colon

Abdominal Wall

Descending Colon

Matured Colostomy

Mesentery Sutured to Peritoneum

Stapled End Removed

A

Construction of End Colostomy

Loop of Colon

Colostomy Rod

JOHN A. CRAIG—AD
©

B

Construction of Loop Colostomy

FIGURE 7-65 Construction of a colostomy (end and loop). (Kodner, I. J., Fry, R. D., & Fleshman, J. W. [1989]. In S. I. Schwartz & H. Ellis [Eds.]. *Maingot's abdominal operations* [9th ed.]. Norwalk, CT: Appleton & Lange.)

Loop colostomy (Fig. 7-65,*B*)
Key steps

1. A loop of transverse colon is brought through the greater omentum and abdominal wall.
2. The abdominal wall and skin are closed snugly around the colon, and a rod is placed to provide support under the loop of the bowel.
3. The colon is opened in a direction that allows the widest separation of functional and nonfunctional limbs.
4. The colon is opened and the stoma is fashioned by suturing full-thickness bowel to full-thickness skin with absorbable sutures.
5. A pouch is applied over the stoma and rod when the construction is complete.

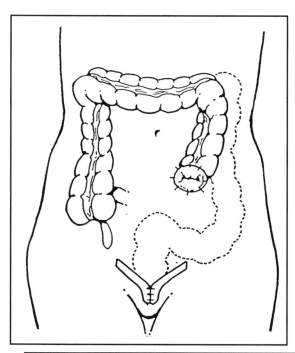

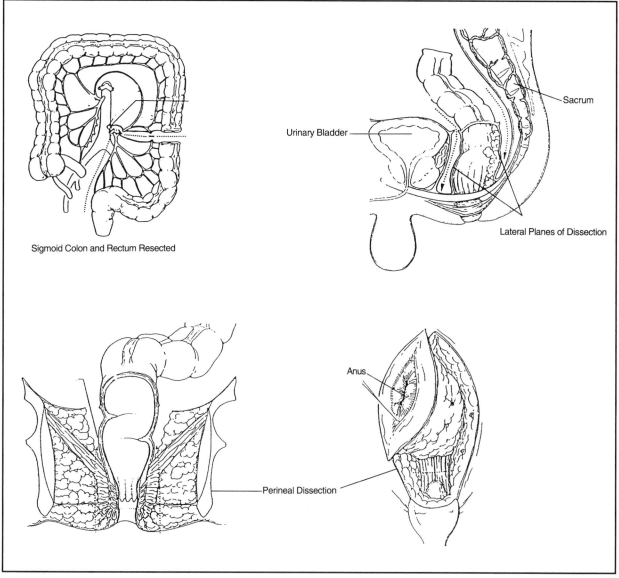

FIGURE 7-66 Abdominal perineal proctectomy. (Kodner, I. J., Fry, R. D., Fleshman, J. W., & Birnbaum, E. H. [1993]. In S. I. Schwartz [Ed.]. *Principles of surgery.* New York: McGraw-Hill. Reprinted with permission of McGraw-Hill.)

FIGURE 7-67 Areas of dissection for abdominal perineal proctectomy. (Kodner, I. J., Fry, R. D., & Fleshman, J. W. [1989]. In S. I. Schwartz & H. Ellis [Eds.]. *Maingot's abdominal operations.* Norwalk, CT: Appleton & Lange.)

Sigmoid Colon and Rectum Resected

Sacrum

Urinary Bladder

Lateral Planes of Dissection

Perineal Dissection

Anus

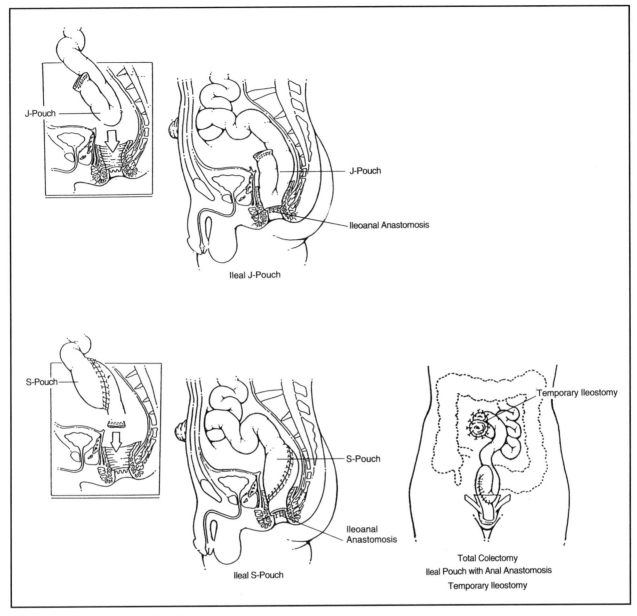

FIGURE 7-68 Restorative proctocolectomy. (Kodner, I. J., Fry, R. D., & Fleshman, J. W. In S. I. Schwartz & H. Ellis [Eds.]. *Maingot's abdominal operations.* Norwalk, CT: Appleton & Lange.)

Abdominal perineal proctectomy (Fig. 7-66)

This proctectomy is performed through combined abdominal and perineal approaches. When the rectum must be removed, it is necessary to divert fecal flow by means of a permanent colostomy. This operation may involve two surgical teams, one performing the abdominal portion and a second performing the perineal portion simultaneously. Two complete instrument setups may be required.

Key steps

1. The left colon is mobilized.
2. A site for the colostomy is determined and the colon is transected. The colon is closed securely, to avoid fecal

contamination during the rectal dissection. This may be accomplished with ties, clamps, or staplers.
3. The rectum is dissected down to the level of the anal sphincters (Fig. 7-67).
4. The perineal incision is made, and the rectum is removed.
5. Abdominal and perineal incisions are closed.
6. The colostomy is created.

Ileal pouch (Fig. 7-68)

The ileal pouch operation is designed to avoid a permanent stoma in patients who have ulcerative colitis or familial polyposis. The intent is to remove the diseased colon, preserve the anal sphincters, and construct a "neorectum" of small intestine (Kodner et al., 1993).

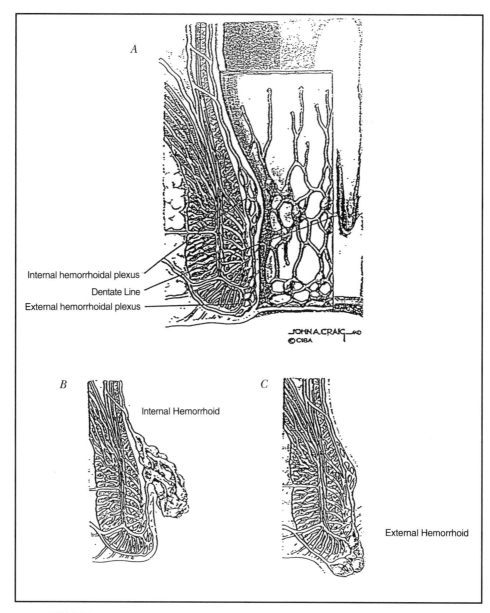

FIGURE 7-69 (*A*) The vascular plexus in relation to the dentate line. (*B*) Internal hemorrhoid. (*C*) External hemorrhoid. (Fry, R. D., & Kodner, I. J. [1985]. *Anorectal disorders.* © 1985 CIBA-GEIGY Corporation. Reprinted with permission from CLINICAL SYMPOSIA, illustrated by John A. Craig, M.D. All rights reserved.)

Key steps

1. The entire colon is mobilized, and major arteries are divided and ligated. The colon is resected down to the proximal rectum.
2. Care is taken to preserve the ileum and its blood supply.
3. The mucosa of the rectum is removed, preserving the pelvic musculature.
4. A pouch is constructed of ileum, taking either an S or a J configuration.
5. The pouch is then placed low in the pelvis, and the distal ileum is anastomosed to the anus with absorbable suture.
6. A temporary ileostomy is constructed to protect the pouch during the healing process (Kodner et al., 1993).

Anal Procedures

Hemorrhoidectomy

Hemorrhoidal tissue is found at the distal end of the rectum within the anal canal (Fig. 7-69). These vascular and connective tissue cushions are usually found in the right anterolateral, posterolateral, and the left lateral position. Internal hemorrhoids are above the dentate line; external hemorrhoids are the vascular complexes under

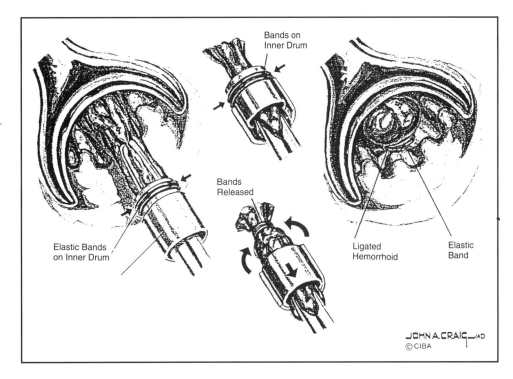

Bands on Inner Drum

Bands Released

Elastic Bands on Inner Drum

Ligated Hemorrhoid

Elastic Band

JOHN A. CRAIG AD
© CIBA

the skin of the anal canal. The function of normal hemorrhoidal tissue is to protect the underlying muscle during defecation and to allow complete closure of the anal canal during rest (Fry & Kodner, 1985).

The pathophysiology of symptomatic hemorrhoids is related to the engorgement of the hemorrhoidal vessels with blood. These vessels then dilate and stretch, causing the tissue to enlarge with straining, lifting, or standing. Bleeding occurs from local trauma to the hemorrhoid complex, usually during defecation (Kodner et al., 1993).

Elastic ligation (Fig. 7-70)

Key steps

1. The internal hemorrhoid is grasped and pulled into the cylinder of a rubber band applicator.
2. The rubber bands are placed at the base of the hemorrhoidal tissue.
3. The rubber bands fall off after 5 to 10 days with tissue necrosis and sloughing. A scar forms in the area of the vascular pedicle (Fry & Kodner, 1985).

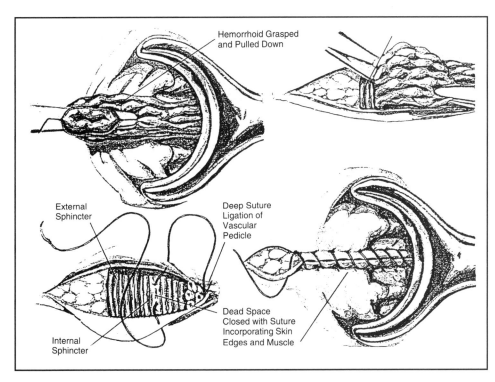

Hemorrhoid Grasped and Pulled Down

External Sphincter

Deep Suture Ligation of Vascular Pedicle

Dead Space Closed with Suture Incorporating Skin Edges and Muscle

Internal Sphincter

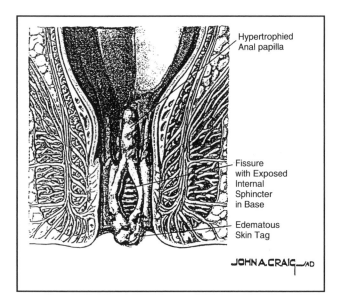

Hypertrophied
Anal papilla

Fissure
with Exposed
Internal
Sphincter
in Base

Edematous
Skin Tag

JOHN A. CRAIG ˍᴀᴅ

FIGURE 7-72 Anal fissure. (Fry, R. D., & Kodner, I. J. [1985]. *Anorectal disorders.* © 1985 CIBA-GEIGY Corporation. Reprinted with permission from CLINICAL SYMPOSIA, illustrated by John A. Craig, M.D. All rights reserved.)

3. The mucosal defect is then closed with a running absorbable suture.
4. Hemostasis is obtained with this suture, the laser, or electrocautery (Fry & Kodner, 1985).

An anal sphincterotomy is an incision into the lower third of the internal anal sphincter. This is done to relieve sphincter spasm in treatment of anal fissure (Fig. 7-72) or ulcer, or in conjunction with hemorrhoidectomy (Fry & Kodner, 1985).

Excisional hemorrhoidectomy (Fig. 7-71)

Key steps

1. A scalpel, scissors, laser, or electrocautery is used to elliptically incise the external and internal portions of hemorrhoidal tissue.
2. The incision avoids the underlying internal sphincter muscle as the hemorrhoid is dissected from the surface of the muscle.

Anal sphincterotomy (Fig. 7-73)

Key steps

1. An incision is made laterally to the anus.
2. The lower one third of the anal sphincter is pulled up through the incision and divided with a knife or electrocautery.
3. Bleeding is controlled by electrocautery, and the incision is left open.

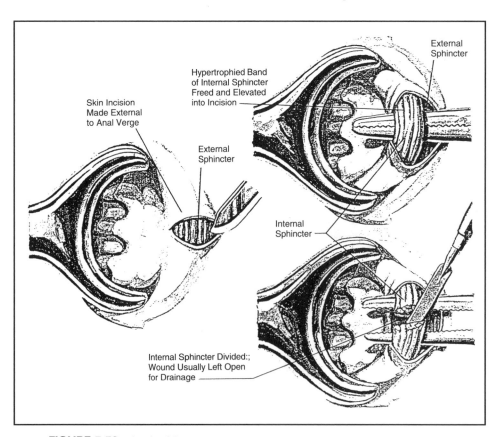

Skin Incision
Made External
to Anal Verge

Hypertrophied Band
of Internal Sphincter
Freed and Elevated
into Incision

External
Sphincter

External
Sphincter

Internal
Sphincter

Internal Sphincter Divided:;
Wound Usually Left Open
for Drainage

FIGURE 7-73 Anal sphincterotomy. (Fry, R. D., & Kodner, I. J. [1985]. *Anorectal disorders.* © 1985 CIBA-GEIGY Corporation. Reprinted with permission from CLINICAL SYMPOSIA, illustrated by John A. Craig, M.D. All rights reserved.)

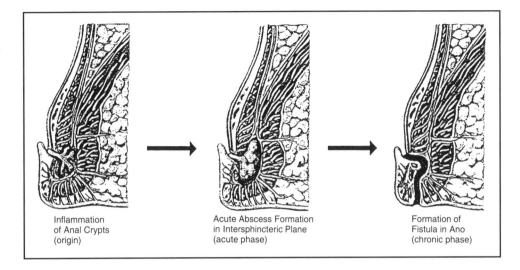

Inflammation of Anal Crypts (origin)

Acute Abscess Formation in Intersphincteric Plane (acute phase)

Formation of Fistula in Ano (chronic phase)

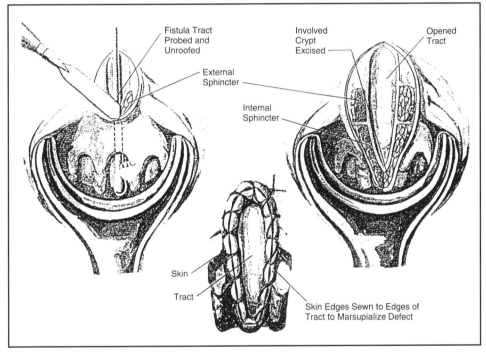

Fistula Tract Probed and Unroofed

External Sphincter

Internal Sphincter

Involved Crypt Excised

Opened Tract

Skin

Tract

Skin Edges Sewn to Edges of Tract to Marsupialize Defect

Drainage of anorectal abscess

Acute infection of an anal gland leads to an anorectal abscess. The anal glands lie in the space between the muscle layers of the anal canal and empty into anal crypts at the level of the dentate line. This infection leads to the formation of a local abscess in the area between the sphincter muscles. As the abscess enlarges, it spreads in one of several possible directions to form a perianal abscess. This can involve the space between the muscles or can expand into the fat of the soft tissue. Acute abscesses are operated upon immediately (Fry & Kodner, 1985).

Key steps

1. The abscess is identified by digital examination.
2. The abscess is drained by placing a drain through a skin incision.

A perianal abscess may be resolved through drainage alone, or it can form a fistula in the anal canal (Fig. 7-74). This fistula consists of a chronically infected tract with an internal opening located in the rectum and an external opening located at the drainage site of the earlier abscess. Treatment depends on the location of the tract (Fry & Kodner, 1985).

Anal fistulotomy (Fig. 7-75)

An anal fistulotomy is one component of the procedure. It can be accompanied by placement of additional drains in the areas of extension of the fistula (Fry & Kodner, 1985). Anorectal probes (Fig. 7-76) are used to identify the tract.

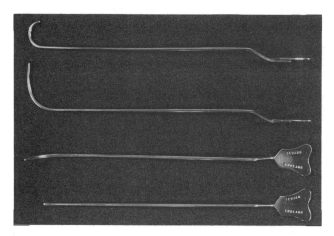

Figure 7-76 Anorectal probes.

Key steps

1. The fistula tract is identified by placing a probe from the external opening in the skin to the internal opening in the mucosa of the rectum.
2. The tissue overlying the probe is then incised.
3. The involved anal crypt is excised, and the tract is opened.
4. The fistula may be left open to heal by excising the skin edges, or the skin edges may be sewn to the edges of the tract (marsupialization).

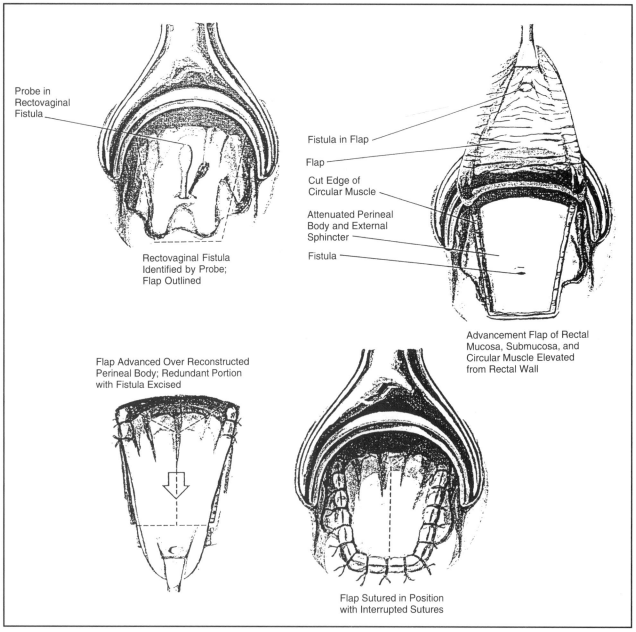

Probe in Rectovaginal Fistula

Rectovaginal Fistula Identified by Probe; Flap Outlined

Fistula in Flap

Flap

Cut Edge of Circular Muscle

Attenuated Perineal Body and External Sphincter

Fistula

Advancement Flap of Rectal Mucosa, Submucosa, and Circular Muscle Elevated from Rectal Wall

Flap Advanced Over Reconstructed Perineal Body; Redundant Portion with Fistula Excised

Flap Sutured in Position with Interrupted Sutures

FIGURE 7-77 Sliding flap repair of rectovaginal fistula. (Fry, R. D., & Kodner, I. J. [1985]. *Anorectal disorders.* © 1985 CIBA-GEIGY Corporation. Reprinted with permission from CLINICAL SYMPOSIA, illustrated by John A. Craig, M.D. All rights reserved.)

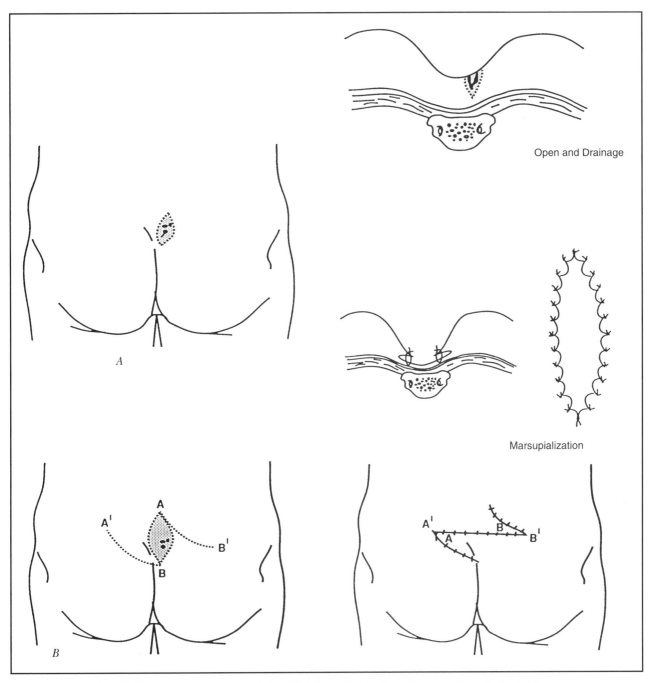

Open and Drainage

Marsupialization

FIGURE 7-78 (*A*) Excision of pilonidal sinus. (*B*) Z-plasty for complicated pilonidal disease. (Karulf, R. E. [1992]. In D. E. Beck and S. D. Wexner. *Fundamentals of anorectal surgery.* New York: McGraw-Hill. Reproduced with permission of McGraw-Hill.)

Sliding flap repair of anorectal or rectovaginal fistula (Fig. 7-77)

A rectovaginal or anorectal fistula may be repaired by sliding a flap of rectal mucosa to cover the internal fistula opening. Preoperative bowel preparation is necessary to enhance healing of the flap (Fry & Kodner, 1985).

Key steps

1. Exposure is gained using an operating anoscope.
2. An anorectal advancement flap consisting of mucosa, submucosa, and circular muscle is created, including

the rectal opening of the fistula in the flap.
3. The flap is advanced over the defect, and the apex of the flap containing the fistulous defect is excised.
4. The perineum is reconstructed with absorbable sutures. The flap is sutured in place.

Excision and drainage of pilonidal sinus (Fig. 7-78,*A*)

A pilonidal cyst is a hair-containing sinus or abscess that involves the skin and subcutaneous tissues in the area of the sacrum, between the buttocks. The sinus is superficial to the fascia overlying the sacrum and may be single or have multiple fistulous extensions. When the sinus is infected, it is treated with a drainage procedure (Karulf, 1992).

Key steps

1. The sinus is identified by placing a probe along the infected tract.
2. The tissue above the probe is incised, and the tract is curretted to remove the infected tissue and hair.
3. The tissue is left open for secondary healing or is excised and the wound closed primarily.

When the pilonidal disease is extensive or recurrent, this treatment may not be effective. Excision of the sinus followed by a Z-plasty to obliterate the intergluteal cleft has been utilized to eliminate complicated recurrent pilonidal disease (Fig. 7-78,*B*) (Karulf, 1992).

SUMMARY

For abdominal surgery, the desired outcome includes not only a favorable result from the surgery in terms of repair or excision, but the physiological and psychological aspects as well. According to AORN Standards, surgical patients share expected outcomes. When determining expected outcomes for each patient, the statements must be individualized to ensure continuity of care. Specific outcomes for abdominal surgery patients may include the following:

* The patient is free from infection.
* Fluid and electrolyte balances are maintained or corrected.
* The patient is free from injury related to positioning.
* The patient shows no signs or symptoms of hypothermia.
* Skin integrity is maintained.
* Adequate gas exchange is maintained.
* Nutrition and immunity are maintained or improved.
* The bowel elimination pattern is restored.

Outcomes that may be evaluated later in the postoperative phase may include the following:

* The patient is free from pain related to physiological disturbance.
* Nutritional status is improved.
* The patient returns to a normal level of activity and self-care.
* The sleep cycle is restored.
* The patient accepts the change in body image.

The evaluation of patient outcomes reflects not only the patient's ability to adapt to changes but also the ability

of the perioperative nurse to individualize patient care within the scope of responsibility.

The wide scope of desired patient outcomes following "abdominal" surgery (this chapter) reflects the broad scope of this specialty and the large areas of the body involved.

This chapter discussed pertinent information that the perioperative nurse must know to provide effective patient care: anatomy, preparation of the patient, special considerations, and procedural steps of the surgeries.

Abdominal surgery is often referred to as "general" surgery, but general surgery is now more often referred to as a specialty in and of itself.

REFERENCES

Association of Operating Room Nurses (1994). *AORN standards and recommended practices.* Denver: Author.

Bagnato, V. J. (1992). Laparoscopic Nissen fundoplication. *Surgical Laparoscopy and Endoscopy, 2,* 188–196.

Ball, P. (1986). Pancreatic transplantation: Perioperative nursing care. *AORN Journal, 43,* 632–637.

Becker, J. M. (1992). Pancreatic pseudocysts. In J. L. Cameron (Ed.). *Current surgical therapy* (pp. 423–426). St. Louis: Mosby–Year Book.

Beckermann, S., & Galloway, S. (1989). Elective resection of the liver: Nursing care. *Critical Care Nurse, 9,* 41–47.

Braasch, J. W., & Gasbarro, K. A. (1990). Fibrous bile duct obstructions: Diagnosis, treatment, prognosis. *AORN Journal, 52,* 818–826.

Braasch, J. W., & Rossi, R. L. (1982). Liver, gallbladder, biliary tract, pancreas and spleen. In O. H. Beahrs and R. W. Beart (Eds.). *General surgery: Therapy update service, update 8.* New York: John Wiley & Sons.

Brayman, K. L., Najarian, J. S., & Sutherland, D. E. R. (1992). Transplantation of the pancreas. In J. L. Cameron (Ed.). *Current surgical therapy* (pp. 458–475). St. Louis: Mosby–Year Book.

Broadwell, D. B., & Jackson, B. S. (1982). *Principles of ostomy care.* St. Louis: C. V. Mosby.

Campra, J. L., & Reynolds, T. B. (1988). Hepatic circulation. In I. M. Arias, W. B. Jakoby, H. Popper, D. Schacter, and D. A. Shafritz (Eds.). *The liver: Biology and pathology.* New York: Raven.

Carrico, C. J., & Stevenson, J. K. (1987). Stomach. In J. H. Davis (Ed.). *Clinical surgery* (pp. 1435–1473). St. Louis: C. V. Mosby.

Chassin, J. L. (1980). *Operative strategy in general surgery,* (Vol. I). New York: Springer-Verlag.

Condon, R. E. (1989). The anatomy of the inguinal region and its relation to groin hernia. In L. M. Nyhus and R. E. Condon (Eds.). *Hernia.* Philadelphia: J. B. Lippincott.

Condon, R. E., & Telford, G. L. (1991). Appendicitis. In D. C. Sabiston (Ed.). *Textbook of surgery: The biological basis of modern surgical practice* (14th ed.) (pp. 884–898). Philadelphia: W. B. Saunders.

Corbitt, J. D. (1992). Preliminary experience with laparoscopic-guided colectomy. *Surgical Laparoscopy & Endoscopy, 2,* 79–81.

Corman, M. L. (1993). Crohn's disease and indeterminate colitis. *Colon and rectal surgery* (pp. 1012–1076). Philadelphia: J. B. Lippincott.

Dafoe, D. C. (1991). Pancreatic and islet cell transplantation. In G. D. Zuidema and J. G. Turcotte (Eds.). *Shackelford's surgery of the alimentary tract* (pp. 126–133). Philadelphia: W. B. Saunders.

Eisenberg, P. (1987). The surgical patient. In N. M. Matheny (Ed.). *Fluid and electrolyte balance: Nursing considerations.* Philadelphia: J. B. Lippincott.

Ellis, H. (1989). Incisions and closures. In S. I. Schwartz and H. Ellis (Eds.). *Maingot's abdominal operations* (pp. 181–197). Norwalk, CT: Appleton & Lange.

Fry, R. D., & Kodner, I. J. (1985). Anorectal disorders. *Clinical Symposia, 37,* 2–32.

Gadacz, T. R. (1991a). Cholecystectomy and cholecystostomy. In G. D. Zuidema and J. G. Turcotte (Eds.). *Shackelford's surgery of the alimentary tract* (pp. 186–199). Philadelphia: W. B. Saunders.

Gadacz, T. R. (1991b). Treatment of common duct stones. In G. D. Zuidema and J. G. Turcotte (Eds.). *Shackelford's surgery of the alimentary tract* (pp. 210–217). Philadelphia: W. B. Saunders.

Gadacz, T. R. (1991c). Laparoscopic cholecystectomy. In J.L. Cameron (Ed.). *Current surgical therapy* (pp. 330–334). St. Louis: Mosby–Year Book.

Gliedman, M. L., & Gold, M. S. (1989). Choledochoduodenostomy. In S. I. Schwartz and H. Ellis (Eds.). *Maingot's abdominal operations* (pp. 1451–1462). Norwalk, CT: Appleton & Lange.

Gordon, R. D., Teperman, L., Iwatsuki, S., & Starzl, T. E. (1989). Orthotopic liver transplantation. In S. I. Schwartz and H. Ellis (Eds.). *Maingot's abdominal operations* (pp. 1291–1312). Norwalk, CT: Appleton & Lange.

Gray, S. W., & Skandalakis, J. E. (1988). *Atlas of surgical anatomy.* Baltimore: Williams & Wilkins.

Guyton, A. C. (1986). *Textbook of medical physiology* (7th ed.). Philadelphia: W. B. Saunders.

Hansen, V. A., Johnson, M. B., & Rappaport, W. D. (1991). Splenic salvage vs splenectomy: Care of the trauma patient. *AORN Journal, 53,* 1519–1528.

Harmel, R. P. (1989). Umbilical herniorrhaphy. In L. M. Nyhus and R. E. Condon (Eds.). *Hernia* (pp. 354–360). Philadelphia: J. B. Lippincott.

Hermann, R. E., & Vogt, D. P. (1991). Anatomy of gallbladder. In J. H. Davis (Ed.). *Clinical Surgery* (p. 1638). St. Louis: C. V. Mosby.

Hinder, R. A., & Filipi, C. J. (1992). The technique of laparoscopic Nissen fundoplication. *Surgical Laparoscopy & Endoscopy, 2,* 265–273.

Hoerr, S. O., & Hermann, R. E. (1987). Cystic duct cholangiogram. In L. W. Way and C. A. Pelligrini (Eds.). *Surgery of the gallbladder and bile ducts.* Philadelphia: W. B. Saunders.

Jackson, B. T. (1987). Abdominal wall and hernias. In J. H. Davis (Ed.). *Clinical surgery* (pp. 1743–1783). St. Louis: C. V. Mosby.

Jones, W. G., Reilly, D. M., & Barie, P. S. (1991). Pancreatic injuries: Diagnosis, treatment. *AORN Journal, 53,* 917–933.

Karulf, R. E. (1992). Hidradenitis suppurativa and pilonidal disease. In D. E. Beck and S. D. Wexner (Eds.). *Fundamentals of anorectal surgery* (pp. 183–191). New York: McGraw-Hill.

Keith, R. (1987). Pancreas. In J. H. Davis (Ed.). *Clinical surgery* (pp. 1681–1743). St. Louis: C. V. Mosby.

Kirk, R. M. (1989). Drainage procedures. In S. I. Schwartz and H. Ellis (Eds.). *Maingot's abdominal operations* (pp. 667–679). Norwalk, CT: Appleton & Lange.

Kittur, O. S., & Smith, G. W. (1991). Techniques of liver resection. In G. D. Zuidema and J. G. Turcotte (Eds.). *Shackelford's surgery of the alimentary tract* (pp. 477–494). Philadelphia: W. B. Saunders.

Kodner, I. J. (1978). Colostomy and ileostomy. *Clinical Symposia, 30,* 2–36.

Kodner, I. J., Fry, R. D., & Fleshman, J. W. (1989a). Total proctectomy for malignancy. In S. I. Schwartz and H. Ellis (Eds.). *Maingot's abdominal operations* (pp. 1131–1141). Norwalk, CT: Appleton & Lange.

Kodner, I. J., Fry, R. D., & Fleshman, J. W. (1989b). Intestinal Stomas. In S. I. Schwartz and H. Ellis (Eds.). *Maingot's abdominal operations* (pp. 1143–1172). Norwalk, CT: Appleton & Lange.

Kodner, I. J., Fry, R. D., Fleshman, J. W., & Birnbaum, E. H. (1993). Colon, rectum, and anus. In S. I. Schwartz (Ed.). *Principles of surgery.* New York: McGraw-Hill.

Kortz, W. J., & Sabiston, D. C. (1987). Hernias. In D. C. Sabiston, Jr. (Ed.). *Essentials of surgery.* Philadelphia: W. B. Saunders.

Lewis, F. R. (1987). Appendectomy. In J. H. Davis (Ed.). *Clinical surgery* (pp. 1581–1600). St. Louis: C. V. Mosby.

Mittal, V. K., & Toledo-Pereyra, L. H. (1986). Pancreatic transplantation: The surgical process. *AORN Journal, 43,* 620–629.

Morrow, M., & Jaffe, B. M. (1987). Small intestine. In J. H. Davis (Ed.). *Clinical surgery* (pp. 1473–1519). St. Louis: C. V. Mosby.

Morton, J. H. (1989). Abdominal wall hernias. In S. I. Schwartz, G. T. Shires, and F. C. Spencer (Eds.). *Principles of surgery* (pp. 1525–1544). New York: McGraw-Hill.

Murray, G., & Keagy, B. (1987). Esophagus. In J. H. Davis (Ed.). *Clinical surgery* (pp. 1393–1471). St. Louis: C. V. Mosby.

Nyhus, L. M. (1989). The preperitoneal approach and ileopubic tract repair of femoral hernia. *Hernia* (pp. 189–199). Philadelphia: J. B. Lippincott.

Nyhus, L. M., Klein, M. S., Rogers, F. B., & Kowalczyk, S. (1990). Inguinal hernia repairs: Types, patient care. *AORN Journal, 52,* 292–394.

Partain, N. (1991). *Laparoscopic surgery and the O.R. nurse.* Somerville, NJ: Ethicon.

Pelligrini, C. A., & Way, L. W. (1987). Anatomy of esophagus. In L. W. Way (Ed.). *Current surgical diagnosis and treatment* (p. 401). Norwalk, CT: Appleton & Lange.

Pemberton, J. H. (1991). Anatomy and physiology of the anus and rectum. In G. D. Zuidema and R. E. Condon (Eds.). *Shackelford's surgery of the alimentary tract* (pp. 242–275). Philadelphia: W. B. Saunders.

Quinlan, R. M. (1991). Operations on the spleen. In G. D. Zuidema and J. G. Turcotte (Eds.). *Shackelford's surgery of the alimentary tract* (pp. 539–544). Philadelphia: W. B. Saunders.

Quinlan, R. M. (1991). Anatomy and embryology of the pancreas. In G. D. Zuidema and J. G. Turcotte (Eds.). *Shackelford's surgery of the alimentary tract* (pp. 3–19). Philadelphia: W. B. Saunders.

Redwine, D. B., & Sharpe, D. R. (1991). Laparoscopic segmental resection of the sigmoid colon for endometriosis. *Journal of Laparoendoscopic Surgery, 1,* 217–220.

Rossi, R. L., & Schirmer, W. J. (1991). Chronic pancreatitis. In *Current surgical therapy* (pp. 431–440). St. Louis: Mosby–Year Book.

Rout, W. R. (1991). Abdominal incisions. In G. D. Zuidema and W. P. Ritchie (Eds.). *Shackelford's surgery of the alimentary tract* (pp. 284–326). Philadelphia: W. B. Saunders.

Schoenfield, L. J. (1982). Gallstones and other biliary diseases. *Clinical Symposia, 34,* 2–32.

Schultz, L., Graber, J., Pietrafitta, J., & Hickok, D. (1990). Laser laparoscopic herniorrhaphy: A clinical trial preliminary results. *Journal of Laparoendoscopic Surgery, 1,* 41–45.

Schultz, L. S., Pietrafitta, J. J., Graber, J. N., & Hickok, D. F. (1991). Retrograde laparoscopic appendectomy: Report of a case. *Journal of Laparoendoscopic Surgery, 1,* 111–114.

Schwartz, S. I. (1989a). Appendix. In S. I. Schwartz, G. T. Shires, and F.C. Spencer (Eds.). *Principles of surgery* (pp. 1315–1326). New York: McGraw-Hill.

Schwartz, S. I. (1989b). Gallbladder and extrahepatic biliary system. In S. I. Schwartz, G. T. Shires, and F. C. Spencer (Eds.). *Principles of surgery* (pp. 1381–1412). New York: McGraw-Hill.

Schwartz, S. I. (1989c). Liver. In S. I. Schwartz, G. T. Shires, and F. C. Spencer (Eds.). *Principles of surgery* (pp. 1326–1379). New York: McGraw-Hill.

Schwartz, S. I. (1989d). Spleen. In S. I. Schwartz, G. T. Shires, and F. C. Spencer (Eds.). *Principles of surgery* (pp. 1441–1457). New York: McGraw-Hill.

Sessler, D. I. (1990). Temperature monitoring. In R. D. Miller (Ed.). *Anesthesia* (pp. 1227–1241). New York: Churchill Livingstone.

Silen, W. (1964). Surgical anatomy of the pancreas. *Surgical Clinics of North America, 44,* 1253.

Silen, W., & Steer, M. L. (1989). Pancreas. In S. I. Schwartz, G. T. Shires, and F. C. Spencer (Eds.). *Principles of surgery* (pp. 1413–1440). New York: McGraw-Hill.

Skinner, D. B. (1991). Hiatal hernia and gastroesophageal reflux. In D. C. Sabiston Jr. (Ed.). *Textbook of surgery: The biological basis of modern surgical practice* (pp. 704–715). Philadelphia: W. B. Saunders.

Starzl, T. E., Bell, R. H., Beart, R. W., & Putnam, C. W. (1975). Hepatic resections. *Surgery, Gynecology & Obstetrics, 41,* 429–437.

Steuer, K. (1990). Hepatic resection: Indications, procedures, patient care. *AORN Journal, 52,* 230–250.

Turcotte, J. G., Campbell, D. A., Merion, R. M., Burtch, G. D., & Ham, J. M. (1991). Hepatic transplantation. In G. D. Zuidema and J. G. Turcotte (Eds.). *Shackelford's surgery of the alimentary tract* (pp. 494–509). Philadelphia: W. B. Saunders.

Way, L. W. (1987). Anatomy of stomach. In *Current surgical diagnosis and treatment* (p. 461). Norwalk, CT: Appleton & Lange.

Zinner, M. J. (1992). *The atlas of gastric surgery.* New York: Churchill Livingstone.

Chapter 8

Breast Surgery

Key Concepts
Introduction
Anatomy
Nursing Considerations
Surgical Procedures
Summary

Key Concepts

- The mammary glands undergo physiologic changes during four major life periods: puberty, onset of menstruation, pregnancy and lactation, and menopause.
- The breast is the number one site of cancer in women.
- Three methods of screening and early diagnosis of cancer are physical examination, mammography, and breast self-examination.
- *Staging* is the categorization of cancer according to the extent of the disease.
- The patient with breast disease may experience anxiety and anticipatory grieving, because of possible loss of the breast.
- Mastectomy patients experience an alteration in body image owing to the loss of the breast.
- During breast surgery, the patient is at risk for potential blood loss owing to the vascularity of the breast.
- Invasive diagnostic procedures include fine-needle aspiration, percutaneous core needle biopsy, and incisional or excisional breast biopsy.
- Lumpectomy with axillary node dissection has an outcome at least as favorable as that of more radical treatments, such as modified radical mastectomy.
- Results of identification of estrogen receptors are used to plan adjuvant therapy.
- Adjuvant therapy is given to eliminate circulating microscopic cancer cells before they "seed" other vital organs.

INTRODUCTION

This chapter includes discussions of breast disease; diagnosis of lesions; various surgical treatment modalities; and the perioperative nursing care planning. Also included are nursing diagnoses particularly important in breast patients and used to organize care. Screening and early diagnosis of breast disease are explained.

ANATOMY

Anatomic Structure

The mammary gland, or breast, lies within the superficial fascia of the anterior chest wall. It extends from the second to the sixth rib and from the lateral border of the sternum to the anterior, or midaxillary, line. It is surrounded by subcutaneous connective tissue and adipose tissue and is molded within a conical pocket of skin. The largest portion of the mammary gland lies anteriorly on the connective tissue of the pectoralis major and laterally on the serratus anterior. The suspensory structures that support the breast are known as Cooper's ligaments. Additional mammary tissue, known as the axillary tail or tail of Spence, extends upward and laterally into the anterior axillary fold.

Each mammary gland is composed of 15 to 20 lobes containing ducts, ductules, and lobular-alveolar units (lobules containing the secreting cells, or alveoli) separated by fibrous connective tissue, or septa, and surrounded by fibrofatty tissue. Each lobe radiates away from the nipple, spoke-like. Each lobe of the mammary gland ends in a lactiferous duct that drains, through a constricted opening, from the nipple. The nipple is surrounded by the areola, which is pigmented and somewhat wrinkled (Fig. 8-1).

Blood Supply

The breast is supplied with blood from three major arterial systems: (1) branches of the internal thoracic, or internal mammary, artery; (2) lateral branches of the anteroposterior intercostal arteries; and (3) branches from the axillary artery (Bland & Copeland, 1991). The veins of the breast follow the same course as the arteries. Three major groups of veins are responsible for venous drainage of the thoracic wall and the breast: (1) branches of the internal thoracic vein; (2) tributaries of the axillary vein; and (3) branches of posterior intercostal veins. Metastatic emboli that travel through any of these routes pass through the venous return to the heart and are arrested when they reach the capillary bed of the lungs. This provides a route for direct venous metastasis of breast cancer to the lungs (Bland & Copeland, 1991).

Lymphatic Drainage

The lymph drainage system of the breast runs parallel to the venous pathways. The lymphatics in the lateral part of the mammary gland drain into the anterior axillary, or pectoral, nodes. The medial part drains into nodes aligned with the internal thoracic artery. The posterior intercostal nodes receive some drainage from lymph vessels along the posterior intercostal arteries. Through this system of lymphatic drainage, malignant cells are disseminated to the lymph nodes.

Lymph nodes are most commonly identified in the following groupings:

1. The axillary vein, or lateral, group
2. The external mammary, or anterior or pectoral, group
3. The scapular, or posterior or subscapular, group
4. The central group
5. The subclavicular, or apical, group
6. The interpectoral, or Rotter's, group.

In addition, surgeons identify the axillary lymph nodes in relation to the pectoralis minor muscle (Fig. 8-2). Level I includes the external mammary, axillary vein, and scapular lymph node groups, which lie lateral to or below the lower border of the pectoralis minor. Level II includes the central lymph node group and some of the subclavicular lymph node group, which lie behind the pectoralis minor. Level III includes the subclavicular lymph node group, which lies above the upper border of the pectoralis minor. The term "prepectoral" is used to identify a rare single lymph node that is found only in the subcutaneous tissue (Bland & Copeland, 1991).

Nerve Supply

The superior portion of the breast receives its nerve supply from the supraclavicular nerves from the third and fourth branches of the cervical plexus. Skin on the medial portion of the breast is innervated by the anterior cutaneous divisions of the second through the seventh intercostal nerves. Nipple sensation derives from the lateral cutaneous branch of the fourth intercostal nerve (Smith, 1991).

Physiologic Changes

The female mammary glands undergo physiologic alterations during major life changes: growth and development at the onset of puberty, cyclic events related to the menstrual cycle, and pregnancy and lactation. At puberty, the rise in the estrogen level promotes the development of glandular tissue, the growth of the ductal structures, and the pigmentation of the areola and nipple. Progesterone affects the development of the alveoli. The monthly cyclic changes in estrogen and progesterone during the menstrual cycle may cause enlargement, tenderness, or pain of the breasts. During pregnancy, the breasts enlarge owing to secretion of large amounts of estrogen, progesterone, and lactogen by the placenta (Thompson & Rock, 1992). At menopause, the shutdown of estrogen production may increase the risk of a woman developing breast cancer. Therefore, the prognosis for breast cancer may be better for estrogen users than for nonusers (Scott et al., 1990).

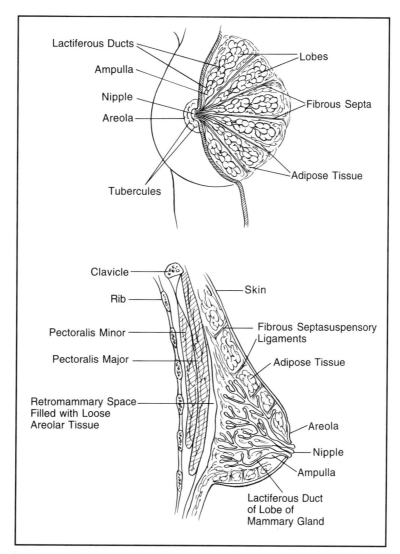

FIGURE 8-1 Mature mammary gland in the female. (A), Anterior view with skin partially removed to show internal structure. (B), Sagittal section. (From *Clinical anatomy for medical students* [3rd ed], Snell, R. S. [1986]. Published by Little, Brown and Company. Adapted with permission.)

Abnormalities

The most common physical breast abnormality of both males and females is an accessory nipple (polythelia). Other breast anomalies include hypoplasia (underdevelopment); amastia (congenital absence); and amazia (deficient breast tissue in the presence of a nipple) (Harris et al., 1991).

NURSING CONSIDERATIONS

Breast Disease

According to the American Cancer Society, the breast is the number one site of cancer in women. About one of nine women develops breast cancer during her lifetime (American Cancer Society, 1992). Early detection is the

primary objective for controlling breast cancer. Three methods are physical examination, mammography, and breast self-examination. "Screening" is the implementation of these techniques in *asymptomatic* women (Miaskowski, 1990). The goal of screening is to detect occult lesions before they might otherwise be found (Harris et al., 1991).

Diagnosis

Physical examination and screening

The American Cancer Society recommends a clinical physical examination of the breast every 3 years for women aged 20 to 40 years, and every year after age 40. In addition, women between the ages of 35 and 40 should have a baseline mammogram, followed after age 40 every 1 to 2 years by another study, and annually after age 50.

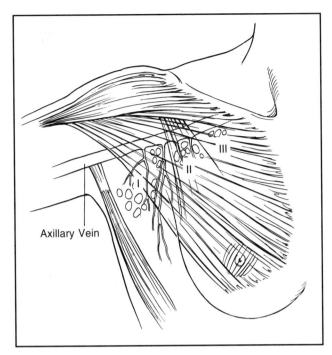

FIGURE 8-2 Axillary lymph node levels: I (low axilla); II (midaxilla); and III (apex of axilla) in relationship to pectoralis minor muscle (fan-shaped muscle superficial to level II nodes). (Adapted from Harris, J., Hellman, S., Henderson, I., and Kinne, D. [1991]. *Breast disease* [2nd ed]. Philadelphia: J. B. Lippincott.)

Discovering cancers at the earliest stage possible is related directly and positively to the survival rate (Baird, McCorkle, & Grant, 1991).

Mammography

Mammography is most valuable when it detects breast cancer even before a lump can be felt, as by abnormal-looking densities and calcium deposits, which can be as small as 3 to 10 mm in diameter. In addition, mammography is used to evaluate questionable lumps found on examination and nodular or very large breasts, which are difficult to examine.

Usually, two pictures are made of the breast, one from above (the craniocaudal view) and one from the side (the mediolateral view). Each breast is inserted into a compression device to improve the picture and reduce the amount of radiation required. This technique results in a lower amount of radiation to the patient (Smeltzer & Bare, 1992). Accuracy of the mammogram depends on precise operator technique as well as the size, structure, and density of the breast. The mammogram should be evaluated by a radiologist and the results reported to the patient's physician.

Biopsy

Malignancy is determined by surgical biopsy. When a lesion is too small to be palpated, a mammogram may be done immediately prior to surgery to mark the location of the lesion located previously on mammogram. A needle is inserted into the localized lesion and then a wire may be inserted into the needle. Once the localization is confirmed, the needle may be removed, leaving the wire to be taped to the patient's skin. In the operating room, the tape is removed, leaving the wire in the lesion, the skin is prepped with the wire in place, and the localized area is removed by surgical biopsy. The tissue can then be sent for radiographic validation of the suspicious tissue before the pathologic examination.

Breast self-examination

The American Cancer Society recommends that women aged 20 years and older examine their breasts once a month. During a woman's reproductive years, the best time to examine the breasts is 7 to 10 days after the onset of menstruation, when the breast swelling and tenderness have subsided. Women who are past menopause should perform breast self-examination (BSE) at any regular, convenient time, on a monthly basis.

The nurse can play an important role in screening and early detection of breast cancer by participating in efforts to educate women, their families, and the general public about the benefits of early detection. The nurse can motivate patients to perform BSE by building awareness and understanding of the risks of cancer, emphasizing the warning signs and symptoms for early recognition, and stressing the importance of regular screening and early detection (Bland & Copeland, 1991). Teaching the BSE technique with return demonstration from the patient enhances the patient's ability to perform the examination and helps motivate repeated use.

Signs and Symptoms

- Palpable lump or thickening in the breast, usually painless
- Nipple discharge, bloody or serous
- Dimpling or change in the skin
- Breast asymmetry
- Nipple retraction or scaliness
- Late signs, including pain, ulceration, and edema

Risk Factors

- Age: The longer a woman lives, the greater are her changes of developing breast cancer (Stein & Zera, 1991).
- Family history: A woman whose mother or sister (first-degree relative) has had breast cancer is at two to three times greater risk than the general population (Stein & Zera, 1991).
- Hormonal influences: Onset of menses before age 12 and nulliparity, or a first full-term pregnancy after age 35, or late onset of natural menopause, or a menstruation history longer than 40 years.
- Benign breast disease: The term "fibrocystic disease of the breast" covers a wide range of histologic diagnoses, some of which carry no added risk of breast cancer.

• Radiation exposure: It is well-documented that high doses of radiation are directly correlated with increased risk of breast cancer, especially through studies conducted on victims of atomic bombing (Harris et al., 1991). Few people will ever be exposed to doses experienced in like circumstances. The use of diagnostic radiography, including mammography, however, has not been shown to increase risk.

Once a breast lump is discovered, it is evaluated for one of three possibilities: (1) a cyst, (2) a benign tumor, or (3) a malignant tumor. A cyst is usually aspirated and, if the effort is successful, it shrinks or disappears. Ultrasound can be used to distinguish between a fluid-filled cystic lump and a solid one (Baird et al., 1991). If a tumor is suspected, mammography is performed. Pathologic diagnosis is ascertained from a fine-needle aspiration, core-needle biopsy, or incisional or excisional biopsy (Baird et al., 1991).

Staging

Staging categorizes patients' disease both clinically and pathologically according to its extent. Staging helps determine an individualized treatment regimen and estimate the prognosis, and it provides a basis for comparison with different treatment programs (Harris et al., 1991). The most widely used system for identifying staging comes from the American Joint Commission on Cancer Staging and End Results Reporting. It is referred to as the TNM (tumor, nodes, metastases) system: T, tumor size, determines the extent of cancer; N denotes axillary lymph node involvement; and M indicates the presence or absence of metastases (see Table 8-1).

Nursing Diagnoses and Care

Preoperative

Although only about two of every ten breast lumps discovered are malignant, a woman's fear of losing her breast, along with the effects of the disease and illness, are very powerful. Emotional support and understanding during the preoperative phase can help alleviate some of those fears. The patient may experience anxiety and anticipatory grieving over possible loss of a body part resulting in alteration of body image. The desired patient outcome is for the patient to acknowledge and verbalize her fears and anxieties. The preoperative period is reported to be the most psychologically stressful time of the breast treatment experience. It is recognized that critical thinking and information-processing abilities of patients who anticipate diagnosis or have been diagnosed with breast cancer are severely impaired during this time. Patients experience terror and anxiety, become disoriented, wonder if they will survive, and have difficulty evaluating and deciding on treatment options because of their distress (Harris et al., 1991).

The nurse works effectively during this phase by providing information and support, giving direction to help the patient, spouse, and family process the information and strengthen their coping mechanisms and come to terms with decision-making (Baird et al., 1991).

The nursing diagnosis is knowledge deficit related to breast cancer and its subsequent diagnosis and treatment. The desired patient outcome is for the patient to acquire the knowledge needed to make informed decisions about her perioperative care. The nurse provides information, oral and written, for the patient to consider and share with her support group. In addition, the nurse serves as a referral source, informing the patient of various commu-

TABLE 8-1   TNM Classification of Breast Cancer

T (tumor)	T0	No evidence of tumor
	Tis	Carcinoma in situ
	T1	Tumor 2 cm or less at greatest dimension
	T2	Tumor greater than 2 cm but not larger than 5 cm at greatest dimension
	T3	Tumor is larger than 5 cm at greatest dimension
	T4	Tumor of any size that extends into the chest wall or skin, including ribs, intercostal muscles, and serratus anterior muscle, but not pectoral muscle
N (nodes)	N0	No regional lymph node metastasis
	N1	Metastasis to movable ipsilateral axillary nodes
	N2	Metastasis to ipsilateral axillary lymph nodes fixed to each other or to other structures
	N3	Metastasis to ipsilateral internal mammary lymph nodes
M (metastasis)	M0	No distant metastases
	M1	Distant metastases including ipsilateral supraclavicular nodes

(Adapted from Harris, J., Hellman, S., Henderson, I., & Kinne, D. [1991]. *Breast disease* [2nd ed.]. Philadelphia: J. B. Lippincott.)

nity support services for persons affected by cancer, and breast cancer in particular.

Intraoperative

The nursing diagnosis is risk for potential injury related to the use of electrosurgery. The expected patient outcome is that there will be no injury from electrosurgery. The circulating nurse is responsible for checking the function of the electrosurgical equipment before the procedure, for correct placement of the dispersive pad, and for keeping the power setting as low as possible to achieve the desired results. The dispersive pad contact and all connections should be checked after changing the patient's position or on requests for increased power. The scrub person is responsible for preventing inadvertent contact of the electrosurgery tip and skin or tissue by placing the electrode in a protective holder when it is not in use.

The patient is at risk for potential blood loss, owing to the vascularity of the breast. The expected patient outcome is that she will not experience postoperative difficulties related to fluid loss. The amount of irrigation fluid used should be documented in order that blood loss may be distinguished from irrigation fluid collection. Surgical sponges should be weighed and the findings reported to the surgeon and anesthesia provider. In addition, fluid loss through direct evaporation from the open surgical cavity may partially account for an immediate postoperative fluid deficit (Carpenito, 1989).

The patient is at risk for potential brachial plexus injury due to positioning. The expected patient outcome is that the patient will not sustain a brachial plexus injury. After the anesthesia induction is complete and the patient is positioned, the nurse reassesses the patient's position to make sure that the arms are not being abducted more than 90 degrees on the armboard.

Postoperative

The patient is at risk for potential postoperative wound infection. The desired patient outcome is for the patient to understand what steps are necessary to help prevent infection. It is important for the patient to learn and participate in postoperative wound care. She should also be aware of the importance of reporting any sensory changes to the health care provider as soon as they are noticed.

The patient is at risk for potential impaired mobility due to intolerance to activity, decreased strength and endurance, pain and discomfort, and musculoskeletal impairment. The desired patient outcome is for the patient to participate in activities to prevent impaired mobility. The patient should be encouraged to balance rest with activity, participate in a defined postmastectomy arm exercise program, and progressively increase activity as healing advances.

The patient will experience an alteration in body image due to the loss of the breast. The desired patient outcome is that the patient will receive the support she needs from family and other systems designed to help her cope with this loss. Many patients are referred to recovery pro-

grams, where they receive information, often from women who have themselves been through mastectomy and recovery.

SURGICAL PROCEDURES

Biopsy of Breast Tissue

When a breast mass or thickening is discovered on physical examination, a biopsy is performed to determine the histologic nature of the tissue.

Fine-needle aspiration

Indications The purpose of fine-needle aspiration (FNA) of a breast lesion is to determine the consistency of a palpable mass, either fluid or solid, or to discover and diagnose a malignancy.

The physician may attempt to aspirate any palpable lesion simply by using a Luer-lok syringe with a disposable 22- or 23-gauge needle. The aspirate is submitted for cytologic examination to determine the presence of malignant cells. It is recommended that FNA be performed before the mammogram, to evacuate the fluid if the mass is cystic. This prevents the fluid from obscuring other tissue on the mammogram and reduces any pain the patient may experience from compression of the breast during the procedure. Advantages of FNA include its simplicity and low cost (it can be performed in the physician's office with no anesthesia), and its accuracy (Harris et al., 1991). Complications include hematoma, mastitis, and possible pneumothorax.

Key steps

1. The skin is gently cleansed, not vigorously scrubbed, with an antimicrobial solution.
2. The mass is grasped and held securely between the fingers of one hand.
3. The disposable needle is inserted into the mass, and the plunger of the syringe is retracted as far as possible, creating a vacuum, while the needle is plunged in a straight line through the mass.
4. This is repeated four or five times, if necessary moving the needle back and forth within the lesion while continuing to aspirate, until sufficient material for examination is collected.
5. The needle is removed after releasing the retraction on the plunger so the pressure is released.
6. The needle is disconnected from the syringe, the syringe is filled with air, the needle is reconnected, and the contents are expelled onto a glass slide.
7. The aspirate is smeared, using a second glass slide. Half of the smears are wet fixed with 95% ethyl alcohol and stained according to Papanicolaou; the other half can be allowed to air dry and are stained immediately (Harris et al., 1991).

Percutaneous core needle biopsy

A percutaneous core needle biopsy is done for diagnosis of solid tumors.

A large-bore trocar containing a cutting needle is used to remove the solid tissue. It produces slender, cylindrical fragments, or cores, of tissue that can then be processed as a frozen as well as a permanent section (Harris et al., 1991). Like FNA, core needle biopsy is relatively simple and inexpensive, and it can be performed conveniently in the surgeon's office using a local anesthetic. Diagnosis can then be confirmed before surgery under general anesthesia.

Key steps

1. The skin is gently cleansed with an antimicrobial solution.
2. The skin and surrounding area are injected with a local anesthetic.
3. The mass is grasped firmly between the fingers and thumb of one hand.
4. The trocar is advanced in the open position into the tumor.
5. The hand holding the trocar remains stationary while the hand grasping the tumor moves to advance the cutting sheath.
6. The instrument is removed with the specimen intact within the specimen notch.
7. Bleeding is controlled with pressure.
8. Specimens are either sent immediately for frozen section or placed in a fixative solution and sent for permanent section diagnosis.

Incisional or excisional biopsy

Indications   Diagnosis of a solid breast mass when FNA or percutaneous needle biopsy is not definitive, when a mass is detected by palpation, mammography, nipple discharge, or skin changes.

Incisional biopsy   Incisional biopsy is the excision of a portion of a breast mass when the entire mass is too large to remove in toto. It can be performed using local anesthesia, or under general anesthesia if the mass is large and suspicious for carcinoma.

Excisional biopsy   Excisional biopsy is the excision of the entire palpable mass or suspicious area. It is the preferred method of surgery for small lesions that may be curable by total excision. It is also indicated for suspected benign masses, to ensure total removal and provide tissue for histologic examination. In patients with suspected malignant disease, a margin of grossly normal breast tissue is removed. The specimen is inked and oriented to save time and provide an accurate reference should the need arise to reexcise a particular margin.

Key steps

1. The patient is positioned supine with the arm on the affected side secured at less than a 90-degree angle on a padded armboard.
2. The skin is gently cleansed with an antimicrobial solution.
3. When a malignancy is suspected, a curvilinear incision is made over the lesion. For central lesions, or clearly benign lesions, a circumareolar incision is made for best cosmetic results.
4. The surgeon explores the location of the mass with a finger, determines the exact location, and tunnels to the mass if it is not located directly beneath the incision.
5. The lesion is retracted with holding forceps or a grasping instrument. If small enough, it is excised entirely with a circumferential edge of normal tissue. If the mass is large, a small portion is excised.
6. The tissue specimen is evaluated by frozen section for immediate diagnosis while the patient remains in the surgical suite, under either local or general anesthesia.
7. Hemostasis is controlled with electrosurgery.
8. Skin closure. For a benign lesion, a small drain may be inserted. The subcutaneous breast tissue is approximated with an absorbable suture. The skin may be closed with fine sutures, subcuticular closure, or skin staples. A firm pressure dressing is applied. For a malignant lesion the skin is closed tightly with a continuous locking suture on a cutting needle. A firm pressure dressing is applied.
9. If more extensive surgery is indicated, it can be performed immediately or can be scheduled for later.

Incision and Drainage of Abscess

Indications   For treatment of an inflamed and suppurative area of the breast, usually the result of infection in a lactating breast, incision and drainage are in order. *Staphylococcus aureus*, the most common pathogen, enters the breast through abrasions or lacerations in the nipple area or through the lactiferous ducts.

Key steps

1. An incision is made over the point of maximum tenderness, usually a radial incision extending outward from the nipple or a circumareolar incision.
2. Once pus is encountered, the cavity is explored with a curved instrument to determine its extent. Cultures are taken for aerobic and anaerobic organisms.
3. Loculations are broken up by examining the cavity with the index finger to verify resolution of the abscess. The cavity is thoroughly drained.
4. The cavity is irrigated with warm saline solution, and hemostasis is achieved through coagulation or ligation with absorbable sutures.
5. The wound is either packed open or closed loosely over a drain brought out through a separate incision.
6. The wound is allowed to close by granulation.

Lumpectomy (Partial Mastectomy, Tylectomy, Segmental Resection, Quadrant Resection, Wedge Resection)

Lumpectomy is a breast-preserving technique designed to retain a cosmetically acceptable breast after complete excision of the tumor. The tumor mass is completely excised with at least a 1-inch margin of surrounding normal breast tissue. A standard lumpectomy includes a partial mastectomy in conjunction with axillary node dissection and postoperative radiation therapy. Tumors in situ are treated with excision alone and postoperative radiation therapy.

Indications Lumpectomy is an alternative for women who have small, peripheral, infiltrating tumors (defined as less than 4 cm in the greatest diameter) and "clinically negative axillae." This approach appears to have comparable results to that of more radical procedures, and the breast is preserved (Baird et al., 1991).

Key steps

1. The procedure for excisional biopsy is followed. Margins of normal breast tissue measure 1 inch.
2. The specimen is inked and oriented to minimize reexcision if on frozen section diagnosis, a margin is narrow, or marginal tissue is involved by disease.

Axillary Node Dissection

Axillary node dissection is removal of the axillary nodes through an incision in the axilla separate from that of the primary lesion. The incisions would overlap in the case of a lesion of the axillary tail. The dissection includes all nodes from at least axillary levels I and II (Bland & Copeland, 1991) (see Fig. 8-2).

Indications Axillary node dissection provides information on lymph node involvement with tumor. The information is used to determine the patient's prognosis, for staging and planning of adjuvant chemotherapy, and for local or regional control (Bland & Copeland, 1991).

Key steps

1. A curvilinear incision is made just below the axillary hairline, or a longitudinal incision is placed along the lateral margin of the pectoralis major muscle.
2. Anatomic structures are identified for delineation of the dissection: the latissimus dorsi muscle, the axillary vein, and the medial border of the pectoralis minor muscle.
3. Major blood and lymphatic vessels are clamped and ligated, avoiding the use of electrosurgery around the axillary vessels and nerves.
4. The nerves to the serratus anterior and latissimus dorsi muscles are identified and preserved.
5. The axillary vein is identified, and tissue over the vein is excised.
6. The lymph nodes between the pectoralis major and pectoralis minor muscles are dissected. Care is taken to avoid injuring the nerves of the pectoralis major muscle.
7. All nodes are removed within the delineated structures (expected average, 15 or more nodes) (Bland & Copeland, 1991).
8. The wound is closed with absorbable suture and skin staples. A suction drain is placed in the wound, exiting out a separate stab wound for lymphatic drainage. A dressing is applied.

Modified Radical Mastectomy

A modified radical mastectomy includes removal of the entire affected breast, the pectoralis minor muscle, and a total axillary lymph node dissection removing all three levels of lymph nodes.

Indications Most patients with operable breast cancer at Stage I, II, or III that is not fixed to the pectoralis major muscle by extensive axillary lymph node involvement undergo modified radical mastectomy. The procedure is done with the objective of decreasing the spread of malignancy.

Key steps

1. The patient is positioned supine, and the entire breast, axilla, and arm are prepared and draped free within the sterile field.
2. A slightly oblique, elliptical incision extending somewhat into the axilla is made with a minimum 4-cm skin margin outlined around the tumor. This technique produces a good cosmetic result that facilitates subsequent breast reconstruction.
3. Hemostasis is obtained using hemostats and suture ligatures or electrosurgery.
4. Thin skin flaps are dissected to the outer edges of the breast in all directions. Cutting instruments must be very sharp, to ensure flawless dissection.
5. The fascia and breast are resected from the pectoralis major.
6. Axillary node dissection of all three levels is completed en bloc.
7. The specimen is removed and sent immediately to the pathology department to be analyzed for estrogen receptors.
8. Bleeding sites are ligated or coagulated. The entire wound is irrigated with warm saline solution. Closed wound suction catheters are inserted through separate stab wounds and secured to the skin with nonabsorbable suture.
9. The subcutaneous tissue is approximated with absorbable suture, then the skin is closed with interrupted nonabsorbable suture or staples.
10. The dressing may consist simply of gauze, or a bulky dressing can be held in place by a surgical bra or secured with a gauze or elastic bandage wrap.

Estrogen receptors The breasts are subject to hormonal influences stimulated by hormones produced in the endocrine glands. The presence of estrogen receptors in tumor cells affects cellular metabolism. Tests have been developed that determine the ability of breast cancer to bind with estrogen and progestins, identifying patients with hormone-dependent tumors. Therapeutic hormonal stimulation may delay recurrence or spread of the disease. For patients whose tumor contains estrogen receptors, anti-estrogen medications, in addition to surgery and chemotherapy, can prolong the disease-free interval. The resected tissue specimen should not be placed in a fixative solution but should be sent immediately to the pathology department for processing for estrogen receptors.

Total (Simple) Mastectomy

Simple mastectomy is the removal of the entire involved breast, including the nipple and areolar complex. The axillary lymph nodes are not dissected.

Indications

- Carcinoma in situ with no suspicious axillary involvement
- Prophylactic mastectomy, often of the contralateral breast (in selected patients)
- Recurrence after lumpectomy and axillary dissection
- Palliation for advanced malignancy (Harris et al., 1991).

Key steps

1. An elliptical incision is made, and the skin edges are dissected away from the fascia.
2. Bleeding vessels are clamped and ligated, or coagulated.
3. The breast tissue is retracted with grasping instruments and dissected away from the underlying pectoral fascia.
4. The specimen is removed and hemostasis is reestablished.
5. A closed wound drainage system is inserted and anchored.
6. The fascia is approximated with absorbable suture. The skin is sutured or stapled, and an appropriate dressing is applied.

Radical Mastectomy

A radical mastectomy involves removal, en bloc, of the breast and skin overlying the tumor, the pectoralis major and minor muscles, plus complete axillary node dissection.

Indications The radical mastectomy is performed mainly for debulking of advanced tumors attached to the pectoralis muscle or for bulky axillary node involvement.

Key steps

1. The dissection technique is similar to that of the modified radical mastectomy.
2. The breast and pectoralis major and minor muscles are removed.

3. Preoperatively, the anterior thigh may be prepared and draped, in the event a skin graft is needed to close the defect.

Immediate Reconstructive Breast Surgery Following Mastectomy

Nursing considerations

The appropriate timing of breast reconstruction following mastectomy varies with the magnitude of the tumor at the time of diagnosis. One of the major factors in influencing reconstruction is the patient's desire. Immediate reconstruction is performed at the time of mastectomy. This option is available for patients with very small tumors that have not spread to the lymph nodes. If a breast tumor is discovered while very small, usually less than 2 cm in size, the new breast can be rebuilt at the time the diseased one is removed (Barton & Rutherford, 1987).

The type of reconstructive surgery chosen for a patient is largely determined by the extent of the mastectomy and the amount of remaining skin and muscle available at the completion of the surgical procedure. The surgeon's goal in breast reconstruction is to surgically produce a mound that resembles a normal breast. In order for this to occur, the mound must be pendulous and form an inframammary fold when the patient is standing. In addition, the mound should move freely when the patient is moving or reclining. The rebuilt breast should feel soft and natural to the touch and should be capped with a nipple/areola complex (Barton & Rutherford, 1987).

The transverse rectus abdominis myocutaneous (TRAM) flap is a reconstructive procedure chosen for bringing in extra muscle and skin for the reconstruction. The abdominal tissue is threaded under the skin on the torso and onto the chest wall. Redundant skin and fatty tissue are often available in the abdominal region, which allows the surgeon to build a breast mound without the addition of an implant.

Indications

The TRAM flap is indicated for patients who have large defects in the mastectomy area. Patients who have a fair amount of surplus skin and fatty tissue in lower abdominal area are ideal candidates. Other indications include patients who refuse to have an implant or those who have experienced contracture, disfigurement, or pain caused by a previous implant.

Advantages

According to Knobf (1990), immediate reconstruction may spare the patient some psychological distress. The patient does not have to wake up without a breast. The greatest advantage of the TRAM flap transfer is that the surgeon can create a breast mound composed of autogenous tissue without the need of an artificial prosthesis, and the patient receives an abdominal lipectomy in the donor area (Smith, 1991). Two teams of surgeons and nurses can work simultaneously in order to be ready to transfer the flap at the completion of the mastectomy.

Disadvantages

Immediate breast reconstruction lengthens the operative time as well as the hospital stay. Immediate reconstruction has also been linked to delayed wound healing (Knobf, 1990). Complications following immediate reconstruction include skin loss, hematoma, seroma, infection, and asymmetry. The TRAM procedure is quite extensive, and the patient may experience an appreciable blood loss, resulting in the need for blood replacement.

Patients with chronic pulmonary disease, severe cardiovascular disease, uncontrolled hypertension, and insulin-dependent diabetes are not recommended as candidates for the TRAM procedure (Hartrampf, 1988).

Preoperative preparation

Much planning is done prior to surgery. The patient may give and store autologous blood, usually two units, prior to surgery. The surgeon marks the patient's skin preoperatively, after measuring the breast to be removed and anticipating the amount of tissue deficit to be filled by the TRAM flap tissue. An elliptical mark is drawn on the abdomen similar to that for an abdominal lipectomy.

Key steps

1. The abdominal panniculus is raised, using a circumferential type incision.
2. The location of the deep superior epigastric vessel is determined, using a sterile Doppler. Intravenous fluorescein dye is injected to enable the surgical team to evaluate circulation to the flap with the use of an ultraviolet lamp.
3. The dissection continues from the anterior abdominal wall to the subcostal margin and then to become continuous with the mastectomy incision site.
4. An incision is made in the anterior rectus sheath 1.5 cm on each side of the deep superior epigastric vessel.
5. The rectus muscle fibers are incised just outside of the anterior rectus sheath incision, which should result in a portion of muscle undisturbed laterally and a portion of muscle undisturbed medially (Hartrampf, 1988).
6. The rectus muscle is raised from the underlying posterior rectus sheath along with its attached abdominal island flap.
7. The flap is tunneled through the continuous dissected area under the chest wall and delivered through the submammary incision in the anterior chest wall.
8. The remaining medial and lateral segments of the rectus muscle are repaired, leaving a small space (one to two fingerbreadths) unrepaired around the vascular pedicle. This first portion of the repair serves to approximate the muscle and close the anterior wall dead space (Hartrampf, 1988).
9. The anterior rectus sheath is then closed with strong, permanent suture material.
10. To balance the anterior abdominal wall and center the umbilicus, the opposite anterior rectus sheath is plicated to match the harvested side.
11. The patient is flexed at the waist to allow for the transverse incision repair, which produces the abdominoplasty effect.
12. The flap is rotated 80 to 90 degrees (clockwise for a right chest defect and counterclockwise for a left chest defect) into place. This is the best rotation for shaping the breast when the patient has a standard modified radical defect where the vertical dimensions are larger than the width of the defect.
13. The flap is carefully molded and shaped into a breast form. The edges are temporarily stapled or sutured together, and the patient is placed into a sitting position for the surgeon to evaluate the size, placement, and symmetry of the reconstructed breast with the opposite remaining breast.
14. When the size and placement have been finalized, the temporary staples or suture are removed and the flap is sutured into place.
15. Suction drains are positioned in the abdomen as well as in the reconstructed breast.
16. Antibiotic ointment may be applied to wound edges, and no dressings may be used. Dressings prevent regular examination of the flap and abdominal wall for changes in color, temperature, and capillary circulation of the flap and the anterior abdominal wall (Dinner & Coleman, 1985).
17. The patient is kept in Fowler's position for 24 hours postoperatively and then is ambulated in a semiflexed position.

Adjuvant Therapy

Adjuvant therapy is chemotherapy or hormonal therapy subsequent to surgery. Tamoxifen, an estrogen-blocking agent, is the drug most commonly used in hormonal therapy for breast cancer. It binds to the estrogen-receptive tissue and can prevent cell growth.

Chemotherapy may be used preoperatively, especially for Stage III cancers, to ''downstage'' tumors before surgery. In addition, preoperative chemotherapy may be given to patients with Stage I and II malignancies, to optimize postoperative cosmetic results.

Postoperative adjuvant chemotherapy is given to eliminate circulating microscopic cancer cells before they multiply and travel to other vital organs. Research shows that patients who receive adjuvant chemotherapy, whether they had positive or negative lymph nodes, have a longer disease-free period and higher survival rate overall than those who are treated with surgery or radiation alone (Stein & Zera, 1991).

SUMMARY

This chapter has included the various surgical treatment modalities for breast disease. Adjuvant therapy subsequent to surgery is also discussed. Perioperative nursing care of the patient with breast disease includes safety and aseptic clinical expertise as well as supportive therapy.

REFERENCES

American Cancer Society. (1992). *Cancer facts and figures.* Atlanta: Author.

Baird, S. B., McCorkle, R., & Grant, M. (1991), *Cancer nursing: A comprehensive textbook.* Philadelphia: W. B. Saunders.

Barton, F. E., & Rutherford, S. (1987). Reconstructive breast surgery following mastectomy: Techniques and options. *Dallas Medical Journal,* Feb., 31–33.

Bland, K., & Copeland, E. M. (1991). *The breast, comprehensive management of benign and malignant diseases.* Philadelphia: W. B. Saunders.

Carpenito, L. (1989). *Nursing diagnosis, application to clinical practice* (3rd ed.). Philadelphia: J. B. Lippincott.

Dinner, M., & Coleman, C. (1985). Breast reconstruction: Use of autogenous tissue. *AORN Journal, 42,* 490–496.

Harris, J., Hellman, S., Henderson, I., & Kinne, D. (1991). *Breast diseases* (2nd ed.). Philadelphia: J. B. Lippincott.

Hartrampf, C. R., Jr. (1988). The transverse abdominal island flap for breast reconstruction: A 7-year experience. *Clinics in Plastic Surgery, 15,* 703–716.

Johnson, J. R. (1994). Caring for the woman who's had a mastectomy. *American Journal of Nursing,* 94:24–31.

Knobf, M. T. (1990). Early-stage breast cancer: The options. *American Journal of Nursing,* 90:28–30.

Miaskowski, C. (guest ed.) (1990). Advances in oncology nursing. *The Nursing Clinics of North America,* 25:10–18.

Scott, J., DiSaia, P., Hammond, C., & Spellacy, W. (1990). *Danforth's obstetrics and gynecology* (6th ed.). Philadelphia: J. B. Lippincott.

Smeltzer, S., & Bare, B. (1992). *Brunner and Suddarth's textbook of medical surgical nursing* (7th ed.). Philadelphia: J. B. Lippincott.

Smith, J. (1991). In S. Aston, *Plastic surgery* (4th ed.). Boston: Little, Brown & Co.

Smith, J., & Sherrell, J. (1991). *Grabb and Smith's plastic surgery* (4th ed.). Boston: Little, Brown & Co.

Stein, P., & Zera, R. T. (1991). Breast cancer, risks, treatment, perioperative patient care. *AORN Journal, 53*(4), 935–964.

Thompson, J., & Rock, J. (1992). *Te Linde's operative gynecology* (7th ed.). Philadelphia: J. B. Lippincott.

ADDITIONAL READINGS

Ariel, I., & Cleary, J. (1987). *Breast cancer: Diagnosis and treatment.* New York: McGraw-Hill.

Atkinson, L. (1991). *Berry & Kohn's Introduction to operating room technique* (7th ed.). St. Louis: Mosby–Year Book

Fowble, B., Goodman, R., Glick, J. & Rosato, E. (1991). *Breast cancer treatment, a comprehensive guide to management.* St. Louis: Mosby–Year Book.

Groenwald, S. (1993). *Cancer nursing principles and practice* (3rd ed.). Boston: Jones and Bartlett.

Nielsen, B. (1990). Advances in breast cancer, implications for nursing care. *Nursing Clinics of North America,* 25, 365–375.

Redfield, C. (1991). *Medical-surgical nursing concepts and clinical practice* (4th ed.). St. Louis: Mosby–Year Book.

Snell, R. (1973). *Clinical anatomy for medical students* (3rd ed.). Boston: Little, Brown & Co.

Strombeck, J., & Rosato, F. (1986). *Surgery of the breast.* New York: Thieme.

Chapter 9

Gynecologic Surgery

Key Concepts

- Many procedures in gynecologic surgery that formerly were accomplished through abdominal incisions are now done using minimally invasive techniques.

- Proper care, inspection, and assembly of the scopes and associated instrumentation are essential components of this specialty.

- Additional skills in operating equipment and in using new technology are imperative, as the amount and variety of equipment used for procedures increase.

- The amount of carbon dioxide gas instilled into the abdominal cavity and the pressure at which it is instilled should be carefully monitored.

- Patient support is essential for procedures done under local anesthesia or on a same-day surgery basis.

- Body image concerns or embarrassment may be encountered since the specialty deals with the female reproductive and sexual organs.

- Care must be taken when positioning the patient in stirrups to avoid neuromuscular injury.

- The use of lasers contributes to the efficiency and cost effectiveness of gynecologic surgery.

- The personal values and beliefs of some perioperative nurses may not allow them to participate in certain gynecological procedures, such as termination of pregnancy, tubal ligation, or in vitro fertilization.

INTRODUCTION

Gynecologic surgery is surgery of the female reproductive system performed to treat pathological conditions, for diagnosis of disease, and for diagnosis or treatment of conditions that affect fertility. Surgical procedures are also performed to repair anatomical structures weakened or injured as a result of pregnancies and childbirth or from normal aging.

This chapter reviews normal anatomy of the female external genitalia and pelvic cavity and presents considerations for the perioperative nurse in caring for patients undergoing gynecologic surgical procedures. The most common surgical procedures are described in a conceptual manner so that the nurse will also be able to plan care for patients having similar surgical procedures. Instrumentation, supplies, and equipment needed are identified and discussed.

While most surgical specialties treat primarily pathological conditions, gynecologic surgery also attempts to treat functional problems related to fertility. This difference presents the perioperative nurse with a variety of patients undergoing similar procedures for quite different reasons. For example, a woman who has determined that she does not want to bear more children may undergo a laparoscopic procedure for a tubal ligation. A second woman may undergo laparoscopic surgery to determine the cause of her inability to conceive, whereas a third woman may undergo laparoscopy for retrieval of ovum for in vitro fertilization, and yet another for excision of a tubal pregnancy. One woman may have vulva surgery to ablate condylomata, while another will have vulva surgery for cancer in situ. Identifying the psychosocial needs of each woman is paramount as the perioperative nurse plans care to support the woman through surgery.

The concept of caring is considered by many to be synonymous with nursing. Caring addresses a specific social relationship consisting of affection and service, which is an integral part of a process that provides for and maintains physical and mental health. It reflects feelings of concern and interest in others that are inherent to nursing (Pepin, 1992).

Women have long been socialized into a caring role in society. In the past nurse midwives were the gynecologists, obstetricians, and confidants of women. Today women often are more comfortable discussing problems of the reproductive organs with another woman. Since most nurses are women, they are looked to for caring, support, and understanding of these personal and private health care issues.

Change in social customs, advances in all aspects of surgery, and vast changes in technology have continually influenced gynecologic surgery in the twentieth century. Culposcopy, pelviscopy, and hysteroscopy are diagnostic tools routinely used since the development and refinement of endoscopic equipment. The refinement of the laparoscope has allowed surgeons to examine the abdominal/pelvic cavity with minimal surgical assault. Pathology or structural problems can be easily identified. The minimally invasive surgery allows women to recover quickly from the procedure, which today is generally performed on an outpatient basis. The development of the surgical laser, often used through the laparoscope, has provided the surgeon with a precision tool for hemostasis and lysis of adhesions that leaves less scar tissue and edema than other methods.

Knowledge of fertility, and of the causes of infertility, and the ability to perform in vitro fertilization or gamete intrafallopian transfer technique (GIFT) have helped develop a new subspecialty of gynecology.

ANATOMY

External Genitalia (Vulva)

The external genitalia of the female include several structures that are referred to as the vulva. These structures are the labia majora and minora, the mons pubis, the clitoris, the vestibule, the urethral orifice, the hymen, and Bartholin's glands and ducts (Fig. 9-1). The external genitalia cover and protect the urethral and vaginal openings.

The mons pubis is a rounded mound of tissue that covers the anterior portion of the pubic bone. Extending downward and backward from the mons pubis are two folds of skin called the labia majora. Within the labia majora are two additional folds called the labia minora, the lateral parts of which form the prepuce of the clitoris. The clitoris is a small, sensitive, densely vascular erectile structure. The vestibule is surrounded by the labia minora and contains the urethral and vaginal openings. The urethra, which connects the bladder to the urethral meatus, is located posterior to the clitoris and anterior to the vagina. The vaginal orifice extends through the hymen, a piece of tissue that partially covers the opening. Bartholin's glands are located on either side of the vagina; the ducts open into the vaginal orifice. The glands provide lubrication to the mucous membranes.

Bony Pelvis

The ilium, symphysis pubis, ischium, sacrum, and coccyx make up the bony pelvis. The lower part forms the true pelvis, which is the passageway for the fetus during childbirth. The true pelvis is divided into the inlet, cavity, and outlet. It is lined with muscles that give shape and support to the cavity. The floor of the pelvis, the pelvic diaphragm, supports the abdominal pelvic viscera. It separates the pelvic cavity from the perineum and consists of the levator ani and coccygeal muscles.

Pelvic Cavity

The remaining female reproductive organs are contained in the pelvic cavity. They include the uterus, fallopian tubes, ovaries, vagina, and cervix (Fig. 9-2).

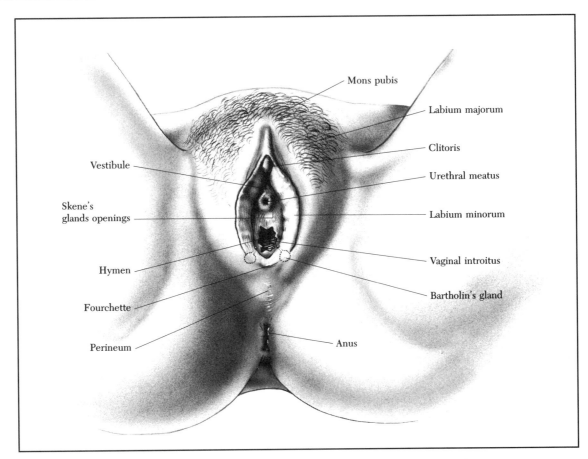

FIGURE 9-1 Anatomy of the vulva. (From Grimes, J. and Burns, E. [1992]. *Health Assessment in Nursing Practice* [3rd ed.]. Boston: Jones and Bartlett Publishers.)

The uterus

The uterus is a pear-shaped hollow organ that lies between the urinary bladder and the rectum. It is supported and maintained in this position by several paired ligaments, the round, broad, cardinal, and uterosacral ligaments. The fallopian tubes enter the uterus at its uppermost points, the uterine cornua. The upper rounded portion of the uterus is the fundus; the lower portion, which joins the vagina, is the cervix. The cervical os connects the uterus to the vagina. The upper and lower portions are separated by a narrowed portion called the isthmus.

The uterine wall has three layers. The outer one is formed by peritoneum, the middle is a muscular layer called myometrium, and the inner layer is endometrium, which lines the cavity. The endometrial layer undergoes changes during the menstrual cycle and is sloughed off as menstrual flow when pregnancy does not occur. When pregnancy does occur, the uterus houses the products of conception until the time of childbirth.

The fallopian tubes

The fallopian tubes enter the uterus at its upper lateral portion and extend laterally from it. The ends farthest from the uterus are wider and have fringelike projections called fimbriae, located just below the ovaries. These musculomembranous tubes form the canal through which the ova travel to the uterus. Fertilization takes place in the fallopian tube, but this can also be the site for an ectopic pregnancy. The fallopian tubes are in close proximity to the ureters, and clear identification of each is a critical step in gynecologic surgery.

The ovaries

The almond-shaped ovaries are located at the sides of the uterus. They are attached to the back of the broad ligament and suspended from it by the ovarian ligament (Fig. 9-3). The outer layer of the ovary is the cortex, and the inner vascular layer is the medulla. Ovarian (graafian) follicles of varying maturity are in the cortex. The ovaries are covered by epithelium.

NURSING CONSIDERATIONS

General Information

The perioperative nurse who cares for the gynecologic patient will be aware of the potential impact of the surgery on the woman's body image and self-esteem. The

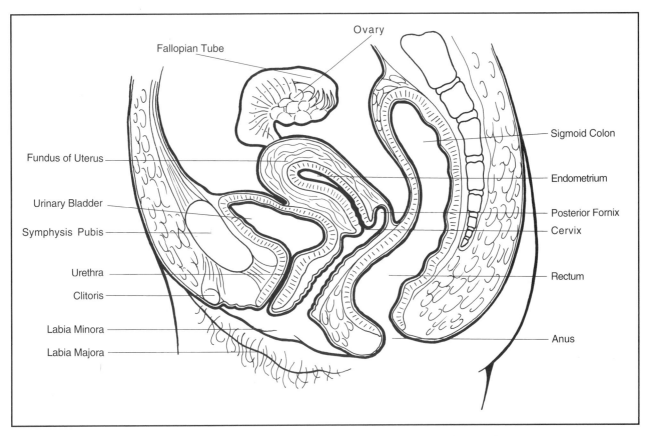

FIGURE 9-2 Anatomy of the pelvic cavity (median sagittal section).

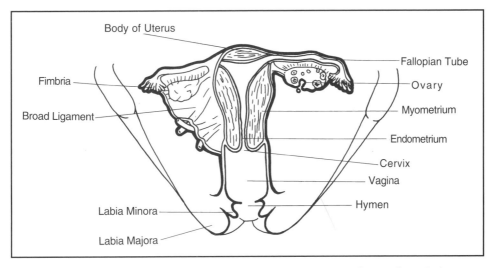

FIGURE 9-3 Reproductive organs of the female (uterus, tubes, and ovaries).

woman may fear rejection by loved ones if she faces removal of a body part related to her sexuality. A woman having infertility surgery may fear rejection if she is unable to bear children. Other women may be grieving for a lost pregnancy or the fact that they will be unable to bear more children.

Gynecologic surgery is performed for diagnosis or treatment of pathology of the vulva, vagina, cervix, uterus, tubes, or ovaries. Pathology can be abnormal bleeding, malignant or benign lesions, or infection. Surgery is also performed to diagnose or treat infertility and problems of pregnancy such as an incompetent uterus, abortion or miscarriage, retained placenta, or ruptured uterus. Another category of gynecologic procedures are performed to correct an injured or weakened anatomical structure.

Many of the gynecologic surgical procedures are performed on an outpatient basis. Often, they are performed on women who have children at home. These factors may necessitate arrangements for assistance in the home after discharge. Preadmission screening can identify these needs, and staff can assist with planning. A follow-up phone call will determine whether further intervention is required.

Signs and symptoms of pathology may be overt or covert. Abnormal bleeding or vaginal discharge, palpable masses, structural weaknesses (cystocele or rectocele), and signs of an infection such as pain and fever will often cause a woman to seek medical advice. Other pathology may not produce symptoms but may be seen on routine examination of the vulva, vagina, or cervix. Some pathology will be identified in a physician's office when colposcopy is done as a follow-up to an abnormal Papanicolaou smear.

Diagnostic studies

In addition to studies that are routine for all surgical patients, gynecologic patients may have diagnostic studies related to their particular diagnosis. Urinary tract studies such as an intravenous pyelogram may be done for a differential diagnosis. Ultrasound is used to diagnose ectopic pregnancy and to visualize masses of the uterus, such as uterine fibroids, or of the adnexa, such as ovarian masses or cysts. Computed tomography (CT) or magnetic resonance imaging (MRI) may be used to determine involvement of lymph nodes or bone when malignancy is suspected.

A *hysterosalpingogram* is done to determine uterine or tubal causes of infertility. The procedure is generally done in a physician's office or clinic. The results will indicate where an obstruction, if any, exists.

Colposcopy is performed in a physician's office or clinic as a follow-up to an abnormal Papanicolaou smear. It is used to identify areas of preinvasive lesions. Biopsy (punch or cone) or endometrial curettage may be done in connection with a colposcopy.

Nursing Diagnoses

Information commonly obtained from a woman having gynecologic surgery will include her menstrual history and a description of her menstrual cycle. If the woman is of child-bearing age it is important to verify the possibility of a pregnancy. Some physicians request a pregnancy test routinely when scheduling certain procedures. The woman should be asked about any urinary tract disorders because they often accompany gynecologic problems. Stress incontinence is associated with a cystocele, for example. The nurse will also observe for surgical scars, since adhesions from previous surgery may complicate a laparoscopic procedure.

Nursing diagnoses commonly identified for gynecologic surgical patients are anxiety, high risk for infection, high risk for injury, high risk for impaired skin integrity, and high risk for alteration in sexuality.

Anxiety

Anxiety may be related to fear of the surgical procedure, lack of understanding of the disease process, concern over sexuality and body image, and concerns about outcomes of surgery that may affect future relationships with a sex partner. Women with young children may have concerns about child care issues or be anxious about leaving their children when they enter the hospital. Nursing interventions involve listening to and discussing concerns and correcting misconceptions related to the surgery and outcomes of surgery.

High risk for infection

Though infection is a concern for all surgical patients, patients who have their normal lines of defense compromised are more at risk. Gynecologic surgery often requires the placement of an indwelling Foley catheter, which bypasses the normal defense mechanisms of the urinary system. Scrupulous care is necessary when inserting and handling the catheter. Some patients may have received preoperative radiation treatment, which renders the skin more friable and susceptible to damage and infection.

High risk for injury

Risk for injury may be related to positioning, equipment, skin prep solution, or retention of a foreign body. The lithotomy position, frequently used for gynecologic surgery, carries potential for nerve and muscle injury or hypotension due to a fluid shift. (See Chapter 28, Vol. 1 on positioning.) The lithotomy position also provides an opportunity for prep solutions to pool under the buttocks. Use of electrical equipment and lasers creates the potential for patient burns.

Slowly lifting and lowering legs into and out of lithotomy position, padding stirrups used for positioning, and using blotting towels to collect the prep solution help to avoid muscle or nerve injuries and chemical burns. Checking equipment and following safety measures for laser and electrical equipment also reduce the potential for injury. Counting instruments, sponges, needles, and other small items is the intervention used to avoid retention of a foreign body.

High risk for impaired skin integrity

Alteration in skin integrity may occur when the patient is debilitated, elderly, or immunocompromised. Skin injury may also result from positioning, even when the positioning is done correctly. Padding of the sacral area when the patient is in lithotomy position helps relieve pressure in this area. Padding bony areas and maintaining proper body alignment during positioning decrease the potential for tissue injury.

High risk for alteration in sexuality

Alteration in sexuality is associated with a change in or loss of a body part. Contributing factors may be the result of physiological limitations or psychological issues related to the patient's feelings of being female. Listening to patients' concerns and providing emotional support and education when necessary are common interventions needed initially. Depending on the problem, additional psychological counseling may be recommended.

PROCEDURES INVOLVING THE EXTERNAL GENITALIA

Only a few procedures are performed on the female genitalia. The simplest is removal of venereal warts (condylomata). The most extensive is radical vulvectomy. Vulvectomy is the treatment for intraepithelial cancers. The extent of the vulvectomy—simple, skinning, or radical—depends on how invasive the cancer is. A skinning vulvectomy is selected most often. This procedure removes the external skin from the affected area. Being less radical than other procedures, it minimizes anatomical deformity and psychosocial consequences without compromising the cure rate. Increasingly, a laser is used for this procedure. Simple and radical vulvectomies are still performed when necessary, but they have been modified to preserve anatomical structures and sexual function. Before any vulvar surgery, the patient is examined and the tumor is classified according to the Tumor Node Metastasis (TNM) System (Table 9-1). The classification helps to determine the procedure performed.

Perioperative Nursing Considerations

The instrumentation for vulva surgery consists of vaginal instruments and soft tissue instruments. A laser and a microscope may be used for removal of condylomata. If extensive dissection is required for vulvectomy, supplies and equipment for skin grafting should be available. A separate specimen container is needed for each node that is removed during node dissection. Standard equipment such as an electrosurgical unit, sutures, and suction, and irrigation and dressing materials are also required.

The patient is placed in a low lithotomy position for procedures of the external genitalia. A standard surgical prep with an approved antimicrobial solution is used to cleanse the area. The patient is then draped in the usual manner for patients in lithotomy position. The exposed area varies according to the procedure. Laser safety measures, such as moist drapes and a moist sponge placed in the rectum, should be followed when a laser is used.

Surgical Procedures

Vulvectomy

Several types of vulvectomy are performed. The procedure selected depends on the stage of the cancer as identified according to the TNM classification (see Table 9-1). A skinning vulvectomy is simple removal of the external skin from the affected area. In a simple vulvectomy the labia majora and minora are removed. Sometimes the cli-

TABLE 9-1 TNM Classification of Vulvar Carcinoma

Classification	Description
T—Primary Tumor	
T1	Tumor confined to the vulva, 2 cm or less in largest diameter
T2	Tumor confined to the vulva, more than 2 cm in largest diameter
T3	Tumor of any size with adjacent spread to the urethra, vagina, perineum, or anus
T4	Tumor of any size infiltrating the bladder mucosa, the rectal mucosa, or both, including the upper part of the urethral mucosa, or fixed to the bone
N—Regional Lymph Nodes	
N0	No lymph node metastasis
N1	Nodes palpable in one or both groins, not enlarged, mobile (not clinically suspicious of neoplasm). Proved by biopsy.
N2	Nodes palpable in one or both groins, enlarged, firm, and mobile (clinically suspicious of neoplasm). Proved by biopsy.
N3	Fixed or ulcerated nodes
M—Distant Metastases	
M0	No clinical metastases
M1a	Palpable deep pelvic lymph nodes
M1b	Other distant metastases

toris and perianal tissue must also be dissected. The most extensive procedure is radical vulvectomy with groin lymphadenectomy. In this procedure the following structures are removed: skin from the abdomen and groin, the labia majora and minora, clitoris, mons veneris, portions of the urethra, and vagina. Additional structures that may be removed include the inguinal lymph nodes, sections of the round ligaments, and sections of the saphenous veins. Figure 9-4 indicates lines of incision for a vulvectomy.

The following nursing considerations are specific to patients undergoing vulvectomy:

1. Patients who undergo vulvectomy require emotional support from the nurse to help deal with the anxiety and fear associated with cancer and with body image adjustments resulting from the surgery.
2. If skin grafting is anticipated, the nurse will be prepared to prep and drape two surgical sites.
3. Sutures, use of a closed drainage system, dressings, and vaginal packing are determined by the surgeon's preference.
4. If lymph nodes are dissected, the nurse will ensure that a separate specimen container, precisely labeled, is used for each node.
5. The nurse will prepare a Foley catheter for insertion at the end of surgery.

Ablation of condylomata

Sexually transmitted venereal warts (condylomata) are removed from the vulva and sometimes from the lower

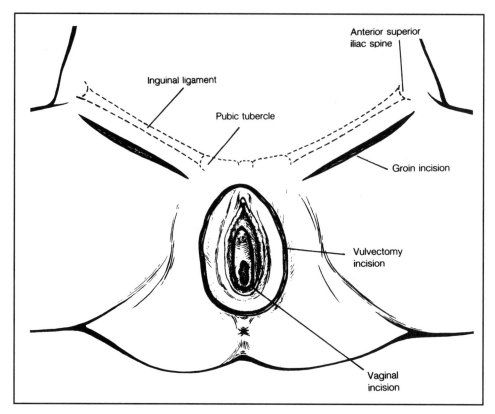

FIGURE 9-4 Incision lines for simple and radical vulvectomy.

portion of the vagina. This is most commonly achieved by laser ablation. The laser is often attached to the microscope for better control of the beam and for better visualization, especially in the vaginal area. This procedure may be done in the operating room suite, physician's office, or clinic.

The following nursing considerations are specific to patients undergoing ablation of condylomata:

1. The nurse ensures that the patient is not unduly exposed during the procedure, and that her privacy is respected, by monitoring the number of personnel who enter the room and by covering windows.
2. The procedure is generally done under general anesthesia as an outpatient procedure.
3. The procedure is done with the patient in lithotomy position. The nurse must ensure that proper measures are taken to prevent nerve and muscle injury.
4. Few instruments are used. A vaginal speculum may be used to provide exposure to determine the extent of the affected area. A microscope may be used to magnify the area and to stabilize a laser.
5. If a laser is used, the nurse must follow laser safety protocols. If the patient is awake, the patient must also wear eye protection.
6. The nurse ensures that a smoke evacuator is used to capture the laser plume, which contains chemical by-products as well as biological materials that may be hazardous (see Chapter 22 in Volume 1).
7. Discharge instructions include information on cleansing the operative site.

8. Laser treatment produces little edema, mild pain (controlled with a mild analgesic), and rapid healing.

Key steps

1. The patient is placed in lithotomy position, prepped, and draped.
2. The surgeon moves the laser beam across the tissue in a pattern that treats all perimeters of the affected area.
3. A sponge moistened with a solution of 3% to 5% acetic acid (vinegar) is used periodically to wipe the affected area. This causes the affected tissue to be more prominent, which then allows treatment to deeper layers.
4. An antibiotic ointment is used to cover the area. The wound is generally left uncovered, but a perineal pad can be placed loosely for coverage.

VAGINAL PROCEDURES

Vaginal procedures refer to procedures performed on the vagina and to those done through a vaginal approach. Vaginal procedures can be done with either general or spinal anesthesia. Some may be done with regional block. Many procedures are done in a same-day surgery setting, clinic, or physician's office. Procedures using the vaginal approach create special problems for the scrubbed person. Most surgeons sit during the procedure, often holding a sterile tray in their lap to hold the instruments to be reused. The scrubbed person must stand behind the surgeon and place the instruments on the tray, being careful to maintain asepsis from this awkward position.

Perioperative Nursing Considerations

The equipment needed for these procedures varies with the technique and its complexity. Some examples are laser, electrosurgery unit, vacuum aspirator, suction, and stirrups for positioning. Padding is needed for the stirrups. Dressing material may include vaginal packing and usually includes a perineal pad. Topical solutions and vaginal creams are commonly used. A Foley or suprapubic cystostomy catheter is used for postoperative urine drainage. The instrumentation usually begins with a dilatation and curettage (D&C) set. Additional soft tissue instruments and retractors are added, according to the procedure planned. Most operating rooms have a special instrument set for vaginal hysterectomy, and special clamps for an anterior–posterior vaginal repair. Heavy suture material and a specially designed needle are needed for Shirodkar's procedure (vaginal instruments are shown in Figure 9-5).

The patient is placed in lithotomy position. The level of the stirrups may vary according to the surgeon's preference. The patient's legs must be level and padded well to avoid pressure areas, especially during long procedures. The legs should be raised and lowered together, to prevent injury to the hip joint. The legs should be lowered slowly to avoid a sudden drop in blood pressure when the blood rushes back into them. For simple procedures like a D&C, hair removal is often not required. The perineum and vagina are cleansed with an approved antimicrobial solution, and the patient is then draped. Draping usually includes three diagonally folded towels placed around the

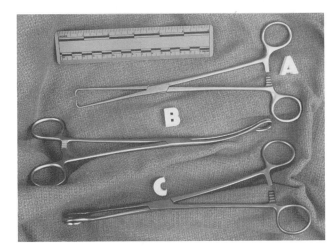

B

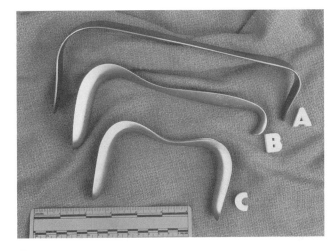

C

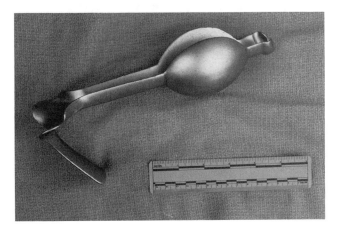

A

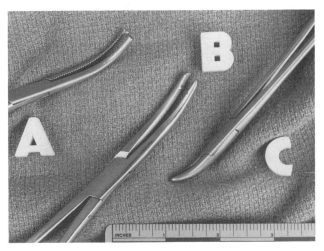

D

FIGURE 9-5 Vaginal instruments. (*A*) Auvard vaginal weighted speculum. (*B*) A: Single toothed cervical tenaculum; B: curved and C: straight sponge forceps. (*C*) Vaginal retractors. A: Heaney, B: single-ended Sims, and C: double-ended Sims. (*D*) A: Curved Kocher forceps, B: curved Heaney forceps, and C: Heaney needle holder.

labia. Leggings cover the stirrups and legs, and half sheets are used under the buttocks and over the abdomen.

Surgical Procedures

Vaginal hysterectomy

Vaginal hysterectomy is the procedure by which the uterus is removed through the vagina. A D&C and anterior and posterior repair are often done at the same time.

The following nursing considerations are specific to patients undergoing a vaginal hysterectomy with or without an anterior and posterior repair of the vagina.

1. The nurse is aware that loss of the uterus may be an emotional event and provides appropriate support to the patient.
2. Protection of privacy and modesty is accomplished by preventing undue exposure, limiting traffic in the operating room, and covering windows, if necessary.
3. Appropriate interventions are provided by the nurse to prevent the hazards associated with the lithotomy position.

Key steps

1. A weighted speculum is first placed in the vagina. Additional retractors are placed on either side of the vagina to provide proper exposure.
2. The cervix is grasped with a tenaculum to provide retraction, and an incision is made in the anterior vaginal wall (Fig. 9-6).
3. Sharp and blunt dissection is used to separate the bladder from the cervix (Fig. 9-7) so the peritoneum can be entered (Fig. 9-8).

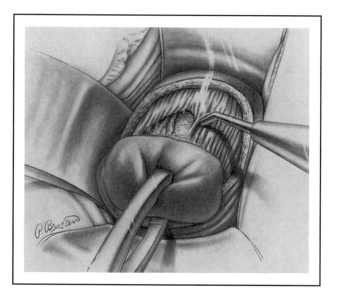

FIGURE 9-6 Vaginal hysterectomy. Incision is made with the ESU blade into the anterior vaginal wall. (From Thompson, J. D., & Rock, J. A. [1992]. *TeLinde's operative gynecology* [7th ed.]. Philadelphia: J. B. Lippincott.)

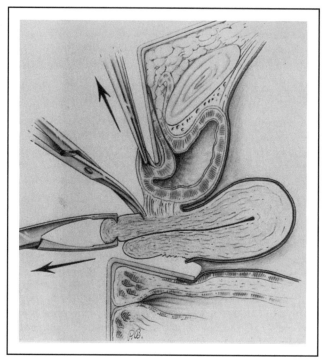

FIGURE 9-7 Vaginal hysterectomy. Retraction allows the bladder to be separated from the cervix. (From Thompson, J. D., & Rock, J. A. [1992]. *TeLinde's operative gynecology* [7th ed.]. Philadelphia: J. B. Lippincott.)

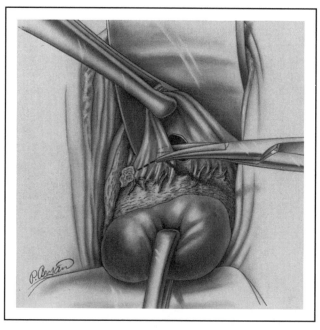

FIGURE 9-8 Vaginal hysterectomy. Entering the peritoneal cavity. (From Thompson, J. D., & Rock, J. A. [1992]. *TeLinde's operative gynecology* [7th ed.]. Philadelphia: J. B. Lippincott.)

4. The uterosacral ligaments are clamped, cut, tied, and tagged with a clamp.
5. The uterus is pulled downward, so that the cardinal ligaments and uterine arteries can be clamped, cut, tied, and tagged.

6. The uterus is pulled down farther, so that the round ligament, ovarian ligament, and fallopian tubes can be clamped, cut, and tied, allowing the uterus to be totally extracted through the vagina.

7. The round, cardinal, and uterosacral ligaments previously tagged with different clamps for identification purposes are approximated (Fig. 9-9).

8. The area is checked for bleeding, and the peritoneum is closed.

9. At this point, if indicated, anterior and posterior repair is done. If a repair is not done, vaginal packing is inserted and either a Foley or suprapubic catheter is inserted for urinary drainage.

Anterior and posterior repair of the vagina

A vaginal repair is done to correct a weakness in the walls of the vagina that allows the bladder or rectum to protrude into the vagina, causing pressure and difficulties in voiding and defecating. Vaginal repair is commonly done in conjunction with vaginal hysterectomy, though it can be done independently. If the weakness in the vaginal wall is isolated, an anterior or posterior wall repair alone may be done.

Key steps

1. If a weighted speculum is not already in place, one is placed in the prepped vagina. Right-angled retractors are placed to retract the lateral walls of the vagina.

2. The anterior vaginal wall is incised and separated from the underlying areolar tissue with sharp and blunt dissection.

3. The urethra and bladder neck are freed up (Fig. 9-10), and sutures are placed that, when tied, narrow the bladder neck (Fig. 9-11).

4. The cardinal ligament is shortened by suturing tissue into the cervix from the lateral aspect.

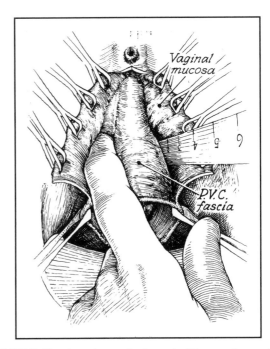

FIGURE 9-10 Anterior vaginal repair. The urethra and bladder neck are freed up. (From C. R. Wheeler, Jr.: *Atlas of Pelvic Surgery.* Philadelphia, Lea & Febiger, 1981. Reprinted with permission.)

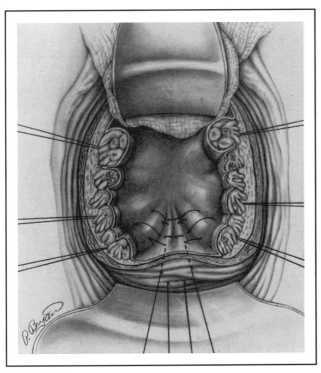

FIGURE 9-9 Vaginal hysterectomy. Vaginal vault after removal of uterus with ligaments tagged. (From Thompson, J. D., & Rock, J. A. [1992]. *TeLinde's operative gynecology* [7th ed.]. Philadelphia: J. B. Lippincott.)

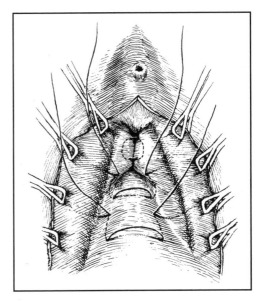

FIGURE 9-11 Anterior vaginal repair. Sutures are placed that, when tied, narrow the bladder. (From C. R. Wheeler, Jr.: *Atlas of Pelvic Surgery.* Philadelphia, Lea & Febiger, 1981. Reprinted with permission.)

5. The edges of the incision are trimmed, and the anterior vaginal wall is sutured closed (Fig. 9-12).
6. The posterior vaginal wall is incised, and the tissue is separated from the muscles beneath by sharp and blunt dissection.
7. The perineum and rectal muscles are strengthened by suturing the levator ani muscle and Colles' fascia together over the perineum.
8. Bleeding is controlled as needed.
9. Excess skin is trimmed, and the tissues are sutured together.
10. A vaginal pack may be left in place, and a Foley or suprapubic catheter is inserted for drainage of urine.

Dilatation and curettage

Dilatation and curettage is a procedure in which the cervical os is enlarged by using dilators of graduated size (Fig. 9-13). Once the os is dilated enough to allow passage of the curettes, a curette is inserted and the inside wall of the uterus scraped, and the tissue is removed for examination (Fig. 9-14). Curettes come in several sizes and with a sharp, cutting edge or smooth edge. This procedure is done for diagnostic purposes and as a treatment for abnormal uterine bleeding and incomplete abortion. It is often combined with other vaginal procedures. Figure 9-15 shows instruments used for this procedure.

Suction curettage

Suction curettage is the procedure done to remove the products of conception from the uterus. This technique is used only during the first trimester of pregnancy. It is essentially the same procedure as dilatation and curettage, except that the cervical os must be dilated enough to accept the suction curettes (Fig. 9-16). These curettes

are connected to a suction pump, which produces 70 mm Hg pressure and airflow of 100 ml per minute. This pressure causes the products of conception to separate from the walls of the uterus (Fig. 9-17). Positive aspects of this

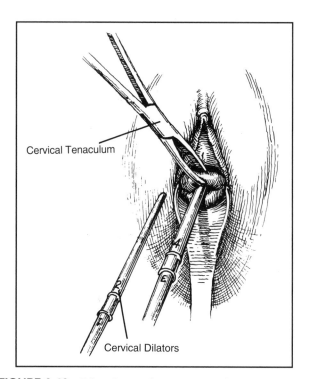

FIGURE 9-13 Dilatation and curettage. Dilators, graduated in size, are used to enlarge the cervical os. (From C. R. Wheeler, Jr.: *Atlas of Pelvic Surgery.* Philadelphia, Lea & Febiger, 1981. Reprinted with permission.)

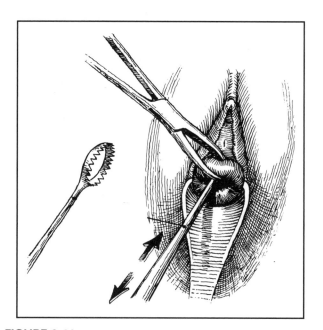

FIGURE 9-14 Dilatation and curettage. The inside wall of the uterus is scraped (curettaged), using a curette in motion indicated. (From C. R. Wheeler, Jr.: *Atlas of Pelvic Surgery.* Philadelphia, Lea & Febiger, 1981. Reprinted with permission.)

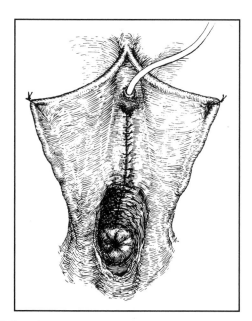

FIGURE 9-12 Anterior vaginal repair. The anterior wall is sutured closed. (From C. R. Wheeler, Jr.: *Atlas of Pelvic Surgery.* Philadelphia, Lea & Febiger, 1981. Reprinted with permission.)

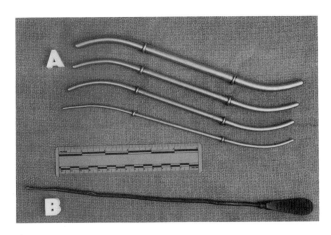

A

FIGURE 9-15 Vaginal instruments. (*A*) Various-size Hanks uterine dilators. A: Double-ended; B: Sims uterine sound. (*B*) A: Sims uterine curette (sharp); B: serrated uterine curette; C: Thomas uterine curette (blunt).

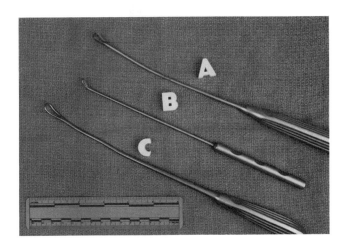

B

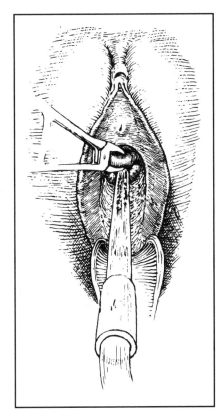

FIGURE 9-16 Suction curettage. Curette entering the cervical os. (From C. R. Wheeler, Jr.: *Atlas of Pelvic Surgery*. Philadelphia, Lea & Febiger, 1981. Reprinted with permission.)

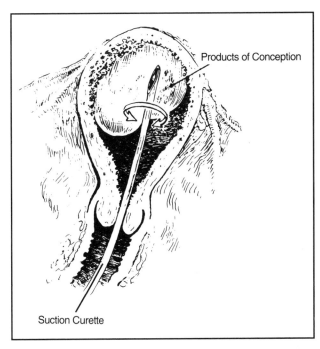

FIGURE 9-17 Suction curettage. Curette in uterus. Arrows indicate motion used. (From C. R. Wheeler, Jr.: *Atlas of Pelvic Surgery*. Philadelphia, Lea & Febiger, 1981. Reprinted with permission.)

procedure include a lower incidence of uterine perforation, decreased blood loss, and a reduction in the need for excessive curettage. This procedure can be performed on an outpatient basis with cervical block anesthesia.

Shirodkar's procedure

A Shirodkar procedure is done early during pregnancy to support an incompetent cervix. Without this procedure the fetus could not be carried to term. A heavy purse-string suture is placed around the cervical tissue at the level of the internal os, to close it and keep it closed until term, when it is removed and labor is initiated and progresses in a normal fashion.

Cervical conization

Cervical conization can be done for either diagnostic or therapeutic purposes. As a diagnostic measure it is

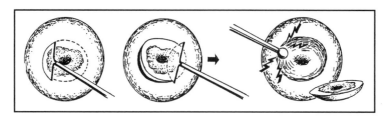

FIGURE 9-18 Steps in LLETZ procedure. (*Left*) The large loop electrode moves from left to right or right to left. (*Center*) A 5-mm margin is taken beyond the lesion. (*Right*) A ball electrode is used for coagulation. (From C. R. Wheeler, Jr.: *Atlas of Pelvic Surgery*. Philadelphia, Lea & Febiger, 1981. Reprinted with permission.)

done for further evaluation of patients with abnormal Papanicolaou smears. It is also a treatment for conditions such as cervical dysplasia and cervicitis. Several conization techniques are in use today. Conization can be accomplished with a scalpel, electrocautery, or laser. The most recent technique is the large loop excision of the transformation zone (LLETZ). Electrosurgical generators that combine cutting and coagulation, in association with the use of new wire loops that can withstand these complex radiofrequency blended currents, are used to remove the cervical tissue (Fig. 9-18).

Hysteroscopy

Hysteroscopy is endoscopic visualization of the uterine cavity and tubal openings after distention of the uterine cavity with 70% dextran in 10% dextrose, dextrose 50% in water, or carbon dioxide gas. Lactated Ringer's solution may also be used. It can be a diagnostic procedure for evaluation of abnormal uterine bleeding, infertility, or recurrent miscarriages. Indications for operative hysteroscopy include division of the uterine septum, myomectomy, removal of endometrial polyps, and endometrial ablation for menorrhagia.

The osmolality of fluids used to distend the uterus during tissue resection may cause electrolyte changes when absorbed, which can lead to severe complications. Therefore, glycine may be used. The nurse must monitor and record the precise amount of fluid that is instilled and recovered. The surgeon should be notified when 500 ml of fluid have been instilled and when each subsequent 500 ml have been instilled. Some surgeons will not instill more than 2000 ml, even if the procedure is not completed.

ABDOMINAL PROCEDURES

Abdominal procedures include simple ones such as hysterectomy and extensive ones such as pelvic exenteration. Any of a number of approaches may be used. Pfannenstiel's incision is often used, to avoid having a noticeable scar on the abdomen. A low midline incision is used if large tumors must be excised, and the surgeon may have to extend the incision to achieve better exposure. A midline incision may be selected if an extensive procedure is planned or there was a previous incision.

Perioperative Nursing Considerations

The instrumentation for abdominal procedures includes a major instrument set with the addition of gynecologic, vascular, and intestinal instruments according to what procedure is planned. Often a dilatation and curettage is done first, so those instruments should be available on a separate table. The bladder is kept empty during the procedure by insertion of a Foley catheter at the start of the procedure. A perineal pad is applied postoperatively. The sutures used are heavy No. 1 or 1-0. Standard dressing supplies should be available, as well as skin staples for closure if this is the surgeon's preference. Multiple specimen containers are needed if nodes are removed for evaluation. An electrosurgical unit and suction are standard for most cases.

The patient is placed in the supine position for standard abdominal procedures. The legs may be placed in low stirrups if access to the perineum is necessary, as in pelvic exenteration. Hair removal may not be necessary on the abdomen, though a small amount of pubic hair usually is removed. A standard antimicrobial is used to prep the abdomen and vagina. Draping is done according to hospital protocol.

Surgical Procedures

Total abdominal hysterectomy with bilateral salpingo-oophorectomy

Total abdominal hysterectomy with bilateral salpingo-oophorectomy removes the cervix, fallopian tubes, and ovaries. If cancer is suspected, lymph nodes can be removed for examination.

The following nursing considerations are specific to patients undergoing a total abdominal hysterectomy.

1. The loss of the uterus or concern over the diagnosis necessitating the surgery may be a highly emotional event for the patient. The nurse helps to allay anxiety and offers emotional support.

2. Patient privacy and modesty are maintained by the nurse by preventing undue exposure.

3. Often, methylene blue is used to identify ureters. This should be available in the operating room to prevent unnecessary delay during surgery.

4. Confine and contain technique is used when excising the uterus so that organisms found on the mucous membranes are not introduced into the abdominal cavity.

Key steps

1. An abdominal incision is made and extended through the fat, fascia, and muscle to the peritoneum. The peritoneum is then opened.

2. The abdominal organs are moved aside, and the posterior peritoneum is opened, exposing the uterus and ovaries.

3. If the ovaries are to be removed, the round ligament and ovarian vessels are clamped, cut, and tied with suture ligature. This is done bilaterally (Fig. 9-19).

4. The dome of the uterus is grasped with a tenaculum and traction is applied. The uterus is moved from side to side, to expose the ligaments and vessels to be divided.

5. The broad ligament on each side is clamped, cut, and tied in sections (Fig. 9-20).

6. The uterine artery is clamped. A second set of clamps is placed on the uterosacral ligaments. The vessels and ligaments are then cut and tied (Fig. 9-21).

7. The bladder and adjacent tissue are separated from the cervix by sharp and blunt dissection. The vagina is opened below the cervix, and the cervix and uterus are completely separated from the vagina (Fig. 9-22).

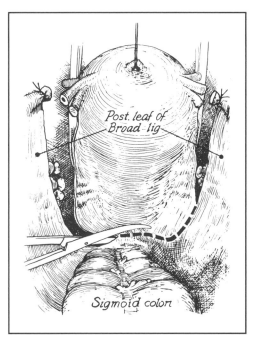

FIGURE 9-20 Abdominal hysterectomy. The broad ligaments have been divided. (From C. R. Wheeler, Jr.: *Atlas of Pelvic Surgery.* Philadelphia, Lea & Febiger, 1981. Reprinted with permission.)

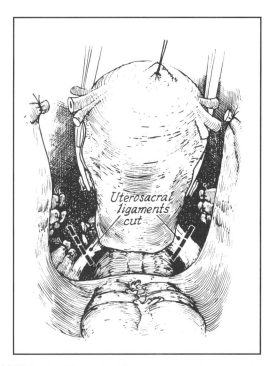

FIGURE 9-21 Abdominal hysterectomy. Uterosacral ligaments are cut. (From C. R. Wheeler, Jr.: *Atlas of Pelvic Surgery.* Philadelphia, Lea & Febiger, 1981. Reprinted with permission.)

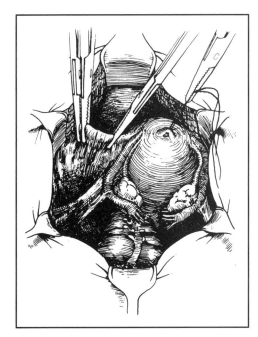

FIGURE 9-19 Abdominal hysterectomy. Clamping of the round ligament. (From C. R. Wheeler, Jr.: *Atlas of Pelvic Surgery.* Philadelphia, Lea & Febiger, 1981. Reprinted with permission.)

8. The edges of the vagina are grasped with Allis forceps while the vault is repaired and the vagina closed.

9. The posterior peritoneum is closed. The bowel and omentum are adjusted in the abdomen, and a routine abdominal closure is accomplished.

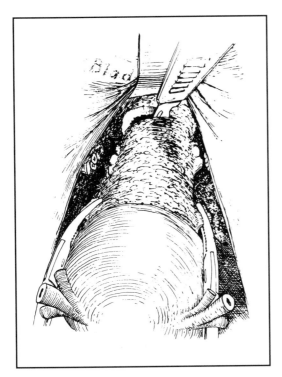

FIGURE 9-22 Abdominal hysterectomy. Cervix and uterus are separated from the vagina. (Thompson, J. D., & Rock, J. R. [1992]. *TeLinde's operative gynecology* [7th ed.]. Philadelphia: J. B. Lippincott.)

10. An abdominal dressing and a perineal pad are applied.

Radical hysterectomy (Wertheim's procedure)

In a radical hysterectomy the lymph nodes, supporting ligaments, upper portion of the vagina, ureters, and bladder are removed, in addition to the uterus, ovaries, and tubes.

Pelvic exenteration

Pelvic exenteration is extensive surgery involving en bloc excision of the rectum, distal sigmoid, bladder, distal ureters, internal iliac vessels and their lateral branches, all reproductive organs, and lymph nodes in the pelvis. The pelvic floor, pelvic peritoneum, levator muscles, and perineum are also removed. Marlex or Teflon mesh is sometimes used to form a pelvic floor. Radiation therapy that often precedes this procedure leaves tissues friable and susceptible to bleeding.

Oophorocystectomy

Oophorocystectomy is removal of an ovarian cyst. It may involve only enucleation of the cyst or include excision of a portion of the ovary.

Myomectomy

Myomectomy is a procedure by which uterine fibroids are excised without the associated removal of the uterus, so that fertility is maintained. Myomas may be found inside or outside the uterus. Usually they are not malignant.

PROCEDURES THAT AFFECT FERTILITY

Procedures that affect fertility are those that prevent or enhance fertility. Several of the procedures can be accomplished through a laparoscope or an open abdominal incision. The choice is the surgeon's. However, the use of the laparoscope is becoming much more commonplace.

Perioperative Nursing Considerations

Open abdominal approach

Depending on the procedure, the instrumentation may include a major instrument set with microsurgical instruments or a minor instrument set. Common equipment consists of a microscope, electrosurgery unit (monopolar and bipolar), laser, smoke evacuator, and video system. Supplies may include microscope and camera drapes, standard dressings, fine to heavy suture, methylene blue, and heparinized lactated Ringer's solution.

Laparoscopic approach

The laparoscopic approach requires a scope and all associated instrumentation for making the incision, such as trocars, and operating instruments that pass through the scope, such as holding, cutting, coagulating, suturing, suctioning, and irrigating instruments. The camera and light source that afford visualization of the abdominal structures are also attached to the scope. Additional equipment needed to allow the instrumentation to work include the light source, video cassette recorder, camera control unit, monitor, carbon dioxide insufflator, suction, and electrosurgical unit. The instrumentation used, the scope, and the trocars may be disposable or reusable. Some facilities use filtered tubing for carbon dioxide insufflation to ensure no particles from the tank enter the abdomen and no blood from the abdomen backflows to the insufflator (Chapter 1 in this volume has many illustrations of instruments and equipment used for laparoscopic surgery).

An abdominal approach requires that the patient be placed in a standard supine position. The laparoscopic approach requires a supine position with the patient's legs in low stirrups. Newer stirrups have been developed that are designed like riding boots. The foot and calf are placed in a supporting piece. Other stirrups support the leg under the knee as well as having a boot for the foot to rest in. Prepping is done with a standard antimicrobial solution. The vagina may or may not be prepped depending on the planned procedure. Draping involves a standard abdominal protocol or a combination abdominal and vaginal protocol, according to the procedure planned.

The following nursing considerations are specific to patients undergoing laparoscopic surgery.

1. When laparoscopic surgery is performed, many pieces of equipment are in the operating room. The nurse explains the equipment to the patient to help alleviate anxiety.
2. Often the procedure is performed as a same-day surgery procedure. The nurse provides discharge instructions related to pain relief and care of the incision.
3. The reusable instruments used must be handled and cleaned carefully since they are fine and delicate. The nurse ensures that competent personnel prepare the instruments.

Surgical Procedures

Tubal ligation

Laparoscopic tubal occlusion is one technique used to ligate the fallopian tubes. Often a dilatation and curettage is performed, followed by the insertion into the cervix of Hulka forceps or a uterine dilator. The forceps or dilator is used to manipulate the uterus during laparoscopy.

Key steps

1. A small incision is made in the abdomen at the lower margin of the umbilicus. A Veress needle is inserted into the peritoneal cavity, and carbon dioxide gas is instilled via tubing that connects the insufflator and the needle (Fig. 9-23). About 2 to 3 liters of gas is instilled while the patient is closely monitored. It is important not to overdistend the abdomen and to ensure that the gas is flowing properly.
2. The needle is removed, and a trocar with a sleeve large enough to accept the scope is inserted (Fig. 9-24). Insufflation is continued, if necessary.
3. The trocar is removed and replaced with the laparoscope, which may or may not be attached to a camera.
4. Under direct vision, a second incision is made and a trocar with a sleeve is inserted suprapubically. Through this sleeve additional instruments are introduced (Fig. 9-25).
5. For tubal ligation, additional instruments are either an electrosurgical unit cauterizing tip to coagulate and cut the tube or an instrument that grasps the fallopian tube and occludes it with a plastic ring (Fig. 9-26, *1* to *3*).
6. Once both tubes have been ligated, the instruments are removed and the carbon dioxide gas is allowed to escape through the scope. The scope and sleeves are removed, and the small incisions are closed and covered with an adhesive bandage.

Chapter 18 in this volume contains extensive information and illustrations that are helpful in understanding laparoscopic surgery and the equipment involved.

Minilaparotomy tubal ligation

The minilaparotomy is another approach to tubal ligation. It is used if the ligation is to be done within 24 hours after the woman gives birth. The tubes are easily accessible at this time because the uterus is still enlarged.

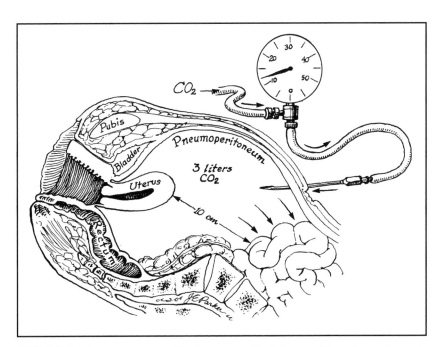

FIGURE 9-23 Laparoscopy. The Veress needle is inserted into the peritoneal cavity and gas is instilled. (From C. R. Wheeler, Jr.: *Atlas of Pelvic Surgery.* Philadelphia, Lea & Febiger, 1981. Reprinted with permission.)

Key steps

1. A small transverse incision is made above the pubic hairline.
2. A Babcock clamp is placed into the incision, and the fallopian tube is brought out through the incision.
3. The tube is folded over and tied with a heavy ligature.

4. The portion of the tube above the ligature is excised and sent to the laboratory.
5. The same procedure is repeated for the other tube.
6. The incision is closed with a subcuticular stitch, and a small dressing is applied.

Microscopic reconstruction of the fallopian tube

This procedure requires a microscope, very fine and delicate microsurgical instruments, and sometimes a laser.

The following nursing considerations are specific to patients undergoing reconstruction of the fallopian tube.

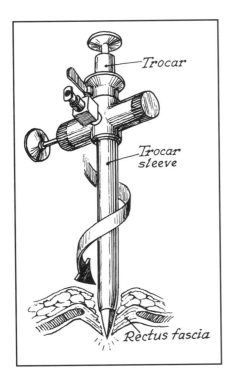

FIGURE 9-24 Laparoscopy. A trocar with sleeve is inserted. (From C. R. Wheeler, Jr.: *Atlas of Pelvic Surgery*. Philadelphia, Lea & Febiger, 1981. Reprinted with permission.)

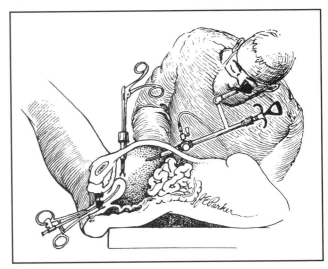

FIGURE 9-25 Laparoscopy. A second incision is made for additional instruments. (From C. R. Wheeler, Jr.: *Atlas of Pelvic Surgery*. Philadelphia, Lea & Febiger, 1981. Reprinted with permission.)

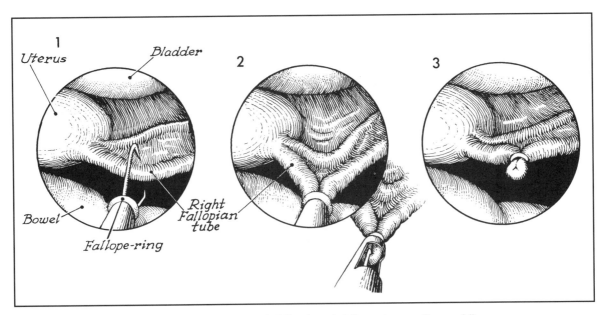

FIGURE 9-26 Laparoscopic tubal ligation. A fallope-ring applicator (*1*) grasps the tube, (*2*) folds the tube on itself, and (*3*) occludes the tube with the ring. (From C. R. Wheeler, Jr.: *Atlas of Pelvic Surgery*. Philadelphia, Lea & Febiger, 1981. Reprinted with permission.)

1. The woman undergoing microvascular reconstruction will have had many diagnostic procedures and tests prior to surgery. She may have anxiety as to the outcome of the surgery that can be reduced, but perhaps not relieved, by the nurse.
2. Laser safety precautions must be followed. The nurse will ensure that the patient's eyes are protected.
3. The microvascular instruments require special handling to preserve their precision.

Key steps

1. A standard abdominal incision is made through all layers to expose the uterus and fallopian tubes.
2. The scarred ends of the tubes are located, and with microsurgical instruments or laser (to minimize trauma) the scar tissue is excised.
3. Patency of the tube is determined by retrograde lavage.
4. The ends of the tubes are then carefully anastomosed with fine suture to ensure that the lumen remains open.
5. The abdominal wound is closed in layers, and a dressing is applied.

Removal of tubal ectopic pregnancy

Removal of an ectopic pregnancy can be performed through an abdominal incision or endoscopically. It involves opening the fallopian tube and removing the conceptus, which remained in the tube after fertilization instead of attaching to the uterine wall.

In vitro fertilization and embryo transfer

In vitro fertilization is achieved by stimulating follicular development and oocyte maturation to obtain a mature oocyte. Oocyte aspiration is done before spontaneous ovulation. The oocyte is placed in an incubator, where within 6 to 24 hours insemination is carried out. Between 36 and 40 hours after insemination, the embryo is placed into the uterine cavity.

Gamete intrafallopian transfer

Gamete intrafallopian transfer (GIFT) is another technique being used. This technique differs from in vitro fertilization in that the oocyte is aspirated, mixed with sperm, and then immediately placed within the fimbriated end of one of the fallopian tubes.

Cesarean section

Cesarean section is delivery of the fetus through an abdominal incision. This technique is used when the mother's condition could cause fetal distress or when fetal distress has developed. Some of the more common conditions are fetal malposition, placenta previa, maternal diabetes, and maternal-fetal cephalopelvic disproportion. Cesarean section may be an elective or an emergency procedure. Basic laparotomy instruments and additional obstetrical instrument are used.

Obstetrical instruments include heavy bandage scissors to cut the cord, Pennington clamps to clamp the edge of the uterine incision, ring forceps to remove the placenta, cord clamps to clamp the umbilical cord, delivery forceps to extract the fetal head, and a bladder retractor. A bulb syringe is needed to clear the infant's nose and mouth of amniotic fluid.

Usually spinal or epidural anesthesia is preferred for cesarean section. If general anesthesia is chosen, prepping and draping is completed before induction to reduce the depressive effect of the anesthetic on the fetus.

Most hospitals require a sponge count as the uterine cavity is closed, in addition to routine counts. The responsibility of the circulating nurse is generally to the mother and the surgical team, with another assigned professional caring for the infant.

Key steps

1. The abdomen is opened and the uterus is identified. The bladder is separated from the cervix by blunt and sharp dissection and a bladder flap is created.
2. An incision is then made into the uterus. The location of the incision depends on fetal position and previous scars.
3. Opening of the uterus and removal of the infant proceeds rapidly. Suctioning is critical as the uterus is opened and the infant delivered.
4. The cord is clamped and the infant passed to a nurse or pediatrician.
5. The surgeon removes the placenta, blood, and amniotic sacs from the uterus and closes the uterine wall in two layers.
6. After the serosa of the bladder and uterus are reapproximated, the abdomen is closed.

SUMMARY

The perioperative nurse who cares for women undergoing gynecologic surgery is continuously challenged by the ever-changing modalities and surgical techniques used for these procedures. The use of minimally invasive surgery means that many patients will have little opportunity to discuss with a nurse their fears, emotions, and anxieties prior to the day of surgery. The nurse must be prepared to provide support to the patient and also manage sophisticated technology used for surgery. This chapter has described certain commonly performed procedures and the equipment, supplies, and instruments used for each. It has also described the nursing care considerations for gynecologic surgical patients.

The female patient often looks to the nurse for caring and understanding of issues related to reproduction and reproductive organs. Providing emotional support and caring can be rewarding for the gynecologic perioperative nurse.

REFERENCES

Anderson, P. D. (1984). *Basic Human Anatomy and Physiology: Clinical Implications for the Health Professions.* Boston: Jones and Bartlett Publishers.

Association of Operating Room Nurses. (1994). *Standards and recommended practices.* Denver: Author.

Jones, H.W. III, Wentz, A. C., & Burnett, L. S. (1988). *Novak's Textbook of Gynecology.* Baltimore: Williams & Wilkins.

Kistner, R. (1990). *Kistner's Gynecology Principles and Practices.* Chicago: Year Book.

Meeker, M. H., & Rothrock, J. C. (1991). *Alexander's care of the patient in surgery.* St. Louis: Mosby–Year Book.

Parsons, C. L., & Ulfelder, H. (1968). *Atlas of pelvic operations* (2nd ed.). Philadelphia: W. B. Saunders.

Pepin, J. I. (Summer 1992). Family caring and caring in nursing. *Image: Journal of Nursing Scholarship, 24,* 127–131.

Rothrock, J. C. (1990). *Perioperative nursing care planning.* St. Louis: C. V. Mosby.

Thompson, J. D., & Rock, J. A. (1992). *TeLinde's operative gynecology* (7th ed.). Philadelphia: J. B. Lippincott.

Wheeler, C. R. (1981). *Atlas of pelvic surgery.* Philadelphia: Lea & Febiger.

Chapter 10

Neurosurgery

Key Concepts

- The patient undergoing neurosurgery is at risk for injury related to changes in intracranial pressure (ICP) and associated neurologic dysfunction.
- The patient has an increased risk of air embolus related to surgical positioning.
- Depending on the site of the lesion, the patient is at risk for alterations in sensoriperceptual functions.
- The anatomic site of the neurologic lesion and the length of the surgical procedure may place the patient at an increased risk for hypothermia.
- The patient has a potential for infection related to foreign bodies implanted during the procedure.
- The highly vascular nature of cerebral aneurysms and arteriovenous malformations (AVM) places the patient at risk for blood loss and decreased perfusion of other organs.
- The patient may experience a deficit of self-care related to the loss of function in a given anatomic region.
- The perioperative nurse combines a knowledge of anatomy and neurosurgical supplies and equipment with a knowledge of the individual patient into an organized plan of care that minimizes complications and maximizes outcomes for the neurosurgical patient.

INTRODUCTION

Development of neurosurgical technique largely took place over the past century. Progress has been made in the past few decades with advances in tumor classification, microsurgical technique, diagnostic modalities, trauma care, and improved instrumentation and technology. New procedures are constantly evolving. Lesions that were once believed to be inoperable are now treated surgically. As neurosurgery has developed, a better prognosis for patients with neurologic disorders has been afforded by the introduction of the operative microscope and microneurosurgical instrumentation, hemostasis via bipolar cautery, computed tomography (CT scan), magnetic resonance imaging (MRI), radiologic techniques, stereotaxis, sonography, intracranial pressure monitoring, shunting techniques, the carbon dioxide (CO_2) laser, high-speed drills, and the development of other equipment and instrumentation. This development in technology dictates an elevation in the perioperative nurse's knowledge and skills to achieve optimal patient outcomes.

Information in this chapter is intended to serve as a basic guideline for commonly performed neurosurgical procedures. Surgical and nursing practices advance rapidly and require constant and curious attention. Areas such as neurosurgical endoscopy and spinal stereotaxis are in the early stages of development. Institutions vary in practice, and specialized neurosurgical centers may perform procedures not within the scope of this chapter. Pediatric neurosurgical procedures are also described in this chapter. General considerations regarding surgery of the infant and child are found in Chapter 18 of this volume.

ANATOMY

The Nervous System

The complexity of the nervous system has caused many nurses to avoid studying it (Snyder, 1991). Perioperative nurses participating in the care of patients undergoing surgical intervention of the nervous system can ill afford to shy away from a basic understanding of its anatomy. Anatomically, the nervous system consists of the central nervous system (CNS), consisting of the brain and spinal cord, and the peripheral nervous system, composed of nerves outside the brain and spinal cord and including the cranial and spinal nerves. Considerations of anatomy and related functions are paramount in the nurse's ability to assess a patient's preoperative status, plan intraoperative care, and identify deviations that may occur preoperatively or postoperatively.

The Head

External structures

The skull is a rigid cavity consisting of eight main bones that enclose and protect the brain. The cranium, or roof of the skull, consists of the frontal bone, the right and left parietal bones, the right and left temporal bones, and the sphenoid and ethmoid bones (Fig. 10-1). The interior of the skull is divided into the anterior, middle, and posterior fossae.

The scalp covers the bony structures of the skull and consists of skin, soft tissue, galea, and muscle. The blood

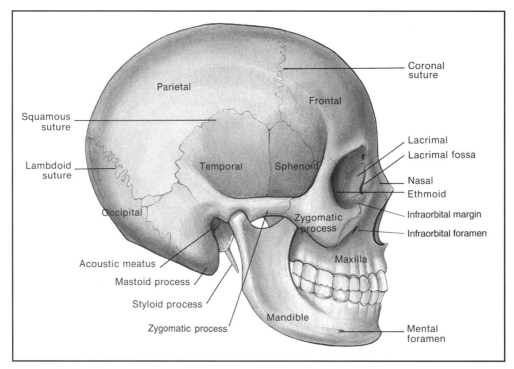

FIGURE 10-1 Bones of the skull (From Anderson: *Basic Human Anatomy and Physiology* [1984]. Jones and Bartlett Publishers, Boston.)

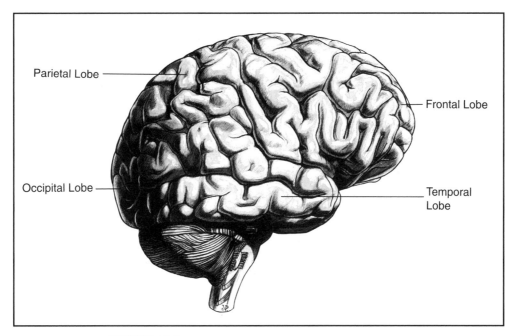

FIGURE 10-2   Lobes of the brain. (Artist: Vincent Perez)

supply to the highly vascular scalp originates from the external carotid arteries and is located above the galea.

Internal structures

The brain is divided into three main areas: the cerebrum, brain stem, and cerebellum. Additional areas include the thalamus, hypothalamus, and basal ganglia.

The *cerebrum* consists of right and left hemispheres, each of which is divided into lobes: frontal, parietal, temporal, and occipital (Fig. 10-2). Control of bodily functions is mediated by the phenomenon of contralateral control, that is, the left side of the brain mediates functions of the right side of the body and vice versa. Basic functions of the lobes of the cerebral hemispheres are listed in Table 10-1.

The *brain stem* is located medial to the cerebrum and is divided into the midbrain, the pons, and the medulla oblongata. The midbrain is composed of nerve fibers passing to and from the cerebrum, the cerebellum, and the spinal cord. The pons is a bridge between the two hemispheres of the cerebellum. The medulla oblongata contains the cardiac and respiratory centers, as well as vasomotor and reflex centers for vomiting, coughing, sneezing, and swallowing. The nuclei of ten of the twelve paired cranial nerves originate in the brain stem (Fig. 10-3). Major functions and innervations of the cranial nerves are outlined in Table 10-2.

The *cerebellum* consists of two lobes that lie directly below the cerebrum. The main functions of the cerebrum are to assist with the maintenance of posture and balance, coordination of fine muscle movement, and maintenance of muscle tone. Stimulation of the cerebellum can produce epilepsy (Sinclair, 1991).

The *thalamus* is located in the center of each cerebral hemisphere and acts as a relay station for impulses for sensing temperature, pain, pressure, and touch.

TABLE 10-1   Functions of the Lobes of the Cerebral Cortex

Function	Lobe
Personality	Frontal
Abstract thinking	Frontal
Judgment	Frontal
Movement	Frontal
Speech	Frontal
Sight	Occipital
Hearing	Temporal
Taste	Temporal
Smell	Temporal
Memory	Temporal
Touch	Parietal
Pain	Parietal
Pressure	Parietal
Emotions	Limbic

The *hypothalamus* lies below the thalamus and influences the autonomic nervous system. It regulates the sensing of thirst, appetite, temperature, and the need for sleep. The hypothalamus also plays a role in cerebrovascular and endocrine functions through its connections to the pituitary gland.

The *basal ganglia* are a relay station for motor activity. Their influence on motor activity and posture is evident in the symptomatology of Parkinson's disease, which is a disorder of the basal ganglia.

TABLE 10-2 Functions of the Cranial Nerves

Name	Origination	Function
Olfactory (I)	Ethmoid	Smell
Optic (II)	Retina	Sight
Oculomotor (III)	Midbrain	Eye movement Pupil response
Trochlear (IV)	Midbrain	Downward gaze
Trigeminal (V)	Pons	Mastication Corneal reflex
Abducens (VI)	Pons	Eye movement
Facial (VII)	Pons	Taste Facial expression
Acoustic (VIII)	Medulla	Hearing Balance
Glossopharyngeal (IX)	Medulla	Taste Parotid gland
Vagus (X)	Medulla	Swallowing Cardiac muscles Pancreas Gastrointestinal tract
Spinal accessory (XI)	Medulla	Swallowing Speaking Shoulder movement
Hypoglossal (XII)	Medulla	Tongue movement

The meninges and ventricular system

Three membranes cover the brain to protect its structures and the underlying blood vessels. The thick outer covering, closely adherent to the periosteum of the skull, is the *dura mater*. The *pia mater* is a delicate, vascular membrane that is adherent to the brain itself. The *arachnoid membrane* is an impermeable membrane that lies between the dura mater and the pia mater. Cerebrospinal fluid (CSF) is manufactured in the ventricles of the brain and circulates in the space between the dura mater and the arachnoid (Fig. 10-4). CSF functions to cushion the brain, to maintain a constant external environment for the brain, and to provide a pathway for transport of certain drugs. CSF, a clear and colorless liquid, is manufactured at a rate of 700 ml per day, although only approximately 150 ml circulates at any one time (Snyder, 1991).

Vascular supply

Because of its need for a constant supply of oxygen and other nutrients, the brain receives about 20% of the cardiac output. The arterial supply to the face, neck, and scalp is from the right and left external carotid arteries. The internal carotid arteries supply the eye and the brain. The *circle of Willis* (Fig. 10-5) is located at the base of the brain and provides several routes of circulation to brain structures. The vertebral arteries join to form the basilar artery, which divides to form the posterior cerebral arter-

ies. These anastomose with the middle and anterior cerebral arteries to complete the circle of Willis.

Venous drainage of the brain is accomplished via venous sinuses, which are thick-walled channels formed by the dura mater. The sinuses communicate with the jugular vein.

The Back

External structures

The vertebral column, consisting of 33 vertebrae, protects the spinal cord and provides the support to maintain an upright position (Fig. 10-6). The first two cervical vertebrae allow for rotation of the head. The remaining five cervical vertebrae provide for attachment of the muscles to keep the head erect. The twelve thoracic vertebrae provide for attachment of the ribs. The bodies of the five lumbar vertebrae are large because they must support the weight of the body. The five bones of the sacrum and the four bones of the coccyx are fused together to form two separate units.

Each vertebra consists of two main parts, the body and the neural arch (Fig. 10-7). The posterior elements of the neural arch are the pedicles and the lamina. Each neural arch has two transverse processes and a spinous process of attachment of muscles. The spinal nerve roots leave the spinal cord through the intervertebral foramina, which lie above and below the pedicles. Cartilaginous tissue, the intervertebral disc, lies between the bodies of the cervical, thoracic, and lumbar vertebrae. The discs consist of the annulus on the outside and the soft nucleus pulposus in the inner portion, and they function as shock absorbers for the body.

Internal structures

The *spinal cord* is an extension of the medulla and extends to the level of the second lumbar vertebra (Snyder, 1991). At its inferior end, the spinal cord tapers into the conus medullaris, which is a prolongation of the pia mater. The cord consists of H-shaped gray matter in the center surrounded by white matter that contains long ascending and descending tracts. The posterior horns of the gray matter are the termination points for many sensory fibers, whereas the motor cells lie in the anterior horn. The main function of the spinal cord is the transmission of impulses from the periphery to the brain and from the brain to the periphery.

Membranes. The spinal cord, like the brain, is covered by three meningeal layers: dura mater, arachnoid mater, and pia mater. CSF circulates around the cord to protect it and provide metabolic nutrients.

Vascular supply. The arterial supply to the spinal cord arises from the radicular arteries and the anterior and posterior spinal arteries, which originate from the carotid and vertebral arteries. Unlike the brain, however, the vas-

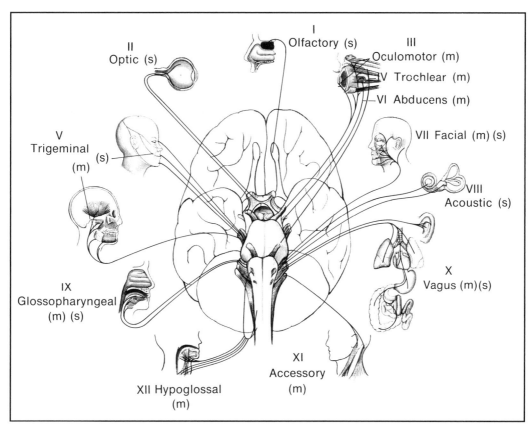

FIGURE 10-3   Cranial nerves. Twelve pairs of nerves arise from the undersurface of the brain to supply the head and neck and most viscera. They are sensory (s), motor (m), or mixed in function.   (From Anderson: *Basic Human Anatomy and Physiology* [1984]. Jones and Bartlett Publishers, Boston.)

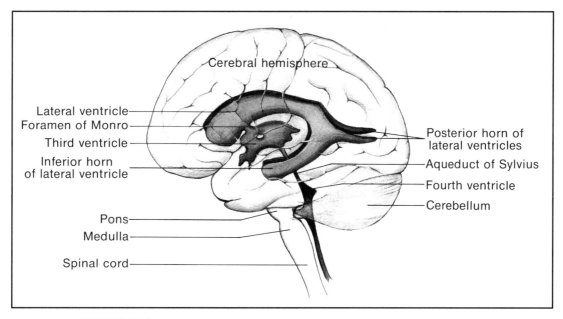

FIGURE 10-4   The brain ventricles, lateral aspect.   (From Anderson: *Basic Human Anatomy and Physiology* [1984]. Jones and Bartlett Publishers, Boston.)

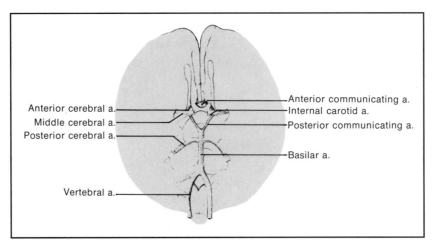

FIGURE 10-5 Circle of Willis showing communicating branches from the basilar and internal carotid arteries. (From Anderson: *Basic Human Anatomy and Physiology* [1984]. Jones and Bartlett Publishers, Boston.)

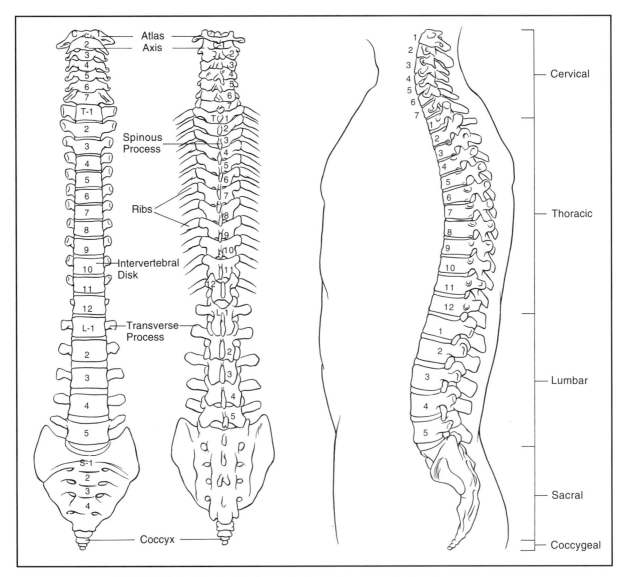

FIGURE 10-6 Vertebral column. *A,* Posterior aspect. *B,* Anterior aspect. *C,* Lateral aspect. (Adapted from Anderson: *Basic Human Anatomy and Physiology* [1984]. Jones and Bartlett Publishers, Boston.)

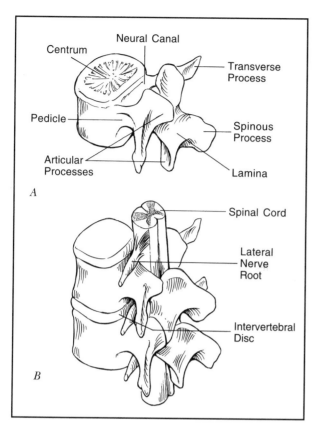

FIGURE 10-7 *A*, Diagonal view from the top of a typical vertebra. *B*, Two vertebrae held in position by an intervertebral disc to show position of the spinal cord and its peripheral nerves. (Adapted from Anderson: *Basic Human Anatomy and Physiology* [1984]. Jones and Bartlett Publishers, Boston.)

TABLE 10-3 Spinal Nerves

Cervical plexus	Muscles of the neck and shoulder Phrenic nerve to the diaphragm
Brachial plexus	Biceps and brachialis Sensation to hand Flexing of fingers
Lumbosacral plexus	Muscles of the lower limbs and lower abdominal wall
Thoracic nerves	Intercostal muscles Oblique and rectus muscles of the abdominal wall

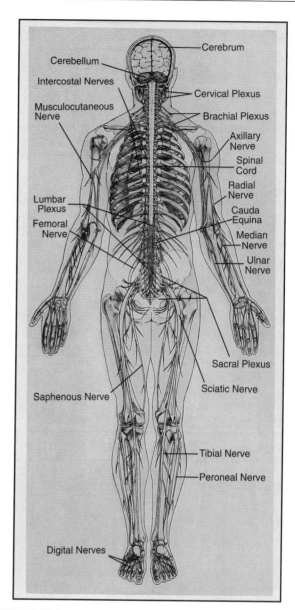

FIGURE 10-8 Peripheral nervous system. (Artist: Vincent Perez)

cular system of the spinal cord does not develop collateral circulation and therefore can be easily compromised.

The Peripheral Nerves

The *peripheral nervous system* is composed of the twelve pairs of cranial nerves outside the cranial cavity, the thirty-

one pairs of spinal nerves outside the vertebral canal, and the autonomic nervous system (Fig. 10-8).

The spinal nerves pass through the intervertebral foramina and divide into motor and sensory branches. In the cervical, lumbar, and sacral regions, the anterior branches join to form a mass of nerves known as a plexus. Major innervations of spinal nerves are found in Table 10-3.

The autonomic nervous system (ANS) controls involuntary function of the internal organs such as the heart, blood vessels, parts of the gastrointestinal and genitourinary tracts, and the exocrine and endocrine glands (Sinclair, 1991). The autonomic nervous system is divided into two parts that complement and antagonize each other. The sympathetic nervous system helps the body adapt to stress, while the parasympathetic nervous system is concerned with controlling functions that are related to rest.

NURSING CONSIDERATIONS

General Information

The perioperative nurse assigned to assist in a neurosurgical procedure is presented with a complex, technology-intensive, and challenging task (Moak, 1992). However, a knowledgeable perioperative nurse will quickly realize the similarities in supplies, equipment, and interventions required during neurosurgical procedures. Armed with a basic understanding of neuroanatomy and the pathology of the individual patient with related function deficits, the perioperative nurse can construct an organized plan of care that will ensure optimal outcomes for the patient.

The perioperative neurosurgical nurse must plan for potential alterations in the patient's body temperature and fluid and electrolyte balance; potential injury to the patient related to surgical positioning, especially in the sitting position; and potential for alteration in the patient's cardiovascular and/or respiratory status related to anatomic deviations and/or surgical intervention. In the following sections, common aspects of categories of procedures will be discussed, as well as unique aspects of individual procedures and patient responses.

SURGICAL PROCEDURES

Cranial Surgery

Perioperative Nursing Considerations

Cranial procedures may be performed to diagnose or remove tumors, drain excess fluid or blood, treat abscesses, resect arteriovenous malformations or aneurysms, relieve pain or seizures, repair congenital anomalies, revascularize tissue, or evaluate and repair injuries.

Regardless of the underlying conditions, access to the brain through the anterior or middle fossa of the skull is similar. Management of the technology required for the patient undergoing cranial surgery can be facilitated by conceptualization of the general principles and understanding the similarities of supplies and equipment needed for the procedures rather than by focusing on the differences. Procedural and physician preferences can be mastered as the perioperative nurse gains experience in the specialty.

Craniotomy

Perioperative nursing care for the patient undergoing a craniotomy is similar to that for many other procedures. However, the unique rationale in neurosurgery warrants reiteration of some of the basic concepts.

A urinary catheter is inserted prior to positioning the patient. Diuretics and hypoosmolar agents, such as Mannitol, are used to decrease brain size to facilitate exposure for the procedure. Sequential pressure devices or an-

tiembolic stockings are used to facilitate venous return. For most craniotomies the entire head is shaved. Hair removal is often performed in the operating room or anesthesia induction room after the patient is anesthetized. Hair is considered the property of the patient and should be saved according to institutional policy.

Organization of supplies and equipment is essential prior to the procedure to ensure safe patient positioning and prioritization of activities throughout the procedure. Placement of equipment is based on knowledge of the surgical approach and orientation of the surgical bed in the room. A monopolar electrosurgery unit (ESU) is used for incision of the scalp and procurement of the bone flap. Bipolar cautery (Fig. 10-9) is used extensively for fine dissection of cerebral tissue and surrounding vessels because of the ability to control the flow of current between the tips and avoid damage to surrounding neural tissue. Additional equipment required may include fiberoptic headlights, an operating microscope (Fig. 10-10) with appropriate lenses, and sterile drapes. Attachment of the

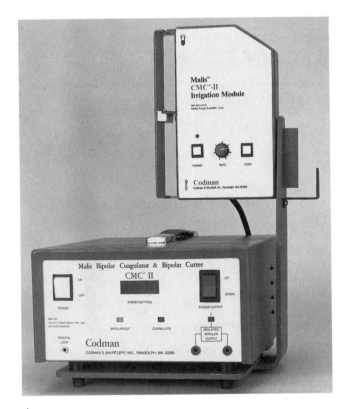

A

FIGURE 10-9 *A*, Malis bipolar coagulator and bipolar cutter with irrigation. *B*, Bipolar forceps. (Courtesy of Johnson & Johnson Professional, Raynham, MA.)

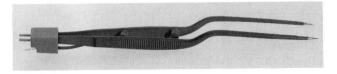

B

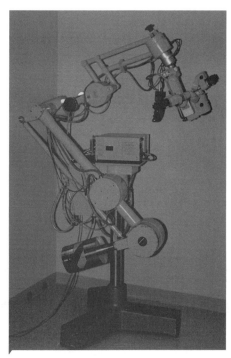

FIGURE 10-10 Operating microscope.

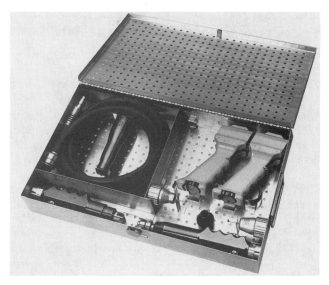

FIGURE 10-11 Craniotome. The craniotome has various attachments that can be used to make burr holes or to carve out bone. (Courtesy of Johnson & Johnson Professional, Raynham, MA.)

microscope to a video system will facilitate anticipation of the surgeon's need by the scrub person and participation of other members of the team. The microscope's primary function is not to illuminate and magnify, but to allow stereoscopic vision within a small depth of field by bringing the operator's interpupillary distance closer together. Instruments must be placed in the surgeon's hand in the position of use because the surgeon's movement and vision are restricted by the microscope. A high-speed drill or drills (Fig. 10-11) will be used to incise the bone of the

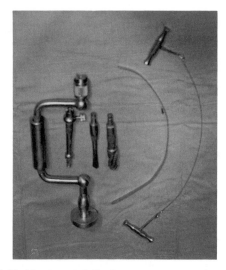

FIGURE 10-12 Hand drill, dura protector, and Gigli saw. Burr holes and a bone flap can be created using these instruments if power equipment is not available.

cranium. Drills should always be tested in advance of prepping and draping the patient, especially in an emergency procedure. A hand-powered Hudson brace drill and Gigli saw should always be readily available in case of failure of the power equipment (Fig. 10-12). A CO_2 laser may be used for dissection and hemostasis in microsurgical procedures to minimize tissue damage and/or metastasis during excision of tumors or vascular anomalies. The ultrasonic surgical aspirator (Fig. 10-13) may be used to fragment large tumors or those that are greatly calcified.

Planning must also include provision of equipment required by other members of the health care team who may support the surgical team. Diagnostic ultrasound may be used to localize and characterize deep brain lesions. The probe is applied to the surface of the dura and is especially useful in highly vascular lesions, where it functions similarly to Doppler ultrasound.

Equipment for measurement of evoked potentials may be used. Evoked potentials are small electrical currents from nerve tissue in response to sensory stimulation. Peripheral nerves are stimulated and elicit responses in the cortical areas that provide information about the integrity of the central nervous system. Monitoring evoked potentials during retraction and dissection of tissue provides an ongoing assessment of neurologic status in an effort to minimize deficits.

Radiologic image intensification may be required for some procedures, such as stereotaxis or insertion of stimulator electrodes.

Various pharmacologic and hemostatic agents should be made available in the operating room at all times. Gelfoam, thrombin, Surgicel, and Avitene may all be used during craniotomies. Bone wax is used on bony surfaces to provide hemostasis and a seal for prevention of air embolus. Cottonoid sponges are available in various sizes and are used for visualization and hemostasis. Cottonoid sponges are less abrasive than gauze sponges and are used around delicate tissue of the brain.

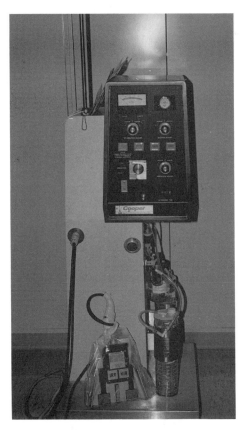

FIGURE 10-13 Ultrasonic surgical aspirator. This equipment allows removal of tumor and other material through gentle ultrasonic action which fragments tumor and calcified material and continuously aspirates material.

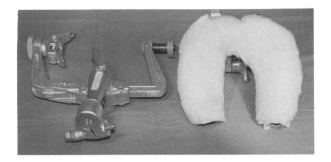

A
FIGURE 10-14 *A*, Three-pin Mayfield and horseshoe headrest. *B*, Horseshoe headrest attached to operating room bed.

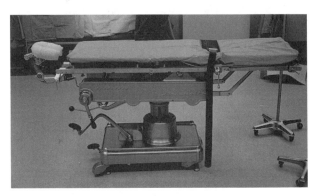

B

Anticonvulsant agents such as Dilantin (phenytoin) may be used prior to stimulation of the brain by instrumentation. Antibiotic irrigation may be used to soak the bone flap during the procedure and for closing. Lactated Ringer's or normal saline solution (NSS) is used for irrigation once the dura is opened. The type of solution used is determined by physician preference and/or the specific requirements of monitoring equipment such as for evoked potentials, as the ions in NSS may interfere with conduction. The solution should be at body temperature.

Successful preoperative planning allows the perioperative nurse to assist anesthesia personnel with intubation and placement of monitoring equipment. Functional suction equipment is essential because patients may have decreased ability to swallow due to cranial nerve involvement or muscular weakness. Based on patient history and the planned surgical procedure, monitoring equipment may include central venous catheter, intracranial pressure line, arterial line, Swan-Ganz catheter, and cerebral blood flow measurement instruments. The patient may be anesthetized on a bed or stretcher and then positioned onto the operating room bed. Due to changes in vascular dynamics following induction of anesthesia, changes in the patient's position must be made slowly with adequate assistance and under the direction of both anesthesia and surgical personnel.

For most craniotomies in the anterior or middle fossae,

the patient is supine with the bed flat. The patient's head may be secured in a square foam headrest or in a Mayfield headrest (Fig. 10-14). This commonly used neurosurgical headrest has a horseshoe attachment as well as an attachment for 3-pin fixation of the skull. Insertion of the pins is performed using sterile technique, and the clamp is applied to the patient's head before the headset is secured to the operating room bed. Antibiotic ointment is applied around the pin as an infection prevention measure and to provide an airtight seal to reduce the risk of air embolus. The lateral and sitting positions may also be used for craniotomies. For additional information on positioning, see Chapter 28 in Volume I. Prior to prepping and draping, a warming blanket is placed on the patient. Draping and establishing a sterile field may be complex due to the location of the surgical site and the shape of the head. Drapes may be stapled or sutured in place in order to obtain maximum conformity to the head. Overhead instrument tables are often used and must be draped into the sterile fields. Standing stools and high back tables are used to maintain the level of the sterile field. Figure 10-15 illustrates the basic instrumentation for a craniotomy. The set-up includes the following groups of instruments:

Scalp instruments

Hemostatic scalp clips (Adson, Raney)

Clip appliers

Clip remover

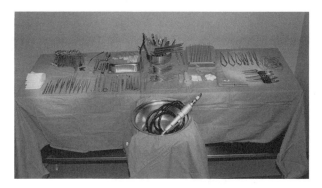

10-15 Back table set up for a craniotomy.

Dull rake retractors

Dull self-retaining retractors (Weitlaner, cerebellar, mastoid)

Malleable brain retractors

Self-retaining brain retractors (Fig. 10-16)

Dura hook

Soft tissue instruments

Towel clips

Mosquito hemostats

Crile forceps

Pean forceps

Kocher forceps

Allis forceps

Needle holder set

Tissue forceps, smooth and toothed

Scissors set, Metzenbaum and Mayo

Bipolar forceps with cord

Hemostatic clip applier and titanium clips (allows for postoperative magnetic resonance imaging)

Ruler

Nerve hooks

Nerve root retractors (Fig. 10-17)

Bayonet forceps, smooth

Gerald forceps

Frazier suction tips, various sizes

Neurosurgical bone instruments

High-speed drill

Hudson brace drill and attachments

Gigli saw, handles, and dura guard

Rongeurs, double and single action

Penfield dissectors, no. 1, 2, 3, and 4

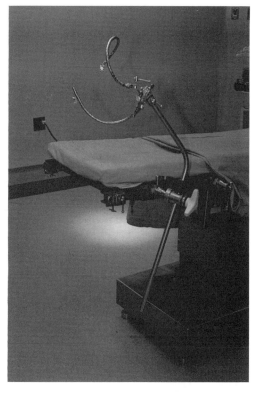

FIGURE 10-16 Yasergil Leyla self-retaining retractor. The retractor attaches to the operating room bed.

Bone curettes, straight and curved

Periosteal elevator set

Dura separator

Freer dissectors

Pituitary rongeurs (Fig. 10-18)

Kerrison rongeurs (Fig. 10-19)

Microsurgical instruments

Key steps

1. The skin and galea are incised and hemostasis achieved with electrosurgery and application of scalp clips (Figure 10-20 shows commonly used incisions for craniotomies.).
2. Soft tissue is removed from the periosteum, and a scalp flap is retracted and secured. The scrub person must keep account of the number of radiopaque sponges, which may be retracted with the scalp.
3. If a free bone flap is developed, the muscle and periosteum are stripped away from the bone. Burr holes are made in the cranium, using an automatic or hand-held drill with perforator. Burr hole debridement is done with a curette, dental instrument, and/or Penfield dissector (Fig. 10-21).
4. The bone is split between the burr holes with a Gigli saw or automatic drill. The bone flap is lifted off the dura mater with periosteal elevators, the edges are

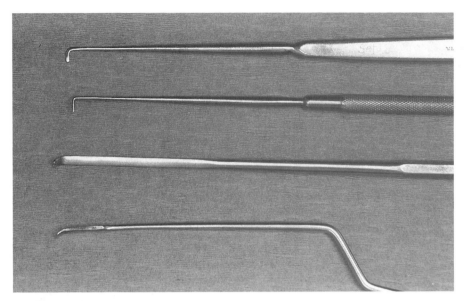

FIGURE 10-17 Nerve root dissectors are used to gently retract the nerves coming directly out of the spinal cord. (Kneedler and Dodge, *Perioperative Patient Care* [1994]. Jones & Bartlett Publishers, Boston. Reprinted by permission.)

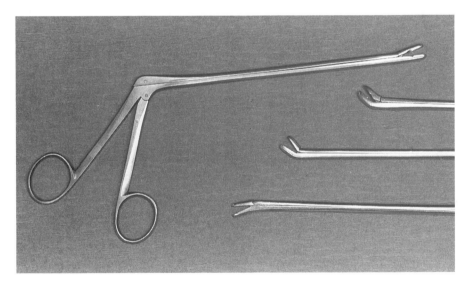

FIGURE 10-18 Pituitary rongeurs come in various cup sizes and angles. They are used to remove brain tumor or tissue or herniated disc material. (Kneedler and Dodge. *Perioperative Patient Care* [1994]. Jones & Bartlett Publishers, Boston, Reprinted by permission.)

smoothed with a rongeur, and the flap is either retracted or removed.

5. The dura is opened with a dural hook and knife and extended with a scissors. Traction sutures are placed at the edge of the dura. Dural veins are ligated using bipolar cautery. Cottonoid sponges are arranged according to size on a fluid-resistant surface and placed within the visual field of the surgeon.

6. Dissection of the brain is carried out to the surgical area, and retractors are placed.

7. The lesion is treated (see individual procedures).

8. Prior to closure, exact hemostasis is obtained because the closed cavity of the skull cannot accommodate even a small hematoma. A drain may or may not be placed subdurally.

9. Either the dura is closed primarily or a synthetic graft is used.

10. The bone flap is replaced and secured with sutures or surgical wire with the assistance of a dural protector. Methylmethacrylate may be used to fill in the defect of the burr holes. If extensive swelling is anticipated, the flap may not be replaced.

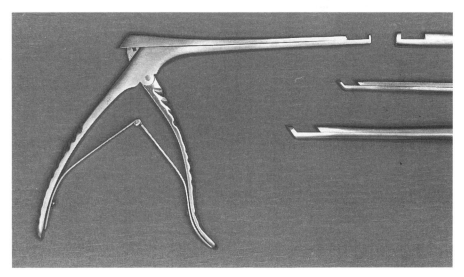

FIGURE 10-19 Kerrison rongeurs are used to remove lamina during a lumbar laminectomy. A variety of angled jaws are available. (Kneedler and Dodge, *Perioperative Patient Care* [1994]. Jones & Bartlett Publishers, Boston. Reprinted by permission.)

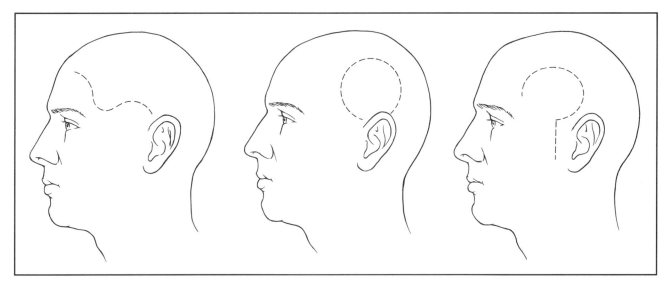

FIGURE 10-20 Commonly used incisions for craniotomies.

11. Periosteum and muscle are reapproximated.
12. Skin closure is accomplished, and dressings are applied.

Excision of intracranial tumor

Tumors may be either malignant or benign. Diagnosis is made by history, neurologic examination, and diagnostic studies. Symptoms result from an increase in intracranial pressure caused by the mass of the tumor or by obstruction of the flow of CSF causing hydrocephalus. Bleeding into the tumor may occur, causing a further increase in size and additional symptoms. Tumors may also cause a deterioration or loss of function in the part of the brain that is affected by the tumor. For example, a left frontal temporal tumor may cause aphasia.

Key steps

1. Depending on its size, the tumor may initially be debulked by using a loop tip on a monopolar cautery, a ring curette, the ultrasonic aspirator, or a CO_2 laser.

Excision of pituitary tumors

Some tumors exert their effect via a hyperactive function. Pituitary adenomas may cause overproduction of one or more hormones, resulting in uncontrollable diabetes or Cushing's syndrome. Approaches to the pituitary gland may be through a traditional craniotomy via a bifrontal or unilateral frontal or frontotemporal incision or through the transsphenoidal approach.

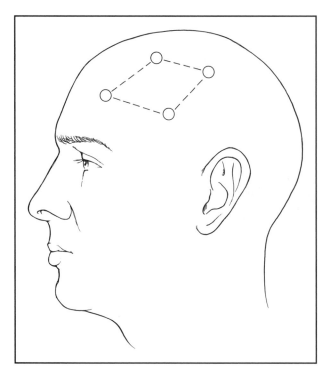

FIGURE 10-21 Location of burr holes for creation of bone flap.

Key steps: traditional approach

1. Using the traditional approach, wet brain retractors padded with moist cottonoid sponges are used to expose the optic chiasm and pituitary gland.
2. The operating microscope is brought to the field for resection of the tumor. Microsurgical instruments and microvascular clips are available.
3. The tumor contents may be aspirated with a syringe and needle. The tumor capsule is coagulated and removed. Pituitary rongeurs, suction, curettes, bayonet forceps, and angled scissors may be used.

Key steps: transsphenoidal approach

1. The entire face, mouth, and nasal cavity are prepped and draped with an impervious drape.
2. An incision is made in the mouth's upper gum margin.
3. The soft tissue of the upper lip and nose is retracted, and the nasal mucosa is elevated.
4. A portion of the cartilaginous septum and osseous vomer plate is resected.
5. The floor of the sella turcica (formed by the sphenoid bones) is identified and opened.
6. The dura is incised, and dissection of the tumor and gland is carried out.
7. The cavity is packed with a muscle graft that is procured at the beginning of the procedure.
8. The nasal cartilage is used to reconstruct the floor of the sella turcica.
9. Nasal packing is inserted, and the gingival incision is closed.

Radical Skull Base Surgery

Lesions at the base of the skull, such as acoustic neuromas and berry aneurysms, require access to the brain via the posterior fossa. Since a flap cannot be turned here, excision of the bony cranium is achieved through craniectomy. A single burr hole is made and enlarged using various sizes and types of rongeurs. Patient positioning for access to the posterior fossa is either in the prone or sitting position.

Air embolus is a potentially lethal complication that may occur when veins are open at a level greater than 5 cm above the right atrium (Temple & Katz, 1987). Air may enter the circulation through the venous sinuses and produce an obstruction in the heart or vascular system. Temple and Katz write of one early study that reported a 25% occurrence rate of air embolus when patients were operated on in the sitting position. Meticulous attention to hemostasis is essential to the prevention of air embolus. Additional monitoring equipment may be used to diagnose and treat potential air embolus. The anesthesia provider may monitor gas exchange through mass spectrometry and/or capnography. Echocardiography and Doppler ultrasound may also be used. Placement of a right atrial line at the junction of the superior vena cava and the right atrium allows for rapid aspiration of air through an attached syringe. The classic "mill-wheel" murmur caused by the mixture of air and blood in the atrium can be heard with a precordial stethoscope but is a late sign (Temple & Katz, 1987).

Acoustic neuroma

An acoustic neuroma arises from the Schwann cells of the eighth cranial nerve. Although it is usually benign, symptoms may be produced as the tumor grows in size (Vaiden, 1991).

Key steps

1. A nerve stimulator may be used to identify the facial nerve, which is in close proximity to the acoustic nerve.
2. A two-team approach with an otolaryngologist and a neurosurgeon may be used.
3. A high-speed drill with irrigation is used for access to the auditory canal.

Trigeminal rhizotomy

This procedure is performed for tic douloureux, severe facial pain of the fifh cranial nerve. Treatment of the neuralgia can be performed peripherally through percutaneous radiofrequency ablation or glycerol injection. Microvascular decompression is achieved through an incision in the temporal bone.

Key steps

1. For radiofrequency ablation, a needle is placed lateral to the oral commissure and aimed toward the inner

canthus of the eye to enter the foramen ovale. An electrode is placed and the ablation is performed.

2. For glycerol injection, a needle is located in the trigeminal cistern and confirmed radiologically. Glycerol (0.2–0.4 ml) is injected. The patient must remain in the sitting position for 1 hour to retain the glycerol in the cistern.

3. For microvascular decompression, an incision is made in the temporal bone over the zygomatic process.

4. The dissection continues through the temporal muscles to the periosteum.

5. A burr hole is made with a hand drill or high-speed drill following stripping of the periosteum from the bone.

6. The dura is retracted and elevated.

7. The middle meningeal artery is clipped and resected. Packing is placed in the foramen spinosum.

8. The trigeminal ganglia are identified and stripped from the temporal lobe.

9. Sections of the ganglion root may be injected or alcohol injected into the nerve root to destroy the root.

Cerebral aneurysm

Intracranial berry aneurysms are thin-walled outpouchings occurring at the bifurcation of large vessels at the base of the brain. Aneurysms may be congenital or caused by degenerative changes and consist of a base, a neck, and a dome. Patients may present with subarachnoid hemorrhage and neurologic deterioration. Patients may experience sudden onset of severe headache associated with a change in level of consciousness. Accumulation of blood may cause sterile meningitis, which produces a stiff neck, fever, and photophobia or retinal hemorrhage. Patients who survive the first rupture are at risk for a second bleed and vasospasm. About half the patients bleed within 6 months if the aneurysm is untreated. Vasospasm with associated decreased cerebral blood flow is manifested by cerebral ischemia and/or stroke in about 60% of patients. Surgery is generally performed one to two weeks after the initial bleed (Kassell & Boarinin, 1985).

Key steps

1. After induction of anesthesia and prior to positioning, the patient is placed in the lateral position for insertion of a lumbar drain attached to a three-way stopcock and an external collection system. The stopcock is opened after the bone flap has been removed to facilitate exposure through retraction of the brain (Fode, 1986).

2. A set of microvascular aneurysm clips, both temporary and permanent, as well as appliers are added to the craniotomy set-up (Fig. 10-22).

3. Following exposure of the aneurysm, the attached veins are coagulated using bipolar cautery.

4. The arachnoid is dissected from the aneurysm.

5. The base of the aneurysm is ligated with a temporary metal clip, while maintaining continuity with the parent vessel.

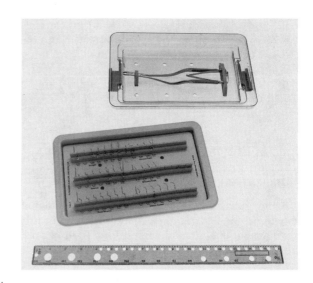

A

FIGURE 10-22 *A,* Aneurysm clips and applier. *B,* Clip applier. (Courtesy of Johnson & Johnson Professional, Raynham, MA.)

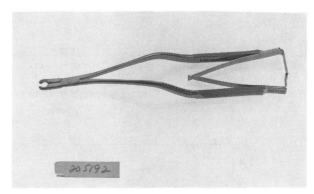

B

6. Once the aneurysm is isolated in its entirety, the dome can be shrunk and shaped with bipolar coagulation.

7. The temporary clip is removed and the permanent clip is placed across the neck of the aneurysm.

8. Surrounding vessels may be covered with Gelfoam soaked in papaverine to decrease vasospasm.

9. An intracranial pressure monitoring device may be inserted.

Arteriovenous malformation (AVM)

An AVM is a coiled mass of arteries and veins that does not supply oxygen to the brain because it lacks capillaries. Treatment of the AVM is necessary when patients experience intractable headaches, uncontrollable seizures, bleeding, or ischemic steal (Fode, 1986).

Key steps

1. Embolization may be carried out preoperatively to reduce the blood supply prior to surgery.

2. If excessive bleeding is expected during surgery, the surgeon may expose the carotid artery in the neck in order to place a temporary tourniquet.
3. Following dissection to the AVM, arteries that drain into the AVM are identified. The arteries are cauterized using bipolar forceps, and the AVM is resected.

Special Cranial Procedures

Craniocerebral injuries

Acute, subacute, and chronic subdural and epidural hematomas may require evacuation of blood and CSF. Acute hematomas generally result from trauma. Subacute and chronic hematoma may be due to epilepsy or coagulopathies.

Head injuries are present in more than 50% of trauma-related deaths. A positive finding of subdural hematoma is a surgical emergency. Figure 10-23 demonstrates how the force of a blow to one part of the head can cause injury to another part.

Key steps

1. In many cases only one or two burr holes are needed instead of a craniotomy with bone flap (Fode, 1986).
2. Irrigation and suction are used to evacuate the hematoma. If bleeding and swelling continue, a craniotomy may be necessary.

3. A subdural drain or intracranial pressure monitoring device may be placed.

Ventriculostomy

Burr holes may also be used for placement of a ventriculostomy needle to initiate external drainage of CSF. Indications in the adult include dementia, headache, intraventricular bleed, or hydrocephalus secondary to subarachnoid hemorrhage. Special instrumentation and equipment include one of a variety of available ventriculostomy systems.

Key steps

1. Bilateral burr holes are made, and the ventricular drainage tubes are placed in the lateral ventricles.
2. The ends of the drains are brought out through separate stab wounds and connected to an external collection system.
3. An intracranial pressure monitoring device may be placed under the dura.

Ventricular shunting

Hydrocephalus occurs when either the flow or absorption of CSF is impaired. In order to relieve the compression, the fluid must be shunted away from the ventricles. The most common sites for diversion are the peritoneal cavity and the right atrium of the heart. Additional equip-

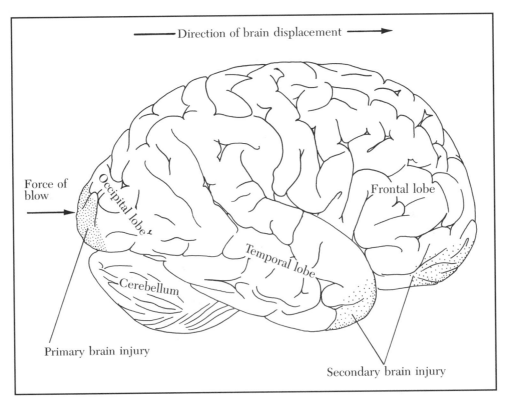

FIGURE 10-23 Mechanism of injury to frontal and temporal poles of brain following blow to back of head. (Crowley, *Introduction to Human Disease*, 3rd edition. [1992]. Jones & Bartlett Publishers, Boston. Reprinted by permission.)

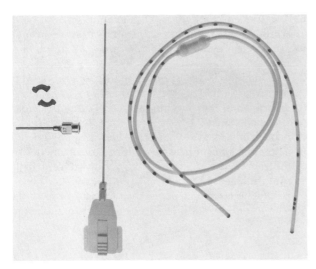

FIGURE 10-24 Ventriculostomy system (blunt needle, tunneler, catheter). (Courtesy of Johnson & Johnson Professional, Raynham, MA.)

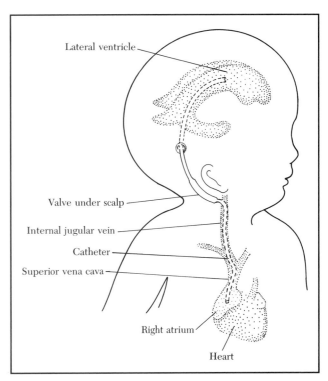

FIGURE 10-25 Principle of shunting fluid from dilated ventricle to right atrium. (Crowley, *Introduction to Human Disease,* 3rd edition [1992]. Jones & Bartlett Publishers, Boston. Reprinted by permission.)

ment required includes a ventricular catheter, a one-way valve to prevent reflux of fluid, a manometer, an appropriate tunneler, and an assortment of connectors and blunt needles (Fig. 10-24).

Key steps

1. A single burr hole or trephine hole is made in the skull.
2. If creating a ventriculoperitoneal shunt, subcutaneous tunneling is done from the head to the abdomen for passage of the catheter. An incision is made above the umbilicus, and the rectus fascia is opened.
3. If creating a ventriculoatrial shunt, a cutdown to the jugular vein is done. Radiographic confirmation is done to ensure proper catheter placement. (Figure 10-25 illustrates the principle of shunting fluid from a dilated ventricle to the right atrium.)

Intracranial revascularization

Extracranial to intracranial bypass procedures are performed for occlusions of major vessels that result in transient ischemic attacks (TIAs). The procedure cannot reverse damage to the infarcted area of the brain but may prevent further damage. The most common site of anastomosis is the superficial temporal artery to a branch of the middle cerebral artery.

Key steps

1. A craniotomy is performed, and the artery to be grafted is identified. Dissection is also carried out to the donor vessel.
2. A branch of the artery to be grafted is developed for anastomosis, and its flow is occluded with a microvascular clip. In order to decrease the metabolic needs of

the brain during occlusion, a dose of intravenous barbiturate is given 1 minute prior to occlusion (Fode, 1986).
3. The operating microscope is used to accomplish anastomosis.

Treatment of epilepsy

Surgical treatment of epilepsy is considered for patients who have incapacitating seizures in spite of medication, a focal origin of the seizure activity, or seizures occurring in an area that can be sacrificed without deficit or if there is adequate neurologic function in other areas (Fode, 1986).

Craniotomies for epilepsy are often carried out under local anesthesia with monitored anesthesia care so the patient can report symptoms and deficits during stimulation of the brain. Excellent preoperative preparation of the patient is essential to ensure cooperation of the patient during the uncomfortable procedure.

Key steps

1. A baseline electroencephalogram (EEG) is obtained preoperatively.
2. Cortical electrodes are placed on the exposed area of the brain, and depth electrodes are used to record EEG tracings and plan the area of resection.
3. An en bloc resection or ablation of the area or areas where the seizures originate is carried out.

Stereotactic procedures

Stereotactic procedures provide detailed information of a patient's brain by combining the information from computed tomography scan, magnetic resonance imaging, and angiography (Fode, 1986). A head frame and localizing system are applied to the patient's head for imaging, and the information gathered is set to a computer to establish a "map" of the brain prior to the definitive procedure. The accurate location of a specific area of the brain is identified by moving probes or electrodes along three separate planes formed by the stereotactic apparatus. The probes are moved until a point where they intersect. Each plane then follows a measured course that coordinates with certain external points of the skull (Koch & Poisson, 1989). The apparatus (Fig. 10-26) may be applied in the operating room or radiology suite.

Key steps

1. A peripheral intravenous line is started for radiopaque dye instillation. If the procedure is performed in the radiology suite, the nurse must ensure that suctioning equipment is available because vomiting may occur if dye leaks into the subarachnoid space.
2. A local anesthetic agent is injected into the skin and periosteum at the site of insertion for the four pins that will hold the frame in place.
3. The frame is secured to the skull with metal drill bits passed through outer sleeves.
4. Outer sleeves are advanced into the skin, and a hand drill is used to seat the drill bits into the skull.
5. The metal drill bits and sleeves are removed and replaced with carbon fiber pins.

6. The frame is applied, and the patient is placed on the scanning table. During the scan, the *xyz* coordinates are ascertained and confirmed on a sterile phantom frame.
7. The patient is transported to the operating room from the radiology area with the frame in place.
8. A local anesthetic is administered because the patient is usually awake.
9. A burr hole is made, and the dura is opened.
10. The indicated surgical procedure is performed. Common procedures include biopsy, third ventriculostomy, thalamotomy, and ablation for relief of chronic pain. The laser may be used for certain procedures.
11. The frame is removed, and dressings are applied.

Spinal Surgery

Spinal surgery is performed to correct congenital malformation, treat injuries, debulk or resect tumors, excise herniated or degenerative discs, drain abscesses, insert shunts, relieve stenosis, or treat intractable pain. Many spinal procedures are performed by either orthopaedic surgeons or neurosurgeons. Additional information about spinal surgery can be found in Chapter 12 of this volume.

There are many variations of surgical approaches and operative procedures to achieve desired outcomes. In some institutions, percutaneous lumbar discectomy may be used to aspirate the nucleus pulposa as an alternative procedure to a traditional lumbar discectomy. Only the open procedures will be discussed in this chapter.

Supplies, equipment, and instrumentation for spinal surgery are similar regardless of the anatomic region of the procedure; only the size of the instruments may differ.

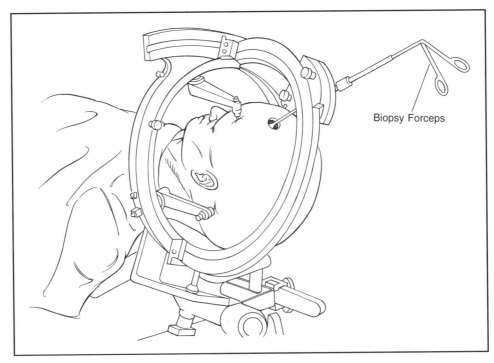

Biopsy Forceps

FIGURE 10-26 Biopsy carried out with a stereotactic guidance system.

In addition, many of the principles of care that apply to craniotomies also apply to surgery of the spine. The need to excise the bony covering to expose the neural tissue is the same in procedures on the spine as in those on the skull. The perioperative nurse can transfer knowledge of principles and procedures, such as use of bipolar cautery or the use of cottonoid sponges to protect neural tissue, when caring for any neurosurgical patient.

Spinal surgery instrumentation includes basic soft tissue and neurosurgical instruments, and may include the following:

Self-retaining retractors

Set of straight and curved pituitary rongeurs

Set of periosteal elevators

A bone cutter

Set of Kerrison rongeurs

Set of single-action and double-action rongeurs

Nerve root retractors

Set of curettes

Microsurgical instruments

Straight and curved osteotomes and gouges (required if bone for a bone graft is to be procured)

Other supplies and equipment for spinal surgery include:

Topical hemostatic agents, such as bone wax, thrombin, Gelfoam

Cottonoid sponges

Evoked potential monitoring equipment

An ultrasonic aspirator

CO_2 laser

An operating microscope with appropriate lens and ocular attachments

A high-speed drill with attachments for both burrs and blades

Laminectomy

Laminectomy is performed for spinal stenosis, herniated disc, and tumor excision. When the spine is unstable, a fusion is done with bone graft, usually from the patient's iliac crest, allograft bone, and/or spinal instrumentation.

Spinal cord tumors are less frequent than intracranial tumors, and a large percentage are benign (Fode, 1986). They may occur at any level of the spinal cord. Tumors occur in three regions in the spine: extradural neoplasms, which are usually malignant; intradural extramedullary tumors, which occur between the dura and the spinal cord and are usually benign; and intramedullary tumors such as gliomas. Spinal cord tumors cause pain by pressing on the nerve roots, and the pain is referred to the distribution of the nerves. Intradural tumors cause pain by distention of the dura, and the pain is usually localized. Metastatic tu-

mors in the spine are usually rapid growing and may cause sufficient swelling to result in paralysis within a few hours (Fode, 1986). These cases constitute a surgical emergency and require immediate decompression.

Key steps

1. Baseline as well as intraoperative evoked potential measurements may be obtained.
2. A midline incision is made over the spinous processes of the affected area, and the paraspinous muscles are dissected.
3. Self-retaining retractors are placed, and the lamina are identified.
4. The spinous processes are removed with a bone cutter or high-speed drill. The lamina are excised using a variety of rongeurs.
5. The dura is identified and opened if the tumor is intradural. Retraction sutures are placed on the cut edges of the dura. A microscope may be used for enhanced visualization during tumor excision.
6. The tumor may be aspirated with a needle and debulked with a CO_2 laser or ultrasonic aspirator prior to fine dissection with microsurgical instruments.
7. The wound may be irrigated with antibiotic solution and is closed in layers beginning with reapproximation of the dura. A dressing is then applied.

Lumbar laminectomy

Proper positioning is essential to ensure adequate exposure during the procedure. The patient may be positioned in the lateral or knee–chest or prone position. When in the prone position, the patient is placed on either chest rolls or a spinal frame such as the Wilson frame (see Fig. 12-42; orthopaedic surgery). The purpose of either is to prevent distention of the intervertebral veins, thus decreasing bleeding, and to prevent compression of the abdominal veins. Compression of the abdominal veins results in hypotension by preventing venous return from the lower extremities (Fode, 1986). Sequential compression devices may be used on the legs and thighs to assist in venous return.

Key steps

1. An intraoperative X-ray film is taken to confirm the proper level for the laminectomy.
2. The surgical exposure down to the lamina is the same as described above for tumor excision.
3. The lamina and ligamentum flava are excised, and bone wax is applied to the cut edges to decrease bleeding and the risk of air emboli.
4. If the intravertebral disc is to be excised, the nerve root is retracted, an incision is made in the annulus, and disc fragments are removed with a pituitary rongeur.
5. To decompress the nerve root, a lateral foraminotomy or a medial facetectomy may be carried out using a curette and/or Kerrison rongeur.

Lumbar laminectomy with fusion

Spinal fusion is indicated when instability results from decompression, for congenital anomalies, or spondylolithiasis (forward displacement of a vertebra over a lower segment). This procedure describes fusion with autograft bone from the patient's iliac crest. (Bone from bone banks may also be used.)

Key steps

1. The donor site is prepped and draped separately from the laminectomy incision site.
2. The soft tissue is stripped away from the facet joints and transverse processes of the affected levels.
3. The donor site is identified, and the iliac crest is identified using sharp dissection.
4. The bone is procured using osteotomes or a high-speed drill and gouges.
5. Gelfoam is placed to decrease bleeding at the donor site, and a drain is placed prior to closing.
6. The graft is placed in the prepared site, and a drain may be placed prior to closure.

Cervical Surgery

Anterior cervical discectomy with fusion

Anterior cervical decompression may be performed for spinal cord or nerve root compression or secondary to trauma. The patient is placed in the supine position. The patient may be placed in a traction apparatus attached to a chin strap for distraction of the disc space during fusion. Various techniques for fusion are available, including autograft iliac crest, allograft, or anterior cervical fusion plates. Additional instruments required include anterior cervical (Cloward) instrumentation and retractors (Fig. 10-27).

Key steps

1. A transverse incision is made above the sternal notch.
2. The platysma muscle is divided, and a fascial plane is made between the trachea and esophagus medially and the carotid sheath laterally.
3. Dissection is carried out down to the spine.
4. The prevertebral fascia is opened, and a needle is placed for radiologic confirmation.
5. Self-retaining retractors are placed, and the disc space is opened. Disc material is removed using curettes and a pituitary rongeur.
6. A laminar spreader may be used to increase distraction for placement of the bone graft. The depth of the space is measured to determine size of the graft.
7. A high-speed drill may be used to prepare the site for an exact fit of the bone plug.
8. The bone is secured using a bone tamp and mallet, and a drain may be placed prior to closure.
9. A cervical collar may be applied.

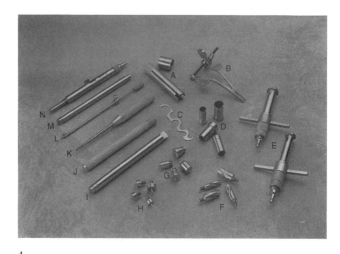

A

FIGURE 10-27 *A*, Anterior cervical fusion kit. A: Drill guard and cap; B: Vertebra spreader; C: Spanner wrench; D: Dowel cutters; E: Drill shafts; F: Cervical drill tips; G: Dowel holders; H: Dowel cutter center pins; I: Codman guard guide; J: Dowel ejector; K: Periosteal elevator; L: Depth gauge; M: Codman dowel cutter shaft; N: Dowel cutter shaft. *B*, Posterior cervical fusion kit. A: Lumbar lamina retractor body; B: Puka chisel handle; C: Lumbar lamina spreader; D: Dural retractor; E: Lumbar lamina retractor blades; F: Spanner gauge; G: Square punch; H: Dowel impactor; I: Depth gauge; J: Bone punch; K: Codman-Harmon chisel; L: Puka (hole) chisels. (Courtesy of Johnson & Johnson Professional, Raynham, MA.)

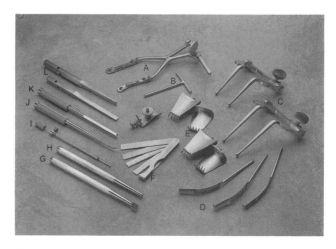

B

Posterior cervical laminectomy

Posterior cervical laminectomy is performed for relief of cord or nerve root compression, for trauma, or for instability due to injury or degeneration. In cases of instability, the patient may be placed in a 3-pin Mayfield headrest with cervical tongs prior to positioning. Posterior cervical laminectomy may be performed with or without fusion. If a fusion is to be performed, bone graft, stainless steel wire, and/or mesh may be used.

Key steps

1. The procedure is similar to lumbar laminectomy, described previously.
2. Postoperatively, the patient may be placed in a halo device until the fusion is complete.

Cordotomy

Cordotomy is performed for treatment of intractable pain. It is the division of the spinothalamic tract. The procedure may be performed under local anesthesia in order to determine the amount of pain relief achieved. An alternative to local anesthesia is "wake-up" anesthesia. During this type of general anesthesia, the patient is allowed to wake up during the procedure to ascertain the success of the procedure and then is reanesthetized for closure. The procedure is generally performed in the cervical or upper thoracic region (Poletti, 1982).

Key steps

1. A midline incision is made over the vertebrae.
2. Self-retaining retractors are placed between paraspinous muscle and the intralaminar space between the desired vertebra.
3. The dura is exposed and opened.
4. The dentate ligament is identified and elevated, and the cord is cut with a cordotomy knife.
5. The wound is irrigated and closed.

Peripheral Nerve Procedures

Peripheral nerve procedures are performed for injury repair, for relief of pain, or for correction of anomalies of nervous tissue outside the brain and spinal cord.

Supplies, equipment, and instrumentation required are a combination of neurosurgical supplies and those required for surgery on an extremity. Additional information may be obtained in Chapter 12 of this volume.

Repair of traumatic injuries

Peripheral nerve injuries may result from blunt or penetrating trauma or may be due to denervated tissue occurring as a result of overstretching, pressure, thermal injury, or immobilization. Following injury, function distal to the nerve is lost. Regeneration must occur from the proximal nerve for function to occur.

Key steps

1. A basic dissecting set, microsurgical instruments, and microloupes or a microscope are required.
2. Dissection of the affected area is carried out, and the injured area is explored. Nerves may be isolated with vessel loops or umbilical tape.
3. Nerve ends are dissected, neuromas excised, and nerve ends anastomosed using microsuture.

4. Evoked potentials may be monitored prior to closure.
5. A splint may be applied for immobilization.

Carpal tunnel release

Carpal tunnel syndrome results from compression of the median nerve by an enlarged carpal ligament at the wrist. It is common among people who work with their hands in a repetitive motion. The syndrome is also discussed in Chapter 12 of this volume. The patient usually presents with pain, paresthesia, and burning in the palm on the radial aspect. Progressive weakness and inability to perform some routine activities of daily living may result. New endoscopic instruments have been developed that may allow the procedure to be performed arthroscopically.

Key steps

1. A circumferential skin prep is performed on the affected extremity following placement of a pneumatic tourniquet.
2. A curvilinear incision is made on the thenar aspect of the wrist, and dissection is carried out to the level of the palmar fascia.
3. The transverse volar carpal ligament is isolated and excised.
4. A single-level closure is performed, and a compression dressing is applied.

Nerve transpositions

Transposition of nerves is performed for traumatic injuries or compression from mechanical obstruction, tension, or scarring. The patient is usually positioned supine with the affected extremity isolated.

Key steps

1. A long skin incision is made over the affected area, and dissection to the affected nerves is accomplished.
2. Vessel loops, umbilical tapes, or small Penrose drains may be used to isolate the nerves.
3. A nerve stimulator may be used to ascertain the function of the nerves.
4. A fascial flap is cut and elevated.
5. The affected nerve is transposed under the fascial flap, and closure is accomplished.
6. Dressings and an immobilization splint are applied.

Sympathectomy

Sympathectomy is most often performed to treat intractable pain or vascular disorders. It consists of excision of part of the sympathetic chain of the autonomic nervous system. Surgical approach varies depending on the area to be resected. This section will discuss a low cervical, high thoracic approach.

Key steps

1. An incision is made above the clavicle, and the platysma muscle is divided.

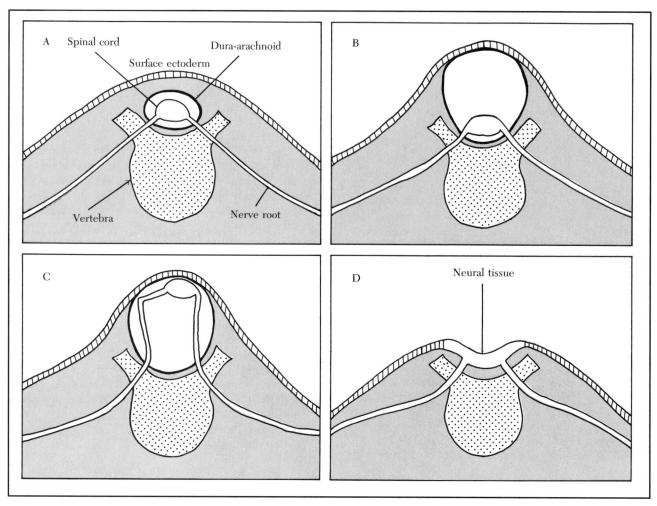

FIGURE 10-28 Various types of spina bifida. *A,* Occult spina bifida. Failure of formation of vertebral arches. No protusion of meninges. *B,* Meningocele. Meninges protrude through the defect in the vertebral arches. Cord and nerve trunks are not present in the sac. *C,* Meningomyelocele. Protrusion of both meninges and nerve tissue. The spinal cord and nerve trunks are frequently incorporated in the wall of the sac. *D,* Failure of the neural tube to form and separate from the surface ectoderm. The neural tissue is continuous with the adjacent skin. (Crowley, *Introduction to Human Disease,* 3rd edition [1992]. Jones & Bartlett Publishers, Boston. Reprinted by permission.)

2. The external jugular vein is ligated and divided.
3. Dissection is carried out to the phrenic nerve, which is carefully retracted.
4. Dissection continues to the stellate ganglion, and the sympathetic chain is followed to the thoracic nerve roots.
5. The cervical ganglia are divided, and wound closure is accomplished.

Pediatric Neurosurgery

Pediatric neurosurgery may be performed for congenital malformations, excision of tumors, or trauma. Specific considerations for the perioperative care of pediatric patients can be found in Chapter 18 in this volume. The supplies, equipment, and instrumentation for pediatric neurosurgery are the same as for adult cranial or spinal surgery. Size of the instrumentation may have to be adjusted based on the age and size of the child. Unique aspects of pediatric neurosurgery will be discussed in this section.

Meningocele

The most common congenital lesion in neurosurgery is the meningocele or meningomyelocele (Vaiden, 1991). The neural elements may be on the exterior of the body (Fig. 10-28) due to a failure of the vertebral arches to unite *in utero.* Meningoceles most often occur in the lumbosacral region. Neurologic deficits vary with the severity of the defect. The goal of surgery is to close the deficit without increasing the existing deficit.

Key steps

1. The lesion must be protected against pressure during intubation.
2. The patient will be positioned prone on small rolls for the procedure.
3. Antimicrobial scrub and paint solution should not be applied to neural tissue. A mild aqueous preparation may be used safely (Amachar, 1982).
4. Excision of the sac and dissection to the nerve roots are accomplished using microloupes or an operating microscope.
5. A watertight closure and reinforcement of the dura are performed.
6. If the defect is large, primary closure may be difficult and a flap of surrounding tissue may be required.

Management of hydrocephalus

Hydrocephalus is an excess accumulation of cerebrospinal fluid in the intracranial space. Hydrocephalus is rarely the result of increased fluid production but rather it is caused by impeded absorption of the fluid (Epstein, 1982).

Key steps

1. The procedure for relief of hydrocephalus is similar to the procedure for adult ventricular shunting.
2. Positioning for the patient is an important step and may be complicated by the large head often associated with hydrocephalus.
3. Extending the neck of the patient with rolls under the shoulders or dropping the head of the operating bed may help with the passing of the shunt tubing through the neck.

Correction of craniosynostosis

Premature closing of the cranial sutures requires that the resulting defect be corrected. The procedure is not done for purely cosmetic reasons but is necessary to protect the growing brain (Wallman, 1982).

Key steps

1. A traditional craniotomy is performed over the area(s) of fused suture lines.
2. Depending on the size and age of the infant, a knife may be used as the starting point for removal of the bone.
3. A burr hole may be made with a Hudson brace drill.
4. Small pieces of bone are removed with a rongeur. A high-speed drill may facilitate excision of a strip of bone and will result in less bleeding than when a scissors or rongeur is used (Wallman, 1982).
5. Closure is as for craniotomy.

SUMMARY

For the patient undergoing surgery of the neurologic system, outcomes can be grouped into two categories. All patients can expect to share the physiologic and psychologic outcomes as outlined in the *AORN Standards and Recommended Practices* (1994). In addition, patients undergoing surgical intervention for neurologic problems can expect to achieve outcomes later in the postoperative period, as outlined by the Association of Neuroscience Nursing (Mitchell, Hodges, Muwaswes, & Walleck, 1988).

Specific outcomes for patients following neurosurgery include:

- The patient is free of infection.
- The patient is free of injury related to positioning.
- Skin integrity is maintained.
- The patient exhibits no signs and symptoms of hypothermia.
- The patient has relief of neurologic symptoms.
- The patient has relief of pain.
- The patient has a decreased risk of secondary brain injury from rebleeding of an intracranial lesion.
- The patient will maintain a normal intracranial pressure.
- The patient will have decreased seizure activity.
- The patient will have return of neurologic function in the affected area.
- The patient's family and significant others demonstrate an understanding of the patient's behavior and/or limitations.
- The patient and family verbalize realistic expectations as a result of the surgical procedure.

The evaluation of patient outcomes reflects the perioperative nurse's ability to plan and implement an individual plan of care for the patient undergoing surgical intervention. In order to assist the perioperative nurse to develop expertise in neurosurgical nursing, this chapter discussed the anatomy and basic function of various components of the nervous system, common practices and procedures in various surgical procedures of the cranium and spine, and special considerations and procedural steps for commonly performed neurosurgical procedures.

REFERENCES

Amachar, A. L. (1982). Surgical management of meningoceles and myelomeningeceles. In Schmidek, H. H. *Operative neurosurgical techniques: Indications, methods, and results* (Vol. 1). New York: Grune & Stratton.

Ellis, H. (1992). *Clinical anatomy: A revision and applied anatomy for clinical students* (8th Ed). Oxford: Blackwell Scientific Publications.

Epstein, M. H. (1982). Surgical management of hydrocephalus. In Schmidek, H. H., & Sweet, W. H. *Operative neurosurgical techniques: Indications, methods, and results* (Vol. 1). New York: Grune & Stratton.

Fode, N. (1986). Common neurosurgical procedures. In Lundgren, J. *Acute neuroscience nursing: Concepts and care.* Boston: Jones & Bartlett.

Kassell, N. F., & Boarinin, D. J. (1985). Timing of aneurysm surgery. In R. H. Wilkins & S. S. Rengachary (Eds.). *Neurosurgery* (Vol. 2). New York: McGraw-Hill.

Koch, F., & Poisson, C. (1989). Targeting cerebral tumors: Combining image-guided stereotactic endoscopy with laser therapy. *AORN Journal, 49*(3), 741–757.

Mitchell, P. H., Hodges, L. C., Muwaswes, M., & Walleck, C. A. (1988). *AANN's neuroscience nursing.* Norwalk, CT: Appleton & Lange.

Moak, E. (1992). Perioperative care of the craniotomy patient: An overview. *Today's OR Nurse,* January, 9–14.

Poletti, C. E. (1982). Open cordotomy: New techniques. In *Operative neurosurgical techniques: Indications, methods, and results* (Vol. 2). New York: Grune & Stratton.

Sinclair, G. M. (1991). *Nursing the neurosurgical patient.* Oxford: Butterworth-Heinmann Ltd.

Snyder, M. (1991). Anatomy and physiology: An overview. In Snyder, M. (Ed.). *A guide to neurological and neurosurgical nursing* (2nd ed.). Albany: Delmar Publishers.

Temple, A. P., & Katz, J. (1987). Air embolism: A potentially lethal surgical complication. *AORN Journal, 45*(3), 387–400.

Vaiden, R. E. (1991). Neurosurgery. In Meeker, M. H., & Rothrock, J. C. *Alexander's care of the patient in surgery* (9th ed.). St. Louis: Mosby–Year Book.

Wallman, L. J. (1982). Surgical management of craniosynostosis. In Schmidek, H. H., & Sweet, W. H. *Operative neurosurgical techniques: Indications, methods, and results* (Vol. 1). New York: Grune & Stratton.

ADDITIONAL READINGS

Agur, A. M. R. (1991). *Grant's Atlas of anatomy* (9th ed.). Baltimore: Williams & Wilkins.

Albin, M. S. (1985). Neuroanesthesia. In R. H. Wilkins & S. S. Rengachary (Eds.). *Neurosurgery* (Vol. 1). New York: McGraw-Hill.

Arand, A. G., & Sawaya, R. (1985). Intraoperative use of topical hemostatic agents in neurosurgery. In R. H. Wilkins & S. S. Rengachary (Eds.). *Neurosurgery* (Vol. 1). New York: McGraw-Hill.

Association of Operating Room Nurses, Inc. (1994). *Standards and recommended practices.* Denver: Author.

Borozny, M., Gray, E., & Ratel, M. (1993). Nursing concerns associated with radical skull base surgery: A case study. *Journal of Neuroscience Nursing, 25*(1), 45–51.

Butler, V. M., Dean, L. D., & Little, J. R. (1984). Positioning the neurosurgical patient in the operating room: a team effort. *Journal of Neurosurgical Nursing, 16*(2), 89–95.

Cerullo, L. F. (1985). Application of the laser to neurosurgery. In R. H. Wilkins & S. S. Rengachary (Eds.). *Neurosurgery* (Vol. 1). New York: McGraw-Hill.

Clark, D. C. (1990). Neurosurgery. In J. C. Rothrock (Ed.). *Perioperative nursing care planning.* St. Louis: C. V. Mosby.

Cloward, R. B. (1992). Anterior cervical discectomy and fusion: The Cloward technique. In S. S. Rengachary & R. H. Wilkins (Eds.). *Neurosurgical operative atlas* (Vol. 2). Baltimore: Williams & Wilkins.

Cooper, P. R. (1985). Traumatic intracranial hematomas. In R. H. Wilkins & S. S. Rengachary (Eds.). *Neurosurgery* (Vol. 2). New York: McGraw-Hill.

Cotler, H. B., & Kaldis, M. G. (1990). Anatomy and surgical approaches of the spine. In J. M. Cotler & H. B. Cotler (Eds.). *Spinal fusion: Science and technique.* New York: Springer-Verlag.

Cravens, G. F. III (1993). Personal communication.

Epstein, C. M., & Boor, D. R. (1988). Principles of signal analysis and averaging. In R. Gilmore (Ed.). *Neurologic clinics: Evoked potentials.* Philadelphia: W. B. Saunders.

Epstein, F. (1985). Ultrasonic dissection. In R. H. Wilkins & S. S. Rengachary (Eds.). *Neurosurgery* (Vol. 1). New York: McGraw-Hill.

Fick, J., & Tew, J. M. (1991). Percutaneous radiofrequency rhizolysis for trigeminal neuralgia. In S. S. Rengachary & R. H. Wilkins (Eds.). *Neurosurgical operative atlas* (Vol. 1). Baltimore: Williams & Wilkins.

Gennarelli, T. A., & Thibault, L. E. (1985). Biomechanics of head injury. In R. H. Wilkins & S. S. Rengachary (Eds.). *Neurosurgery* (Vol. 2). New York: McGraw-Hill.

Greenberg, I. M. (1985). Self-retaining retractors. In R. H. Wilkins & S. S. Rengachary (Eds.). *Neurosurgery* (Vol. 1). New York: McGraw-Hill.

Hargadine, J. R. (1985). Intraoperative monitoring of sensory evoked potentials. In R. Rand (Ed.). *Microneurosurgery* (3rd Ed.). St. Louis: C. V. Mosby.

Harkey, H. L., Caspar, W., & Tarassoli, Y. (1992). Caspar plating of the cervical spine. In S. S. Rengachary & R. H. Wilkins (Eds.). *Neurosurgical operative atlas* (Vol. 2). Baltimore: Williams & Wilkins.

Heilbrun, M. P., & T. S. Roberts (1985). CT stereotactic guidance systems. In R. H. Wilkins & S. S. Rengachary (Eds.). *Neurosurgery* (Vol. 3). New York: McGraw-Hill.

Hitchon, P. W., & Traynelis, V. C. (1991). Lumbar hemilaminectomy for excision of herniated disc. In S. S. Rengachary & R. H. Wilkins (Eds.). *Neurosurgical operative atlas* (Vol. 1). Baltimore: Williams & Wilkins.

Hoff, J. T. (1985). Cervical disc disease and cervical spondylosis. In R. H. Wilkins & S. S. Rengachary (Eds.). *Neurosurgery* (Vol. 3). New York: McGraw-Hill.

Hudgins, W. R., & Jacques, D. S. (1985). The laser in microneurosurgery. In R. Rand (Ed.). *Microneurosurgery* (3rd ed.). St. Louis: C. V. Mosby.

Humphreys, R. P. (1985). Spinal dysraphism. In R. H. Wilkins & S. S. Rengachary (Eds.). *Neurosurgery* (Vol. 3). New York: McGraw-Hill.

Iacono, R. P., & Nashold, B. S. Jr. (1993). Stereotactic neurosurgery. In D. C. Sabiston & H. K. Lyerly (Eds.). *Textbook of surgery pocket companion.* Philadelphia: W. B. Saunders.

Kelly, P. J. (1991). Computer-directed stereotactic resection of brain tumors. In S. S. Rengachary & R. H. Wilkins (Eds.). *Neurosurgical operative atlas* (Vol. 1). Baltimore: Williams & Wilkins.

Kempe, L. G. (1968). *Operative neurosurgery* (Vol. 1): *Cranial, cerebral, and intracranial vascular disease.* Berlin: Springer-Verlag.

Kempe, L. G. (1968). *Operative neurosurgery* (Vol. 2): *Posterior Fossa, Spinal Cord, and Peripheral Nerve Disease.* Berlin: Springer-Verlag.

Levesque, M. F. (1991). En bloc anterior temporal lobectomy for temporolimbic epilepsy. In S. S. Rengachary & R. H. Wilkins (Eds.). *Neurosurgical operative atlas* (Vol. 1). Baltimore: Williams & Wilkins.

Lunsford, L. D. (1985). Trigeminal neuralgia: Treatment by glycerol rhizotomy. In R. H. Wilkins & S. S. Rengachary (Eds.). *Neurosurgery* (Vol. 3). New York: McGraw-Hill.

Malis, L. I. (1985). Surgical resection of tumors of the skull base. In R. H. Wilkins & S. S. Rengachary (Eds.). *Neurosurgery* (Vol. 1). New York: McGraw-Hill.

Marinari, B. (1984). Stereotaxis. *Journal of Neuroscience Nursing, 16*(3), 140–144.

McCullough, D. C. (1985). Hydrocephalus: Treatment. In R. H. Wilkins & S. S. Rengachary (Eds.). *Neurosurgery* (Vol. 3). New York: McGraw-Hill.

McCullough, D. C. (1991). Ventriculoperitoneal shunting. In S. S. Rengachary & R. H. Wilkins (Eds.). *Neurosurgical operative atlas* (Vol. 1). Baltimore: Williams & Wilkins.

McLone, D. G. (1993). Repair of the myelomeningocele. In S. S. Rengachary & R. H. Wilkins (Eds.). *Neurosurgical operative atlas* (Vol. 3). Baltimore: Williams & Wilkins.

Moller, A. M. (1990). Intraoperative monitoring of evoked potentials. In R. H. Wilkins & S. S. Rengachary (Eds.). *Neurosurgery Update I: Diagnosis, operative technique, and neuro-oncology.* New York: McGraw-Hill.

Nashold, B. S. Jr. (1993). Neurosurgical treatment of epilepsy. In D. C. Sabiston & H. K. Lyerly (Eds.). *Textbook of surgery pocket companion.* Philadelphia: W. B. Saunders.

Nugent, G. R. (1985). Trigeminal neuralgia: Treatment by percutaneous electrocoagulation. In R. H. Wilkins & S. S. Rengachary (Eds.). *Neurosurgery* (Vol. 3). New York: McGraw-Hill.

Oakes, W. J. (1993). Congenital malformations of the central nervous system. In D. C. Sabiston & H. K. Lyerly (Eds.). *Textbook of surgery pocket companion.* Philadelphia: W. B. Saunders.

Ojemann, G. A. (1985). Surgical treatment of epilepsy. In R. H. Wilkins & S. S. Rengachary (Eds.). *Neurosurgery* (Vol. 3). New York: McGraw-Hill.

Ommaya, A. K. (1985). Spinal arteriovenous malformations. In R. H. Wilkins & S. S. Rengachary (Eds.). *Neurosurgery* (Vol. 2). New York: McGraw-Hill.

Piatt, J. H., & Burchiel, K. J. (1991). Technique of ventriculostomy. In S. S. Rengachary & R. H. Wilkins (Eds.). *Neurosurgical operative atlas* (Vol. 1). Baltimore: Williams & Wilkins.

Post, E. M. (1991). Shunt systems. In R. H. Wilkins & S. S. Rengachary (Eds.). *Neurosurgery Update II: Vascular, spinal, pediatric, and functional neurosurgery.* New York: McGraw-Hill.

Post, K. D., & McCormick, P. C. (1990). Trigeminal neurinomas. In R. H. Wilkins & S. S. Rengachary (Eds.). *Neurosurgery Update I: Diagnosis, operative technique, and neuro-oncology.* New York: McGraw-Hill.

Prolo, D. J. (1985). Cranial defects and cranioplasty. In R. H. Wilkins & S. S. Rengachary (Eds.). *Neurosurgery* (Vol. 2). New York: McGraw-Hill.

Rand, R. W., & Kleinberg, L. K. (1985). The surgical microscope: Its use and care. In R. Rand (Ed.). *Microneurosurgery* (3rd ed.). St. Louis: C. V. Mosby.

Rengachary, S. S. (1992). Lumbar-peritoneal shunting. In S. S. Rengachary & R. H. Wilkins (Eds.). *Neurosurgical operative atlas* (Vol. 2). Baltimore: Williams & Wilkins.

Rengachary, S. S. (1992). Carpal tunnel syndrome. In S. S. Rengachary & R. H. Wilkins (Eds.). *Neurosurgical operative atlas* (Vol. 2). Baltimore: Williams & Wilkins.

Ryken, T. C., & Loftus, C. M. (1992). Surgical management of anterior communicating artery aneurysms. In S. S. Rengachary & R. H. Wilkins (Eds.). *Neurosurgical operative atlas* (Vol. 2). Baltimore: Williams & Wilkins.

Simeone, F. A. (1985). Lumbar disc disease. In R. H. Wilkins & S. S. Rengachary (Eds.). *Neurosurgery* (Vol. 3). New York: McGraw-Hill.

Stein, B. M. (1985). Spinal intradural tumors. In R. H. Wilkins & S. S. Rengachary (Eds.). *Neurosurgery* (Vol. 1). New York: McGraw-Hill.

Stewart, D. H. Jr., & Krawchenko, J. (1985). Patient positioning. In R. H. Wilkins & S. S. Rengachary (Eds.). *Neurosurgery* (Vol. 1). New York: McGraw-Hill.

Temple, A. P. (1984). Stereotactic surgery: An alternative to craniotomy. *AORN Journal, 40*(4), 543–550.

Tew, J. M. Jr., & Steiger, H. J. (1985). Instrumentation for microneurosurgery. In R. H. Wilkins & S. S. Rengachary (Eds.). *Neurosurgery* (Vol. 1). New York: McGraw-Hill.

Tew, J. H. Jr., & Steiger, H. J. (1985). Aneurysm clips. In R. H. Wilkins & S. S. Rengachary (Eds.). *Neurosurgery* (Vol. 2). New York: McGraw-Hill.

Tindall, G. T., & Tindall, S. C. (1985). Hypophysectomy. In R. H. Wilkins & S. S. Rengachary (Eds.). *Neurosurgery* (Vol. 3). New York: McGraw-Hill.

Tindall, G. T., Woodard, E. J., & Barrow, D. L. (1991). Transsphenoidal excision of macroadenomas of the pituitary gland. In S. S. Rengachary & R. H. Wilkins (Eds.). *Neurosurgical operative atlas* (Vol. 1). Baltimore: Williams & Wilkins.

Weir, B. (1985). Intracranial aneurysms and subarachnoid hemorrhage: An overview. In R. H. Wilkins & S. S. Rengachary (Eds.). *Neurosurgery* (Vol. 2). New York: McGraw-Hill.

Wilkins, R. H. (1985). History of neurosurgery. In R. H. Wilkins & S. S. Rengachary (Eds.). *Neurosurgery* (Vol. 1). New York: McGraw-Hill.

Wilkins, R. H. (1985). Principles of neurosurgical operative technique. In R. H. Wilkins & S. S. Rengachary (Eds.). *Neurosurgery* (Vol. 1). New York: McGraw-Hill.

Wilkins, R. H. (1993). Intraspinal tumors. In D. C. Sabiston & H. K. Lyerly (Eds.). *Textbook of surgery pocket companion.* Philadelphia: W. B. Saunders.

Wilkins, R. H. (1993). Ruptured lumbar intervertebral disc. In D. C. Sabiston & H. K. Lyerly (Eds.). *Textbook of surgery pocket companion.* Philadelphia: W. B. Saunders.

Wilkins, R. H. (1993). Cervical disc lesions. In D. C. Sabiston & H. K. Lyerly (Eds.). *Textbook of surgery pocket companion.* Philadelphia: W. B. Saunders.

Wilkins, R. H., & Gaskill, S. J. (1991). Cervical hemilaminectomy for excision of herniated disc. In S. S. Rengachary & R. H. Wilkins (Eds.). *Neurosurgical operative atlas* (Vol. 1). Baltimore: Williams & Wilkins.

Winston, K. R. (1985). Craniosynostosis. In R. H. Wilkins & S. S. Rengachary (Eds.). *Neurosurgery* (Vol. 3). New York: McGraw-Hill.

Wirth, F. P. (1990). High speed drills. In R. H. Wilkins & S. S. Rengachary (Eds.). *Neurosurgery Update I: Diagnosis, operative technique, and neuro-oncology.* New York: McGraw-Hill.

Young, R. F. (1992). Stereotactic surgical ablation for pain relief. In S. S. Rengachary & R. H. Wilkins (Eds.). *Neurosurgical operative atlas* (Vol. 2). Baltimore: Williams & Wilkins.

Young, R. F. (1991). Percutaneous trigeminal rhizotomy. In S. S. Rengachary & R. H. Wilkins (Eds.). *Neurosurgical operative atlas* (Vol. 1). Baltimore: Williams & Wilkins.

Chapter 11

Genitourinary Surgery

Key Concepts

- Urologic surgery is a minimally invasive specialty. Many procedures are accomplished through an endoscope.
- Proper care, inspection, and assembly of the delicate instruments are essential parts of this specialty.
- Organizational skills are essential, owing to the increasing use of additional cumbersome equipment, such as laser, video, and fluoroscopy.
- Because a large volume of fluid is used to distend the bladder during the procedure, attention must be paid to the solution's temperature. The pressure at which the solution is instilled into the bladder is controlled by the level of the bag above the patient.
- The correct solution for the particular procedure must be used, to avoid hemolysis.
- For many procedures the patient is awake or having a same-day procedure, so patient and family support is essential for the entire perioperative period.
- The amount of solution collected during a transurethral resection of the prostate (TURP) should equal the amount instilled into the bladder during surgery.
- Body image concerns or embarrassment may be encountered, as this specialty deals with sexual function and sex organs.
- Infection is a devastating complication for patients receiving transplants or a prosthesis. Many nursing interventions are aimed at reducing the risk of infection.

INTRODUCTION

Genitourinary surgery is surgery of the urinary system and of the male reproductive system to treat pathological conditions, to diagnose disease, and to diagnose or treat conditions that affect male fertility.

This chapter reviews normal anatomy of the urinary system and of the male reproductive system, and presents considerations for the perioperative nurse who cares for patients undergoing genitourinary surgery. Commonly performed surgical procedures and associated instrumentation and equipment are described in a conceptual manner to assist the nurse in transferring knowledge of one procedure to others that are similar.

As early as 1876 endoscopes were used in genitourinary surgery to allow physicians to view the inside of the bladder. This surgical specialty has remained one that treats many conditions nonsurgically or with minimally invasive procedures. This is exemplified by the various lithotripsy techniques designed to disintegrate renal calculi where they lie, within the body. In many cases it obviates an open surgical procedure that exposes the patient to the dangers of infection, anesthesia complications, and longer recuperation.

Today, surgeons in all specialties are striving to develop endoscopic techniques in order to keep invasive procedures to a minimum and to decrease length of stay and, thus, cost of health care. Genitourinary surgeons are dedicated to the diagnosis and treatment of disease involving (1) the organs that make, store, and excrete urine and (2) the male reproductive system.

ANATOMY

Urinary System

The kidneys, ureters, bladder, and urethra make up the urinary tract. The kidneys are delicate organs that are easily damaged by handling. They are located in the retroperitoneal space at the level of the twelfth thoracic to the third lumbar vertebra. The function of the kidney is to filter impurities from the blood. The kidney is bean shaped and has three sections. The outer portion is the cortex. The central portion, the medulla, contains the renal pyramids. It is in the pyramids that blood is filtered and urine formed. Several pyramids join to form the major and minor calyces. The major calyces join to form the kidney's pelvis, which is also the enlarged proximal end of the ureter (Fig. 11-1).

The renal vein and artery enter at the hilum of the kidney, a concave section located above the ureter. The ureter connects the kidney to the bladder. It is 27 to 30 cm long with a diameter of 4 to 5 mm. Peristaltic contractions of the ureter move urine from the kidney to the urinary bladder, a hollow sac in the pelvic cavity, behind the symphysis pubis. Its function is to hold the urine until it is voided. On the floor of the bladder, in an area called the trigone, are the openings for the ureters and urethra. The sphincter that controls bladder emptying also lies in this area (Fig. 11-2).

The urethra, the distal structure, starts at the bladder and ends at the urinary meatus. The male urethra is 20 to 25 cm long and 7 to 10 mm in diameter. The female urethra is shorter and narrower, about 4 cm long and 6 mm in diameter.

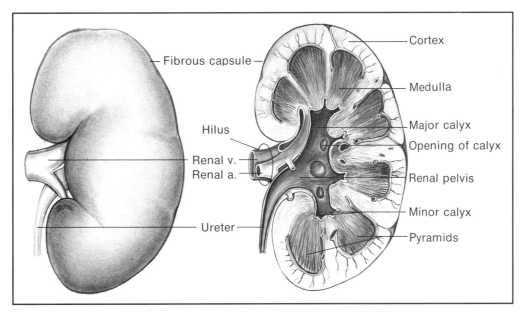

FIGURE 11-1 Internal and external anatomy of the kidney. (Anderson: *Basic Human Anatomy & Physiology: Clinical Implications for the Health Professions* [© 1984]. Boston: Jones and Bartlett Publishers. Reprinted by permission.)

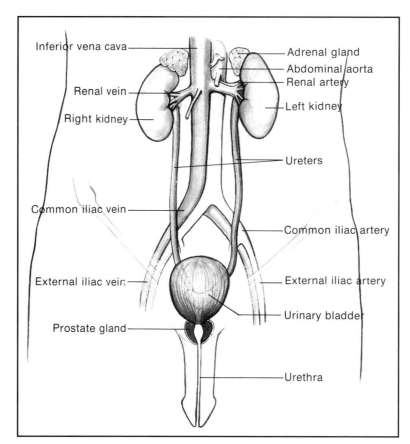

FIGURE 11-2 The urinary system. (Anderson: *Basic Human Anatomy & Physiology: Clinical Implications for the Health Professions* [© 1984]. Boston: Jones and Bartlett Publishers. Reprinted by permission.)

The adrenal glands are included in the urinary system because they rest on top of the kidneys. The adrenal gland is composed of a cortex, which secretes steroids and hormones, and a medulla, which secretes epinephrine. The gland is covered by tough connective tissue.

Male Reproductive System

The testes, epididymis, and a portion of the spermatic cord are held and supported in a loose sac called the scrotum. The two cavities in the scrotum that hold the testes are lined with a tissue called tunica vaginalis, which contains a small amount of fluid. The testes are formed by multiple tubules enclosed in a capsule of connective tissue. It is in these tubules that sperm is produced. Seminal fluid is secreted by a long, twisted duct called the epididymis. This fluid provides the medium and the duct a pathway in which sperm travel from the testes to the ejaculatory duct at the base of the urethra. The portion of the epididymis that passes through the prostate and spermatic cord, ending as the ejaculatory duct, is called the vas deferens. The fibromuscular prostate completely encompasses the urethra at the base of the bladder neck and secretes a fluid that dilutes the seminal fluid. Ligaments suspend the penis from the symphysis pubis. In addition to the urethra, the penis contains three vascular, sponge-

like structures that, when filled with blood, cause an erection (Fig. 11-3).

NURSING CONSIDERATIONS

General Information

With the development and refinement of equipment used for genitourinary surgery, many procedures are now performed on an outpatient basis, and some procedures once done in the operating room are now performed in a physician's office, clinic, or lithotripsy suite. The perioperative nurse will use several approaches for assessing and preparing the patient prior to surgery: telephone interviews, mailed questionnaires, and assessment and teaching on the day of surgery. Follow-up phone calls are routine for many institutions and provide valuable information regarding the patient's function and ability to follow discharge instructions.

Often, patients are sensitive and concerned about the procedure and its effect on their body image and sexuality. Some patients may be embarrassed about surgery that deals with a body function that is considered private. The nurse will be aware of these feelings and provide a sup-

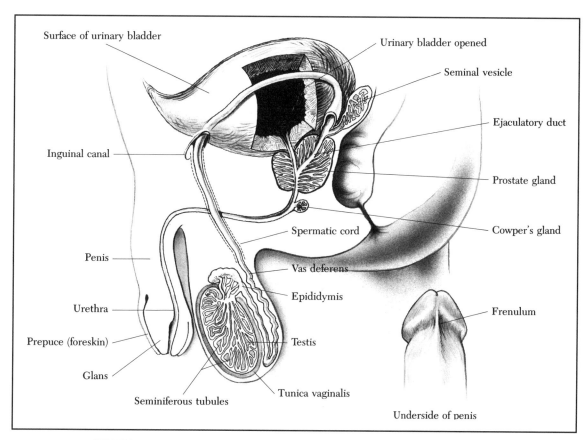

FIGURE 11-3 Anatomy of male genitalia, *side view.* (Grimes, J. Burns, E. *Health Assessment in Nursing Practice,* 3rd edition [© 1992]. Boston: Jones and Bartlett Publishers. Reprinted by permission.)

portive environment. Males having surgery related to fertility will be anxious about the surgical outcome.

Genitourinary problems can be painful, and some patients may be in pain due to bladder or ureteral stones, bladder infection, chronic prostatitis, scrotal injuries, or urinary retention. The perioperative nurse will collaborate with the surgeon or anesthesia provider to ensure that the patient has pain relief.

Diagnostic Studies

Several diagnostic studies may be done prior to genitourinary surgery. An X-ray of the kidney, ureters, and bladder (KUB) is done to reveal size, shape, and position. It can also reveal calculi in the ureters or cysts or tumors. An intravenous pyelogram (IVP) shows dysfunction of the urinary tract through sequential films taken as previously administered dye is excreted. A retrograde pyelogram is an X-ray examination of the upper urinary tract done to confirm findings of an IVP. Catheters are inserted through a cystoscope and into the ureters. Contrast dye is injected and films are taken to identify disease of the ureters and renal pelvis.

A cystogram is performed by inserting contrast medium through a catheter into the bladder. X-ray examination shows the anatomy and contour of the bladder. A renal arteriogram is done to identify the arterial supply to

the kidneys. It is utilized in trauma surgery, to evaluate lesions of the parenchyma and other space-occupying lesions, or to detect arteriovenous malformation.

Computed tomography (CT) and magnetic resonance imaging (MRI) are also used to identify and diagnose tumors, cysts, and obstructions. Ultrasound is used to differentiate between cysts and solid tumors.

The perioperative nurse will make sure that any diagnostic films are available at the time of surgery.

Nursing Diagnoses

Nursing diagnoses commonly identified for patients having genitourinary surgery are anxiety, high risk for injury, high risk for infection, high risk for impaired skin integrity, and high risk for fluid volume excess.

Anxiety related to the surgical procedure or body image

Anxiety may stem from fear of the surgical procedure, ignorance of the disease process, diagnostic tests, body image concerns, or embarrassment. The problem of impotence or any sexually related problem can cause embarrassment or body image concerns. Females faced with surgery of the sexual organs may be embarrassed or concerned about body image. Encouraging patients to express feelings, avoiding unnecessary exposure during the procedure, explaining all activities, and providing an accepting, supportive atmosphere all help patients cope with anxiety.

Embarrassment, fear of having an erection, and, if regional or local anesthesia is used, pain, may make a patient anxious. A nurse with a calm, unhurried manner, who is concerned with the patient's dignity and is supportive in this often embarrassing situation, helps reduce anxiety. If time allows, relaxation techniques may be helpful. If the patient is awake, music from a radio or personal headphones offers distraction.

High risk for injury

Risk for injury may be related to positioning, equipment, or retention of a foreign body. Interventions aimed at avoiding injury through positioning include maintaining proper body alignment and padding of bony prominences, as necessary. Slowly lifting and lowering legs into and out of lithotomy position reduces the chance of hip injury or hypotension due to a fluid shift. To place a patient in the lateral position sufficient personnel are needed. Antiembolic stockings and other antiembolism devices are used, especially if the patient is at risk for developing deep vein thrombosis.

Interventions to prevent injury from equipment such as the electrosurgical unit include checking equipment to ensure there is no damage to the plug, cord, or switch. Laser safety activities depend on the type of laser being used. The safety activities also include personnel. Common safety practices for all lasers include wearing eye protection appropriate for the wavelength, using moist drapes, and putting the laser in standby mode when it is not in use (see Chapter 22, Vol. 1). Counting all instruments, sponges, needles, and other small items that could be left in the wound is the universal intervention for preventing injury from a retained object.

High risk for infection

Infection can occur whenever the body's first line of defense, the skin, is penetrated. Often, it is the patient's own microorganisms that cause the infection and not an organism introduced by the surgical team. In any case, for a patient who has had a prosthesis inserted or an organ transplanted an infection is devastating and expensive. Interventions to avoid infection include strict adherence to aseptic technique and appropriate antimicrobial prophylaxis. A prosthesis to be implanted must be free of contaminants such as lint, powder, or oils from the skin. Routine antibiotic irrigations are often utilized in these procedures.

Maintaining the integrity of closed urinary drainage systems and assuring reflux of urine into the bladder does not occur will help decrease the risk of bladder or urinary tract infection.

High risk for impaired skin integrity

Skin breakdown may occur in any surgical patient during surgery, especially if the patient is elderly, immuno-

suppressed, or otherwise debilitated as a result of the disease process. Skin breakdown may occur even with proper positioning and appropriate preventive measures.

Interventions include maintaining proper body alignment during positioning, padding of bony areas, and meticulous care of the skin around stoma sites.

High risk for fluid volume excess

This diagnosis most often pertains to patients undergoing transurethral resection of the prostate (TURP) because the irrigating solutions have the potential to be absorbed into the vascular system. Only nonhemolytic and nonelectrolytic solutions should be used to distend the bladder during TURP. Irrigation flow is continuous, and fluid returned is measured to ensure that input equals output. Sterile water is acceptable for cystoscopy as no cutting is done and there is no access to the vascular system.

SURGICAL PROCEDURES

Transurethral Procedures

Perioperative nursing considerations

In transurethral procedures, an endoscope is passed through the urethra to visualize the bladder, urethra, bladder neck, and ureteral orifices. The ejaculatory ducts and prostate in the male can also be examined in this manner. Many genitourinary procedures can be performed through an endoscope, from instillation of contrast medium for X-rays to insertion of stents for removal of stones.

Diagnostic cystoscopy is often done in the physician's office, under local anesthesia, before patients are admitted to the hospital for more extensive procedures.

Older operating room suites often have a dedicated room, equipped with a special urology table and sometimes a floor drain, for transurethral procedures. Today, cystoscopy is more frequently performed on a standard operating room table, and since the advent of tandem suction canister setups, floor drains are not necessary.

Many facilities require only a circulating nurse for cystoscopy unless a scrub person is needed to guide catheters for the surgeon. Irrigating solutions are warmed before use, as the large volume of solution used during TURP could lower the patient's body temperature.

Equipment and supplies may include a specially designed urology table with a drawer at the foot that contains a drain opening in the bottom designed to collect the copious volume of fluid. Some older types may even have an X-ray unit attached. These tables are seen less often today, having been replaced with tandem suction setups and special drapes with plastic screens incorporated into them to trap the tissue expelled with the fluid.

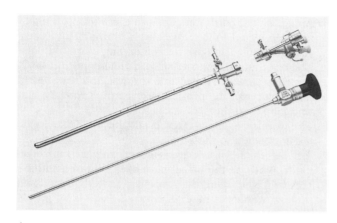

A

FIGURE 11-4   (*A* and *B*) Cystoscope sheath and telescope, separated and together.   (Courtesy of Karl Storz, Endoscopy America Inc., Culver City, CA.)

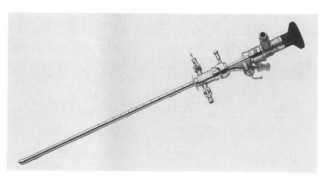

B

An endoscope, telescope, appropriate light source, various attachments, and tubing are used for all procedures. Irrigating fluids are always used to distend the bladder, so the structures can be visualized. The solution generally used for cystoscopy procedures is sterile water. It is supplied in 3000-ml bags and hung 2½ to 3 feet above the level of the patient. For TURP the solution is either 1.5% glycine or 3.3% sorbitol, also supplied in 3000-ml bags.

These solutions are nonelectrolytic, to ensure that the electrical current will not be transmitted through them. They are also nonhemolytic, to prevent hemolysis should some of the solution be absorbed into the circulatory system through the open vessel bed. Several methods can be used to collect irrigating solutions. Most often, the room is equipped with a tandem suction setup, though floor drains are still used in some facilities.

Special Equipment and Supplies

Special equipment and supplies needed for transurethral procedures depend on what procedure is to be done and on the surgeon's preference. An electrosurgical unit is needed if coagulation or cutting with electrical current is to be part of the procedure. A laser may also be used for this purpose. Video equipment may be needed, or fluoroscopy for visualization of internal structures or

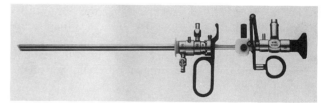

FIGURE 11-5   Resectoscope sheath with telescope in place.   (Courtesy of Karl Storz, Endoscopy America Inc., Culver City, CA.)

placement of stents. Other special equipment and supplies include dilators, catheters, stone basket, contrast medium, and antibiotics.

A basic cystoscopy instrument set includes the cystoscope sheath, obturator, telescope (which comes in 30-, 70-, 90-, 120-, and 0-degree angles), the fiberoptic light cable for the telescope, and an Albarran bridge, an attachment used to guide ureteral catheters (Fig. 11-4).

It is critical to check these instruments before the procedure, to ensure that they are in proper working order. The telescope lens should be checked to determine that it is not scratched or fogged and that the cable is not broken. All parts should be assembled to ensure they fit together easily and that moving parts move. Force should never be used to connect one part to another. The basic instrument for TURP, a resectoscope, has a sheath, obturator, and telescope (Fig. 11-5). The shape of the tip is different from that of a cystoscope because it must accommodate the operating element and associated cutting loops. The other unique piece of equipment for TURP, the Ellik evacuator, is used to express clots and the small pieces of prostatic tissue from the bladder.

For transurethral procedures the patient is placed in the lithotomy position. The stirrups used for genitourinary procedures are a little different from those used in gynecologic procedures: they are lower and support the patient's legs at the knees. The perineal area and urinary meatus are cleansed with a standard antimicrobial solution before draping.

Detailed information pertaining to positioning the patient in lithotomy can be found in Chapter 28 in Volume 1.

Cystoscopy

Cystoscopy is the procedure that examines the inside of the bladder and associated structures, after the bladder has been distended with fluid.

Key steps

1. The irrigation tubing, suction, and light cord are attached to the instrument, and the other ends are passed off the field.
2. The surgeon lubricates the tip of the cystoscope and, with obturator in place, inserts the sheath into the urethra. The cystoscope is carefully advanced until the tip enters the bladder.

3. The bladder is filled with fluid, and the obturator is replaced with the telescope. The bladder is then examined visually.
4. A 70- or 30-degree telescope may be used to examine the bladder. Each angle offers a different view of the bladder wall.
5. The surgeon may conclude the procedure, or, depending on what was found, may do additional procedures: injection of contrast medium, placement of stents, removal of stones, or another procedure.

Transurethral resection of the prostate

A resectoscope is passed through the urethra into the bladder to perform TURP. Small pieces of prostate tissue are removed with the special operating element and cutting loops.

Key steps

1. The resectoscope, with obturator in place, is inserted into the urethra (Fig. 11-6).
2. The irrigating tubing, suction tubing, and light cord are attached, and the other ends are passed off the field.

3. An additional cord is attached to the working element and connected to an electrosurgical unit. The electrical current is necessary for the cutting loops.
4. The obturator is removed and the telescope and working element are inserted into the resectoscope sheath.
5. Small pieces of the prostate are removed with the cutting loop, and the area is coagulated.
6. The working element is removed, and the Ellik evacuator is attached to the scope.
7. The pieces of prostate are removed with the Ellik evacuator. When all the pieces have been removed and the bleeding is stopped, the scope is removed and a 30-ml three-way Foley catheter is inserted.
8. The Foley catheter is attached to a closed irrigation drainage system.
9. All pieces of prostate tissue are collected and sent to the pathology department.

Stone basketing

Stone basketing removes small stones from the lower third of the ureter. A catheter-like instrument with a wire basket on the end is passed into the ureter. As the instrument is withdrawn, the stone is caught in the basket.

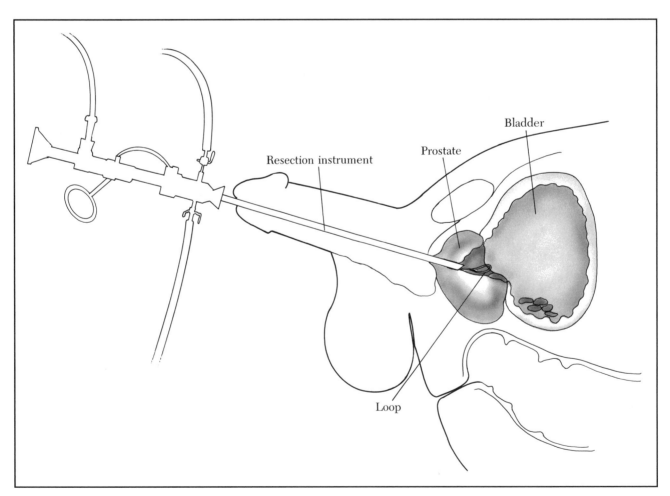

FIGURE 11-6 Principles of TURP. (Crowley, L.: *Introduction to Human Disease,* Second Edition [© 1988]. Boston: Jones and Bartlett Publishers. Reprinted by permission.)

Ureteral stent insertion and removal

Insertion or removal of special ureteral catheters is accomplished under fluoroscopic visualization. The purpose of the stents is to allow drainage of urine past an obstruction in the ureter, most commonly a stone.

Fulguration

Fulguration is a procedure that controls bleeding in the bladder or removes bladder tumors by coagulation with the electrosurgery unit.

Urethral dilatation

Urethral dilatation widens the urethral passage with metal dilators of graduated sizes.

Balloon dilatation of the prostatic urethra

Balloon dilatation of the prostatic urethra is an alternative to procedures that remove the prostate gland. A special balloon is inserted into the urethra. Once in position, at the level of the prostatic urethra, it is inflated for a designated period of time.

Transurethral resection of a bladder tumor

Transurethral resection of a bladder tumor (TURB) is the procedure by which tumors in the bladder are removed in small pieces using the resectoscope and cutting loops as in TURP.

Procedures on Male Genitalia

Perioperative nursing considerations

Procedures on the male genitalia can be as simple as a circumcision or as complicated as transsexual surgery. Feelings of anxiety, body image concerns, and embarrassment are common, especially if impotence is a possibility.

Male genitalia procedures do not routinely require special equipment or supplies, but there are a few exceptions. A laser may be used for excision of condylomata. A prosthesis is needed for surgery for impotence or replacement of the testes. A microscope and microsuture are used for a vasovasostomy. A scrotal support is commonly used. A minor or plastic instrument set is used, as the instruments need to be small with fine tips.

Male genital procedures are done on a standard operating room bed with the patient in the supine position. A scrotal or inguinal incision is used, depending on the procedure. The external genitalia and lower abdomen are prepped with a standard antimicrobial solution, and the patient is draped. The genitalia often are draped free. The patient with condylomata, depending on the extent, may be placed in the lithotomy position for easier access to all affected areas.

Orchiectomy

Key steps

1. A scrotal incision is made, and bleeding is controlled with electrosurgical pencil or clamps and ties.
2. The skin is retracted. The fascia and tunica vaginalis are incised to expose the testes.
3. The spermatic cord is identified and ligated and then the testes are removed.
4. If the patient is young, testicular implants may be inserted to maintain body image.
5. The tissue layers and skin are closed, and all bleeding is controlled.
6. A drain may be placed with a stab wound. The wound is dressed and a scrotal support is applied.

If both testes are removed they are collected in separate containers and correctly labeled *right* and *left*.

Penile implant

A penile implant is inserted to enable a man who is impotent to have an erection. There are two types of implants, rigid and inflatable.

Key steps

1. For placement of the prosthesis in the shaft of the penis an incision is made on the dorsal side, down to the corpus.
2. The corpus is dilated, and a prosthesis of appropriate size is placed.
3. If the prosthesis is the inflatable type, a reservoir is placed in the prevesical space, a pump in the scrotum, and inflatable rods in the penis.
4. To decrease the chance of postoperative bleeding and facilitate healing the prosthesis may be left partially inflated.

Ablation of condylomata

Condylomata, venereal warts, are sexually transmitted lesions. The treatment is usually laser ablation. The patient is placed in lithotomy position, and moist towels are placed over the unaffected areas. The warts are then ablated.

Testicular detorsion

Testicular detorsion is performed to untwist the testicle, spermatic cord, and vascular pedicle. This condition occurs occasionally in young adults. It is extremely painful and should be treated as urgent. If correction is delayed necrosis of the testis will result, which requires orchiectomy.

Key steps

1. An incision is made in the scrotum on the affected side.

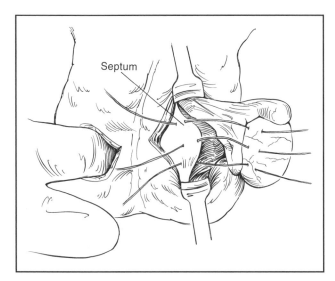

FIGURE 11-7 Testis delivered through scrotal incision for detorsion of testicle. (Marshall, F. F. *Operative Urology*, [© 1991]. Philadelphia, W. B. Saunders Co. Reprinted with permission.)

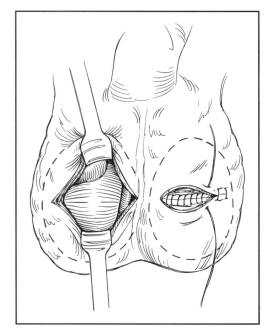

FIGURE 11-8 Testis fixed to septum. (Marshall, F. F. *Operative Urology*, [© 1991]. Philadelphia, W. B. Saunders Co. Reprinted with permission.)

2. The tunica vaginalis is opened, and the testis is brought out through the incision and untwisted (Fig. 11-7).
3. To prevent recurrence of torsion either the tunica vaginalis is sutured loosely back over the cord or the testis is sutured to the scrotal wall or septum.
4. The unaffected testis is also exposed and fixed in place to obviate torsion.
5. The incision is then closed with small absorbable suture (4-0) (Fig. 11-8).
6. Finally, a dressing and scrotal support are applied.

Hydrocelectomy

A hydrocele is a fluid-filled sac inside the scrotum. To remove a hydrocele the tunica vaginalis is excised, the fluid drained, and the sac removed.

Vasectomy

Vasectomy is bilateral excision of the vas deferens for the purpose of sterilization. Reversal of the procedure is called vasovasostomy.

Orchiopexy

Orchiopexy is done to correct an undescended testicle in a child. An inguinal incision is used to locate the testicle, which is pulled down into the scrotum and anchored. Left in the abdomen too long an undescended testicle results in sterility, as body temperature kills the sperm.

Circumcision

Circumcision is often performed on infants to excise the foreskin of the glans penis. When it is performed on an adult it is usually because of phimosis, paraphimosis, or balanoposthitis.

Penectomy

Penectomy is the removal of all or part of the penis because of invasive cancer.

Open Urologic Procedures

Perioperative nursing considerations

In open urologic procedures on the kidney, ureter, or adrenal gland, a variety of procedures can be accomplished with similar instrumentation and surgical approaches. The surgical approach is determined by the procedure to be performed and by which approach affords the best exposure. The most common approach is the flank incision. Proper exposure may require removal of the 11th or 12th rib. The transthoracic approach requires entering the chest and removing the 10th and 11th ribs. The standard abdominal incision may be used for some procedures. Sometimes more than one incision is needed to complete the procedure. On occasion a posterior approach is used for adrenalectomy, as when the patient is debilitated and entering the abdomen is to be avoided.

Radical procedures usually involve removal of several lymph nodes, which are sent for frozen section examination to determine the extent of metastasis. A kidney can be removed in total or in part.

Plastic reconstruction can be performed on the kidney or the ureter. If stones cannot be disintegrated with one of the less invasive techniques, an open procedure such as pyelolithotomy (removal of a stone from the renal pelvis) or nephrolithotomy (removal of a stone from the renal calyx) will be necessary.

The electrosurgical unit is used to control bleeding. Drains and catheters are commonly used. Instrumentation basic to all open procedures is a major abdominal instrument set. Drapes, irrigating solutions, positioning materials, and prepping supplies are standard.

Special equipment and supplies

Special equipment varies with the procedure and the position selected. Ice slush or cold saline is needed for procedures that require cooling of the kidney. If a transthoracic or flank incision is used, chest instruments and chest tubes and drainage are required. Long instruments, gastrointestinal, plastic, and vascular instruments are needed if reconstruction is planned. For removal of stones, stone forceps are added to the abdominal instruments. If a cystectomy is planned for a female, abdominal hysterectomy instruments are added. A fluoroscopy unit, multiple specimen containers, laser, video equipment, and endoscopes may be used for specific procedures.

A lateral, supine, or lithotomy position is used, depending on what procedure is to be performed. For cystectomy procedures, with bladder replacement and reanastomosis of the ureters, an abdominal approach is used. If surgery is to be performed on only one ureter, adrenal gland, or kidney, a flank incision and lateral positioning are most likely to be chosen. Procedures such as perineal prostatectomy require that the patient be placed in the lithotomy position. If two incisions are planned for a procedure, such as nephroureterectomy, the patient's position may be changed during the procedure. Reprepping and redraping are required. Otherwise, standard prepping and draping are done.

Prostatectomy approaches

In addition to TURP and balloon dilatation of the prostate, there are two abdominal approaches and one perineal approach for excision of the noncancerous prostate gland. A radical retropubic prostatectomy or radical perineal prostatectomy are the alternative procedures for a cancerous prostate gland.

Retropubic

The retropubic approach removes the hypertrophic prostate through an incision in the capsule. There is excellent visualization of the area with this approach, and minimal bleeding.

Suprapubic

The suprapubic approach uses an abdominal approach, and the prostate is removed from within the urinary bladder. In this technique the bladder is filled with solution before Pfannenstiel's incision is made. Once the level of the bladder is reached and it is opened and drained of the fluid, the surgeon digitally enucleates the prostate tissue. Control of associated bleeding is more difficult with this approach.

Perineal

The perineal approach is not used frequently unless an associated radical prostatectomy is to be performed. An inverted U incision is used, and the patient is placed in an exaggerated lithotomy position. Radical retropubic prostatectomy is also done for metastatic disease. In radical procedures, the entire prostate is removed, along with the capsule and seminal vesicles. Lymph nodes are commonly removed.

Radical nephrectomy with lymphadenectomy

A radical nephrectomy removes the kidney, perirenal fat, adrenal gland, Gerota's capsule, and periaortic lymph nodes.

Key steps

1. A flank incision is made, and bleeding is controlled through the subcutaneous tissue, fascia, and muscle layer.
2. Retraction is applied where necessary, to provide exposure.
3. The ribs are exposed and one or more may be removed to afford access to the kidney.
4. Blunt dissection is used to expose the kidney pedicle, which is ligated.
5. Blunt dissection is continued to free up the kidney and associated tissue for removal.
6. Lymph nodes taken at this time are examined for metastasis.
7. The area is then explored and irrigated, and all bleeding is controlled.
8. Drains and chest tubes are placed as necessary.
9. The incision is closed in layers and the wound is dressed.

Radical cystectomy with bladder replacement

Radical cystectomy removes the bladder and associated structures. In males this includes the prostate, seminal vesicles, and distal ureters. In females, it includes the urethra, distal ureters, uterus, cervix, and the proximal third of the vagina. The ureters can be attached to the abdominal wall as a stoma (ureterostomy), or a new bladder can be designed from a section of bowel and the ureters inserted into it. The right colon, ileal segment, sigmoid colon, or ascending colon can be used to make the reservoir. Most often, the ileal segment is used. A radical retroperitoneal lymphadenectomy, removal of retroperitoneal lymph nodes, including channels and fat around the renal pedicles, vena cava, and aorta, may be done in addition to cystectomy.

Key steps

1. The procedure begins with an abdominal midline incision extended down through the skin, fat, fascia, and muscle.

2. The muscle is retracted to expose the bladder, which is then grasped and, with sharp and blunt dissection, freed up.

3. The distal ureters, prostate, seminal vesicles (and distal vas in the male) are freed up.

4. The urethra is ligated and all the above structures are removed.

5. In females, the bladder is freed up along with the distal ureters. The urethra is removed along with the cervix, uterus, and proximal third of the vagina.

6. If lymphadenectomy is to be included, the iliac and obturator lymph nodes are excised bilaterally, along with the channels and fat around the renal pedicles, vena cava, and aorta.

7. Next, preparation is made for a ureterostomy, ileal conduit, or bladder replacement.

8. If the bladder is to be replaced, the selected portion of the bowel is freed up while its blood supply is maintained.

9. The ends of the bowel are closed and the ureters implanted.

10. A stoma is made in the abdominal wall, through which the urine can be collected in a bag or by intermittent self-catheterization.

Nephroureterectomy

Nephroureterectomy is the removal of the kidney and ureter because of severe hydroureteronephrosis or tumors involving the kidney and ureter.

Pyelolithotomy, nephrolithotomy, ureterolithotomy

Pyelolithotomy, nephrolithotomy, and ureterolithotomy are all open procedures by which stones are removed from the kidney and ureter, respectively. Less invasive stone-disintegrating procedures are preferred; however, an open procedure may be required because of the size or type of stone.

Adrenalectomy

Partial, total, or bilateral adrenalectomy may be done to remove tumors of the gland and control hormone secretion.

Transplant and Reconstructive Procedures

Perioperative nursing considerations

Planning for kidney transplant surgery may involve preparation of two patients, the recipient and a living donor. Though the majority of kidneys for transplant are obtained from cadaver donors, living donors are still used. Kidneys obtained from cadavers may be transported great distances to the recipient. If the kidney is obtained from a living donor, surgery on donor and recipient is done simultaneously.

If the kidney is obtained from a living donor, an antibiotic solution is instilled into the recipient's bladder at the beginning of the procedure. Cold saline is needed for storing the donor kidney until it is transplanted. Heparin is administered to prevent clotting. Equipment such as an electrosurgical unit, suction, and sutures are standard.

Instrumentation used to remove the kidney from the donor includes an abdominal set with vascular instruments and some chest instruments. An abdominal set and vascular instruments are used to transplant the kidney into the recipient.

If a cadaver kidney is to be obtained, a special surgical team is often used to care for and transport it. Heparin and a cold electrolyte solution are needed to perfuse the kidney after it is removed. An insulated container of cold saline and saline slush or a special hypothermic perfusion machine is used to transport the kidney from the point of retrieval to the point of transplantation.

A living donor is placed in a lateral position for kidney removal, and a flank incision made. Standard positioning equipment for the lateral position is used. The patient is prepped and draped in the standard manner.

The cadaver donor is placed in the supine position and a midline abdominal incision is made. Standard prepping, draping, and positioning for an abdominal procedure are used. The recipient is placed in the supine position, and a curved lower-quadrant incision is made. Prepping and draping are standard for an abdominal procedure.

Kidney transplantation

Key steps: removal from a living donor

1. A standard flank incision is made through all tissue layers and bleeding is controlled at each level.

2. The muscle layer is retracted to expose the ribs.

3. One or more ribs may have to be removed to provide proper access to the kidney.

4. Blunt dissection is continued through Gerota's fascia and perirenal fat, to expose the kidney.

5. Careful dissection of the ureter is done to preserve as much length as possible and to avoid damaging the vascular supply.

6. The renal vein and artery are dissected free.

7. Heparin is administered, and the renal artery and vein are double clamped. The kidney and ureter are removed.

8. The kidney is placed in cold saline and flushed with an electrolyte solution.

9. The area is explored and irrigated, and all bleeding is controlled.

10. The muscles, fascia, fat, and skin are closed in layers. Drains, if left in, are sutured in place and a dressing is applied.

Key steps: removal from a cadaver donor

1. A midline incision is made through all levels of tissue, and bleeding is controlled as necessary.

2. The kidney, ureter, and renal artery and vein are exposed and carefully dissected out. Both kidneys may be harvested, as well as other organs.

3. Heparin is administered before removal of the kidney.

4. Once removed, the kidney is placed in cold saline and perfused with an electrolyte solution.

5. After the kidney has been cared for, lymph nodes and the spleen are removed for tissue typing.

6. The incision is closed, and life support is turned off.

Key steps: recipient

1. The kidney recipient is placed in the supine position, and an antibiotic solution is instilled into the bladder.

2. A curved abdominal incision is made in the lower quadrant of the side in which the kidney is to be placed.

3. The incision is carried through all layers, and bleeding is controlled as necessary.

4. The common, external, and internal iliac arteries and the aorta are exposed (Fig. 11-9).

5. The internal iliac artery and vein are prepared to be anastomosed to the renal artery and vein of the donor kidney (Figs. 11-10 and 11-11).

6. The patient's vessels are heparinized just before the anastomosis. During the anastomosis the kidney is placed in a moist stockinette or sponge to protect it from damage.

7. When the anastomosis is completed the vessels are again irrigated with heparin, the stockinette or sponge is removed, and the anastomosis is checked for leaks.

8. An incision is made in the dome of the bladder, where the ureter is sutured into place (Fig. 11-12).

9. A stent is placed from the kidney pelvis to the urethra, to ensure patency. The anastomosis is checked by filling the bladder with saline.

10. The incision is then closed in the usual manner, and a dressing is applied.

11. The bladder is filled with an antibiotic solution and emptied.

Pyeloplasty

Pyeloplasty is plastic repair of the junction where the renal pelvis and ureter meet that has been enlarged owing to obstruction.

Hypospadias and epispadias

Hypospadias is failure of the urinary meatus to extend to the tip of the penis. The opening occurs somewhere on the underside of the penile shaft, scrotum, or perineum.

In epispadias the urethral meatus does not extend to the tip of the penis, owing to the absence of the dorsal wall of the urethra. In either of these conditions, the degree of urethral reconstruction required depends on where the urethra opens on the shaft. Urethral reconstruction can be accomplished by use of a buried skin tube, skin flap, or free graft. Urine is usually diverted during healing.

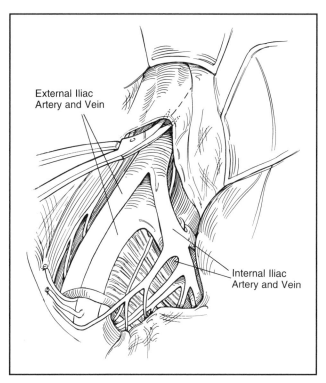

FIGURE 11-9   Internal and external iliac veins and arteries exposed for kidney transplantation. Stewart, B. H. Operative Urology: the kidneys, adrenal glands and retroperitoneum (© 1975) Baltimore, Williams & Wilkins. Reprinted with permission.

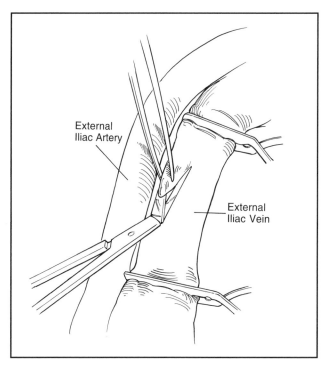

FIGURE 11-10   Iliac artery and vein prepared for anastomosis. Stewart, B. H. Operative Urology: the kidneys, adrenal glands and retroperitoneum (© 1975) Baltimore, Williams & Wilkins. Reprinted with permission.

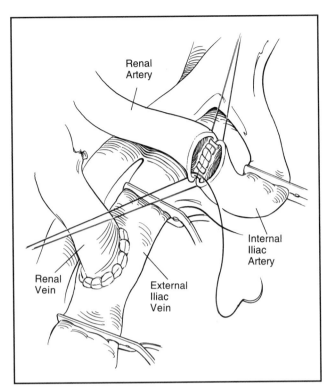

FIGURE 11-11 Anastomosis of donor renal vein and artery to external and internal iliac vein and artery. Stewart, B. H. Operative Urology: the kidneys, adrenal glands and retroperitoneum (© 1975) Baltimore, Williams & Wilkins. Reprinted with permission.

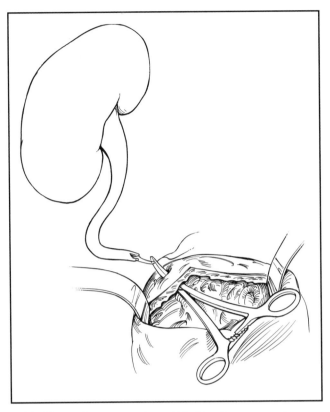

FIGURE 11-12 Preparation of bladder for ureter. Stewart, B. H. Operative Urology: the kidneys, adrenal glands and retroperitoneum (© 1975) Baltimore, Williams & Wilkins. Reprinted with permission.

Stone-Disintegrating Procedures

Perioperative nursing considerations

Three approaches can be used to disintegrate stones in the urinary tract. The first is extracorporeal shock wave lithotripsy (ESWL). The second, transurethral ureteroscopic lithotripsy, accesses the stone by passing an endoscope through the urethra and a second into the ureter to the level of the stone. The third approach, percutaneous lithotripsy, accesses the kidney stone by passing a nephroscope through a percutaneous nephrostomy tract.

The equipment for the *percutaneous approach* includes a fluoroscopy unit or video equipment for visualization of the stone. In addition, the equipment for the preferred method for disintegrating the stone must be ready. The choices are the pulsed-dye laser (Fig. 11-13) and fiber lithotripter and probe (Fig. 11-14), or the ultrasonic lithotripter and sonotrode (Fig. 11-15). A plastic instrument set with the addition of dilators, nephrostomy tubes, nephroscope and light source, electrosurgical unit, and suction should be ready. For this approach the prone position is used.

The patient is placed in the prone position on the operating room bed. If a nephrostomy tract was not established in the X-ray department, one is established in the operating room. Positioning is followed by standard prepping with an antibacterial solution and draping.

The equipment and instrumentation for the *transurethral approach* include the cystoscope, and if the stone is in the ureter, a ureteroscope. Video equipment or fluoroscopy is used to visualize the stone. Ureteral stents, a light source, an electrosurgical unit, fluids for distending the bladder, and a drainage system for retrieving the fluid must be available. The three instruments used to disintegrate the stone are the pulsed-dye laser and associated fiber, the electrohydraulic lithotripter and probe, or the ultrasonic lithotripter and sonotrode. Stirrups and other positioning equipment appropriate for the lithotomy position should be available. This procedure is most likely to be done in a cystoscopy room equipped with a urology table.

The patient is placed in lithotomy position for the transurethral approach, prepped with an antimicrobial solution, and draped in the usual manner.

Percutaneous Lithotripsy

Key steps

1. A small incision is made in the patient's back, over the level of the kidney.
2. A nephrostomy tract is made and dilated under visualization with fluoroscopy.
3. A flexible guide wire is passed down the tract, followed by the flexible nephroscope.

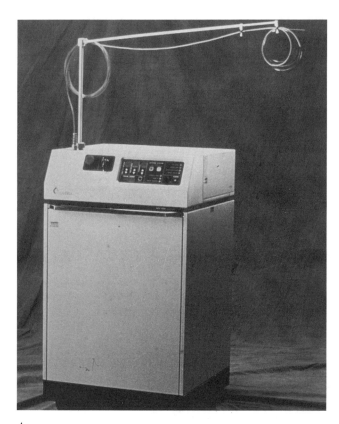

A

FIGURE 11-13 (*A* and *B*) Pulsed-dye laser and fiber.
(Courtesy of Candela Laser Corp., Wayland, MA.)

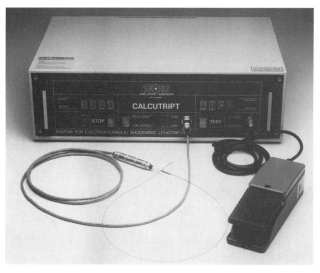

FIGURE 11-14 Electrohydraulic lithotripter and probe.
(Courtesy of Karl Storz, Endoscopy America Inc., Culver City, CA.)

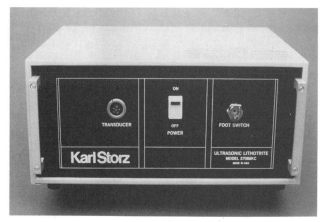

A

FIGURE 11-15 (*A* and *B*) Ultrasonic lithotripter and
sonotrode. (Courtesy of Karl Storz, Endoscopy America Inc.,
Culver City, CA.)

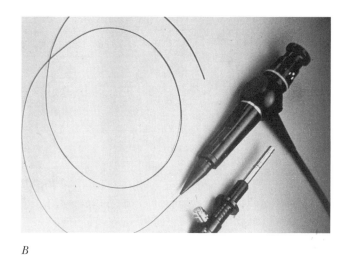

B

4. Once the scope is in the proper position, the laser fiber, sonotrode wand, or electrohydraulic probe is passed down the scope to the level of the stone.
5. The laser is activated to disintegrate the stone.
6. After disintegration of the stone, all instrumentation is removed.
7. The wound is closed.

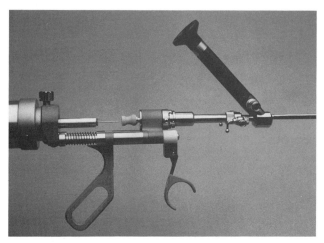

B

Transurethral ureteroscopic lithotripsy

Key steps The patient is prepared as for cystoscopy.

1. The cystoscope is inserted, and all attachments and accessory cords are passed off the field to be attached to the proper equipment.
2. The ureter is dilated before the ureteroscope is passed.
3. The ureteroscope is inserted into the ureter until the stone is visualized.
4. The working element of the selected stone disintegrator is passed through the scope to the level of the stone and the stone is disintegrated.
5. At the conclusion of the procedure all equipment is removed.
6. A ureteral stent may be left in place.

SUMMARY

The perioperative nurse who cares for the patient having genitourinary surgery will be aware that this surgery is often embarrassing for the patient and will provide the patient with privacy and support. Many procedures are now done on a same-day surgery basis, providing a challenge to the nurse for patient preparation and discharge teaching. Often, the patient has undergone many diagnostic studies before arriving in the operating suite and will be anxious about the outcome of surgery.

This chapter has reviewed the anatomy of the urinary system and the male reproductive system. Information related to diagnostic studies, surgical procedures, and the associated equipment and supplies used for surgery has been presented.

REFERENCES

Anderson, P. D. (1984). *Basic human anatomy and physiology: Clinical implications for the health professions.* Boston: Jones and Bartlett Publishers.

Association of Operating Room Nurses. (1994). *Standards and recommended practices.* Denver: Author.

Atkinson, L. J., & Kohn, M. L. (1992). *Berry and Kohn's introduction to operating room technique* (7th ed.). St. Louis: Mosby–Year Book.

Brooks Tighe, S. M. (1989). *Instrumentation for the operating room: A photographic manual.* St. Louis: C. V. Mosby.

Calne, R., & Pollard, S. G. (1992). *Operative surgery.* London: Gower.

Cubler-Goodman, A., Devlin, M. A., Dinatale, R. (1993). Endoscopic lithotripsy for urinary calculi: Treatment alternatives. *AORN Journal, 58,* 954–960.

Cumes, D. M. (1993). Transurethral prostate resection: A frustration-free surgical method. *AORN Journal, 58,* 302–311.

Fuller, J. R. (1986). *Surgical technology principles and practice.* Philadelphia: W. B. Saunders.

Grimes, J., & Burns, E. (1992). *Health assessment in nursing practice,* 3rd Edition. Boston: Jones and Bartlett.

Kenney, L. (1993). Extracorporeal shock wave lithotripsy. *AORN Journal, 56,* 251–263.

Kneedler, J. A., & Dodge, G. H. (1994). *Perioperative patient care: The nursing perspective,* 3rd Edition. Boston: Jones & Bartlett.

Marshall, F. F. (1991). *Operative urology.* Philadelphia: W. B. Saunders.

McConnell, E. A. (1987). *Clinical considerations in perioperative nursing preventive aspects of care.* Philadelphia: J. B. Lippincott.

Meeker, M. H., & Rothrock, J. C. (1991). *Alexander's care of the patient in surgery,* 9th Edition. St. Louis: Mosby–Year Book.

Newton, M., Moore, S., Gaehle, K. E. (1994). Prostate cancer: Staging through laparoscopic lymphadenectomy. *AORN Journal, 59,* 823–836.

Reuter, H. J. (1982). *Atlas of urologic endoscopic surgery.* Philadelphia: W. B. Saunders.

Rothrock, J. C. (1990). *Perioperative nursing care planning.* St. Louis: C. V. Mosby.

Stewart, B. H. (1975). *Operative urology: The kidneys, adrenal glands and retroperitoneum.* Baltimore: Williams & Wilkins.

Tiemann, D., Shea, L., Klutke, C. G., Gaehle, K., Moore, S. (1993). Artificial urinary spincter: Treatment of post-prostatectomy incontinence. *AORN Journal, 57,* 1366–1379.

Chapter 12

Orthopaedic Surgery

Key Concepts

- Orthopaedic surgery deals with structures of the musculoskeletal system including the bones, muscles, tendons, ligaments, cartilage, and articulating surfaces (joints) of the body.

- Orthopaedic surgery encompasses a wide range of instruments, power tools, fixation devices, and prosthetic components, all of which may vary dramatically with the specific procedure.

- Special equipment for orthopaedic surgery is cumbersome and includes special operating room tables and beds, video equipment carts, pneumatic tourniquets, fluoroscopy units, cast carts, and personnel protective gear.

- Infection prevention measures are strictly enforced and may include a special air filtration system for the operating rooms and/or the use of air filtration hoods for the operating team.

- Orthopaedic nurses care for patients from all age groups, pediatric to geriatric.

- Musculoskeletal disease almost always produces pain and dysfunction, both of which affect the patient's mobility and activities of daily living. Additionally, musculoskeletal deformities are usually externally obvious and therefore may affect the patient's body image.

- More than any other specialty, surgical treatment of orthopaedic disease requires a multidisciplinary approach. Social services, occupational therapy, and extensive physical rehabilitation are often required.

INTRODUCTION

Perioperative nurses who choose to specialize in orthopaedics are faced with a wide array of challenges. The patient population covers the entire life span, from pediatrics to geriatrics. The perioperative nurse must possess knowledge of the anatomy and physiology of bones, muscles, and joints, as well as the disease processes that afflict them. Instrumentation is greater in both quantity and specificity for orthopaedics than for any other surgical service. Additionally, orthopaedic equipment is bulky and frequently heavy, making orthopaedics a physically demanding service.

Management of an orthopaedic service also presents unique challenges. Adequate storage space and operating room size must be provided. More than any other service, orthopaedics requires relentless and accurate inventory control of supplies, instruments, and implants. The cost of inventory is a manager's nightmare, yet the availability of inventory is essential. In recent years, the collaborative efforts between the manufacturers of orthopaedic implants and perioperative nurse managers have produced creative strategies for meeting these challenges.

ANATOMY

Anatomy that relates to the procedures in this chapter is discussed and illustrated here.

Hip

The hip, a ball-and-socket joint, is the major weight-bearing joint of the body (Fig. 12-1). It is formed by the almost spherical femoral head and the acetabular portion of the innominate bone. The hip is surrounded by a capsule, ligaments, muscles, nerves, and femoral vessels. Arthritic changes of the hip may result from inflammatory, traumatic, or osteoarthritic processes.

Knee

The knee is a diarthrodial or freely mobile, hinge-type joint. It allows flexion, extension, and limited rolling and gliding movements. This joint is the largest, most complex, and probably the most vulnerable in the body.

The knee joint is composed of three articular surfaces. The two articulating surfaces of the femur and the tibia are the medial and lateral tibiofemoral joints, and the articulating surface of the femur and the patella is the patellofemoral joint (Fig. 12-2). The knee joint is protected and stabilized by the medial and lateral collateral ligaments and the anterior and posterior cruciate ligaments. The medial and lateral menisci and joint capsule also help to stabilize the knee (Fig. 12-3, A and B).

Shoulder

The shoulder is a ball-and-socket joint formed by the articulation of the humeral head with the shallow glenoid fossa of the scapula (Fig. 12-4). It is the most freely movable joint of the body and, as such, one of the least stable. The shoulder is primarily stabilized by the muscles and tendons that pass over it (Fig. 12-5). These muscles, collectively referred to as the rotator cuff, include the supraspinous, infraspinsous, teres minor, and subscapular. Additional stabilization comes from the three ligaments surrounding the shoulder.

Vertebral Column

The spine or vertebral column consists of 33 bones called *vertebrae*. There are seven cervical, twelve thoracic, five lumbar, five fused sacral, and five fused coccygeal vertebrae. The vertebrae articulate with each other at the superior and inferior facet joints and are stabilized by the infraspinous ligaments. The most important ligaments of the spinal column are the anterior and posterior longitudinal ligaments and the ligamentum flavum. Spinal nerves pass from the spinal cord to the periphery through the intervertebral foramina.

From the second cervical vertebra to the sacrum, the vertebrae are separated by fibrocartilaginous intervertebral discs which serve to increase flexibility and cushion the stress of movement (Fig. 12-6, A). The intervertebral disc consists of a tough, fibrous outer ring, the annulus, and a softer center, the nucleus pulposus. In Figure 12-6, B, the nucleus pulposus is extruded and is impinging on a spinal nerve.

Carpal Tunnel

The carpal tunnel is a rigid compartment located in the wrist and hand. It is formed by the transverse volar carpal ligament ventrally and the carpal bones dorsally (Fig. 12-7).

Ankle and Foot

The ankle joint is composed primarily of the tibiotalar articulation. The fibula provides lateral stability. A capsular structure surrounds the joint (Fig. 12-8).

The metatarsophalangeal joint of the foot is important, especially in the formation of bunions. Spanning this joint is an intricate structure of flexor, extensor, abductor, and adductor muscle tendons. The joint is composed not only of the first metatarsal in the proximal phalanx of the great toe, but also of two sesamoid bones on the plantar aspect of the first metatarsal head. The muscles pull in a balanced fashion, and the sesamoids are normally well seated under the first metatarsal head.

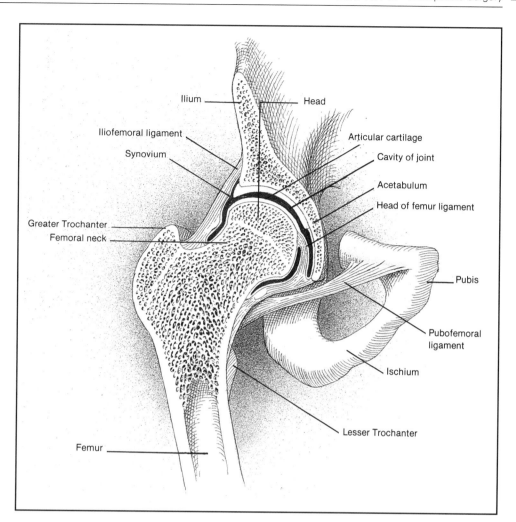

FIGURE 12-1   Structures of the right hip.   (Courtesy of Johnson & Johnson Medical, Inc., Arlington, TX.)

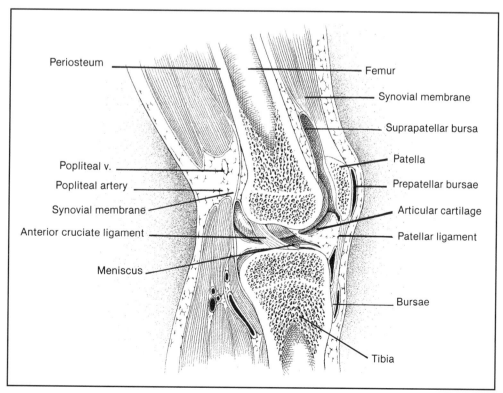

FIGURE 12-2   Sagittal section through the knee joint.   (Courtesy of Johnson & Johnson Medical, Inc., Arlington, TX.)

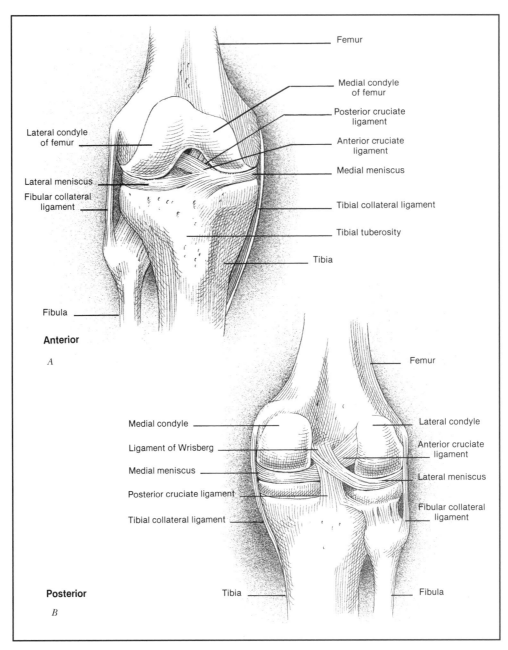

FIGURE 12-3 Structures of the knee joint. (*A*) Anterior view of the right knee. (*B*) Posterior view of the right knee. (Courtesy of Johnson & Johnson Medical, Inc., Arlington TX.)

NURSING CONSIDERATIONS

Mobility and ambulation are mainstays of many of life's activities. Because orthopaedic surgery has an impact on these activities, the outcomes of the surgery are critical. Perioperative nurses, as part of the operating room team, can make a difference in outcomes through assessment of the patient, planning the care through use of the nursing process, knowing the operation's basic steps, and being clinically competent.

Preparation of an orthopaedic operating room can tax even the most ingenious mind. Cumbersome equipment,

drills and hoses, positioning aids, orthopaedic implants, heavy and bulky bone instruments, fixation devices, and the like, all find their way into an orthopaedic procedure.

Patients with injuries or fractures often come to the operating room in their own bed, with attached devices, casts, fixations, and traction. The devices must be carefully removed before the procedure begins. Transfer and positioning of the patient become major procedures because of the personnel needed, the planning required, the devices that are necessary, and the constant consideration of alignment and protection of the patient's musculoskeletal system that is necessary.

(continued on page 242)

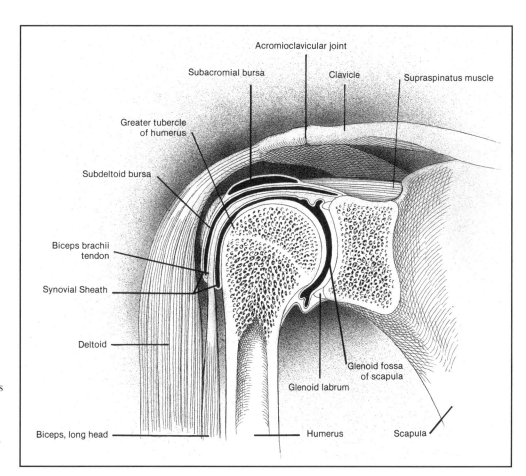

FIGURE 12-4 Structures of the glenohumeral and acromioclavicular joints, right shoulder. (Courtesy of Johnson & Johnson Medical, Inc., Arlington TX.)

Acromioclavicular joint

Subacromial bursa

Clavicle

Supraspinatus muscle

Greater tubercle of humerus

Subdeltoid bursa

Biceps brachii tendon

Synovial Sheath

Deltoid

Biceps, long head

Glenoid labrum

Glenoid fossa of scapula

Humerus

Scapula

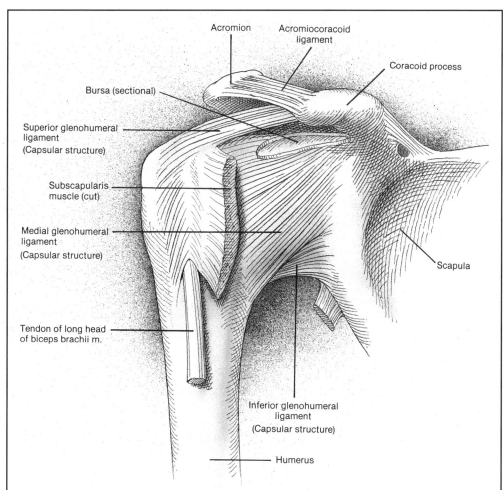

Acromion

Acromiocoracoid ligament

Coracoid process

Bursa (sectional)

Superior glenohumeral ligament (Capsular structure)

Subscapularis muscle (cut)

Medial glenohumeral ligament (Capsular structure)

Tendon of long head of biceps brachii m.

Inferior glenohumeral ligament (Capsular structure)

Scapula

Humerus

FIGURE 12-5 Anterior view of the right shoulder joint. (Courtesy of Johnson & Johnson Medical, Inc., Arlington TX.)

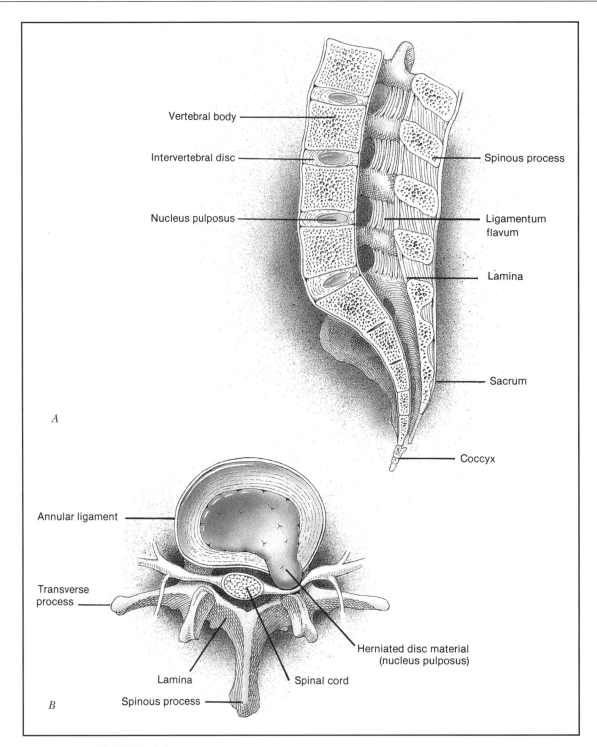

FIGURE 12-6 (*A*) Sagittal section, lumbosacral vertebrae. (*B*) Ruptured annulus with extrusion of nucleus pulposus. (Courtesy of Johnson & Johnson Medical, Inc., Arlington TX.)

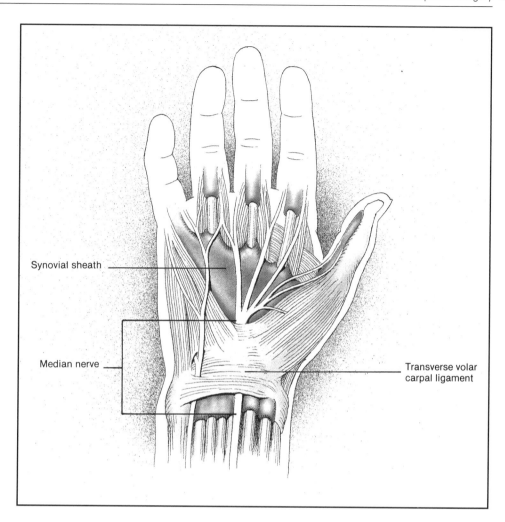

FIGURE 12-7 Structures affected in carpal tunnel syndrome (right wrist and hand). (Courtesy of Johnson & Johnson Medical, Inc., Arlington TX.)

Synovial sheath

Median nerve

Transverse volar carpal ligament

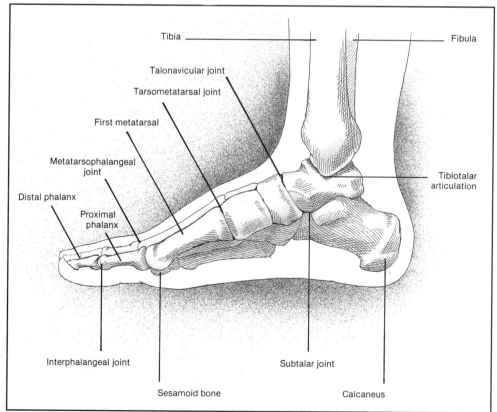

Tibia

Fibula

Talonavicular joint

Tarsometatarsal joint

First metatarsal

Metatarsophalangeal joint

Distal phalanx

Proximal phalanx

Tibiotalar articulation

Interphalangeal joint

Subtalar joint

Sesamoid bone

Calcaneus

FIGURE 12-8 Bones and joints of ankle and foot. (Courtesy of Johnson & Johnson Medical, Inc., Arlington TX.)

Juggling the high regard for asepsis in bone and joint surgery with the amount of required equipment and activity in the room during the surgery is a priority of the operating room staff. Strict adherence to sterile technique is a must, as is keeping air turbulence to a minimum. Some operating rooms are equipped with special air-filtering systems, and a number of surgeons use hoods and air-evacuation systems when doing implant procedures.

Directing traffic and movement, monitoring the team's sterile practices, and verifying implant sizes are high on the agenda for perioperative nurses (Gruendemann & Yocum, 1990).

Care Planning

Assessing, planning, and implementing perioperative care for the orthopaedic patient require a nursing care plan or a critical pathway that may incorporate one or several of the following nursing diagnoses:

High risk for infection

High risk for injury

High risk for impaired skin integrity

Altered role performance

Impaired physical mobility

High risk for peripheral neurovascular dysfunction

Pain

High risk for activity intolerance

New procedures, devices, and techniques for fracture reductions and joint replacements are continuously evolving. In spite of this, orthopaedic surgery often is followed by physical therapy and rehabilitation. The perioperative period and care of the patient are crucial elements in this total course of treatment and rehabilitation for the patient.

Instrumentation and Equipment

Instrumentation for orthopaedic surgery consists of soft tissue and bone instruments. "Small," "basic," and "plastic" refer to instrument sets used in less extensive orthopaedic procedures, and terms such as "major bone" are used to describe instrumentation for more extensive procedures. Figures 12-9 to 12-13 are examples of varied orthopaedic instrument sets.

The use of the pneumatic tourniquet as a device to control bleed is discussed on pages 262–264.

ARTHROSCOPIC SURGERY

Arthroscopy allows the orthopaedist to examine, accurately diagnose, and often treat surgical joint pathology through minimally invasive techniques (also see Chapter

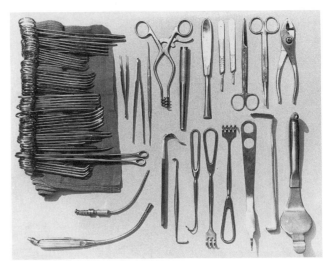

FIGURE 12-9 Small orthopaedic instrument set. *Left, top* to *bottom*: Kocher clamps, mosquito clamps, curved Crile clamps, straight Crile clamps, Allis clamps, Kelly clamps, needle holders, straight Mayo scissors, Metzenbaum scissors, ring forceps for sponge sticks, towel clamps. *Top, left* to *right*: Adson tissue forceps, toothed tissue forceps, Freer elevator, Weitlaner retractor, bone tamp, Cushing periosteal elevator, No. 4 knife handle, No. 3 knife handle, straight Mayo scissors, curved Mayo scissors, pliers. *Bottom, left* to *right*: Yankauer suction tip, Frazier suction tip, Smillie knee retractor, Senn retractor, Lahey retractor, 3-prong rake retractor, 4-prong rake retractor, Hohmann retractor, U.S.A. retractor, Bennett retractor.

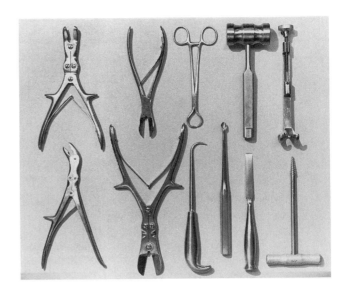

FIGURE 12-10 Orthopaedic bone set. *Top row, left* to *right*: double-action rongeur, single-action bone cutter, Lewin bone-holding clamp, mallet, Lowman 3-prong bone-holding clamp. *Bottom row, left* to *right*: goose neck rongeur, double-action bone cutter, bone hook, curette, osteotome, corkscrew.

17 in this volume). Currently, arthroscopic techniques are most frequently employed with the knee; however, arthroscopic techniques involving the shoulder, ankle, elbow,

wrist, and hip are also gaining acceptance. Arthroscopes range in size from 1.7 mm to 6 mm, with lenses varying from 30 to 90 degrees. These scopes allow the surgeon visual access to narrow spaces through a small incision.

The advantages of arthroscopic surgery include the following:

1. Accurate diagnosis with minimal joint disruption
2. Reduced inflammatory response
3. Reduced morbidity resulting in earlier, more aggressive, and less extensive rehabilitation
4. Reduced length of hospitalization

Perioperative Nursing Considerations

Positioning

Positioning for arthroscopy is usually supine, with the exception of shoulder arthroscopy, which requires lateral positioning. Positioning devices and other special equipment vary depending on the joint involved and the surgeon's preference. (See Chapter 28 in Volume 1 for a detailed discussion of patient positioning.)

Special equipment

Special equipment required for arthroscopy includes the positioning devices previously mentioned, pneumatic tourniquet, size-specific arthroscope and instruments, light source, sterile camera, video system, and instruments specific to the planned procedure. Arthroscopic procedures require constant irrigation. Tandem irrigation and suction systems are employed to eliminate flow disruption. Large amounts of irrigation necessitate the use of numerous strategies to prevent strikethrough and provide

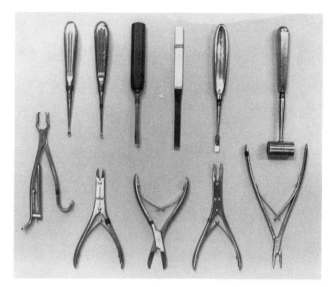

FIGURE 12-12 Orthopaedic plastic bone set. *Top row, left to right*: curettes (0, 3-0), gouges, osteotomes (2), periosteal elevator, mallet. *Bottom row, left to right*: Kern bone-holding clamp, double-action bone cutter, single-action bone cutter, double-action rongeur, single-action rongeur.

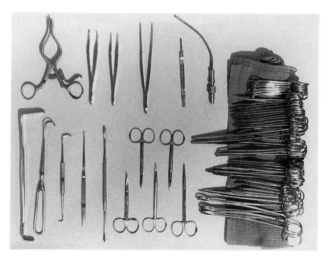

FIGURE 12-13 Plastic instrument set. *Top, left to right*: Weitlaner retractor, Martin forceps, Adson tissue forceps with teeth, jeweler's forceps, No. 3 knife handle, Frazier suction tip. *Bottom, left to right*: U.S.A. retractor, Lahey retractor, Ragnell retractors (2), skin hook, Freer elevator, Stevens scissors, curved iris scissors, Littler scissors, straight iris scissors, straight Metzenbaum scissors. *Instruments on right, top to bottom*: towel clamps, mosquito clamps, Kocher clamps, Allis clamps, needle holders, Metzenbaum scissors, straight and curved Mayo scissors, ring forceps for sponge sticks.

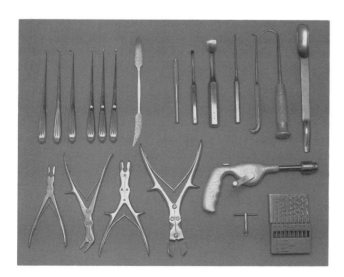

FIGURE 12-11 Orthopaedic major bone set. *Top row, left to right*: bone curettes (6), rasp, tamp, osteotomes (3), bone hooks (2), bone skid. *Bottom row*: double-action rongeurs (3), double-action bone cutter, hand drill with key, drill points.

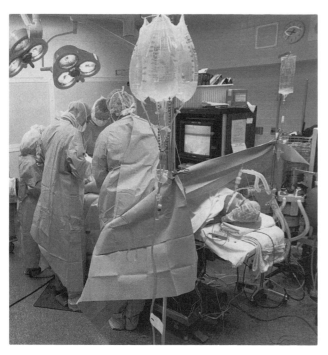

FIGURE 12-14 Room setup for knee arthroscopy. Note tandem irrigation and video rack.

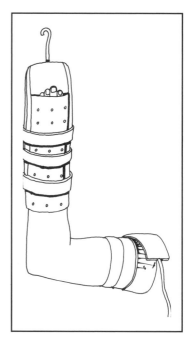

FIGURE 12-16 Arm in gauntlet with tourniquet in place.

a safe environment for both the patient and the surgical team (Fig. 12-14).

Knee procedures

Knee arthroscopy requires flexion of the knee (Fig. 12-15). This may be accomplished by flexing the foot of the table or by elevating the knee with a leg holder or post.

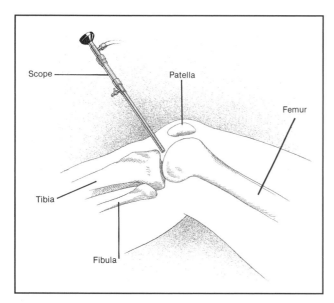

FIGURE 12-15 Knee arthroscopy. (Courtesy of Johnson & Johnson Medical, Inc., Arlington TX.)

There are a variety of "surgical assistant" devices available, which, in addition to initial positioning, provide a stable fulcrum for manipulation of the knee during the procedure.

Anesthesia may be general, local block, or spinal. A pneumatic tourniquet is placed around the thigh. The leg is prepped to just below the tourniquet and draped free using impervious materials.

Elbow procedures

Elbow arthroscopy requires 90-degree flexion of the elbow. This is usually accomplished by placing the forearm in a suspension device called a *gauntlet* (Fig. 12-16). This allows maximum access by allowing the entire arm to be suspended free over the side of the operating room bed. Additionally, this position allows the forearm to be freely manipulated and protects important neurovascular structures of the antecubital fossa. General anesthesia is usually preferred to provide patient comfort and permit total muscle relaxation. A pneumatic tourniquet is applied, and the area is prepped.

Shoulder procedures

Shoulder arthroscopy requires lateral positioning. A traction arm holder is used to suspend the arm in a forward flexed and abducted position. The glenohumeral joint is distracted with 5 to 15 pounds of traction. General anesthesia is employed. The shoulder is prepped and draped free to permit full range of motion during the procedure.

Ankle or wrist procedures

Wrist or ankle arthroscopy requires supine positioning of the patient. A pneumatic tourniquet is placed proximally but is inflated only when excessive bleeding occurs. As with other arthroscopies, the joint is draped for free manipulation and with impervious materials. General anesthesia is preferred.

Arthroscopic Procedures

Indications

Arthroscopy is indicated to aid in the evaluation and diagnosis of joint disease, lesions, or instabilities and in the treatment of certain surgical pathologies. Treatments performed through the arthroscope include repair of torn cartilage, retrieval of loose bodies, synovial biopsy and synovectomy, ligament reconstruction, debridement of arthritic lesions and osteophytes, fixation of chondral or osteochondral defects, decompression for impingement syndrome, and drainage and irrigation of a septic joint.

Arthroscopy of the knee, elbow, shoulder, and ankle or wrist

Key steps

1. The joint is distended with fluid through a Verres needle or irrigation cannula. Fluid may be instilled manually through a syringe or through a pressure-sensitive pump.
2. A stab incision is made to accommodate the arthroscopic sheath.
3. The sheath with the sharp trocar is inserted to a point just through the joint capsule.
4. The sharp trocar is removed and replaced with a blunt trocar, which is advanced within the joint.
5. The blunt trocar is removed and replaced with an arthroscope of the appropriate size, to which the light source, camera, and video attachments are connected.
6. Irrigation tubing is connected to the arthroscope to establish inflow. Another needle is placed to allow egress of fluid.
7. The joint is visually inspected.
8. Additional portals of entry are established under direct visualization.
9. The surgical intervention is performed.
10. The joint is thoroughly irrigated and drained.
11. The portals are closed with single sutures or adhesive strips.
12. An appropriate dressing is applied.

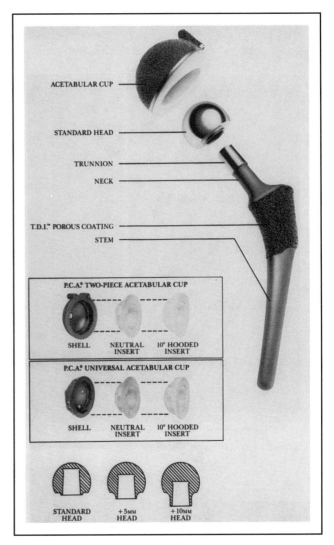

FIGURE 12-17 Components of the P.C.A. (Porous Coated Anatomical) primary total hip system. (Courtesy of Howmedica Inc.)

TOTAL HIP ARTHROPLASTY

Total hip arthroplasty replaces a degenerated or diseased hip joint with an ultra–light-molecular-weight polyethylene cup component and a metallic (chrome-cobalt or titanium) femoral component (Fig. 12-17). In the past, these components were secured in place with cement. Today, however, bone-growth prostheses are an option. These components allow the ingrowth of bone, which theoretically reduces the likelihood of slippage secondary to cement degeneration. The acetabular cup is secured in place with fixation screws, or press-fit, and the femoral component is press-fit into the femoral canal (Fig. 12-18).

Perioperative Nursing Considerations

The patient is placed in the lateral decubitus position (Fig. 12-19). Special equipment required includes positioning aids, power drill and saw (Fig. 12-20), and the

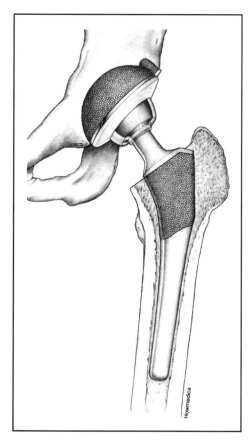

FIGURE 12-18 Hip with prosthetic components in place. (Courtesy of Howmedica Inc.)

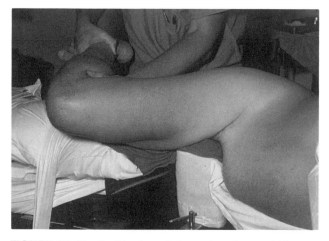

FIGURE 12-19 Positioning of the patient for total hip arthroplasty. (Courtesy of Johnson & Johnson Medical, Inc., Arlington, TX.)

Procedure

Indications

Total hip arthroplasty is indicated when pain with weight bearing and limited range of motion interfere with the patient's activities of daily living. The diagnosis is made after physical examination demonstrates loss of hip rotation and abduction. The anteroposterior and lateral

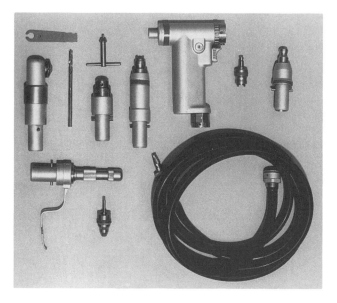

FIGURE 12-20 Air-powered drill/saw set. *Top, left* to *right*: saw blade, saw attachment, drill bit, Jacobs chuck and key, reamer motor, handpiece, reamer adaptor, trinkle attachment. *Bottom, left* to *right*: wire driver, quick coupling device, hose.

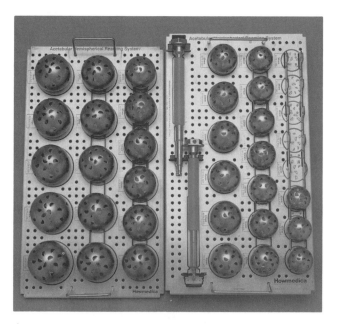

A

FIGURE 12-21 P.C.A. total hip system. (*A*) Acetabular reamers. (*B*) Acetabular instrumentation. (*C*) Acetabular trials. (*D*) Femoral flexible intramedullary reamers. (*E*) Femoral broaches and accessory tray.

total hip system of the surgeon's choice (Fig. 12-21,*A* to *E*). The steps required for cemented total hip replacement and noncemented total hip replacement vary considerably. Presented here are the basic steps common to both types of hip replacement. It is advisable to consult technical manuals provided by the manufacturer for detailed procedural steps involved with the specific total hip replacement system used.

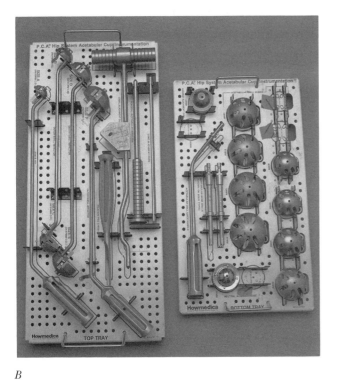

B

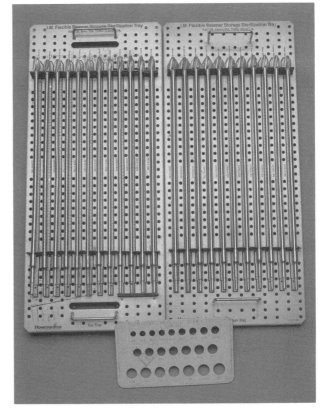

D

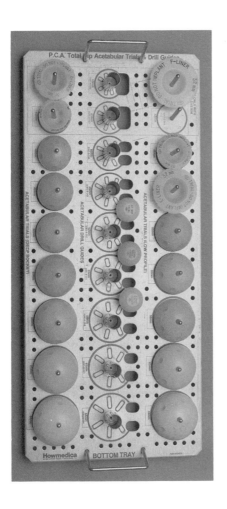

C

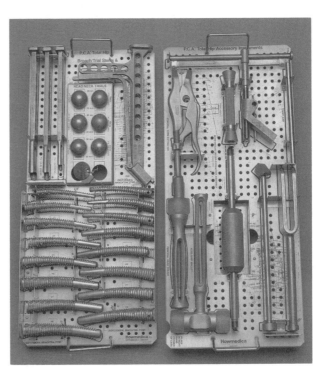

E

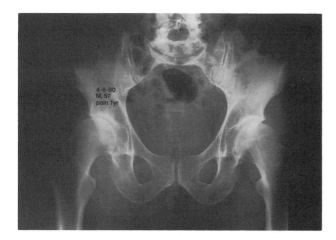

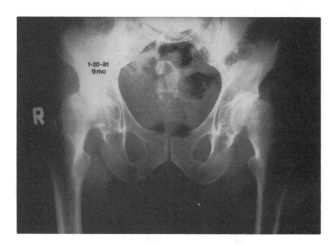

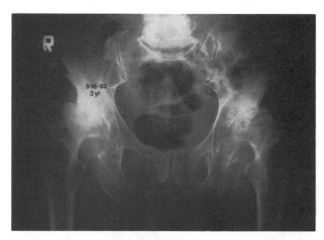

FIGURE 12-22 Diseased hip showing loss of articular space and secondary marginal osteophytes, commonly seen in arthritis of the hip joint. (*Top*) Radiograph of the pelvis showing minimal loss of articular cartilage space in the right hip after the patient had had pain for one year. (*Middle*) Note the marked loss of articular cartilage space in the right hip nine months later. (*Bottom*) Three years later both hips display loss of articular cartilage space and secondary marginal osteophytes. (From Cohen, J. [1990]. *Orthopedic pathophysiology in diagnosis and treatment.* New York: Churchill Livingstone. Reprinted with permission.)

X-ray films of the hip joint in weight bearing often reveal joint space narrowing, cyst formation, sclerosis, and osteophytes (Fig. 12-22, *A*, *B*, and *C*). Congenital hip disease, Legg-Calvé-Perthes' disease, and avascular necrosis may also produce changes that require total hip replacement.

Total hip arthroplasty

Key steps

1. The hip and leg are prepped and draped free.
2. A slightly curved posterolateral incision is made over the greater trochanter and extended distally along the course of the femoral shaft.
3. The subcutaneous tissue is divided down to the fascia lata and gluteus maximus muscle.
4. The joint capsule is incised, and the hip is dislocated.
5. The femoral head is osteotomized with a power saw.
6. The acetabulum is reamed to the appropriate size.
7. Osteophytes, if present, are removed with a bone rongeur.
8. The femoral canal is reamed to the appropriate size.
9. Trial components are used to check that the sizing is correct.
10. The acetabular cup is fixed into place with cement or bone screws, or is press-fit into place.
11. The femoral component is fit into the femoral canal, and a trial reduction is performed. When reduction is adequate, and when range of motion has been verified, the component is secured.
12. The hip is again reduced, and range of motion is evaluated.
13. A closed-suction wound drain is placed.
14. The wound is closed in layers, and a compression dressing is applied.
15. A abduction pillow is secured between the legs to maintain the desired position.

TOTAL KNEE ARTHROPLASTY

Total knee arthroplasty is performed to replace damaged articular surfaces of the knee. Surgery is indicated for painful or dysfunctional conditions that affect activities of daily living. Pain and dysfunction may be secondary to osteoarthritis, rheumatoid arthritis, nonseptic arthropathy, or traumatic degeneration of the articular surfaces. The patient usually presents with pain and loss of motion. Radiography demonstrates joint surface deterioration and a narrowing of the joint space (Fig. 12-23).

Perioperative Nursing Considerations

The patient is positioned supine with a pneumatic tourniquet placed at mid thigh. Special equipment required includes power saw and drill and the total knee system of the surgeon's choice (Fig. 12-24, *A,B*, and *C*). As with other orthopaedic implant systems, instrumentation and procedural steps are specific to the system. The following steps are common to most systems.

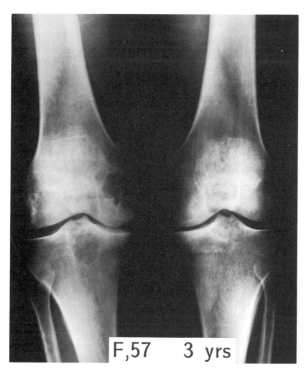

FIGURE 12-23 Radiographs of knees demonstrating joint degeneration and narrowing of medial compartment cartilage space. (From Cohen, J. [1990]. *Orthopedic pathophysiology in diagnosis and treatment.* New York: Churchill Livingstone. Reprinted with permission.)

Procedure

Total knee arthroplasty

Key steps

1. The leg is prepped and draped free.
2. The extremity is exsanguinated, and the tourniquet is inflated.
3. A longitudinal incision curving around the patella or a midline patellar incision is made.
4. The joint is entered through a median parapatellar capsulotomy.
5. The quadriceps tendon is incised longitudinally, allowing eversion and dislocation of the patella.
6. The knee is flexed. Diseased soft tissue and osteophytes are debrided.
7. Alignment devices (calipers, cutting blocks, and rods) and specific cutting jigs are used to make accurate bone cuts for precision fitting of the prosthetic components (Fig. 12-25).
8. Distal femoral cuts are made.
9. Proximal tibial cuts are made.
10. The articular surface of the patella is resected.
11. Tibiofemoral angulation is evaluated using an alignment assembly. Flexion gap is checked with a spacer.
12. Trial components are positioned and trial reduction performed.

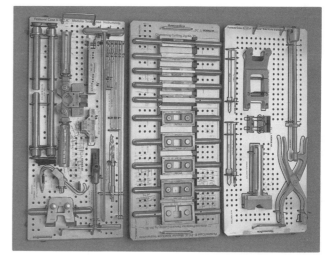

A

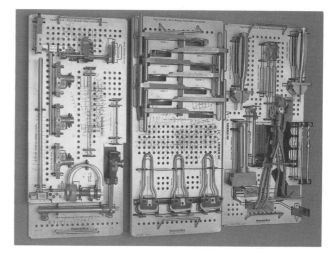

B

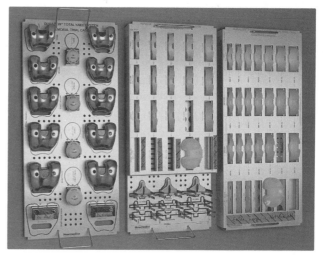

C

FIGURE 12-24 P.C.A. modular total knee. (*A*) *Left* to *right,* trays A and B and P.C.A. accessory tray. (*B*) *Left* to *right,* tibial and patellar instruments. (*C*) Trial components.

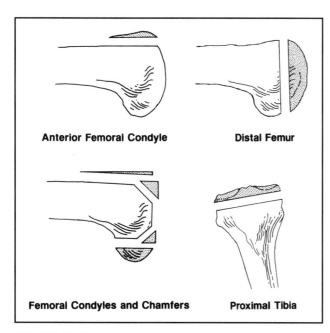

FIGURE 12-25 Bone cuts required during total knee arthroplasty.

(labels in figure:)
Anterior Femoral Condyle

Distal Femur

Femoral Condyles and Chamfers

Proximal Tibia

13. Permanent components are selected and secured into place.
14. Final reduction is accomplished.
15. A closed-suction wound drain is placed.
16. The wound is closed in layers, and a dressing is applied.
17. A knee immobilizer is applied to maintain the desired position.

SHOULDER ARTHROPLASTY

The purpose of total shoulder arthroplasty is to replace the joint structures with prostheses (Fig. 12-26). Indications for surgery include severely comminuted fractures of the humeral head or painful degenerative arthritic conditions with loss of motion. It should be noted that the shoulder is the most difficult joint in the body to rehabilitate. Because of its great range of motion and primarily muscular stabilization, outcome of surgery is inextricably tied to rehabilitation outcomes.

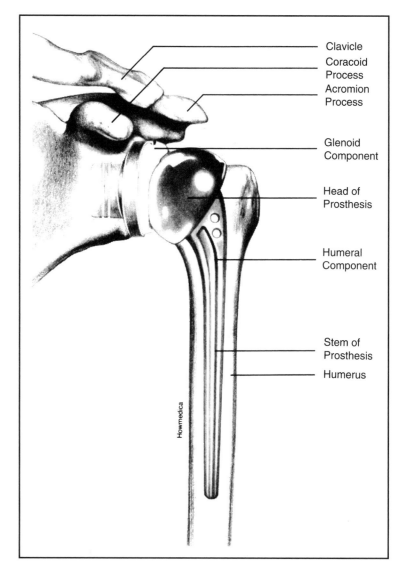

(labels in figure:)
Clavicle
Coracoid Process
Acromion Process
Glenoid Component
Head of Prosthesis
Humeral Component
Stem of Prosthesis
Humerus

Howmedica

FIGURE 12-26 Shoulder with prosthetic components in place. (Courtesy of Howmedica Inc.)

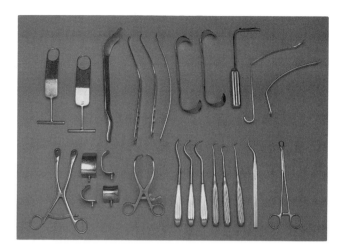

FIGURE 12-27 Shoulder retractor tray. *Top, left* to *right*: Fucuda retractors (2), bone skid, blunt Homan retractors (2), curved spike, Goulet retractors (2), conjoined retractor, humeral head retractor, pitch-fork retractor. *Bottom, left* to *right*: Lynx retractor with four blades, Gelpi retractor, Crego set (3), Rowe shoulder instruments (5).

Perioperative Nursing Considerations

The patient is placed in semisitting or "beach-chair" position, with the arm draped free and abducted slightly on an armboard. A pad may be place under the scapula to elevate relevant structures. Special equipment includes power saw and drill, shoulder retractors (Fig. 12-27), and the shoulder component system of the surgeon's choice.

Procedure

Shoulder arthroplasty

Key steps

1. A curvilinear incision is made, beginning immediately above the coracoid process and extending distally and laterally along the deltopectoral groove, following the anterior border of the deltoid muscle.
2. The cephalic vein is identified and retracted or ligated and cut.
3. With the shoulder abducted 70 to 90 degrees, the anterior deltoid and lateral pectoralis muscles are retracted to expose the humeral head and glenohumeral joint.
4. The coracoacromial ligament is identified and divided.
5. The subscapularis muscle is divided, tagged, and retracted medially, and the humeral head is dislocated, exposing the interior of the joint.
6. The joint is irrigated and debrided.
7. The humeral head is removed.
8. The humeral shaft is prepared with tapered reamers and sized.
9. The glenoid is prepared with a longitudinal slot along its axis in the cancellous bone and with multiple drill holes in subchondral bone.

10. The components may be cemented or press-fit into the humerus and fixed with screws on the glenoid surface.
11. The humeral head is reduced, and range of motion is evaluated.
12. A closed-suction wound drain is placed.
13. The wound is closed in layers, and a dressing is applied.
14. A shoulder immobilizer is used postoperatively until rehabilitation of the shoulder is sufficient for its removal.

REPAIR OF FRACTURES

A fracture is a disruption in the continuity of a bone. Fractures are most commonly caused by trauma, but pathologic fractures of diseased bone may occur from simple muscle tension produced with activities of daily living. The objectives of fracture treatment are (1) to restore normal bone alignment (reduction), (2) to maintain bone reduction until healing occurs, and (3) to preserve and restore musculoskeletal function. Fractures are often complicated by injury to soft tissues and neurovascular structures surrounding the fracture, as well as by the systemic effects sustained during the trauma.

There are two broad groups of fractures: open and closed. A closed fracture does not communicate with the external environment, whereas an open fracture does. Further classification denoting the type and extent of fracture and soft tissue injury is required for determination of the best treatment option available. Russell (1992) notes that extensive classifications of skeletal injuries are currently being developed by both the (Swiss) Association for the Study of Internal Fixation (ASIF) and the Orthopaedic Trauma Association (OTA). The major OTA categories of long bone fractures are shown in Figure 12-28.

Perioperative Nursing Considerations

Patient positioning and special equipment required are determined by the type of fracture and the extremity involved. A fracture table (Figs. 12-29 and 12-30) or arm table may be used. Other required equipment generally includes a power drill and saw, fluoroscopy, and the implants and instrumentation of the surgeon's choice (Figs. 12-31 to 12-34).

Now, more than ever before, the orthopaedic surgeon has a wide variety of options available for treating fractures. Treatment techniques may be categorized as *closed reduction, external fixation,* or *internal fixation.*

Closed Reduction

A simple fracture of a long bone that produces little or no bone displacement can be treated through closed reduction. General anesthesia is usually employed for patient

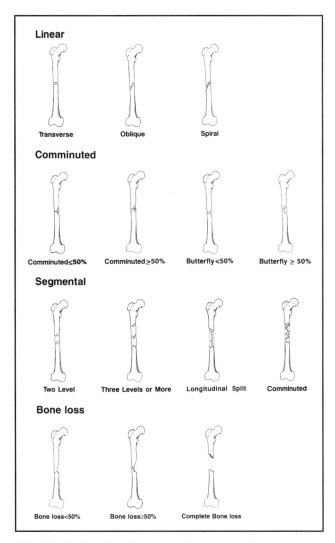

Linear

Transverse   Oblique   Spiral

Comminuted

Comminuted≤50%   Comminuted≥50%   Butterfly<50%   Butterfly ≥ 50%

Segmental

Two Level   Three Levels or More   Longitudinal Split   Comminuted

Bone loss

Bone loss<50%   Bone loss≥50%   Complete Bone loss

FIGURE 12-28 Classifications of long bone fractures as described by the Orthopaedic Trauma Association (OTA).

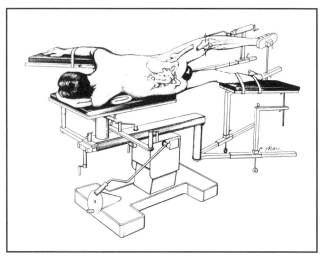

FIGURE 12-29 Patient with fractured femur positioned laterally on fracture table. (Courtesy of Howmedica Inc.)

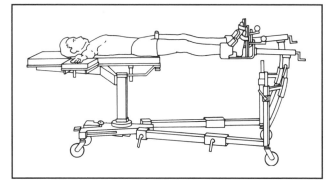

FIGURE 12-30 Patient positioned supine on fracture table. (Courtesy of Howmedica Inc.)

comfort, but regional block or spinal anesthesia is acceptable. The fracture is reduced through manual manipulation, aided by fluoroscopy, and immobilized with a cast (Fig. 12-35). Casting techniques are discussed later in the chapter.

Pins and plaster

There are times when a closed reduction of a forearm or wrist is indicated and the fracture requires the additional stabilization of percutaneous pins. The closed reduction is accomplished with the aid of fluoroscopy. The area is then prepped and a percutaneous placement of a pin or pins is performed. The alignment of the fracture is again assessed with fluoroscopy, and, if alignment is adequate, a plaster or fiberglass cast is applied that incorporates the pins.

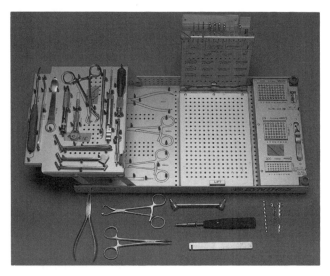

FIGURE 12-31 Synthes mini-fragment set.

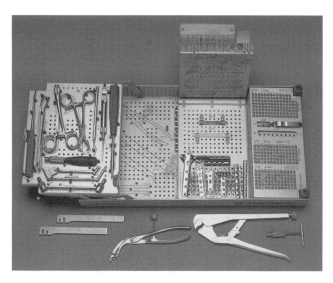

FIGURE 12-32 Synthes small fragment set.

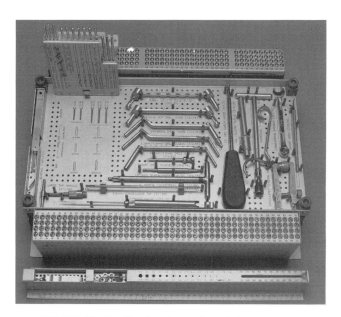

FIGURE 12-33 Synthes basic (large) fragment set.

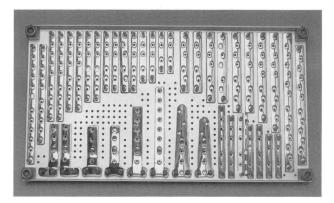

FIGURE 12-34 Synthes large fragment plates.

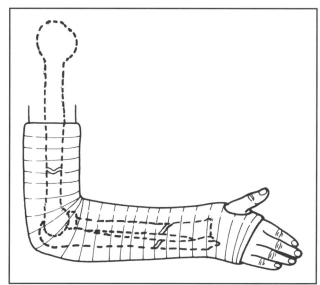

FIGURE 12-35 Long arm cast.

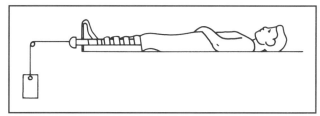

FIGURE 12-36 Buck's skin traction. (Courtesy of Howmedica Inc.)

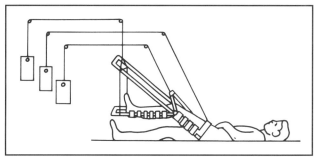

FIGURE 12-37 Skeletal traction. (Courtesy of Howmedica Inc.)

Traction

Simple fractures involving minimal displacement of bone ends and minimal soft tissue damage may be reduced and immobilized through either skin or skeletal traction. Application of skin traction such as Buck's or Russell's traction is a non-invasive procedure (Fig. 12-36). Skeletal traction requires the placement of one or more sterile pins into the bone distal to the fracture site. A traction bow is then attached to the pin, and the desired traction is delivered through a balanced suspension system (Fig. 12-37). While traction techniques reduce the chance of infection inherent with an open procedure, they require prolonged immobilization and increase the risks associated with prolonged bedrest.

External Fixation

External fixation provides rigid stabilization of bones through an external apparatus in circumstances where other forms of immobilization, for whatever reason, are deemed inappropriate. It is most often employed for fractures presenting with a large amount of soft tissue injury. External fixation allows direct surveillance of the limb and wound status and permits simultaneous and aggressive treatment of bone and soft tissue injuries. Early mobilization is allowed, and motion of the immediately proximal and distal joints is not restricted. External fixation is advantageous for use in contaminated wounds because it allows for aggressive management of potential infection. The major complications associated with external fixation devices include pin tract infection, neurovascular impairment, and delayed union.

Perioperative nursing considerations

External fixation devices are composed of a bone anchorage system with three main components: (1) wires or pins that anchor to the bone fragments, (2) articulations in the form of rings or clamps, and (3) longitudinal supports. Three types of external fixation systems are Hoffman, ASIF/AO (Fig. 12-38,*A* and *B*), and Ilizarov (Fig. 12-38,*A*, *B*, *C*). General or regional anesthesia is employed for the application of an external fixation device. Special equipment required includes fluoroscopy (Fig. 12-38,*D* and *E*), suction irrigator, large pin cutter, and the fixation device and instrumentation of the surgeon's choice (Fig. 12-38,*F*).

Indications

Indications most accepted, as reported by Russell (1992), include the following:

1. Severe open fractures
2. Fractures associated with severe burns
3. Fractures requiring flaps, grafts, or other reconstructive procedures
4. Certain fractures requiring distraction to maintain length
5. Limb lengthening
6. Arthrodesis
7. Infected fractures or nonunions

Open Reduction and Internal Fixation

Open reduction and internal fixation (ORIF) is a widely used method of fracture treatment. This method requires open surgical reduction and implantation of pins, screws, wires, nails, rods, and/or plates to maintain the reduction. Internal fixation devices are available in a vast array of sizes and configurations to be used with various bone sizes and fracture types.

Indications

The indications for open reduction and internal fixation generally include the reduction of unstable fractures

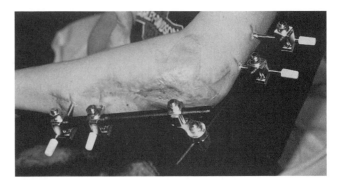

A

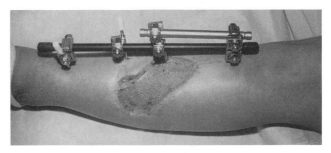

B

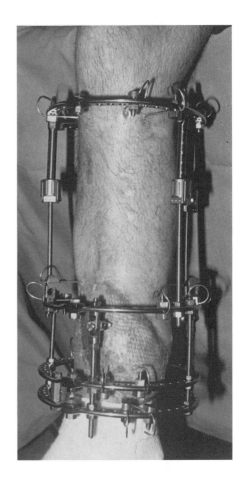

C

FIGURE 12-38 External fixation devices. (*A* and *B*) ASIF/AO external fixation devices. (*C*) Ilizarov external fixation device. (*D*) Fluoroscopy unit (C arm). (*E*) Monitor for fluoroscopy unit. (*F*) Back table setup for Ilizarov application.

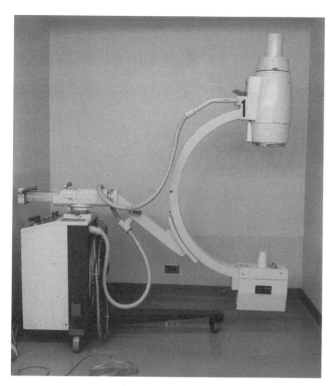

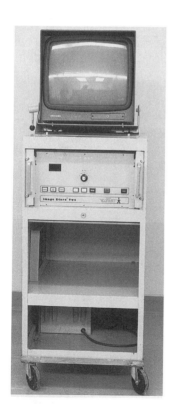

D

E

and those types of fractures for which other treatment methods have demonstrated poor functional results. Included in the latter group are femoral neck fractures, distal forearm fractures, and displaced intraarticular fractures. A third indication is for major avulsion fractures associated with disruption of significant musculotendinous structures.

The ORIF method of fracture treatment allows the surgeon to visually inspect damage to collateral structures, to debride and repair the fracture site as necessary, and to effect an anatomical alignment of a complex fracture. Additionally, prolonged immobility is not required for healing to occur. The disadvantages of ORIF include the need for general anesthesia and the increased risk of infection that comes with any open procedure. Implants frequently require a second surgical procedure for removal. Russell (1992) notes that internal fixation is generally contraindicated in situations where (1) osteoporotic bone is too fragile to anchor an implant, (2) overlying soft tissue is of poor quality, (3) infection is present, or (4) severe comminution prevents successful reconstruction.

Types of internal fixation implants

The wide variety of orthopaedic implants is overwhelming to all but the most seasoned orthopaedic perioperative nurse. Procedurally, most ORIFs are similar. However, the instruments and implants are variable and depend largely upon the type of fracture to be repaired. Knowledge of the different implants and the types of instruments necessary for their implantation will vastly improve the perioperative nurse's ability to plan care effectively.

Pin and wire fixation   Kirschner wires or Steinmann pins are frequently used for fixation of small fractures of the metaphyseal and epiphyseal regions of the distal foot, forearm, and hand. They may also be used in conjunction with closed reduction of displaced metacarpal and phalangeal fractures. Wire(s) and pin(s) may be inserted percutaneously under fluoroscopy, or they may be used in conjunction with other fixation devices during an open procedure.

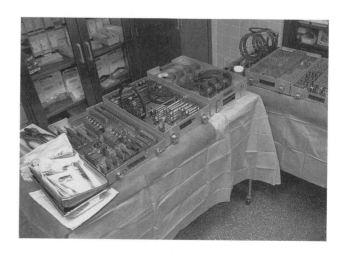

F

Screws There are a wide variety of fixation screws. All screws are composed of four parts: head, shaft, thread, and tip. The head of the screw may be hexagonal, cruciate, slotted, or Phillips in design and determines the type of screwdriver to be employed. The shaft of the screw is the smooth portion between the head and the threads. The thread of a screw is the portion that anchors the fragment and prevents the screw from being pulled out. The tip of the screw may be rounded and require pretapping, or fluted and self-tapping.

Cortical screws are designed for use in cortical bone and are usually threaded their entire length. Cancellous screws, designed to be used in spongy cancellous bone, have larger threads and are threaded for less than their entire length. A malleolar screw is a cancellous-type screw with a self-tapping trephine tip. Surgeons sometimes refer to lag screws. Rather than a specific type of screw, a lag screw is merely a cancellous screw used in a certain way. Specifically, the lag screw is placed so that the screw glides freely through the fragment adjacent to the screw head and engages only the opposite fragment (Fig. 12-39).

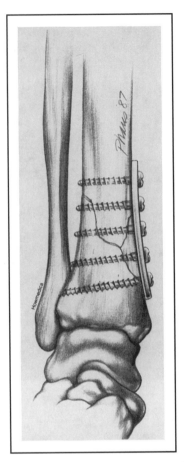

FIGURE 12-40   Plate and screw fixation of right tibial fracture.   (Courtesy of Howmedica Inc.)

Plates Screws may be used alone or with plates to fix various types of fractures. Like screws, plates are available in a wide variety of designs and sizes and may serve one or more of several different functions. Russell (1992) divides the various types of plates into four functional categories: neutralization, compression, buttress, and bridge. The plate must be fixed to bone both above and below the fracture (Fig. 12-40).

Bone grafting

Bone grafting may be used to stimulate the growth of new bone, to fill bone defects, or to stabilize a fusion. It is often used in conjunction with internal fixation techniques. The graft may be obtained from the patient at the time of surgery or from a bone bank. The type, size, and shape of graft used depend on its purpose. A cancellous bone graft is most frequently used to promote bone growth, whereas a cortical graft is employed to help stabilize the fracture.

A cancellous graft is most often taken from the ilium, although the olecranon or distal radius may also be used. The anterior iliac crest usually provides convenient access. The hip may be slightly elevated, and the area is prepped and draped at the beginning of the procedure. An iliac wedge graft provides both cortical bone for stabilization

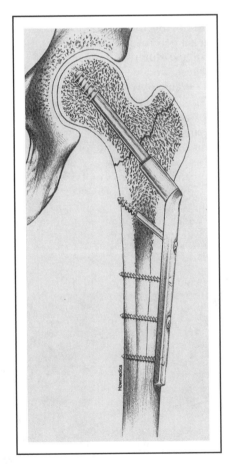

FIGURE 12-39   Internal fixation of left intertrochanteric fracture using the Omega compression hip screw system. A lag screw is used with a side plate anchored by one cancellous and three cortical screws.   (Courtesy of Howmedica Inc.)

and cancellous bone for osteogenic stimulation. Osteotomes or a power saw may be used to obtain the wedge graft. Cancellous chips may be obtained by creating a window into the outer table of the ilium and then scooping out the chips with a curette or gouge.

A cortical graft may be taken from the tibia, fibula, or ribs. The site is prepped and draped at the beginning of the procedure. The graft is then removed with an osteotome or oscillating saw. The cortical graft is then secured within the fracture or fusion site.

Bone growth stimulators

Today, with advanced technology, there are noninvasive devices as well as implantation devices for the treatment of nonunion fractures, failed fusions, and congenital pseudarthrosis. These devices significantly accelerate bone growth and fracture repair by providing artificially applied electrical stimulation to the bones. Bone growth stimulators may be used as an adjunct to fracture treatment where the risk of nonunion is high or in cases involving severe bone loss. The noninvasive units are small, lightweight, and flexible, and may be used with or without a cast.

Implantable bone growth stimulators A bone growth stimulator may be implanted at the time of the open reduction or during a procedure for nonunion. The tibia is the most common site of long bone nonunion. The surgical procedure is as follows:

Key steps

1. The area is prepped and draped.
2. Skin incision is made away from the adherent scar and extended through all tissues to the periosteum.
3. The nonunion site is identified and debrided.
4. A second incision is made away from the fracture site and carried down to the muscle.
5. The intermuscular plane is dissected, and the generator is implanted.
6. A tunnel between the fracture site and the generator site is created, and the electrode is passed through.
7. The electrode is placed in the bone defect and checked.
8. The incisions are closed, and dressings are applied.

Intramedullary Rodding

An intramedullary (IM) rod or nail may be used to treat midshaft fractures of a long bone such as the femur, tibia, or humerus. Chapman (1988) claims intramedullary rodding to be particularly well suited for the treatment of diaphyseal fracture of weight-bearing bones. This is because the rod is placed in the intramedullary canal and thus virtually guarantees proper axial alignment. Additionally, and unlike plates and screws, the IM rod is a load-sharing device.

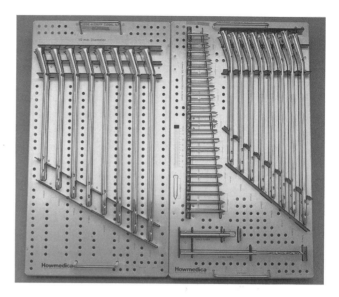

FIGURE 12-41 Grosse-Kempf nails with interlocking screws.

The reamed IM rod (e.g., AO, Kuntscher, Grosse-Kempf) is generally used for unstable fractures (Fig. 12-41). One reason for this is that reaming permits larger nails to be used and thus provides a stronger fixation device. Additionally, these rods allow the use of proximal and/or distal locking screws.

The nonreamed IM rod (e.g., Schneider, Lottes, Sage) is employed for stable fractures and offers the advantage of simple insertion with less disruption of endosteal blood supply. Rush rods are IM nails designed to be used in groups. Chapman (1988) notes that Kirschner wires and Steinmann pins may also be used in this way.

Perioperative nursing considerations

For IM rodding of the lower extremity, the patient is positioned supine on a fracture table. A separate setup is required for insertion of a traction pin prior to the rodding procedure. The traction pin is placed distally, and traction is applied. For femoral rodding, the thigh is draped free, from the iliac crest to the traction pin. For tibial rodding, the lower leg is draped free, from the distal thigh to the traction pin. Other required equipment includes fluoroscopy, powered reamers, and implants of the surgeon's choice.

Procedure

Intramedullary nails are most commonly indicated in closed fractures of the femoral shaft. Other indications for rodding of the femur and tibia include fractures of the proximal or distal third of the shaft, lengthening or shortening osteotomy, and simple transverse or oblique fractures. IM rodding of an open fracture is controversial, and active infection contraindicates use of this procedure.

Key steps

1. A small incision is made, beginning at the greater trochanter. In cases requiring a distal locking nail, a second incision at the distal screw site is performed.
2. Under fluoroscopy, a guidewire is placed into the shaft through the fracture site.
3. The canal is reamed to the appropriate width if necessary.
4. The nail is driven into the canal.
5. Locking screws, if needed, are placed at this time.
6. The incision or incisions are closed, and the wounds are dressed.

LAMINECTOMY (LUMBAR)

Lumbar laminectomy is most often performed for lumbar pathology; however, a laminectomy is also frequently performed in the cervical region. The purpose of spinal laminectomy is to relieve pressure on or impingement of the spinal nerve root(s). Impingement may be secondary to a herniated disc, spinal stenosis, vertebral fractures, spinal tumor, or congenital narrowing of the spine.

Herniated disc, one of the most common disorders of the spine, occurs when the annulus ruptures and the nucleus pulposus extrudes and impinges on a spinal nerve (see Fig. 12-6,*B*).

Perioperative Nursing Considerations

The lumbar spine is most commonly exposed through a direct posterior approach. The patient is positioned prone on positioning devices such as chest rolls or a Wilson frame (Fig. 12-42). In recent years, the Andrews spine table has gained popularity (Fig. 12-43). Particular care must be taken to prevent injury during prone positioning. Other required equipment includes a laminectomy set (Fig. 12-44) and, for fusions, fusion instrumentation.

Procedure

Indications

Surgery is indicated when spinal cord compromise is evident and not relieved by conservative measures. Acute symptoms that do not indicate cord compression or severe compromise usually include numbness, tingling, and weakness over the distribution of the affected nerve root. However, any loss of motion or impairment of bowel or bladder function requires immediate intervention. Chronic symptoms such as sustained lumbar pain, fatigue, and muscle spasms are frequently experienced by patients with arthritic spine changes. A thorough neurological examination and diagnostic studies including spine films, computed tomography (CT) scan, myelogram, and magnetic resonance imaging (MRI) confirm an operative diagnosis.

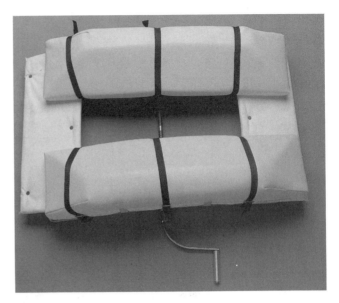

FIGURE 12-42 Wilson frame.

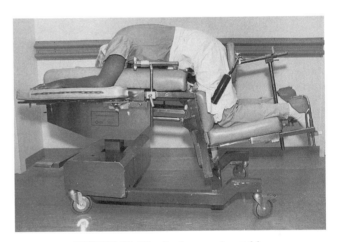

FIGURE 12-43 Andrews spine table.

Lumbar laminectomy

Key steps

1. The lumbar area is prepped and draped.
2. A midline incision is made.
3. The fascia and muscles are dissected and retracted to expose the spinous processes and laminae.
4. Rongeurs are used to produce the laminectomy.
5. The ligamentum flavum is excised.
6. The nerve root is identified and retracted.
7. The annulus is incised, and the herniated disc is removed.
8. Lacking disc involvement, stenotic pathology requires only the removal of bone.
9. If fusion is required, it is performed at this time.
10. After hemostasis is ensured, the wound is closed and a dressing is applied.

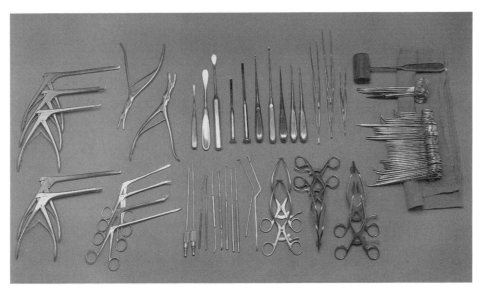

FIGURE 12-44 Laminectomy instruments. *Top, left* to *right*: 45-degree angled Kerrison rongeurs (3), Leksell rongeurs (2), Adson periosteal elevator, Hoen elevator, Cobb elevator, osteotomes (2), curettes (5), Cushing tissue forceps with teeth (2), bayonet tissue forceps (2), Adson tissue forceps (2). *Bottom, left* to *right*: 90-degree angled Kerrison rongeurs (2), pituitary disc rongeurs (4), Frazier suction tubes (2), dissectors (4), nerve hooks (2), nerve root retractors (2), Gelpi retractors (2), unilateral Adson retractors (2), bilateral Adson cerebellar retractors (2). *Right, top* to *bottom*: mallet, various scissors, clamps, needle holders.

CARPAL TUNNEL RELEASE

Carpal tunnel syndrome is a painful condition caused by compression of the median nerve within the carpal tunnel. Compression is usually caused by thickening of the carpal ligament, which then entraps the median nerve in the tendon sheath as it passes under the transverse ligament.

Thickening often occurs secondary to chronic stress or trauma to wrist structures or malpositioning of the wrist. Any activity involving repetitive twisting or turning movement of the hand and wrist, such as driving, knitting, or typing, may produce chronic inflammation of the carpal ligament. Extensive use of the computer keyboard in the workplace has increased the incidence of this syndrome. Its highest incidence occurs in females between 30 and 60 years of age.

Perioperative Nursing Considerations

Carpal tunnel release will generally be done on an outpatient basis and frequently with local or block anesthesia. The patient is positioned supine, with the affected arm extended on an armboard or hand table. Special equipment required generally includes a pneumatic tourniquet and soft tissue or hand instruments.

Procedure

Indications

Carpal tunnel syndrome is characterized by severe pain, burning, and paresthesia (numbness and tingling) in the radial palm, palmar surface of the thumb, the index and middle fingers, and the radial half of the fourth finger. Sensory loss may also occur with decreased sensation to light touch and pinprick on the affected side. Progressive weakness affects the patient's ability to perform some activities of daily living and is most often cited as the indication for surgery.

The physical examination demonstrates decreased sensory and motor function. A positive Tinel's sign, tingling over the median nerve on light percussion, and a positive Phalen's test, which reproduces symptoms with acute flexion of the wrist, are significant diagnostic findings. Diagnosis may be confirmed with electromyography (EMG).

Carpal tunnel release

Key steps

1. Padding and a tourniquet cuff are applied to the upper arm.
2. The hand and lower arm are prepped and draped free.
3. A curvilinear incision is made along the ulnar aspect of

the thenar crease and extended proximally to the wrist flexor crease.

4. Dissection proceeds to the level of the palmar fascia, avoiding the palmar sensory nerve, and distally in that same plane.
5. The transverse volar carpal ligament is isolated and transected.
6. If the epineurium is thickened or the nerve is constricted with pseudoneuroma formation, an epineurectomy is performed.
7. The skin and subcutaneous tissues are closed in a single layer.
8. A "boxing glove" compression dressing is applied to limit both edema and movement.
9. The hand is elevated to reduce pain and swelling.

BUNIONECTOMY

Hallux valgus (Fig. 12-45,*A*) is a common deformity in which the great toe deviates toward the other toes. There is usually a rather painful exostosis (Fig. 12-45,*B*) at the medial side of the metatarsophalangeal joint. Hallux valgus occurs most commonly in women. It may be caused by an anatomical deformity in the musculoskeletal composition of the foot. Bunion development may also be related to rheumatoid arthritis or osteoarthritis.

Perioperative Nursing Considerations

Diagnosis of a bunion is made by physical examination and radiographic studies. The most common presenting complaint is pain. There may also be altered gait, callus formation, and fatigue on ambulation.

Special equipment required for the operative procedure includes a pneumatic tourniquet and an oscillating saw.

Procedure

Bunionectomy

Key steps

1. The tourniquet is applied at mid thigh.
2. The extremity is prepped, and the foot is draped free.
3. An incision is made between the great toe and the second toe, and the adductor tendon is cut.
4. Another incision is made over the first metatarsophalangeal joint, exposing the capsule.
5. The capsule is opened, and the exostosis is exposed.
6. The bony protuberance is osteotomized either with a micro-oscillating saw or with a small osteotome and mallet.
7. One-third of the proximal phalanx is also resected.
8. If pins are to be placed for temporary fixation, they are inserted at this time.
9. The wound is closed, and a dressing is applied.

COMPARTMENT SYNDROME

Compartment syndrome, a potentially severe emergency condition, is an elevation of interstitial pressure in a closed, usually noncompliant osseofascial compartment of an extremity, such as the lateral, anterior, and deep posterior compartments of the leg and the superficial and deep volar compartments of the arm and wrist. Microvascular compromise and local tissue necrosis can result from the increased pressure.

The most common causes of acute compartment syndrome are bleeding from fractures, soft tissue trauma, or burns; arterial injury; and limb compression during altered consciousness. A restrictive bandage or cast can also be the cause.

In compartment syndrome, fluid accumulates in the muscle compartment, but the fibrous fascia cannot expand, so edema increases and pressure rises, leading to ischemia, if not treated. Severe pain and edema are cardinal symptoms but are often associated with the condition that triggers the syndrome, thereby making diagnosis difficult. Frequent neurovascular assessments are of prime importance.

Diagnosis is also very difficult in the anesthetized or unconscious patient and may call for a direct needle measurement of pressure. Compartment pressures greater than 30 mm Hg usually call for surgical intervention.

Compartment syndrome associated with a fracture of either an upper or lower extremity should be treated at the time of fracture stabilization. Fasciotomy is the most common treatment modality and, if done within 25 to 30 hours after onset, the prognosis is good.

A fasciotomy consists of opening the skin, subcutaneous tissue, and fascial envelope over the compartment. The swelling muscles may bulge through the incision, decompressing the compartment and restoring normal perfusion.

More than one incision may be made in a fasciotomy, depending on the size or number of compartments involved. Any necrotic tissue will be removed and the wound may be packed and left open for a period of time, depending on the severity of the tissue damage.

PNEUMATIC TOURNIQUET

Use of the tourniquet as a device to control bleeding has been attributed to the ancient Greeks and Romans. The word *tourniquet* was used by the surgeon Louis Petit, in 1718 for the vice-like device he developed. Petit called the device a "tourniquet," from the French word "tourner" or turning action. In 1864, Lister used a tourniquet to produce a bloodless surgical field. He recommended elevation of the limb for exsanguination prior to application of the tourniquet. In 1873, Johnson von Esmarch introduced a rubber bandage for exsanguination and tourniquet use. Harvey Cushing developed the inflatable (pneumatic) tourniquet in 1904). Today, pneumatic tourniquets are frequently used to reduce bleeding during ex-

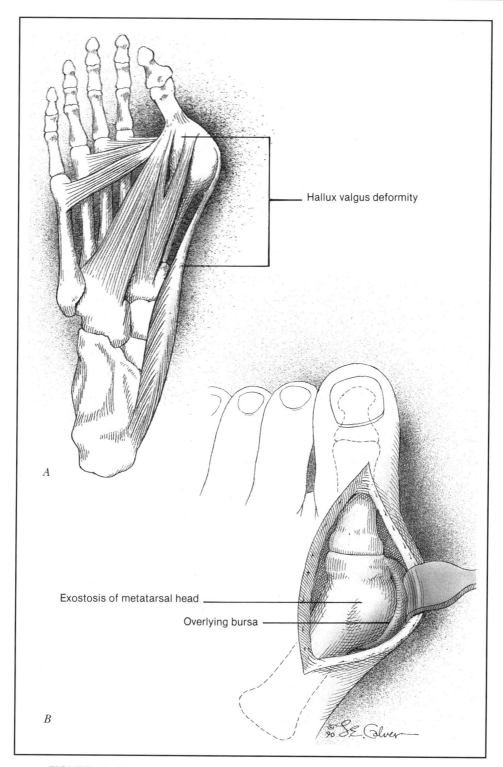

Hallux valgus deformity

A

Exostosis of metatarsal head

Overlying bursa

B

FIGURE 12-45 (*A*) Hallux valgus deformity. (*B*) Exostosis of metatarsal head. (Courtesy of Johnson & Johnson Medical, Inc., Arlington, TX.)

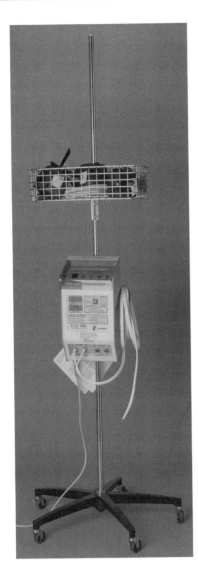

FIGURE 12-46 Pneumatic tourniquet.

correctly calibrated and checked with a manometer before use, the cuff fit properly, minimal effective pressure be used, and the cuff be applied with care and attention.

SUMMARY

Orthopaedic procedures and perioperative care have been discussed in this chapter. Since orthopaedic therapies include a large amount of devices and equipment, it is necessary that operating room staff members have detailed knowledge of equipment, positioning devices, operating room beds and tables, X-ray units, pneumatic tourniquets, and cast materials. The nursing process approach to care is espoused.

Infection prevention protocols receive special emphasis in orthopaedic surgery because of the sometimes disastrous results of bone infections. Special air-filtration systems and air-filtration hoods may be used.

Multidisciplinary care of the patient is required since the orthopaedic patient frequently needs occupational therapy and extensive rehabilitation after the surgery itself. Perioperative nursing care of orthopaedic patients presents special challenges that are outlined in this chapter.

REFERENCES

Aegerter, E., & Kirkpatrick, J. A. Jr. (1975), *Orthopedic diseases: Physiology–pathology–radiology.* Philadelphia: W. B. Saunders.
Aspen Labs, Inc. (1988). *Tourniquet safety home study.* Englewood, CO: Author.
Atkinson, L. J. (1992). *Berry and Kohn's operating room technique.* (7th ed.). St. Louis: Mosby–Year Book.
Biomet, Inc. *Biomodular total shoulder surgical technique.* Warsaw, IN: Author.
Biotechtron, Inc. (1989). *Ortho Pak II.* Hackensack, NJ: Author.
Cahill, M. (Ed.) (1991). *Illustrated manual of nursing practice.* Springhouse, PA: Springhouse Corporation.
Chapman, M. W. (1988). Principles of intramedullary nailing. In M. W. Chapman (Ed.). *Operative orthopaedics.* (pp. 151–161.). Philadelphia: J. B. Lippincott.
Cohen, J., Bonfiglio, M., & Campbell, C. J. (1990). *Orthopedic pathophysiology in diagnosis and treatment.* New York: Churchill Livingstone.
Crenshaw, A. H. (Ed.) (1992). *Campbell's operative orthopedics* (8th ed., Vols. I, II, III, pp. 1769–1856, 1891). St. Louis: Mosby–Year Book.
Duckworth, M., & Marquez, R. A. (1991). Carbon dioxide laser arthroscopy: A new dimension in knee surgery. *AORN Journal, 54,* 4.
EBI Medical Systems (1991). *EBI bone healing system.* Parsippany, NJ: Author.
Everett, C. L., Walker, C., & Dodson, D. K. (1992): Arthroscopic fixation of osteochondritis dissecans: Outpatient treatment for condylar defects. *AORN Journal, 55,* 492–502.

tremity surgery and also for intravenous regional block anesthesia (Zimmer, 1991).

There are two types of tourniquets: one is noninflatable and constructed of rubber or elasticized cloth; the other is pneumatic and has a cuff that is inflated by compressed gas. The pneumatic tourniquet consists of an inflatable cuff, a connecting tubing, a pressure regulator, a timing device, and a source of compressed gas (Fig. 12-46).

The tourniquet cuff with a 3- to 6-inch overlap is applied over padding to the middle of the upper limb or the middle of the thigh. A common pressure for the upper limb should be a preoperative systolic blood pressure plus 70 to 90 mm Hg; for the lower limb the tourniquet pressure should be twice the preoperative systolic blood pressure. The cuff pressure should be high enough to completely occlude blood flow without causing tissue or nerve damage.

For safety reasons it is recommended that tourniquet inflation use should not exceed 2 hours, the pressure be

Gamron, R. B. (1988). Taking the pressure out of compartment syndrome. *American Journal of Nursing, 88,* 1076–1080.

Gates, S. J., & Mooar, P. A. (Eds.) (1989). *Orthopedics and sports medicine for nurses.* Baltimore: Williams & Wilkins.

Goldstein, L. A., & Dickerson, R. C. (1981). *Atlas of orthopedic surgery* (2nd ed.). St. Louis: C.V. Mosby.

Gruendemann, B. J., & Yocum, L. A. (1990). *Inside orthopaedic surgery: An illustrated guide.* Arlington, TX: Johnson & Johnson Medical, Inc.

Insall, J. N. (1978). *Total condylar knee prosthesis surgical technique.* Rutherford, NJ: Howmedica, Inc.

Kaplan, P. E., & Tanner, E. D. (1989). *Musculoskeletal pain and disability.* Norwalk, CT: Appleton & Lange–Prentice Hall.

Lavin, R. J. (1989). The high-pressure demands of compartment syndrome. *RN, 52,* 22–25.

Lilliott, N. (1991). Discharge instructions: Advice for knee, shoulder, arthroscopy outpatients. *AORN Journal, 54,* 5.

Mourad, L. A. (1991): *Orthopedic disorders.* St. Louis: Mosby–Year Book.

North American Nursing Diagnosis Association (1992). *NANDA nursing diagnoses: Definitions and classification 1992–1993.* Philadelphia: NANDA.

Perry, C. R. (1992). Basic principles and clinical uses of screws and bolts. *Orthopedic Review, 21*(6).

Russell, T. A. (1992). General principles of fracture treatment. In A. H. Crenshaw (Ed.). *Campbell's operative orthopaedics.* (8th ed., pp. 725–785). St. Louis: Mosby–Year Book.

Stearns, C., & Brunner, N. (1987). *OpCare: Orthopaedic patient care* (Vols. 1–3). Bridgewater, NJ: Pfizer Hospital Products Group, Inc.

Zimmer, Inc. (1991). Tourniquet safety. Dover, OH: Author.

Chapter 13

Cardiac Surgery

Key Concepts
Introduction
Anatomy
Nursing Considerations
Perioperative Considerations
Surgical Procedures
Summary

Key Concepts

- Modern cardiac surgery was born in 1953; the heart was the last organ to be approached by surgeons.

- An understanding of cardiac anatomy and physiology and abnormalities, attention to detail, curiosity, and a good memory are all characteristics of the excellent cardiac perioperative nurse.

- A host of special supplies, equipment, and instruments is necessary for cardiac surgery. Vascular clamps are designed to cause minimal damage, and vascular tissue forceps cause minimal trauma to fragile structures and tissues. Tubing clamps are designed to occlude pump tubing without damaging the clamp or the tubing.

- Development of the heart–lung machine, allowing for cardiopulmonary bypass (CPB), was the "springboard" for cardiac surgery. CPB provides a means of temporarily bypassing the patient's heart and lungs, and yet substituting for their actions.

- In 1989, there were 368,000 coronary artery bypass graft (CABG) procedures done in the United States, making it the most frequent cardiac surgical procedure performed in this country.

- Pediatric cardiac surgery is a highly specialized area in which perioperative nurses can participate. Earlier correction of pediatric cardiac defects, usually congenital, is accomplished because of better understanding of the advantages relating to cardiac, pulmonary, and cerebral functions.

- Cardiac transplantation is becoming more common. The administration of cyclosporine, introduced in 1980, results in prolonged survival of heart and heart–lung transplant patients.

- Circulatory-assist devices are used for patients who cannot be "weaned" from cardiopulmonary bypass, those with acute myocardial infarction and cardiogenic shock, and candidates for heart transplant awaiting a donor organ.

- Failure of pulse formation or of the cardiac conduction system is the major reason for implanting pacemakers. The purpose of each of many types of pacemakers is to electrically stimulate the heart to beat. Perioperative nurses may be involved with the implantation of permanent pacemakers or procedures to change pulse generators.

INTRODUCTION

It is not surprising that the heart was the last organ to be approached by surgeons (McGoon, 1987). Cardiac surgery has become so commonplace today that we easily forget how "new" this surgical specialty is. Although credit for the beginning of heart surgery is given to Ludwig Rehn, who closed a stab wound of the heart in 1896, many pioneers have contributed to this field of surgery. Modern cardiac surgery was born in 1953, when John Gibbon closed an atrial septal defect while using his invention of the heart–lung machine (McGoon, 1987).

With 898 U.S. hospitals having cardiac surgery programs (American Hospital Association, 1991), this surgical specialty is a challenging arena for perioperative nurses. The knowledge and skills needed are numerous, intricate, and highly refined. Competency in the scrub and circulating roles in general surgery is necessary before advancing to this specialty.

Attention to detail, curiosity, and a good memory are characteristics of the cardiac surgery perioperative nurse. An understanding of cardiac anatomy and physiology underpins the nurse's grasp of the cardiac surgical interventions. Cardiac abnormalities must be understood in order to anticipate the intended surgical procedure and expected outcomes.

ANATOMY

The heart begins its lifelong work at about 22 days of gestation. The heart is the driving force that moves the blood through the vascular system, thereby transporting oxygen, nutrients, and essential substances to all body cells as it removes metabolic waste products. The heart's action has two phases (called the cardiac cycle), (1) systole, when the heart muscle contracts, and (2) diastole, when the heart muscle relaxes.

The heart, which is enclosed in the pericardial sac, is located in the mediastium, or the middle of the thoracic cavity. Approximately two-thirds of the heart is situated to the left of midline. The heart sits at an angle, with the base posterior and the apex anterior and to the left (Fig. 13-1). The heart is slightly rotated, and the right ventricle is the most anterior structure. Surrounding anatomical structures include the sternum; costal cartilages; portions of the third, fourth, and fifth ribs; lungs; diaphragm; esophagus; and descending thoracic aorta (Figs. 13-1 and 13-2).

Three layers of tissue compose the heart wall. The epicardium is the outer layer; the myocardium is the middle layer and is composed of interconnecting muscle fibers; and the endocardium is the smooth, inside lining, which

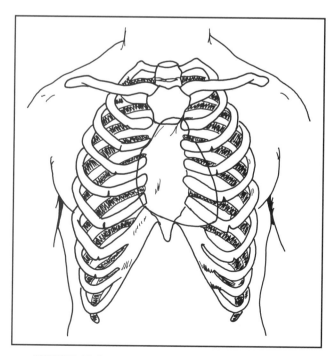

FIGURE 13-1 Location of the heart in the thorax.

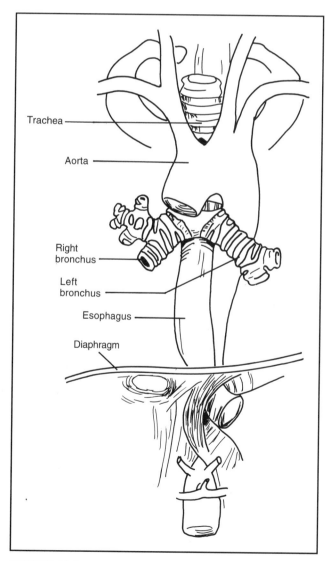

FIGURE 13-2 Anatomical structures surrounding the heart.

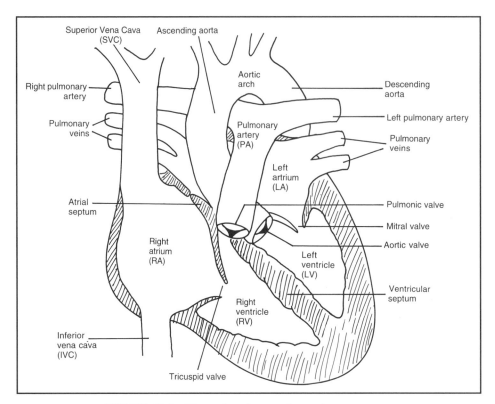

FIGURE 13-3 Heart chambers and vascular structures.

has a negative charge to repel blood elements that could cause clot formation (Reed, 1985).

The right heart is separated from the left heart longitudinally by the atrial and ventricular septum. The right heart atrium receives the venous blood from the inferior vena cava (lower body) and the superior vena cava (upper body) and from the heart itself via the coronary sinus. The blood flows through the tricuspid valve into the right ventricle during diastole. With ventricular contraction (systole) the blood is moved through the pulmonic valve and into the pulmonary circulation (Fig. 13-3). The myocardial layer of the right ventricle is thinner than the left because of the lower resistance in the pulmonary circulatory system (Fig. 13-4).

The gas exchange of carbon dioxide and oxygen occurs in the pulmonary capillaries, and the newly oxygenated blood flows through the pulmonary veins into the left atrium. Again, during diastole the blood flows through the mitral valve into the left ventricle, and during systole through the aortic valve and into the systemic circulatory system.

The heart valves keep the blood flowing through the heart in the correct direction. The pulmonic and aortic valves are called semilunar valves because they are shaped like half moons. The three leaflets of each valve are cup-shaped and support the blood column during diastole. The tricuspid and mitral valves are more complex, with the supporting structures, the chordae tendineae and the papillary muscles, that prevent the valves from opening backward during systole.

Coronary Circulation

The coronary arteries supply the myocardium with oxygenated blood at approximately 220 ml per minute when the heart is at rest and up to 1100 ml per minute with increased activity (Hurst & Schlant, 1990).

The openings, or ostia, for the two major coronary arteries are located just above the aortic valve in the aorta. During diastole the blood column in the aorta exerts backward pressure that closes the aortic valve and forces blood into the coronary arteries.

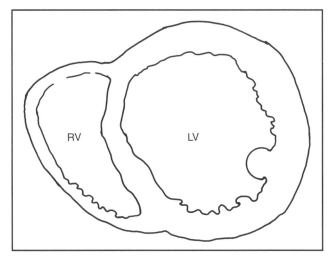

FIGURE 13-4 Cross-section of right (RV) and left (LV) ventricles. Note differences in chamber size and myocardial thickness.

The left main coronary artery branches into the left anterior descending (LAD) and the circumflex arteries. The LAD follows the anterior intraventricular groove and gives off diagonal and septal branches that provide blood to the left ventricular walls and septum. The circumflex artery travels posteriorly around the heart, following the atrioventricular groove. It supplies blood via its marginal branches to the left atrium, left ventricular wall, and 40% to 50% of the time to the sinus node (Hurst & Schlant, 1990; Andreoli et al., 1987) (Fig. 13-5).

The right coronary artery follows the right atrioventricular groove until it branches into the posterior descending artery (PDA), which follows the posterior intraventricular groove. The PDA arises from the right coronary artery 80% to 90% of the time, and this is referred to as a dominant right system. When this artery arises from the circumflex artery, the patient is said to have a nondominant right system. The right coronary system supplies blood to the right atrium, right ventricle, sinus node, atrioventricular node, posterior left ventricle, and the posterior septum (Hurst & Schlant, 1990; Andreoli et al., 1987).

The coronary arterioles branch into arterio-sinusoidal vessels, which may enter directly into the heart cavities or form an interconnecting network with each other or the capillaries. The thebesian veins drain venous blood directly into the heart cavities while other major veins drain the venous blood into the coronary sinus, which empties into the right atrium (Reed, 1985).

Cardiac Conduction System

The spontaneous initiation of cardiac electrical impulses arises from the sinus node, which is located at the junction of the superior vena cava and the right atrium (Fig. 13-6). This impulse is conducted through the atria via internodal tracts to the atrioventricular node. This causes the atria to contract and is seen as the P wave on the electrocardiogram (ECG). Once the electrical impulse reaches the atrioventricular (AV) node it is slowed and is seen as the PR interval on the ECG. The impulse leaves the AV node and rapidly travels to the bundle of His to the right and left bundle branches and terminates with the Purkinje fibers that are distributed to the endocardium of both ventricles. (Fig. 13-6). As the impulse leaves the Purkinje fibers, it stimulates the ventricles to contract (depolarization) and is reflected as the QRS portion of the ECG. The T wave of the ECG represents the repolarization of the ventricles that occurs after contraction. The atrial repolarization wave is hidden in the QRS complex.

The autonomic nervous system regulates the rate of impulse formation, the conduction speed of the impulse, and the contractility of the atria and ventricles. The vagus nerves are the parasympathetic innervation that, when stimulated, decrease the heart rate, contractility, and conduction speed through the AV node. The sympathetic innervation (cardiac, accelerator, augmentor), when stimulated, increases the heart rate, contraction, and conduction through the AV node.

Central nervous system reflex control centers are located in the medulla oblongata and can inhibit or accelerate the heart rate. Stimulation of receptors located in the aortic arch and carotid bodies by increased blood pres-

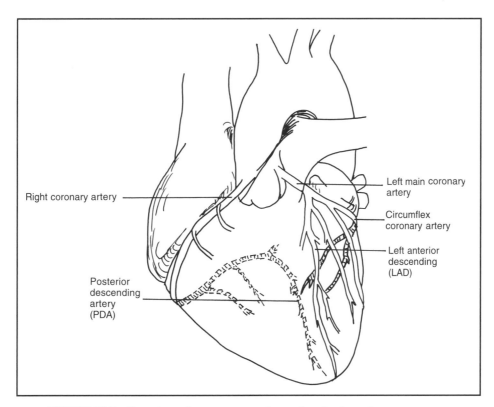

FIGURE 13-5   Location of coronary arteries and major branches.

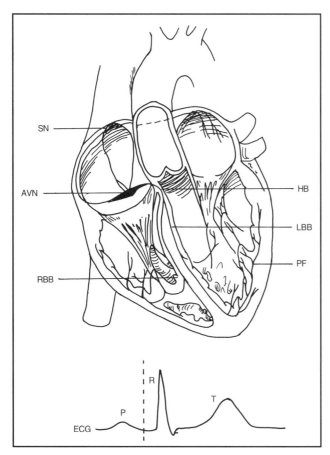

FIGURE 13-6 Cardiac conduction system and its relationship to the electrocardiogram. SN = sinus node; AVN = atrioventricular node; HB = His bundle; LBB = left bundle branch; RBB = right bundle branch; PF = Purkinje fibers.

sure causes stimulation of the cardioinhibitory center and depression of the accelerator center to slow the heart and decrease the blood pressure. Chemoreceptors in these same areas are sensitive to changes in oxygen and carbon dioxide levels in the blood and will stimulate the appropriate center as needed.

There are other intrinsic factors that regulate the heartbeat, such as increased metabolism (can be due to fever, exercise, anxiety, decreased peripheral resistance, or increased carbon dioxide), drugs, electrolyte disorders, and "Starling's law" (when the diastolic volume in the heart increases, the force of the heart contraction is increased, as is the volume delivered with each stroke) (Hurst & Schlant, 1990).

NURSING CONSIDERATIONS

Cardiac Problems

Signs and symptoms

The signs and symptoms of cardiac problems develop when the heart is no longer able to function normally.

Initially, the signs and symptoms may occur only with exertion because of the increased demands on the heart. As problems increase, the signs and symptoms occur at rest as well.

Subjective and objective information about the patient is necessary and can be obtained in a variety of ways. The subjective information is obtained from the patient. Through effective interviewing techniques, the symptoms the patient is experiencing can be determined. The patient's condition and ability to communicate influence the interview outcomes.

Objective information relates to what is observed about the patient on physical examination or assessment. The examination techniques used include inspection, palpation, percussion, and auscultation. Common physical findings for a patient with cardiac problems may include the following:

Pulmonary:
  Dyspnea
  Orthopnea
  Paroxysmal nocturnal dyspnea
  Tachypnea
  Hemoptysis
  Abnormal breath sounds (wheezing, rhonchi, rales)

Cardiac:
  Arrhythmias
  Murmurs
  Abnormal heart sounds
  Venous distention
  Pulse abnormalities
  Hypo/hypertension
  Syncope
  Vertigo
  Enlargement

Skin:
  Cyanosis
  Clubbing of nails on fingers/toes
  Pallor
  Diaphoresis
  Cool/clammy
  Edema

Other:
  Weight gain/loss
  Failure to thrive
  Mental confusion
  Fatigue
  Restlessness
  Pain in chest, arm, leg, back, neck, jaw

Causes

Coronary artery disease Atherosclerotic changes in the walls of the coronary arteries can occur for a variety of reasons. The most common causes or risk factors are hypertension, smoking, hyperlipidemia, male sex, age, diabetes mellitus, and a family history of coronary disease. Other possible causes include obesity, physical inactivity, stress, oral contraceptives, excess coffee consumption, hyperuricemia, impaired glucose tolerance, and air pollution (Kloner, 1990; Hurst & Schlant, 1990). As atherosclerotic changes occur, the lumen of the coronary artery is narrowed until it is totally occluded. This decrease in blood flow to the myocardium leads to injury, scarring, and, if there is extensive damage, death due to cardiac failure. This is the leading cause of death in the United States, with 497,850 deaths in 1989 (American Heart Association, 1992).

Congenital cardiac disease There are two major causes of congenital cardiac disease: genetic and environmental. With certain chromosomal abnormalities (e.g., Down syndrome) there is an increase in cardiac abnormalities. Family history of congenital heart disease is an important factor. Environmental factors could include infectious diseases during the first trimester of pregnancy, especially rubella (Hurst & Schlant, 1990).

Valvular heart disease Deformities of the heart valves can be due to congenital defects; degenerative changes; infectious processes, such as rheumatic fever, bacterial endocarditis, or scarlet fever; myocardial infarctions that affect the papillary muscles; ascending aorta diseases; or trauma. Stenosis (narrowing) or insufficiency (leaking) or a combination of these two problems can occur. Valvular dysfunction can lead to hemodynamic alterations that impair cardiac function and lead to cardiac strain, congestive heart failure, and eventual death (Hurst & Schlant, 1990; Cooley, 1984).

Diagnostic procedures

Several standard laboratory tests can detect cardiac-related problems: complete blood count, electrolytes, glucose, lipids, and arterial blood gases. Serum enzymes are tested to determine myocardial damage (Table 13-1).

Chest X-rays can reveal cardiac and pulmonary changes that occur with certain cardiac diseases.

The 12-lead ECG will indicate conduction abnormalities, abnormal rhythms, chamber enlargement, myocardial ischemia, and myocardial infarctions. For additional information about the ECG, a long-term monitoring device (Holter monitor) can be used for a period up to 24 hours or more.

The exercise stress test (treadmill) ECG is used to determine if ischemic ECG changes occur with exercise. It is also useful for evaluating arrhythmias and cardiac function. During a stress test the ECG, heart rate, and blood pressure are monitored.

There are various radionuclide techniques for evaluating cardiac function and blood flow to the myocardium. Thallium-201 provides myocardial imaging that indicates myocardial viability. Positron emission tomography (PET) assesses myocardial blood flow and metabolism. Technetium-99m pyrophosphate is used to evaluate acute myocardial infarctions. Radionuclide angiography demonstrates left ventricular function. Magnetic resonance imaging (MRI) can give anatomical information and information regarding ventricular function. However, it cannot give any information regarding pressures in the cardiac chambers or pressure gradients (variations across

TABLE 13-1 Serum Enzymes*

Major Enzymes	Isoenzymes (Specific to certain tissues)		
CK = creatinine kinase	CK:	MM	(skeletal muscle)
CPK = creatinine phosphokinase		BB	(brain tissue)
LDH = lactic dehydrogenase		MB	(heart muscle)
SGOT = serum glutamic oxaloacetic transaminase	LDH:	1 2	Heart, rbc's, kidney
(Causes of elevation can be other than myocardial injury)		3	Lungs
		4 5	Liver, skeletal muscle

Enzyme Occurrence Following Myocardial Infarction			
CK:	Occurs at 4–8 hours Peaks at 24 hours (with reperfusion at 12 hours) Normal at 72–96 hours	LDH:	Occurs at 24–48 hours Peaks at 3–6 days Normal at 8–14 days
CK-MB:	Occurs at 4–6 hours Peaks at 24 hours (with reperfusion at 8–12 hours) Normal at 48–72 hours	LDH₁ LDH₂	Occurs at 8–12 hours Peaks at 24–48 hours
SGOT:	Occurs at 8–12 hours Peaks at 18–36 hours Normal at 3–5 days	Flipped LDH: LDH₁ exceeds LDH₂ (Occurs with myocardial infarction)	

*Certain enzymes are released into the bloodstream when myocardial cells are injured (as in a myocardial infarction).

valves). Rubidium-82 and dipyridamole can demonstrate viability of the myocardium (Hurst & Schlant, 1990).

Echocardiography uses ultrasound waves to assess cardiac structures, motion, and function. M-mode echocardiography uses only one ultrasound beam, whereas two-dimensional echocardiography uses a planar beam that gives cross-sectional information about the heart. The Doppler is used for hemodynamic assessment and indicates blood flow and velocity characteristics. There is an auditory and spectral signal. Because the sound waves are reflected by the red blood cells, the introduction of the color Doppler flow gives valuable information about the direction of blood flow. Blood flow toward the transducer is red and blood flow away from the transducer is blue. The transesophageal transducer probe can be inserted into the esophagus and thus posterior to the heart. The views from this position are superior to the usual transthoracic echocardiogram. This technique can be used intraoperatively to assess the results of surgical interventions or to determine left ventricular function. An epicardial probe is also available that can be used directly on the heart during surgery (Docker et al., 1992; Nichols et al., 1991).

Cardiac catheterization continues to be the optimum test for evaluating the heart. This is an invasive procedure in which catheters are inserted through an artery or vein into the heart. This method can be used to obtain information about the hemodynamics, anatomy, and electrophysiology of the heart. Contrast media can be injected through the catheter for X-ray visualization of the cardiac chambers and structures, cardiac function, and blood flow. Special catheters can be connected to transducers for information regarding intracardiac pressures. Cardiac output can also be measured, as well as oxygen levels in the different chambers (Fig. 13-7).

Coronary arteriography is used for a definitive diagnosis of coronary artery disease. Contrast media can be injected directly into the coronary arterial system for fluoroscopic visualization and filming. The arteries must be viewed from several different directions in order to be adequately visualized, and this requires multiple injections of contrast media. Obstructions or stenotic areas within the coronary arteries are identified and reported according to the percentage of obstruction (Fig. 13-8).

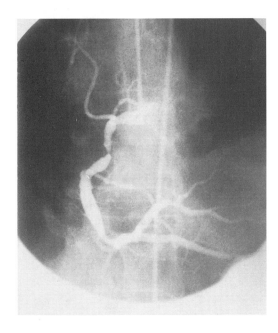

A

FIGURE 13-8 *A,* Obstruction in right coronary artery. *B,* Obstruction in circumflex coronary artery. *C,* Obstruction in left anterior descending coronary artery.

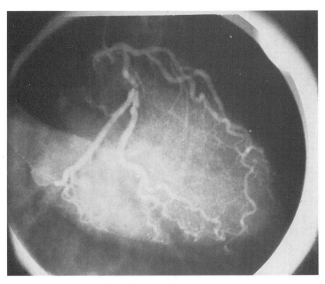

FIGURE 13-7 Normal pressures in cardiac chambers and great vessels.

B

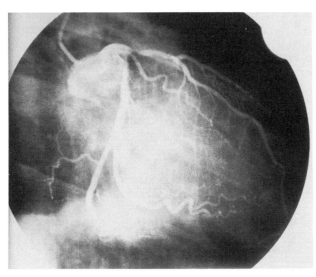

C

Contrast media can be injected directly into the left ventricle in order to determine ventricular function. The performance of the left ventricle with systole is expressed as ejection fraction. This is the stroke volume times the diastolic volume. An ejection fraction of 55% or greater is considered normal. Abnormal ventricular wall motion and aneurysms can be seen. The end-diastolic pressure of the left ventricle is measured during diastole. Elevation in pressure indicates there is increased wall tension. This is another indicator of left ventricular performance.

Injection of contrast media into the ascending aorta is necessary for evaluation of the aortic valve's competency and to determine the presence of aortic aneurysms at this level. Pressures in the aorta above and below a coarctation are necessary to determine the need for surgery.

Preoperative evaluation

An Ad Hoc Committee for Cardiothoracic Surgical Practice Guidelines appointed by the Society of Thoracic Surgeons published guidelines in the *Annals of Thoracic Surgery* in 1992. In these guidelines is a section on a preoperative evaluation. The following minimum evaluation is recommended:

1. Thorough history and physical examination
2. Chest roentgenogram
3. Urinalysis
4. Electrocardiogram
5. Blood sample for typing in all patients and a type and crossmatch for blood products in patients having a risk of significant blood loss. Patients who have previously provided blood via autologous donation may be excused from this requirement.
6. Blood analysis to include complete blood count, platelet count, prothrombin time, partial thromboplastin time, and SMA-18
7. Blood gas determination while the patient is breathing room air, including pCO_2, pO_2, and pH in patients with suspected pulmonary compromise

8. Appropriate medical consultation where indicated
9. Assessment of nutritional status

According to the Association of Operating Room Nurses (AORN) *Standards of Perioperative Clinical Practice* (1994), Standard I: The perioperative nurse collects patient health data. Health data to be collected includes information related to:

- Medical diagnoses and therapies
- Physical/psychological status
- Physiological responses
- Cultural, spiritual, and lifestyle information
- Understanding, perceptions, and expectations regarding the procedure
- Previous responses to surgical procedures
- Results of diagnostic tests

This information is used to plan intraoperative care for the patient.

Depending on the time frame and the patient's condition, the perioperative nurse may have opportunities to provide patient education related to the intraoperative care.

Intraoperative Considerations

Monitoring

Electrocardiogram It is ideal to monitor the patient's ECG during transport to the operating room. Cardiac surgery patients are all considered potentially unstable. The perioperative nurse must be familiar with the normal ECG pattern and the more common atrial and ventricular arrhythmias (Fig. 13-9). The nurse must be able to initiate appropriate emergency interventions.

Blood pressure The blood pressure monitoring equipment must be placed on the patient as soon as the patient is transferred to the operating room bed. Automatic blood pressure machines will determine the patient's blood pressure and display the reading on a regular basis (every 1 to 3 minutes). Blood pressure abnormalities can signal an impending problem.

Pulse oximetry This is a noninvasive method of continuously monitoring the patient's arterial blood oxygen saturation (SaO_2). The sensor may be placed on the patient's finger, toe, nose, earlobe, or forehead. The normal value is 95% to 100%, and a value less than 70% could represent a potentially life-threatening situation. This does not, however, replace the need for arterial blood gas determinations during surgery.

Arterial pressure line This provides a means of continuous measurement of the arterial blood pressure during cardiac surgery and is essential for guiding the perfusionist while the patient is on cardiopulmonary bypass. This is a direct method requiring insertion into an artery (usually the radial or femoral) of a cannula or needle that is

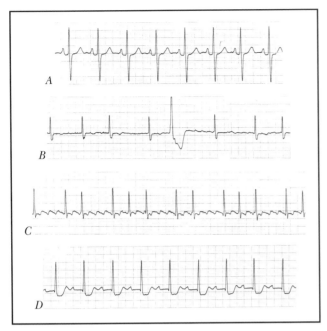

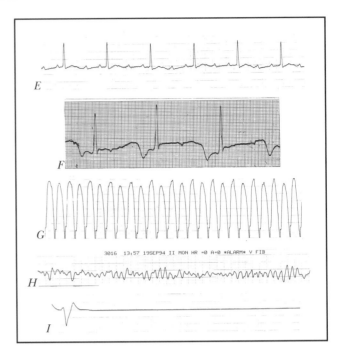

FIGURE 13-9   Electrocardiogram patterns. *A,* Normal sinus rhythm. *B,* Atrial fibrillation (note: no distinct P waves; irregular rhythm). The fifth beat is a premature ventricular complex (PVC) (note the broad QRS complex). *C,* Atrial flutter (note: rapid, regular atrial tachycardia with classic sawtooth pattern; ventricular rhythm may vary). *D,* First-degree atrioventricular block (note: prolonged conduction of P wave by increased PR interval; QRS complex for each P wave). *E,* Second-degree atrioventricular block: Type II (note: more than one P wave for each QRS complex). *F,* Third-degree atrioventricular block (note: complete; no conduction between atria and ventricles; wide QRS; different rates for atria and ventricles). *G,* Ventricular tachycardia (note: usually regular, rapid rhythm). *H,* Ventricular fibrillation (note: rhythm is chaotic; disorganized). *I,* Ventricular standstill: asystole (note: no electrical activity).

connected to a monitoring machine that continually displays the arterial pressure (Fig. 13-10) (Reed, 1985).

Pulmonary artery flow directed catheter (Swan-Ganz)   This catheter is inserted into the internal jugular or subclavian vein and into the right atrium (Fig. 13-11). The catheter balloon is inflated and the catheter is "floated" across the tricuspid valve, into the right ventricle, across the pulmonic valve, and into the pulmonary artery where it "wedges" in a pulmonary capillary (Fig. 13-12). The balloon is deflated and the catheter is secured to prevent dislodgement or accidental change of position. A continuous reading of the pulmonary artery pressure can be recorded on the monitoring machine (see Fig. 13-10). By inflating the balloon, capillary wedge pressure can be determined. This indicates the pressure of the left atrium. The normal pressure is 2 to 7 mm Hg below the mean pulmonary artery pressure, and over 12 mm Hg is considered abnormal. Catheters with thermodilution tips can be used for measuring cardiac output. Normal cardiac output, which is the volume of blood pumped by the ventricle per minute, is 3 to 7 L/minute. By injecting cold

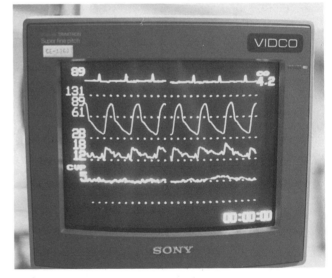

FIGURE 13-10   Monitor display. Bottom line = central venous pressure; second line = pulmonary artery pressure; third line = arterial pressure; fourth line = ECG.

solution into the right atrium or superior vena cava and measuring its arrival in the pulmonary artery by the thermodilution tip, the cardiac output is determined (Andreoli et al., 1987; Nurse's Clinical Library, 1984).

Temperature   The patient's temperature is continuously monitored during cardiac surgery. Hypothermia is usually used during cardiopulmonary bypass, and it is essential to know the patient's temperature before, during, and after bypass. Temperature probes may be placed in the esophagus, rectum, or bladder, or located on the Swan-Ganz catheter. The perfusionist can measure the temperature of the venous and arterial blood while the

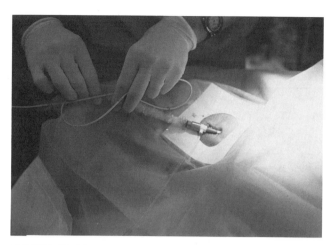

FIGURE 13-11 Insertion of a pulmonary artery catheter into the internal jugular vein.

patient is on bypass. The temperature of the heart can be measured while on bypass with a myocardial temperature probe.

Urinary output A urinary catheter must be inserted for patients undergoing cardiopulmonary bypass. Urine output is measured every 30 minutes and there should be a minimum of 30 ml of urine excreted every hour. Because renal function can be depressed with bypass due to decreased blood flow, diuretic agents may be needed.

Blood loss Measuring blood loss during cardiac surgery is optional. Blood volume status can more accurately be determined by hemodynamic monitoring of pulmonary artery and arterial pressures. Bloody sponges can, however, be weighed in plastic bags and the weight recorded. Contents of suction cannisters are measured and recorded.

Laboratory tests

Activated clotting time (ACT) This test can be done in the operating room and is needed to ensure adequate heparinization of the patient during cardiopulmonary bypass. The normal control is 100 seconds and the level should be at least 400 seconds for bypass in order to prevent clotting. This test is helpful after bypass to determine if adequate reversal of the heparin occurs with protamine (Doty, 1985).

Arterial blood gases It is essential to monitor the arterial blood gases during cardiac surgery in order to provide adequate oxygenation and maintain acid–base balance. Alterations can adversely affect the cardiac patient very rapidly. During cardiopulmonary bypass, arterial blood gases are checked frequently, and the perfusionist makes necessary adjustments to correct any abnormalities (Table 13-2).

Hemoglobin/hematocrit Blood loss during surgery and hemodilution of the blood that occurs with bypass will alter the hemoglobin and hematocrit levels. Because the oxygen-carrying capacity of the blood will be decreased

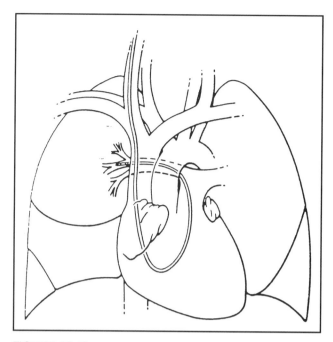

FIGURE 13-12 Location of the pulmonary artery catheter inside the heart and pulmonary artery.

with low levels of hemoglobin, the need for administering red blood cells must be determined to maintain adequate oxygenation.

Blood glucose Blood glucose levels may increase with the stress of cardiac surgery. Many cardiac patients have diabetes and need close monitoring of the glucose levels during surgery. Undiagnosed diabetes may be discovered. Insulin is administered to correct elevated blood glucose.

Electrolytes Alterations in electrolytes can occur during cardiac surgery. This can be due to physiological changes, fluid loss, and/or the composition of intravenous fluids. Abnormal electrolytes affect the cardiac muscle contractility and irritability. This can result in arrhythmias and can impair cardiac function.

Medications

There are several medications that are used during cardiac surgery. Their use will be determined by the patient's condition. The anesthesia provider and/or the surgeon will decide what medications are to be used. The perioperative nurse needs to be familiar with the various medications and how and when they are used (Table 13-3).

Special equipment and supplies

Defibrillator: Sterile and unsterile external paddles and sterile internal paddles (in infant, pediatric, and adult sizes) are needed (Fig. 13-13).

Cell saver: Shed blood in the operative field is suctioned to the machine, where the blood is washed. The retrieved red blood cells are administered to the patient (Fig. 13-14).

TABLE 13-2 Arterial Blood Gases (ABGs)

Normal Values				
pO_2	SaO_2	pH	pCO_2	HCO_3^-
Oxygen	% of hemoglobin saturated with oxygen	Acid–base level	Carbon dioxide	Bicarbonate
80–100 mm Hg	95%–100%	7.35–7.45	35–45 mm Hg	22–26 mEq

Acid–Base Imbalance			
	pH	pCO_2	HCO_3^-
Acidosis			
Respiratory	Decreased	Increased	Normal
Metabolic	Decreased	Normal	Decreased
Alkalosis			
Respiratory	Increased	Decreased	Normal
Metabolic	Increased	Normal	Increased

Compensation of Acid–Base Imbalance

Noncompensation:	Reflected in alteration of pCO_2 or HCO_3^-; pH is abnormal
Partial compensation:	Both pCO_2 and HCO_3^- are abnormal; pH is abnormal
Complete compensation:	Both pCO_2 and HCO_3^- are abnormal; pH is normal

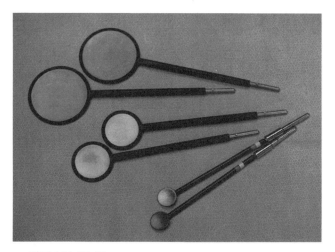

FIGURE 13-13 Various sizes of defibrillator paddles.

Fibrillator: Sterile electrodes or pads are placed on the heart's surface. Electrical current is used to fibrillate the heart when it is hazardous or difficult to operate with the heart beating (Fig. 13-15).

Infusion pumps: Used to administer intravenous solutions (Fig. 13-16).

"Slush" machine: Used to make soft ice to place around the heart (topically) for cooling (Fig. 13-17).

Temporary pacemakers and wires: Temporary atrial, ventricular, or atrioventricular (AV) pacing may be needed (Fig. 13-18).

Scales: For weighing used sponges to determine blood loss.

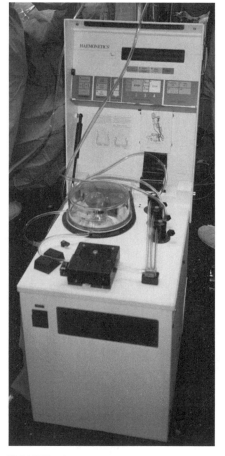

FIGURE 13-14 Haemonetics cell saver.

Table 13-3 Medications Commonly Used During Cardiac Surgery

Hemostatic Agents, Topical		Other Medications (cont'd)	
Absorbable collagen sponges (Hemotene/Instat)		Furosemide (Lasix)	Diuretic
Gelatin sponges (Gelfoam)		Heparin sodium	Anticoagulant
Fibrin glue (cryoprecipitate, thrombin, and calcium chloride)		Hydralazine HCl (Apresoline)	VD, ↓BP, ↑CO, ↑HR
Microfibrillar collagen hemostat (Avitene)		Insulin	Treat hyperglycemia
Oxidized regenerated cellulose (Surgicel)		Isoproterenol HCl (Isuprel)	↑CC, ↑CO, ↑HR, VD
Topical thrombin (Thrombogen/Thrombostat)		Lidocaine HCl (Xylocaine)	AA
Hemostatic Agents: Intravenous		Magnesium sulfate	Maintain Mg balance, AA
Aminocaproic acid (Amicar) (to treat fibrinolysis)		Mannitol	Diuretic
Desmopressin acetate (DDAVP) (to increase Factor VIII activity)		Nitroglycerin (Tridil)	VD, ↑CD
		Norepinephrine (Levophed)	↑CC, ↑BP, VC
Other Medications		Papaverine HCl	VD
Albuterol inhalation aerosol (Proventil/Ventolin)	Treat bronchospasm	Phenylephrine (Neo-Synephrine)	VC, ↑BP
Aminophylline	Treat bronchospasm	Potassium HCl	Maintain K balance
Amrinone (Inocor)	↑CC, ↑CO, ↑BP, VD	Procainamide (Pronestyl)	AA
Atropine SO₄	↑HR	Propranolol (Inderal)	↓HR, ↓CO, ↓BP, AA
Bretylium tosylate	AA, ↑HR, ↑CC, ↑BP, VD	Protamine sulfate	Reverse heparinization
Calcium chloride or gluconate	Maintain calcium balance ↑CC, ↑BP, ↑CO, VD	Quinidine gluconate	AA
Cefazolin	Antibiotic	Sodium bicarbonate	Correct metabolic acidosis (buffer agent)
Cimetidine (Tagamet)	Histamine H₂ receptor antagonist	Sodium nitroprusside (Nipride)	VD, ↑CO
Dexamethasone (Decadron)	Adrenocorticosteroid	Vancomycin	Antibiotic
Digitalis (Cedilanid)	↑CC, ↓HR, AA, ↑BP, ↑CO	Verapamil	VD, AA
Dobutamine HCl (Dobutrex)	↑CC, ↑CO, ↑BP		
Dopamine HCl (Intropin)	↑CC, ↑CO, ↑BP		
Edrophonium (Tensilon)	AA, ↓CC, ↓HR		
Epinephrine (Adrenalin)	↑CC, ↑HR, ↑BP, VC		

Key: AA = antiarrhythmic; BP = blood pressure; CC = cardiac contractility; CO = cardiac output; HR = heart rate; VC = vasoconstriction; VD = vasodilatation.

Electrosurgical units: Two are needed if simultaneous incisions are made (chest and leg).

Suction lines: Three are essential, two for the sterile field, one for anesthesia use.

Heater/cooler machine: Used by the perfusionist to regulate the patient's temperature while on cardiopulmonary bypass (Fig. 13-19).

Thermal pad: Used under the patient to assist with maintaining the patient's temperature.

Intra-aortic balloon pump (IABP) and supplies (Fig. 13-20).

Heart–lung machine and supplies.

Headlights and power sources: Used by the surgeons to increase illumination of the surgical field.

Vascular prosthetic grafts and/or patch material.

Teflon felt material.

Valve prostheses: Tissue (biological) and mechanical valves in various sizes; allografts may be used in some heart centers.

Special sutures: Vascular microsutures, sternal wires, braided synthetics.

Chest tubes and drainage sets (various sizes).

Sternal saws (Fig. 13-21).

Temperature box and probe for measuring myocardial temperature.

Urinary catheters and drainage sets.

Hemostatic agents.

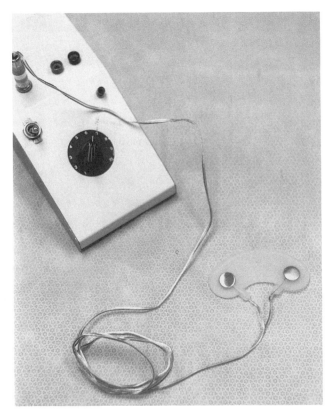

FIGURE 13-15 Fibrillator and fibrillator pad. The sterilized pad is placed on the heart's surface and connected to the fibrillator. Electrical current is conducted through the metal electrodes, and the heart fibrillates.

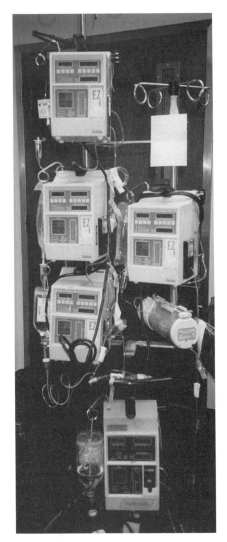

FIGURE 13-16 Infusion pumps.

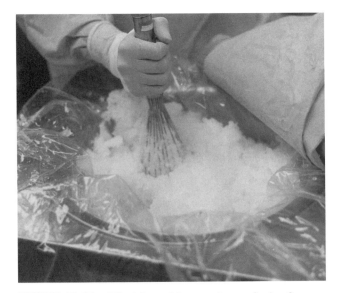

FIGURE 13-17 "Slush" machine used to make ice for topical cooling of the heart.

Cannulas/connectors: Assortment needed (depends on the patient's size and operative procedure). Used for cardiopulmonary bypass (Fig. 13-22).

Special instrumentation

Vascular clamps: Designed to cause minimal damage to vascular structures. Various sizes, shapes, and occlusive surfaces are available. Clamps can be used to totally or partially occlude vessels (Fig. 13-23).

Tissue forceps: Various sizes, shapes, and designs are needed. Microsurgical forceps cause minimal trauma to fragile tissues (Fig. 13-24).

Scissors: Vascular and microvascular scissors are available in various angles, sizes, and designs (Fig. 13-25).

Microsurgical knives: Used for incising small vessels (Fig. 13-26).

Vascular suction tips: Very small tips are designed to cause minimal trauma and can be used on fragile vascular tissues (Fig. 13-27).

Microvascular needle holders: These can be used on the small, delicate needles used with vascular sutures. They

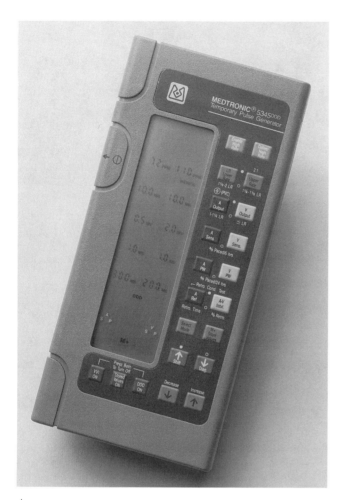

A

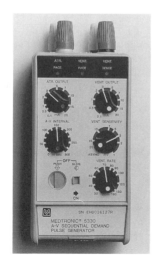

B

FIGURE 13-18   *A*, DDD temporary external pacemaker. (Reprinted with permission from Medtronic, Inc. © Medtronic, Inc. 1992.) *B*, AV sequential demand temporary external pacemaker. (Reprinted with permission from Medtronic, Inc. © Medtronic, Inc. 1992.)

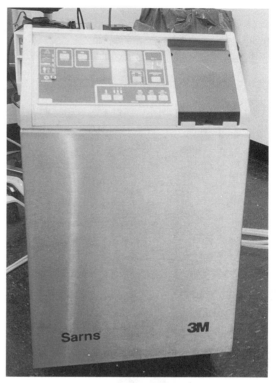

FIGURE 13-19   Heater/cooler machine. The water temperature in the machine is regulated and circulated through hoses to the heart–lung machine. Blood temperature can be altered while the patient is on cardiopulmonary bypass.

are designed to be held like a pencil, so the surgeon has increased control of the needle (Fig. 13-28).

Retractors: Sternal and/or rib retractors of various designs for infant, pediatric, and adult patients (Fig. 13-29). Special retractors for exposing the mitral valve (see Fig. 13-68) and for exposing the internal mammary artery (see Fig. 13-52) are available.

Tubing clamps: Designed for occluding pump tubing without damaging the clamp or the tubing. The tubing can be securely and totally occluded (Fig. 13-30).

Small vascular clamps: Various designs are available. "Bulldog" types are used for small, fragile vessels (Fig. 13-31).

Vessel loops or tapes: Used to encircle vessels for control of blood flow (Fig. 13-32,*A*).

Tourniquets: Used to tighten or secure sutures or tapes (Fig. 13-32,*B*).

Dilators: Used to dilate or calibrate vessels (Fig. 13-33).

Cardiopulmonary bypass (CPB)

Although the perioperative nurse is not responsible for the operation of the heart–lung machine, it is important to understand how it functions. A trained perfusionist, certified by the American Board of Cardiovascular Perfusion (in the United States), is recommended for operat-

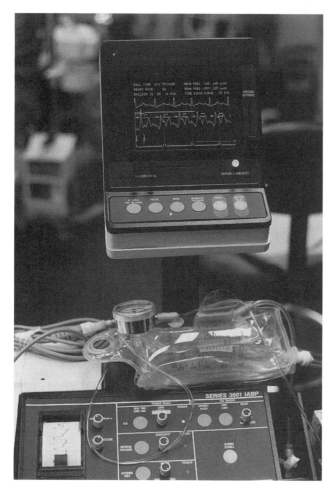

FIGURE 13-20 Intraaortic balloon pump (IABP).

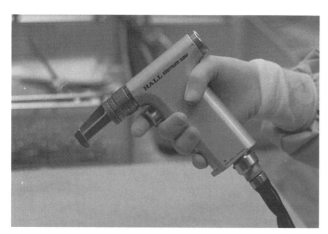

FIGURE 13-21 Sternal saw.

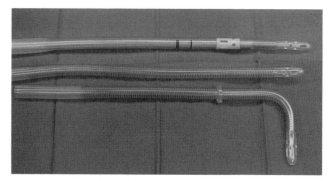

A

FIGURE 13-22 *A*, Venous cannulae: *top*, two-stage; *middle*, straight, single; *bottom*, right angle, single. *B*, Other cannulae: *top*, left ventricular venting cannula; *middle* and *bottom*, various arterial cannulae.

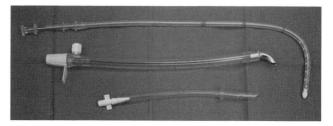

B

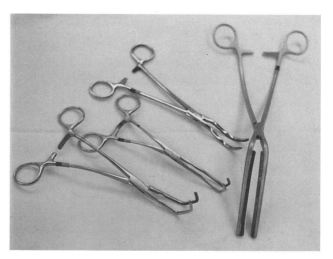

A

FIGURE 13-23 *A*, *B*, Various vascular clamps.

ing the heart–lung machine under the supervision of the cardiac surgeon (*Guidelines for minimal standards of cardiac surgery*, American College of Surgeons, 1991).

Development of the heart–lung machine was the "springboard" for cardiac surgery. Since 1953, the changes in techniques of CPB and refinements in the

heart–lung machine and equipment have contributed to the safety in using CPB today.

The purpose of CPB is to provide a means of temporarily bypassing and yet substituting for the patient's heart and lungs. This allows the heart to be stopped, emptied, and surgically incised. CPB has been modified for use in extracorporeal membrane oxygenation (ECMO) for patients with respiratory distress syndromes and to provide ventricular assist.

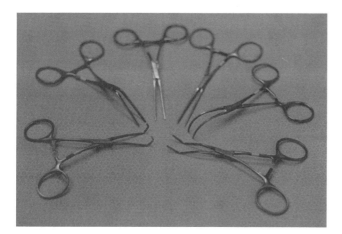

B

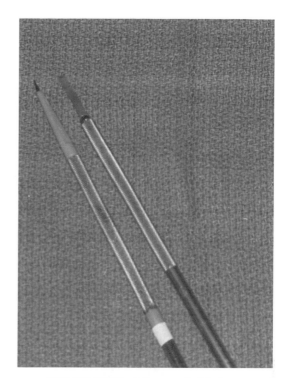

FIGURE 13-26 Microsurgical knives.

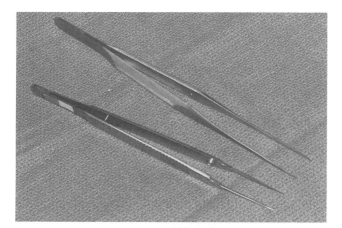

FIGURE 13-24 Microsurgical forceps.

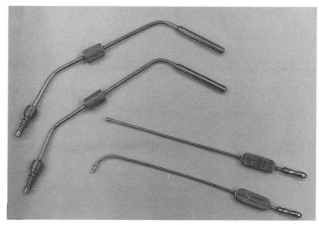

FIGURE 13-27 Suction tips. Upper left: cardiotomy suction tips ("pump" suctions). Bottom right: vascular suction tips.

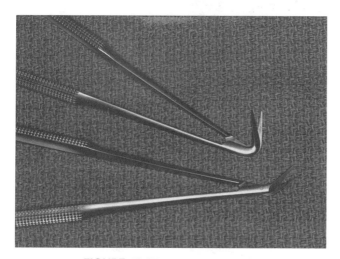

FIGURE 13-25 Vascular scissors.

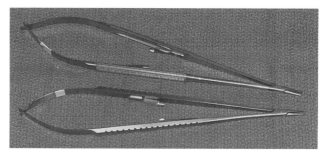

FIGURE 13-28 Microsurgical needleholders.

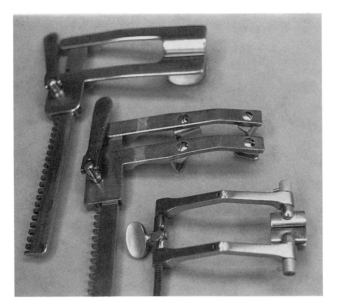

FIGURE 13-29   Sternal retractors.

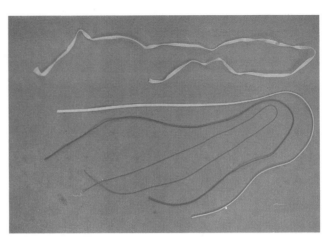

A

FIGURE 13-32   *A*, Umbilical tapes; vessel loops. *B*, Tourniquets and guides for pulling suture or tapes through tourniquet.

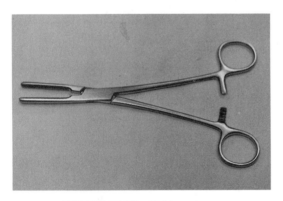

FIGURE 13-30   Tubing clamp.

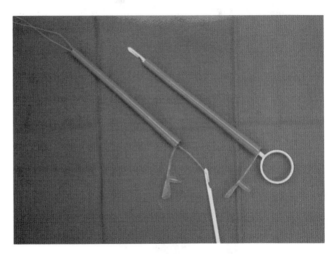

B

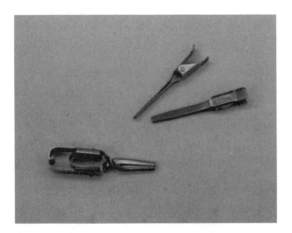

FIGURE 13-31   "Bulldog" type vascular clamps.

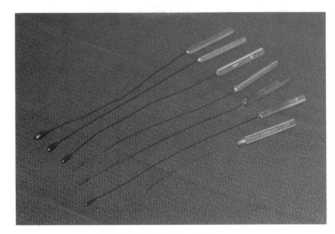

FIGURE 13-33   Dilators.

The major components of the heart–lung machine are the oxygenator (the lungs) and the pump (heart). The oxygenator provides for the exchange of oxygen and carbon dioxide. This must be done with minimal damage to blood components and without introducing emboli into the circulation (Pearson, 1991; Utley, 1990).

Oxygenators There are basically two methods or types of oxygenators: the "bubble" and the "membrane." Several brands of oxygenators are available as sterile, disposable units.

The "bubble" oxygenator consists of three sections. The oxygenation section is where the gas mixture is "bubbled" through the venous blood that is returning from the patient. This oxygenates the blood and causes the elimination of excess carbon dioxide. The defoaming section is where the gas bubbles are removed from the blood. The arterial reservoir collects the defoamed blood prior to its return to the patient. The reservoir is large enough to hold enough blood for 20 to 40 seconds of pumping should the venous return become obstructed. This safety feature is designed for prevention of pumping air into the patient (Reed, 1985). There is concern that the "bubble" oxygenator causes more microemboli than the membrane oxygenator (Pearson, 1990).

The "membrane" oxygenator has a membrane between the blood and the oxygenated gas. The gas can permeate the membrane, but direct contact between the blood and the gas is not allowed. It is easier to manage gas exchange with this type of oxygenator (Utley, 1990) (Fig. 13-34).

Pump The pump is the part of the heart–lung machine that propels the blood through the circulatory system while the patient is on CPB. Occlusive roller type pumps have been used since the 1960s (Utley, 1990). These are called "positive displacement pumps." The pump tubing containing the blood is squeezed by the roller, and the blood is thus forced forward (Fig. 13-35). The occlusiveness of the pump rollers against the tubing

must be set by the perfusionist for each patient in order to prevent backward motion of the blood (Reed, 1985). The speed at which the pump heads turn (RPM) will determine the rate and amount of blood flow. The amount of blood flow is determined by the size of the patient and the patient's temperature. The desired flow is 1.6 $L/m^2/$ minute with a pO_2 of greater than 40 mm Hg. The pump can be modified to provide pulsatile flow by acceleration/deceleration of the pump heads. This type of flow has the advantage of preventing vasoconstriction that occurs with nonpulsatile flow. Normal values of peripheral vascular resistance, improved oxygen consumption by cells, and improved brain capillary circulation also occurs with pulsatile flow (Utley, 1990). Pulsatile flow provides more uniform cooling and rewarming of the patient during CPB (Parenteau et al., 1992).

The vortex type of pump operates by creating a centrifugal force that propels the blood. This type of pump is used primarily for ECMO and ventricular assist devices (Reed, 1985).

Blood filters Blood filters are used to remove microemboli in the blood that can occur with the trauma to the blood during CPB. The most common locations for the filters are between the cardiotomy reservoir and the venous reservoir of the oxygenator; between the arterial pump head and the patient; and between any blood transfusions and cardiotomy reservoir (Reed, 1985).

Heat exchanger The heat exchanger provides a means of maintaining normal blood temperature or of changing it during CPB. Water from a heater/cooler machine is used to regulate the blood temperature. The water is circulated from the machine to the oxygenator, which has an integral heat exchanger system (Fig. 13-36). The temperature of the water, as it circulates through the heat exchanger, is conducted to the blood. There is no direct contact of the water with the blood. Hypothermia is usually used during CPB to lower the metabolism and oxygen consumption by the patient's tissues. For most CPB procedures, moderate hypothermia is used (Table 13-4). Profound hypothermia with total circulatory arrest (the heart–lung machine is stopped) is used for the repair of

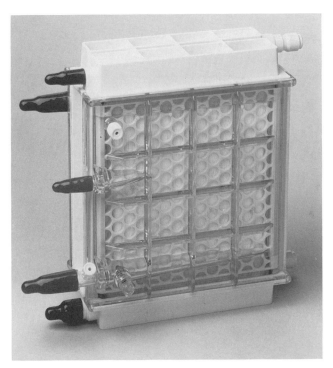

FIGURE 13-34 Membrane type oxygenator. (Courtesy of Bard Cardiopulmonary, a division of C.R. Bard, Inc.)

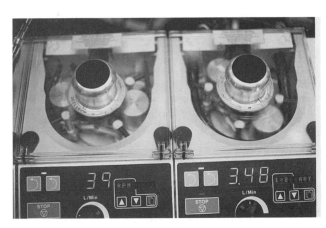

FIGURE 13-35 Roller pump head. Note tubing compressed by rollers.

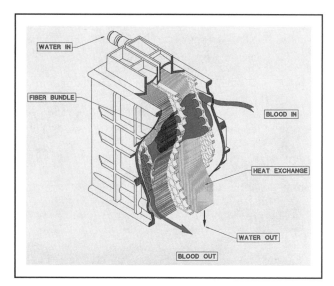

FIGURE 13-36 Integral heat exchanger inside membrane oxygenator. (Courtesy of Bard Cardiopulmonary, a division of C.R. Bard, Inc.)

TABLE 13-4 Hypothermia Ranges for Cardiopulmonary Bypass

Mild	37–32° C
Moderate	32–28° C
Deep	28–18° C
Profound	18–0° C

(Adapted from Reed, C. [1985]. *Cardiopulmonary bypass* [2nd ed.]. Houston: Texas Medical Press.)

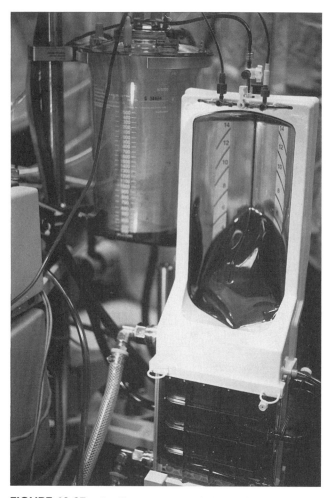

FIGURE 13-37 Cardiotomy reservoir (round chamber). Blood from cardiotomy suctions goes to this chamber, drains into the oxygenator reservoir (bag chamber), and then into the oxygenator.

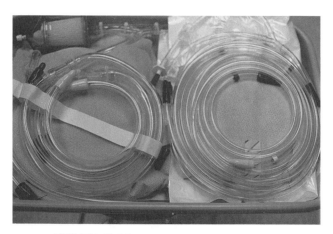

FIGURE 13-38 Sterile pump tubing pack.

some congenital defects and occasionally for selected adult procedures. When rewarming the blood (and the patient), a blood temperature over 42° C will cause destruction to the blood components. Temperature regulators in heat exchangers and heater/cooler machines will not allow the temperature to exceed 42° C (Bell & Diffee, 1991; Reed, 1985).

Cardiotomy suctions Special suction tips (see Fig. 13-27) and/or cannulas are used to return shed blood to the heart–lung machine after the patient has been heparinized. The tips are attached to ¼-inch pump tubing that goes through a pump head in order to provide suction. The minimum amount of suction necessary is used as this is traumatic to the blood. The blood goes to the cardiotomy reservoir before it returns to the oxygenator (Fig. 13-37).

Pump tubing Special, medical-grade tubing is used for the blood as it comes from the patient, goes through the heart–lung machine, and is returned to the patient. Most pump tubing is made of polyvinyl chloride and is available precut and sterile in custom packs (Fig. 13-38).

The size of tubing needed depends on its use and the size of the patient. The tubing size is measured by the inside diameter.

Patient's weight	Arterial line	Venous line
8 kilograms or less	¼″	¼″
8–25 kilograms	¼″	⅜″
25–50 kilograms	⅜″	⅜″ or ½″
50 kilograms or more	⅜″	½″
Cardiotomy suction tubing	¼″	

(Adapted from Reed, 1985)

Perfusate The perfusate solution used to "prime" or fill the heart–lung machine is a balanced salt solution. An example of a prime solution is lactated Ringer's solution, 2500 ml, 25 g mannitol, 50 mEq sodium bicarbonate, and 10,000 units of heparin. This solution is mixed with the patient's blood once CPB is started. This is called hemodilution as the use of blood transfusions is avoided. The hematocrit is maintained between 20% to 25% while on CPB, or blood transfusions may be necessary. If additional volume is needed, crystalloid or albumin may be added (Bell & Diffee, 1991).

Cannulation The venous blood is removed from the patient by one or two venous cannulae that connect to the venous pump line. When the heart is not opened (e.g., coronary artery bypass grafts), a single, two-stage cannula is frequently used. This cannula has a cage-type section that drains the blood from the atrium; the distal tip drains the blood from the inferior vena cava. This cannula is inserted through the right atrium (Fig. 13-39). When two cannulae are needed they are inserted through separate sites on the right atrium and into the superior and inferior venae cavae (Fig. 13-40). If the right heart is opened, umbilical tapes and/or vessel loops around the cavae can be tightened and prevent air from being "sucked" into the cannulae and creating an airlock in the venous line.

The oxygenated blood is returned to the patient from the heart–lung machine through an arterial line that connects to the arterial cannula. The most common site for arterial cannulation is the distal ascending aorta or arch of the aorta (Fig. 13-41). The femoral artery is used when the aorta cannot be used.

Venting the heart Left ventricular venting (removal of blood) is done to prevent overdistention of the left ventri-

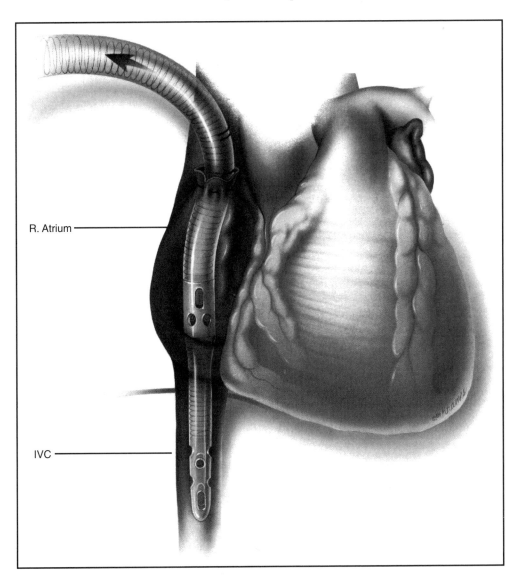

R. Atrium

IVC

FIGURE 13-39 Two-stage venous cannula. (Reprinted with permission of Research Med. Inc.)

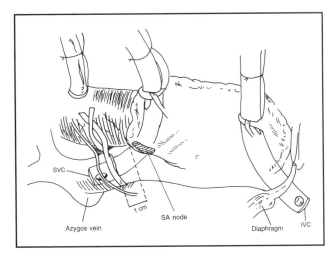

FIGURE 13-40 Venous cannulae through right atrial incision into the inferior and superior venae cavae. Umbilical tapes are around the cavae.

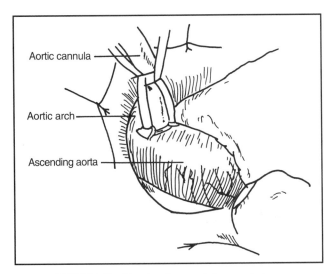

FIGURE 13-41 Aortic arterial cannulation.

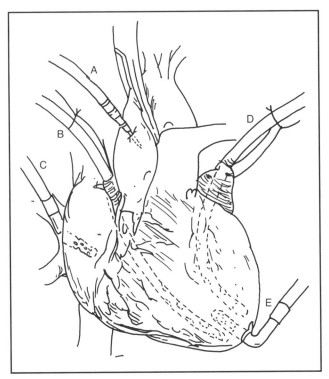

FIGURE 13-42 Various sites for venting the heart: *A*, ascending aorta; *B*, left atrium; *C*, pulmonary vein; *D*, left atrium; *E*, apex of left ventricle.

cle and tension on the left ventricular wall, which can impair its function. Venting also improves subendocardial coronary artery flow during CPB and provides a dry field during coronary artery surgery. Indirect methods of venting are through the aorta or the pulmonary artery, with varying degrees of success. Direct venting is most commonly used. There are several approaches to the left ventricle through the left atrium (Fig. 13-42), but a commonly used approach is through the right superior pulmonary vein, across the mitral valve, and into the left ventricle. The blood is drained from the left ventricle through the cannula by gravity or suction into a cardiotomy suction line that returns to the cardiotomy reservoir (Lundy et al., 1992).

Heparinization Prior to cannulating and establishing CPB, the patient is given heparin, which neutralizes thrombin and prevents clot formation while on CPB. The standard dose frequently is 3 mg/kg of body weight (300 units). The activated clotting time (ACT) is measured be-

fore heparin is administered in order to have a baseline. It is checked again 3 to 5 minutes after the heparin has been given and must be at least 400 seconds. Perfusionists keep the ACT at 480 to 600 seconds. The ACT is checked at least hourly while the patient is on CPB and additional heparin is given if needed. Protamine sulfate is used to neutralize the heparin at 1.3 to 1.5 times the heparin dose (Doty, 1985; Aren, 1990).

Cardioplegia A dry, motionless operative field is desired during cardiac surgery. This is obtained by arresting the heart and stopping blood flow through the coronary arteries. Cross-clamping the aorta proximal to the arterial cannula will stop the blood flow through the coronary arteries. Myocardial protection to prevent ischemic damage is provided by using hypothermia and administering cardioplegic solutions into the coronary circulation.

Hypothermia is accomplished in several ways. The blood circulating through the heart–lung machine is cooled by the heat exchanger. The heart can be topically cooled by surrounding it with iced saline solution, or "slush." Cold cardioplegic solution can be administered at a temperature of 4 to 10° C. A separate heat exchanger is used for the cardioplegia. The myocardial temperature is monitored with a temperature probe, and a temperature of 15° C or less is desired (Lichtenstein & Abel, 1992).

There are two basic types of cardioplegic solutions: blood and crystalloid. It is the high potassium content of either solution that causes a chemically induced electromechanical cardiac standstill. The solution is adminis-

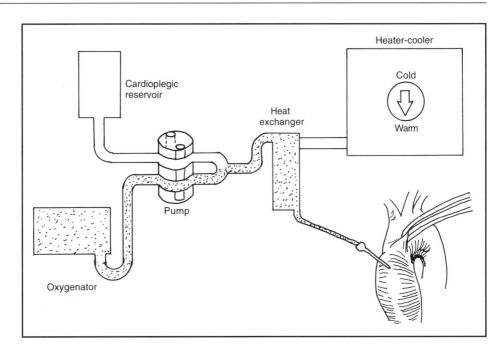

FIGURE 13-43 Cardioplegia administration system.

tered approximately every 20 minutes while the aorta is cross-clamped. The primary advantage of blood cardioplegia is its oxygen-carrying capacity; however, crystalloid solutions are commonly used (Bell & Diffee, 1991; Barner, 1991).

The delivery system may go through a roller head on the heart–lung machine or a pressure bag may be used. There is a system for monitoring the pressure at the delivery site. The pressure for antegrade administration is 80 to 200 mm Hg and for retrograde it is 40 to 50 mm Hg. A flow of 100 to 150 ml/minute is optimal. The cardioplegia solution may be cold or normothermic (Fig. 13-43) (Lichtenstein, 1990).

With antegrade technique, the cardioplegia is administered into the aorta proximal to the aortic cross-clamp and then flows into the coronary arteries. With retrograde technique, the solution is administered into the coronary sinus (Fig. 13-44). The use of the retrograde technique is increasing as it seems to be a more effective method of providing cardioplegia to the myocardium, especially in the presence of coronary artery disease. This method provides increased chamber cooling and avoids possible injury to the coronary ostia. A combined technique of retrograde and antegrade may be used (Menasche & Piwnia, 1991; Arom & Emery, 1992). Direct cannulation of the coronary arteries may be indicated (Fig. 13-45).

Monitoring of serum values While the patient is on CPB, the perfusionist must monitor several serum values, as abnormalities can have adverse effects on the patient. These are checked at least every 15 minutes. Inline gas analyzers are very accurate and can be integrated into the heart–lung tubing circuits. This analyzer provides a quick method of monitoring blood gases and electrolytes (Fig. 13-46).

PERIOPERATIVE CONSIDERATIONS

Incisional Sites

The selection of the incisional site is related to providing optimal exposure and access during the operative procedure.

The median sternotomy incision is the most frequent approach for cardiac surgery. The sternotomy incision may be extended into the neck or abdomen for selected procedures.

An anterolateral or a posterolateral chest incision may be needed for certain cardiac procedures.

Leg incisions following the route of the greater or lesser saphenous veins may be needed for coronary artery bypass surgery. Arm veins are used infrequently, but if needed, incisions follow the cephalic or basilic veins.

Incisions over the femoral arteries may be needed.

Positioning (see Chapter 28 in Volume 1)

Median sternotomy

For this approach the patient is supine. The arms are usually placed at the patient's sides or may be extended on armboards. The legs may be positioned straight, slightly separated, or slightly flexed and externally rotated with adequate supportive devices.

Padding of all bony prominences (head, elbows, sacrum, and heels) is necessary to prevent pressure-related injuries. Cardiac surgeries can be lengthy procedures and peripheral circulation is impaired during the hypothermic conditions of CPB. Elderly patients usually have impaired circulation and more fragile tissues. Special consideration must be given to infants and diabetics.

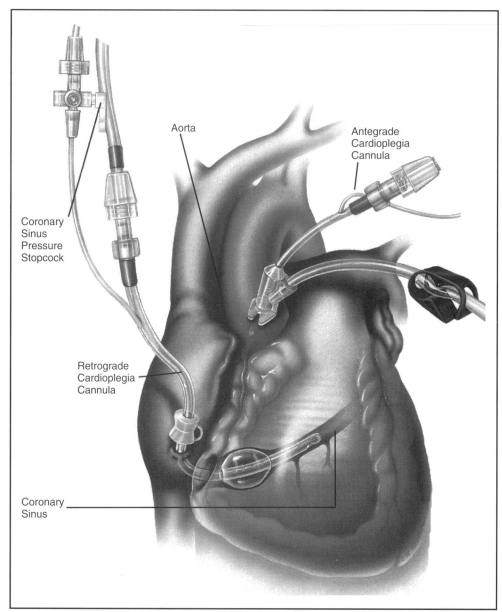

Aorta

Antegrade
Cardioplegia
Cannula

Coronary
Sinus
Pressure
Stopcock

Retrograde
Cardioplegia
Cannula

Coronary
Sinus

FIGURE 13-44 Cardioplegia: antegrade via the aorta or retrograde via the right atrium and into the coronary sinus. (Reprinted with permission of Research Med., Inc.)

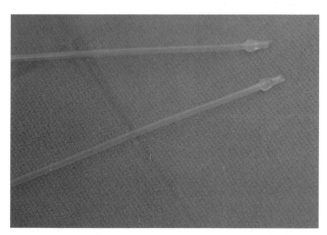

FIGURE 13-45 Cannulae for coronary arteries.

Anterolateral and posterolateral

Positioning for these thoracic incisions is described in the thoracic surgery chapter (Chapter 14 in this volume). Access to the femoral arteries must be considered.

Prepping

Standard prepping procedures are followed (see Chapter 15 in Volume 1). If leg incisions are needed, both legs must be prepped. Circumferential prepping of legs and arms may be desired.

Draping

The upper edge of the drape should be placed 1 to 2 inches above the sternal notch. The side drapes are placed lateral to the nipple line on the chest. The peri-

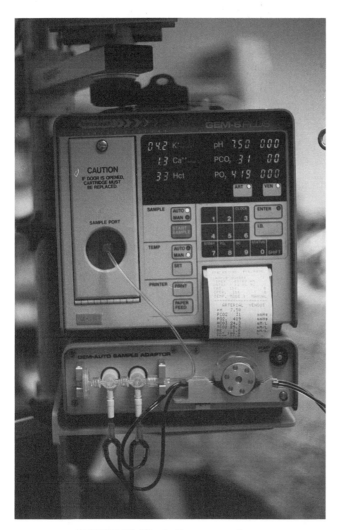

FIGURE 13-46 In-line gas analyzer.

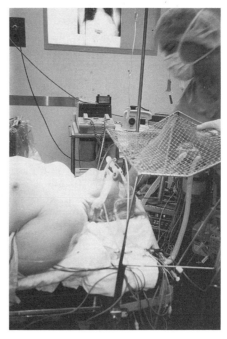

FIGURE 13-47 Overhead screen being positioned over the patient's head.

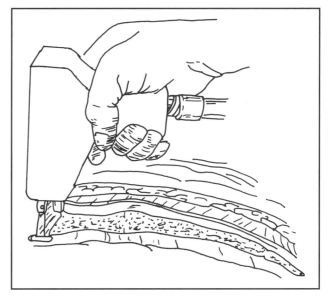

FIGURE 13-48 Cutting sternum with sternal saw.

neal area is covered, allowing access to the femoral arteries. Adhesive barrier drapes may be used. Specially designed overhead screens keep the drapes off the patient's head and allow easy access to the patient by the anesthesia provider (Fig. 13-47).

Sternotomy

The surgeon palpates for landmarks prior to making the skin incision. These landmarks are the sternal notch, the xiphoid process, and the costochondral joints. The incision is made vertically in the middle of the sternum from the sternal notch to just below the xiphoid process. Hemostasis is achieved with electrocauterization. The sternal saw is used to open the sternum (Fig. 13-48). If the patient has had a previous sternotomy, the surgeon may use blunt dissection techniques to free underlying adhesions prior to sawing the sternum. Extreme care must be taken on reoperations to prevent injury to the right ventricle that may be adhered to the sternum. Sternal bleeding is controlled by using bonewax in the marrow cavities and electrocauterization of the periosteum.

Retractor

The sternal retractor is placed under the edges of the sternum. Some surgeons prefer to have the ratchet end of the retractor toward the patient's head so the bar does not interfere with surgical access. The retractor is opened slowly, and care is taken, because sternal, rib, and costal cartilage fractures and/or displacements can occur. Excessive retraction can displace the clavicles posteriorly and cause brachial plexus injuries.

Thymus

In children the thymus is present and is dissected free and removed. Thymic remnants in the adult patient are divided and hemostasis is achieved with cauterization or ligature.

Pericardium

The pericardium is usually divided vertically in the middle, and a "T" is made at the lower end along the diaphragm. The pericardial fluid is suctioned away and the edges of the pericardium are retracted upward by the use of retraction sutures. This facilitates exposure of the heart and forms a "well" for any blood that is lost. Excessive traction upward on the pericardium can interfere with exposure during procedures where the heart must be rotated.

Major Vessels

The surgeon may dissect around and place vessel loops or umbilical tapes around the inferior vena cava, the superior vena cava, the aorta, and/or the pulmonary artery. A right-angled clamp or Semb ligature carrier may be used to go around the vessel and grasp the loop or tape and pull it into place. Sometimes the surgeon uses a double loop for occluding the vessel later or a tourniquet.

Cannulation for CPB

Arterial

The cannula for the arterial line coming from the heart–lung machine is usually inserted in the upper ascending aorta or into the arch of the aorta. One or two pursestring nonabsorbable sutures are placed into the adventitial layer of the aorta. Teflon felt bolsters may be used to prevent tearing of the tissue by the sutures. The suture is secured with a tourniquet. A stab wound incision is made in the aorta and may be dilated with special dilators. The cannula is inserted and secured with the suture as the tourniquet is tightened (see Fig. 13-41). The tourniquet and the cannula are tied together to prevent dislodgment of the cannula. The cannula is allowed to fill with blood from the aorta, and the arterial pump line is filled by the perfusionist as the surgeon connects the two. All air must be removed before connecting the cannula and the arterial line to prevent an air embolus. The arterial line is secured to the drapes without any kinks that would restrict or obstruct flow. Any clamps on the line must be removed prior to CPB. There are several types of cannulae available, and the surgeon determines what type is to be used (see Fig. 13-22).

Femoral artery cannulation may be indicated for procedures involving the ascending, arch, or thoracic aorta or during an emergency when CPB must be established prior to opening the sternum. The artery is exposed and a vessel loop or umbilical tape is placed above the cannu-

lation site. A transverse incision is made in the artery, and the cannula is threaded in very carefully toward the heart. Once in place, the loop or tape is tightened to prevent bleeding and is secured with a clamp (Fig. 13-49). The arterial line and cannula are connected and the line is secured to the drapes to prevent accidental displacement. Any clamps on the line are removed before CPB. Because femoral cannulation is infrequently used, all team members must be aware of its location and use care not to place instruments or hands on the cannula site.

The major risks with arterial cannulation are dislodging atheromatous material (emboli); dissection of the aorta/femoral artery; tearing of the artery; puncturing the opposite wall of the artery; misdirection of the arterial flow, which could damage the intima; and introduction of air into the arterial system (Khonsari, 1988).

Venous

The cannula or cannulae for taking the venous blood from the patient to the heart–lung machine via the venous line are usually placed into the right atrium and then into the inferior or superior vena cava (or both). A pursestring nonabsorbable suture is placed in the atrial wall and secured with a tourniquet. A partial-occlusion vascular clamp may be used to grasp the atrium. The atrium is incised with a knife or scissor and the cannula is inserted as the partial occlusion clamp is opened by the assistant. After proper placement of the cannula into the atrium and cava, the tourniquet is tightened and tied to the cannula. The cannula is filled with saline, as is the venous pump line (above where it has been clamped), and the two are connected securely together. The venous line remains clamped to prevent drainage of the patient's blood into the heart–lung machine. The venous line is secured to the drapes, and enough length is provided to allow repositioning of the line as necessary during the procedure. The venous line must not be allowed to kink or venous blood return to the pump will not occur.

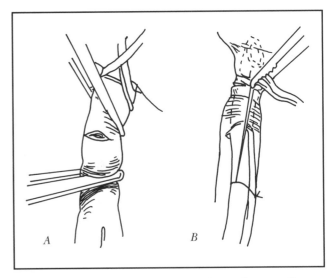

FIGURE 13-49 *A,* Incision into the femoral artery. *B,* Cannula inserted into the femoral artery and secured with a vessel loop, tape, and suture (or tape and suture).

The femoral vein may be used for venous cannulation in select procedures or when CPB must be established prior to opening the chest.

The major risks of venous cannulation are tearing or perforation of the atrium or cava, injury to the sinoatrial (SA) node, accidental clamping of the right coronary artery with the atrial vascular clamp, and trapping of air in the venous line, which creates an air lock and prevents venous return to the heart–lung machine (Khonsari, 1988).

Cardiopulmonary Bypass (CPB)

Once the arterial and venous lines are connected to the cannulae, the surgeon will determine when to advise the perfusionist to "go on pump." Any tubing clamps must be removed from the arterial and venous lines at this time. The heart empties and collapses as blood is drained to the heart–lung machine and the anesthesia provider stops ventilating the lungs.

For most cardiac procedures the surgeon wants the patient's heart to be motionless, and cardiac arrest is induced by ischemia (stopping the blood flow through the coronary arteries) and/or pharmacologically by using potassium cardioplegia (Buckberg, 1987).

For antegrade cardioplegia administration, a pursestring suture is placed on the lower portion of the ascending aorta and secured with a tourniquet. For retrograde administration, the suture is placed on the right atrium (see Fig. 13-44). A stab incision is made, and the cannula is inserted. The suture is tightened with the tourniquet and the cannula and tourniquet are tied together. Any air is removed from the cannula and the cardioplegia administration line coming from the heart–lung machine, and they are connected together. A pressure line is connected to the cardioplegia line in order to measure the pressure used to administer the cardioplegia. The aorta is cross-clamped proximal to the aortic cannula and distal to the antegrade cannula (if used) prior to administering the cardioplegia. The retrograde cannula balloon must be inflated prior to starting the cardioplegia (see Fig. 13-44).

If a left ventricular vent is needed, a pursestring suture is placed at the junction of the right superior pulmonary vein and the left atrium. The cannula is inserted after a stab incision is made and is threaded into the left ventricle (see Fig. 13-42). The suture is tightened with the tourniquet and is tied to the cannula. The cannula is attached to the cardiotomy suction line and primed with saline, and blood is drained from the left ventricle to the heart–lung machine.

If iced slush is used for topical cooling around the heart, a sterile foam pad can be placed behind and to the sides of the heart to protect the phrenic nerves from cold injury and to prevent rewarming of the heart from surrounding structures. The myocardial temperature probe is inserted and the heart temperature is monitored.

Once the operative procedure is completed, the aortic cross-clamp is removed. A hypodermic needle may be inserted if necessary into the aorta to remove any trapped air. The balloon on the retrograde cannula must be de-flated to allow coronary sinus venous blood to return to the right atrium, and the cannula is removed and the suture is tied.

The perfusionist is directed by the surgeon when to "rewarm" the patient, and often the heart will begin to beat as the patient's temperature nears 37° C. Defibrillation may be needed. Once the heart is beating, the left ventricular vent can be removed. The vent cannula is clamped and the left heart is allowed to fill with blood. The pericardial well is filled with saline above the entrance of the vent cannula into the heart. This prevents air from being "sucked" into the heart when the vent is removed and while the suture is tied. The caval tapes, if used, have been loosened.

Temporary pacing wires are usually placed in the event a temporary pacemaker is needed after surgery. Atrial and/or ventricular wires are attached to the surface of the heart (Fig. 13-50), brought out through the chest wall, and attached to a pacing cable that connects to the temporary pacemaker. The surgeon advises the circulating nurse regarding the pacemaker settings and when to turn it on and/or off.

The surgeon determines when the patient is ready to be "weaned" from the CPB. This is done by gradually decreasing the venous return by partially clamping the venous line and allowing more blood to go through the patient's heart. The perfusionist decreases the arterial

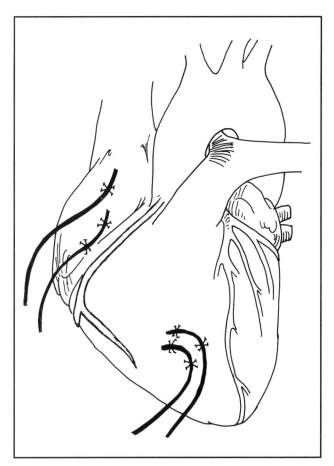

FIGURE 13-50 Location of temporary atrial and ventricular pacing wires on the surface of the heart.

blood flow as the venous return is decreased. Gradually, the patient's heart is allowed to resume the full workload as venous and arterial flows from the heart–lung machine are stopped. The anesthesia provider has resumed ventilating the patient once the "weaning" from CPB has begun. The arterial and venous cannulae are removed once the patient is determined to be hemodynamically stable with satisfactory cardiac function. Protamine is then given to reverse the heparin.

Closure

Obtaining hemostasis after CPB is essential and can be time-consuming. The surgeon may choose to loosely suture portions of the pericardium and thymic tissues together. Chest tubes are placed. One mediastinal tube is usually used, and one or two pleural chest tubes may be needed if the pleural spaces have been opened. The chest tubes are secured to the skin with a suture to prevent dislodgment. Wires or synthetic nonabsorbable sternal sutures are placed through the sternum, and the sternal edges are tightly proximated as the wire/suture is tied. The other tissue layers are closed, and a sterile, occlusive dressing is applied. Incisions in the patient's leg or abdomen are also closed. The chest tubes are connected to underwater chest drainage apparatus.

Transfer

The patient is carefully moved from the operating room bed to the transport bed. All monitoring cables, intravenous lines, pacemakers, chest tubes, and urinary catheters are secured for transport. Continuous monitoring of the arterial pressure and ECG during transport is possible by using a portable transport monitor. Portable defibrillators are available for use during transport. The endotracheal tube is left in place and the anesthesia provider manually ventilates the patient, using portable oxygen. The circulating nurse and the perfusionist assist the anesthesia provider to transport the patient to the recovery area.

Besides the written report of intraoperative activities, the circulating nurse gives a verbal report to the recovery nurse. This report includes information related to the patient's current status, intravenous medications, and an overview of patient responses intraoperatively. The endotracheal tube is connected to the mechanical ventilator, and the ECG and arterial and pulmonary arterial lines are connected to the bedside monitors.

Expected Outcomes of Cardiac Surgery

The expected outcomes for patients undergoing cardiac surgical procedures are individualized based on the patient's condition, the type and extent of the cardiac problem, and the complexity of the surgical technology required for the operative procedure.

The primary expected outcome is survival. The intent of surgical intervention is to survive the procedure in order to benefit from this form of therapy. Understandably, certain operative procedures and patient conditions will carry a higher mortality risk than others. This mortality risk is addressed with the patient, family, and/or significant other prior to the operation.

Improving the patient's quality of life is another expected outcome. By relieving or decreasing the patient's symptoms or stabilizing an unstable condition, this outcome can be achieved. Although many cardiac procedures are palliative rather than curative, the patient's condition may be greatly improved. Complex cardiac problems may require multiple surgical procedures and must be viewed in relation to the overall or long-term goals of surgical intervention.

Another expected outcome may be the prevention or diminishing of events that could be catastrophic. Asymptomatic patients with potentially lethal cardiac lesions/conditions may have difficulty understanding the need for surgical intervention.

A major outcome of perioperative nursing care is the prevention of complications related to the intraoperative period. Many nursing interventions are interdependent with interventions of other members of the surgical team. The perioperative nurse must recognize and understand the importance of all care provided to the patient undergoing cardiac surgery. The "Patient outcomes: Standards of perioperative care" (AORN, 1994) identify key areas that can be evaluated in relation to perioperative nursing interventions.

SURGICAL PROCEDURES

Surgery for Ischemic Heart Disease

Revascularization: coronary artery bypass graft procedure (CABG)

The purpose of a CABG procedure is to provide increased blood flow to a myocardium that is ischemic because of stenotic or obstructive atherosclerotic lesions in the coronary artery or arteries.

Favaloro and Effler at the Cleveland Clinic and Johnson and Lepley of Milwaukee are credited with development of the CABG techniques that became accepted in the United States in 1967 (Cooley, 1984). CABG procedures are done worldwide, but the high cost of these procedures has been a limiting factor in some countries. In 1989, there were 368,000 CABG procedures done in the United States, making this the most frequent cardiac surgical procedure performed in this country (American Heart Association, 1992).

Studies of patient outcomes after CABG procedures over the past 25 years demonstrate that these procedures can relieve ischemic heart disease symptoms (angina) and delay unfavorable events (myocardial infarction [M.I.], return of angina, or death) for many patients.

Recommendations for surgery are made on an individualized basis. *The Guidelines and Indications for CABG Surgery* were developed by a Task Force of the American College of

Cardiology and the American Heart Association in 1991. These guidelines provide information regarding the analytical processes used to decide when surgery is to be recommended to the patient. Studies compare outcomes related to medical therapy, angioplasty, and surgery on patients with comparable risk factors.

The contraindications for CABG procedures are:

1. Absence of any open major coronary artery of less than 1 mm in diameter beyond the obstructing lesion
2. Absence of viable myocardium in the area supplied by the diseased coronary artery
3. Presence of noncardiac conditions with a poor prognosis
4. Extreme debilitation
5. Mental/emotional deterioration
6. Multisystem disease

Changes in the patient population undergoing CABG procedures have occurred in recent years. Patients requiring reoperation are now being seen more frequently. Patients with more complex, multivessel disease are now being offered surgery. Sicker, older patients are also being seen in surgery. Emergency surgery is being done more frequently for patients with unstable angina, acute infarction, or failed angioplasty. These changes are increasing the mortality and morbidity associated with CABG procedures (Jones et al., 1991). Certain risk factors need consideration when surgery is recommended to the patient (Table 13-5).

Conduits Patients who have had incomplete revascularization procedures are at increased risk for premature death. Coronary arteries as small as 1 mm in diameter are now being grafted by some surgeons. Because more grafts are being inserted, various conduits are being used.

The first conduit used for this procedure was the greater saphenous vein. This conduit is still used today, as is the lesser saphenous vein and the short saphenous vein, by some surgeons (Glick et al., 1990).

Because of improved survival rates and higher patency rates of the bypass, the left internal mammary artery is the conduit of choice. Use of the right internal mammary artery is increasing, as is the use of bilateral internal mammary artery grafts. Use of both internal arteries has been reported to increase sternal wound complications. Recent studies show there is a decrease in the blood supply to the sternum when both arteries are used, but this decrease is believed to be transient and reverses within 1 month after surgery. Complications may be due to the increased operative time and increased bleeding, requiring reexploration. Patients at increased risk for sternal wound complications (diabetic) and elderly patients and patients with chronic obstructive pulmonary disease [COPD] should probably not have bilateral mammary grafts (Carrier et al., 1992).

Other conduit choices include the right gastroepiploic artery, the inferior mesenteric artery, and the inferior gastric artery. These are small, fragile arteries and technically more difficult to prepare and use.

The least satisfactory conduits with poor long-term patency rates are the radial artery, arm veins, allograft arteries/veins, and synthetic vascular grafts (American College of Cardiology and American Heart Association Task Force Report, 1991).

The perioperative nurse needs to know what the planned CABG procedure is in order to have the appropriate instrumentation, supplies, and equipment available. Commonly, the internal mammary arteries and saphenous veins are used in combination in order to have an adequate source of conduits.

Special instrumentation, equipment, and supplies

Positioning: Devices are needed to support the legs. Legs may be abducted and rotated laterally.

Prepping: Leg holders may be needed if a circumferential prep is done. Prep legs from groin to ankle or midfoot.

Draping: Legs are draped to expose the inner aspect of the leg from groin to ankle.

Electrosurgical unit: One is needed for the chest and one for the leg incisions.

Instrumentation
    Internal mammary retractor (Fig. 13-51).
    Abdominal retractor if gastroepiploic artery used
    Weitlaner or other self-retaining retractor for leg incision
    Parsonnette epicardial retractor (Fig. 13-52).
    Vessel clips
    Microvascular knives, needle holders, scissors, and tissue forceps (see Figs. 13-24, 13-25, 13-26, and 13-28)
    Coronary artery dilators/probes (see Fig. 13-33)
    Vascular bulldog clamps (see Fig. 13-31)
    Vascular suction tips (see Fig. 13-27)
    Aortic punch (Fig. 13-53)
    Valvulotome to remove valves of vein (if needed)

Sutures
    Fine ties (4-0 or 5-0 silk) for proximal end of vein branches
    Vascular microsutures (6-0, 7-0, 8-0) nonabsorbable, monofilament

Procedure

Key steps

1. A sternotomy incision is made; the internal mammary retractor is attached to the side of the operating room bed. The surgeon dissects the internal mammary artery (see Fig. 13-51) while the assistant removes the saphenous vein (Fig. 13-54). Usually the heparin is given prior to dividing the distal end of the internal mammary artery.
2. CPB: A standard aortic cannula and a two-stage cannula, aorta crossclamped, cardioplegia (retrograde if possible), and left ventricular vent are required.

Table 13-5 Preoperative and Operative Risk Factors for Increasing the Probability of Death Early or Late After a Primary Coronary Artery Bypass Operation*

Risk Factors†

Demographic
Age at coronary bypass operation (older)
Body size (smaller)
Gender (female)

Clinical status
Angina (Canadian class 0 to IV) (more severe)
Unstable angina
Response to stress testing (more severe)
Acute myocardial infarction
Hemodynamic instability (grade 0 to 4) (more severe)
NYHA functional class (I to IV) (higher)

Distribution and severity of coronary artery disease (greater)

Left ventricular dysfunction (grade 0 to 4) (more severe)

Aggressiveness of arteriosclerotic process
Diffusely diseased coronary arteries
Peripheral vascular disease
Cerebrovascular disease
Hyperlipidemia (more severe)
Age at coronary bypass operation (younger)

Coexisting disease
Diabetes
Hypertension
Pulmonary disease (more severe)
Stroke
Smoking

Surgical factors
Date of operation (earlier)
Nonuse of IMA to LAD
Incomplete revascularization
Perioperative myocardial infarction
(inadequate myocardial management)
Surgeon

Institutional factors

*This table is not the result of a specific multivariable analysis, but is a composite depiction of data from many studies. IMA = internal mammary artery; LAD = left anterior descending coronary artery; NYHA = New York Heart Association.
†From American College of Cardiology and American Heart Association Task Force (1991). Guidelines and indications for coronary artery bypass surgery. *Journal of the American College of Cardiology, 17*, 543–509.

The Canadian Cardiovascular Society Function Classifications‡

I Ordinary physical activity, such as walking or climbing the stairs, does not cause angina. Angina may occur with strenuous or rapid or prolonged exertion at work or recreation.

II There is *slight limitation* of ordinary activity. Angina may occur with walking or climbing stairs rapidly, walking uphill, walking or stair climbing after meals or in the cold, in the wind, or under emotional stress, or walking more than two blocks on the level, and climbing more than one flight of stairs at normal pace under normal conditions.

III There is *marked limitation* of ordinary physical activity. Angina may occur after walking one or two blocks on the level or climbing one flight of stairs under normal conditions at a normal pace.

IV There is inability to carry on any physical activity without discomfort; angina may be present at rest.

New York Heart Association Functional Classification‡

I Patients with cardiac disease but without resulting limitation of physical activity. Ordinary physical activity does not cause undue fatigue, palpitation, dyspnea, or anginal pain.

II Patients with cardiac diseases resulting in slight limitation of physical activity. They are comfortable at rest. Ordinary physical activity results in fatigue, palpitation, dyspnea, or anginal pain.

III Patients with cardiac diseases resulting in marked limitation of physical activity. They are comfortable at rest. Less than ordinary physical activity causes fatigue, palpitation, dyspnea, or anginal pain.

IV Patients with cardiac disease resulting in inability to carry on any physical activity without discomfort. Symptoms of cardiac insufficiency or of the anginal syndrome may be present even at rest. If any physical activity is undertaken, discomfort is increased.

‡From Society of Thoracic Surgeons.

---

3. A pericardial pad is positioned around the heart, and a temperature probe is placed into the myocardium while cardioplegia is administered; iced "slush" is placed around the heart.

4. The coronary artery is identified and incised with a microknife distal to the obstructive lesion. The incision is extended with microscissors. Dilators are used to calibrate and evaluate the artery.

5. A conduit is prepared for anastomosis to the coronary artery. If the saphenous vein is used, the assistant has prepared it by distending it with physiologic solution and tying any branches. The internal mam-

mary artery remains attached at the proximal end and is positioned through a pericardial incision.

6. The conduit is anastomosed to the coronary artery (Fig. 13-55). Support sutures are used to suture the internal mammary pedicle to the surface of the heart to prevent tension on the coronary suture line.

7. Cardioplegia is administered every 20 to 25 minutes until the distal anastomoses are completed.

8. The perfusionist is advised when to rewarm the patient's blood; warm blood can be administered through the retrograde cardioplegia line while proximal anastomoses are done, unless the aortic cross-

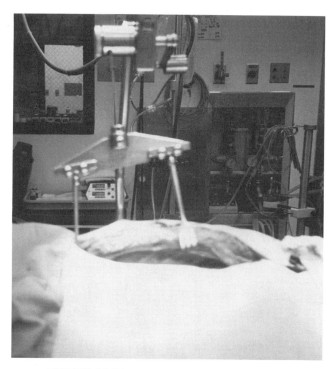

FIGURE 13-51 Internal mammary retractor.

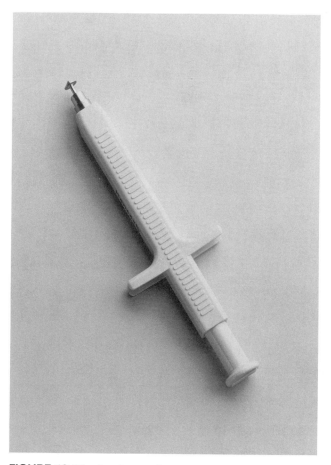

FIGURE 13-53 Aortic punch. (Reprinted with permission from Medtronic, Inc. © Medtronic, Inc., 1992.)

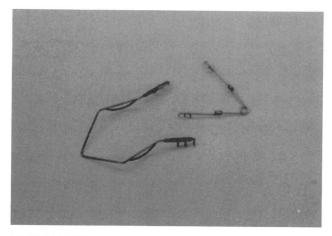

FIGURE 13-52 Parsonnette epicardial retractor: used to expose the coronary artery.

clamp is removed and a partial occlusion clamp is used.

9. The aorta can be cross-clamped with two clamps. The proximal anastomoses sites are incised and an aortic punch is used to make smooth, round openings. Vein grafts are sutured to the aorta.

10. Vascular bulldog clamps are placed on the vein grafts and the aortic clamps are removed.

11. Air is evacuated from the aorta and the vein grafts with a hypodermic needle, and the bulldog clamps are removed; flow is established to the coronary arteries.

12. The cardioplegia cannula and left ventricular vent are removed. Pacing wires are placed and the CPB is discontinued.

Use of gastroepiploic artery (GEA) for coronary artery bypass

Key steps

1. The sternal incision is extended distally to the abdomen.
2. The GEA is identified and dissected free.
3. Fine sutures and/or vessel clips are used to occlude arterial branches.
4. The distal end of the GEA is divided after heparin has been given.
5. The GEA is routed behind or in front of the liver through an incision in the diaphragm and into the pericardial space.
6. The GEA is prepared and anastomosed to the coronary artery. The GEA pedicle is secured with sutures to the heart surface (similar to internal mammary artery [IMA]) to prevent dislodgement (Fig. 13-56).
7. A standard closure is done (see Closure, earlier in this chapter).

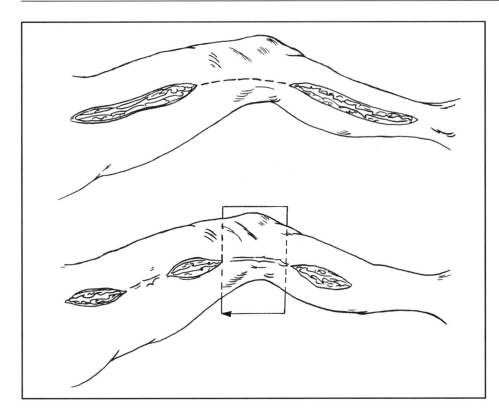

FIGURE 13-54 Incision sites for removing saphenous vein.

Repair of left ventricular aneurysm (LVA)

An aneurysm of the left ventricle is the result of a myocardial infarction that causes scarring and thinning of the myocardium. The degree of myocardial involvement will vary and result in akinesia, dyskinesia, or paradoxical motion of the ventricle. The anteroapical area is the most common site (Khonsari, 1988). Mural thombus may be present inside the aneurysmal area and the ventricle.

The first surgical repair of a LVA was in 1955 by Baily, and Cooley in 1958 was the first to repair a LVA while using CPB (Komeda et al., 1992).

Jantene of Brazil emphasized the importance of left ventricular reconstruction in the 1980s. The goal of the surgical repair is to restore the left ventricular geometry in order to obtain the best left ventricular function (Komeda et al., 1992).

Newer surgical techniques have reduced the mortality rate, but this operation remains a high-risk procedure. The repair may be by plication (taking a tuck in the aneurysmal area) or by excising the aneurysm and closing the ventricle. The septum may be involved, as well as the papillary muscles. Mitral valve replacement may be necessary if the papillary muscle cannot be repaired. Frequently, CABG procedures are done to revascularize myocardium.

Special instrumentation, equipment, and supplies

As for CABG, if necessary

Teflon felt, a large piece

Dacron patch

Sutures for aneurysm repair

Procedure

The usual sternotomy incision is done. The procedure for the CPB is usual, except two venous cannulae may be needed. No left ventricular vent is necessary. Cardioplegia is used.

Conventional resection

Key steps

1. An incision is made into the aneurysm; thrombus is removed if present. Aneurysmal tissue is resected, leaving a rim of fibrous tissue (Fig. 13-57,*A*).
2. The ventricle is closed with interrupted mattress sutures of nonabsorbable suture (braided polyester), using Teflon felt strips along each side of the suture line for reinforcement and to prevent cutting of the tissues by the suture (Fig. 13-57,*B*).
3. A continuous, over-and-over suture is used to reinforce the suture line. Additional felt strip may be used to cover the myocardial edges and prevent cutting by the over-and-over suture.

Reconstruction method

Key steps

1. The aneurysm is incised and excised as in the conventional resection.
2. The left ventricular wall is reconstructed to provide normal configuration and improve function.

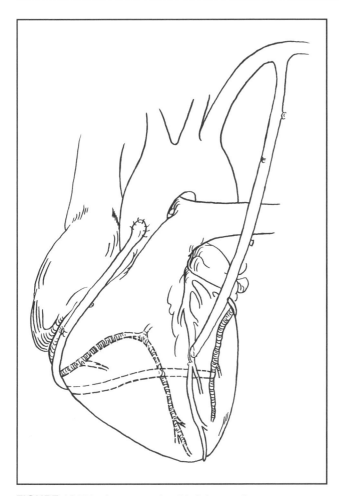

FIGURE 13-55 Anastomosis of left internal mammary artery into the left anterior descending coronary artery. Anastomosis of vein graft to the right coronary artery and circumflex artery.

3. A Dacron patch may be used to reconstruct the left ventricular wall and may be sutured to the endocardium with the left ventricular wall sutured over the patch to provide support (Fig. 13-58). An inverted T repair may be used for the reconstruction if adequate left ventricular myocardium is present (see Fig. 13-57,*C*).
4. The left ventricle is filled with saline or blood, and air is evacuated. A 10-ml syringe with an 18-gauge needle may be needed to aspirate air through the apex of the left ventricle.
5. An air-venting needle is placed in the aorta, and the aortic cross-clamp is removed.
6. Caval tapes have been released to facilitate filling of the heart.
7. Pacing wires are placed.
8. CPB is discontinued.
9. Standard closure is completed.

Repair of ventricular septal rupture

Necrosis of the septum can result from a myocardial infarction. This necrosis can result in perforation and/or

rupture of the septum. The anteroapical area is the most common site. CABG may be necessary to revascularize the myocardium. Repair of septal rupture is a surgical emergency, and if treated prior to the patient becoming compromised by cardiogenic shock, 40% to 60% survival is possible (Calderon & Ott, 1991).

Special instrumentation, equipment, and supplies

As for CABG, if necessary

Teflon felt

Dacron patch

Sutures for septal repair and closure of ventricle

Procedure

Key steps

1. A sternotomy is done.
2. CPB is usual except two venous cannulae are needed.
3. The left ventricle is vented through the ventricular septal defect (VSD).
4. Cardioplegia is accomplished.
5. The infarcted area of the ventricle (or ventricles) is incised. The necrotic area of the ventricular wall and septum is excised.
6. A Dacron patch may be used to repair the VSD; this is usually approached from a left ventricle incision. A transatrial (right) and transtricuspid valve approach sometimes is used to avoid incisional damage to the ventricle.
7. The upper edge of the Dacron patch may be incorporated into the ventricular suture line.
8. Ventricular closure is accomplished as in left ventricle aneurysmectomy (Fig. 13-59).
9. The left ventricle air is removed as with the left ventricle aneurysmectomy.
10. Pacing wires are placed.
11. CPB is discontinued.
12. Standard closure is accomplished.

Surgery for Valvular Heart Disease

The most common causes of heart valvular disease are rheumatic fever, degenerative changes, ischemia, congenital defects, and bacterial endocarditis (Table 13-6).

The valve may be stenotic (narrowed) or regurgitant (leaking, insufficient, incompetent) or a combination of these two problems. Most valvular disease occurs over time and is considered chronic; however, there are situations where there are acute changes requiring urgent attention.

The signs and symptoms that the patient experiences are related to the increased workload and strain on the heart. Common signs and symptoms are arrhythmias, cardiac enlargement, fatigue, chest pain, dyspnea, syncope, pulmonary hypertension, edema, and other indications of congestive heart failure (Hurst & Schlant, 1990).

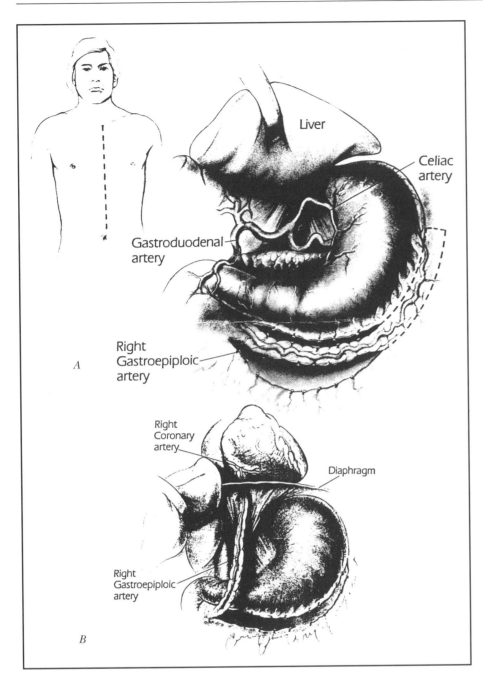

FIGURE 13-56 *A,* Dissection of the right gastroepiploic artery. *B,* Routing of the gastroepiploic artery through the diaphragm and anastomosis to the right coronary artery. (Reprinted with permission of Doty, D. *Cardiac Surgery.* [1985] Mosby-Year Book, Inc., St. Louis, MO.)

Historical perspective

Early interest in treating valvular heart disease began in 1898 when Samway suggested surgical incision of mitral valve stenosis. Early surgical approaches met with limited success until 1948, when Bailey and Harken demonstrated the effective use of mitral valve commissurotomy. A special cutting instrument (valvulotome) or the surgeon's finger was inserted inside the heart and across the valve, where the valve was cut or "fractured" to decrease the stenosis (McGoon, 1987).

Introduction of CPB allowed surgeons to approach heart valvular problems under direct vision, which improved the surgical results. The "closed" technique is still used in some countries, but the "open" technique is the accepted standard in the United States today. The advantages of the "open" technique are the ability to correct subvalvular stenosis, remove calcifications, correct regurgitation, and replace the valve if necessary (Pluth, 1987).

Surgical techniques

Refinements of techniques for repairing heart valves have occurred in recent years. Therefore, the surgeon will choose to repair the valve if that is possible. The introduction of intraoperative echocardiography allows the surgeon to evaluate the effectiveness of the valve repair at the time of surgery. If necessary, the surgeon can proceed with a valve replacement, thereby avoiding a second operation.

Artificial mechanical heart valves were successfully introduced in 1960 by Starr and Harken (Starek, 1987). In 1962, Ross in England and Barrat-Boyes in New Zealand initiated the clinical use of aortic and mitral homografts

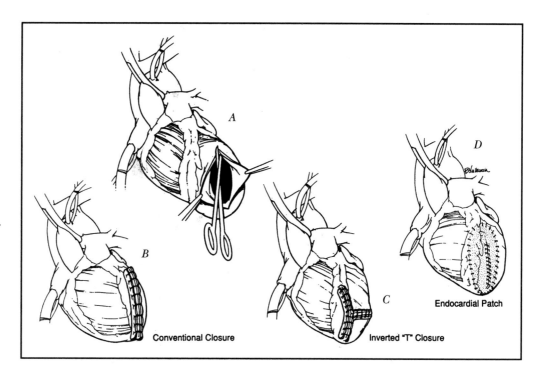

FIGURE 13-57 *A,* Resection of left ventricular aneurysm. *B,* Conventional repair of left ventricle after the aneurysm is excised. *C,* Inverted "T" repair after a left ventricular aneurysm is excised. *D,* Use of endocardial patch. (Reprinted with permission from Komeda, et al. Left Ventricular Aneurysm, The Society of Thoracic Surgeons [*The Annals of Thoracic Surgery,* 1992; 53:229].)

Conventional Closure

Inverted "T" Closure

Endocardial Patch

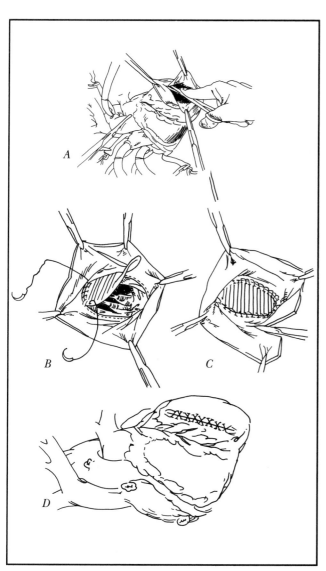

FIGURE 13-58 *A,* Resection of a left ventricular aneurysm. *B,* Suturing of a patch to the left ventricular wall: the epicardium has been retracted. *C,* The patch sutured into place. *D,* Epicardium is positioned and sutured over the left ventricular patch. (Redrawn with permission of *Texas Heart Institute Journal,* 16:73, 1989, Houston, TX.)

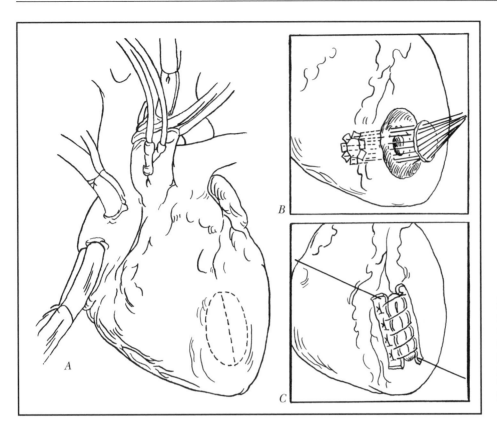

FIGURE 13-59 Repair of ruptured ventricular septum. (Adapted with permission from the illustrator Joan Livermore, CMI, from Khonsari, S. *Cardiac Surgery Safeguards: Pitfalls in Operating Techniques,* 1988, Raven Press, New York, NY.)

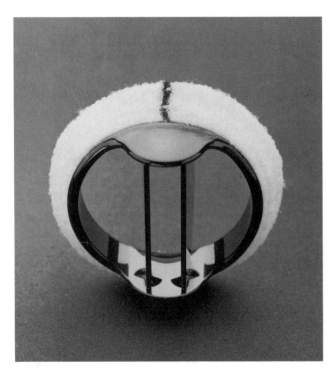

FIGURE 13-60 St. Jude Medical mechanical heart valve. (St. Jude is a registered trademark of St. Jude Medical, Inc.) (Courtesy of St. Jude Medical, Inc., St. Paul, MN.)

(Hopkins, 1989). Homografts are still used in some countries today. Ross also introduced the "Ross" procedure in 1967, in which the patient's pulmonary valve is transplanted to the aortic position: a pulmonary valve autograft. This technique is used today for a select group of patients (Constancia, 1991). Carpentier in Paris introduced the glutaraldehyde-preserved heterograft valve in 1968, and Hancock in the United States introduced the glutaraldehyde-treated porcine xenograft valve in 1970 (Bonchek, 1987). O'Brien, in Australia, developed the techniques of cellular preservation (cryopreservation) and introduced allografts in 1975 (Hopkins, 1989). Carpentier introduced the bovine pericardial aortic valve in Paris in 1980. This valve received Food and Drug Administration (FDA) approval for use in the United States in 1991 (Frater et al., 1991). There are several types of heart valves available worldwide that have not received FDA approval and are not available for use in the United States. Several valves have been removed from the market because of problems or known defects. Those valves used commonly in the United States will be discussed.

Types of heart valves

Basically, there are two types of heart valves: mechanical and tissue.

Mechanical

St. Jude: Bileaflet, pyrolytic carbon discs (Fig. 13-60)

Medtronic-Hall: Single, tilting disc coated with pyrolytic carbon (Fig. 13-61)

TABLE 13-6 Common Causes of Valvular Heart Disease

	Stenosis	Regurgitation
Mitral valve	Rheumatic fever	Mitral leaflet prolapse Congenital
	Congenital	Myxomatous degeneration
	Thrombus	Ischemia
		Papillary muscle
	Atrial myxoma	dysfunction or rupture
		Ruptured chordae tendineae
	Bacterial vegetation	
		Left ventricular dilatation
	Degenerative calcification	Rheumatic fever
		Connective tissue disorders
		(e.g., Marfan's)
		Calcification of annulus
		Congenital
		Systemic lupus erythematosus
		Infective endocarditis
		Trauma
Aortic valve	Congenital (bicuspid or	Rheumatic fever
	unicuspid)	
		Syphilis
	Rheumatic fever	
		Aortitis (Takayasu)
	Degenerative calcification	Aorticoannuloectasis
		Connective tissue disorders
		Congenital
		Arthritic diseases
		Cystic medial necrosis (aorta)
		Hypertension
		Arteriosclerosis
		Myxomatous degeneration
		Infective endocarditis
		Acute aortic dissection
		Trauma
Tricuspid valve	Rheumatic fever	Right ventricular dilatation
	Carcinoid syndrome	Infectious endocarditis
	Endocardial fibro-elastosis	Myocardial infarction
	Endomyocardial fibrosis	Trauma
	Lupus erythematosus	Carcinoid syndrome
	Right atrial myxoma	Congenital
	Tumor	
	Thrombus	
	Congenital	
Pulmonic valve	Congenital	Pulmonary hypertension
	Tumor	Inflammatory lesions
	Carcinoid syndrome	Rheumatic fever
		Endocarditis
		Tumors
		Carcinoid syndrome

Adapted from Hurst, J. W., & Schlant, R. C. (1990). *The heart* (7th ed.). San Francisco: McGraw-Hill.

Starr-Edwards: Silastic ball inside a stellite cage (Figs. 13-62 and 13-63)

Omniscience: Single, pyrolytic carbon disc

Tissue

Carpentier-Edwards: Porcine valve leaflets; preserved and mounted to a frame (Fig. 13-64)

Carpentier-Edwards: Bovine pericardial aortic valves; tailored, preserved, and mounted to a frame (Fig. 13-65)

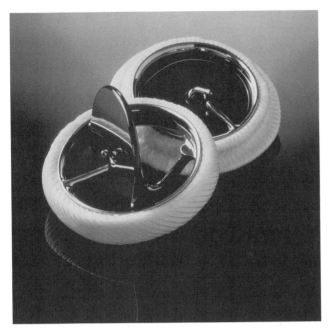

FIGURE 13-61 Medtronic-Hall aortic and mitral valve replacement. (Reprinted with permission from Medtronic, Inc. © Medtronic, Inc., 1992.)

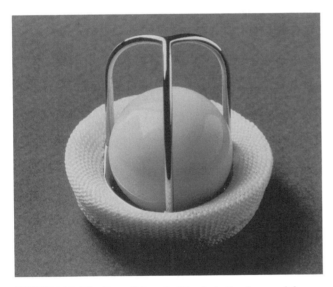

FIGURE 13-62 Starr-Edwards Silastic ball valve model 1260 (aortic) cage. (Courtesy of Edwards CVS Division of Baxter Healthcare Corp.)

Hancock: Porcine valve leaflets; preserved and mounted to a frame

Allografts: Cryopreserved human heart valves (Fig. 13-66)

Autograft: Use of patient's pulmonic valve for aortic valve replacement (Fig. 13-67)

Homografts: Use of fresh human heart valve; antibiotically treated

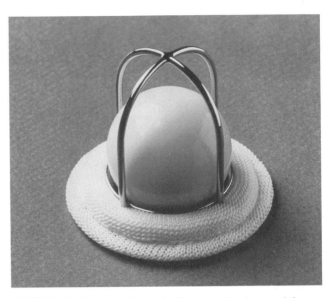

FIGURE 13-63 Starr-Edwards Silastic ball valve model 6120 (mitral). (Courtersy of Edwards CVS Division of Baxter Healthcare Corp.)

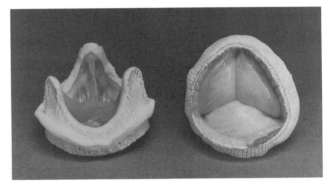

A

FIGURE 13-64 Carpentier-Edwards porcine valves. *A*, Aortic. *B*, Mitral. (Courtesy of Edwards CVS Division of Baxter Healthcare Corp.)

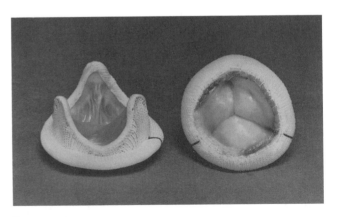

B

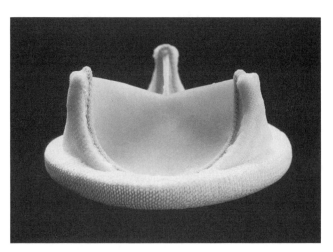

FIGURE 13-65 Carpentier-Edwards bovine pericardial valve. (Courtesy of Edward CVS Division of Baxter Healthcare Corp.)

Selection of a heart valve

The surgeon, patient, and cardiologist are involved preoperatively in the decision regarding the selection of the artificial heart valve. The major considerations are durability and the need for anticoagulants. The mechanical valves are more durable and have a longer life expectancy, whereas the tissue valve may need to be re-replaced in 10 to 15 years because of degenerative changes (perforations, tears in leaflets). Porcine and bovine tissue valves are usually not used in children under 18 years of age because the patient's high serum calcium level will cause the valve leaflets to calcify. The mechanical valves are more thrombogenic, and anticoagulation is a life-long need for almost all patients. For those patients in whom anticoagulation would be contraindicated, the tissue valve would be the valve of choice. Examples of patients who should not take anticoagulants are:

- Patients with medical conditions with the potential for hemorrhage (e.g., ulcers)
- Patients with social or mental conditions that may interfere with compliance related to taking anticoagulants
- Patients who engage in hazardous activities that could result in injury and bleeding into tissues or joints
- Patients who desire future pregnancies

The allograft valves are more durable than other tissue valves but there are problems related to accessibility, preservation, and storage techniques, as well as technical difficulty with their surgical implantation (Starek, 1987; Hopkins, 1989).

Mitral valve surgery

Special instrumentation, equipment, and supplies

Retractor for exposing the mitral valve (Fig. 13-68)

Allis clamps for grasping the valve

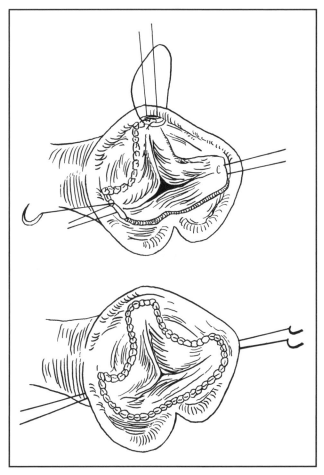

FIGURE 13-66 Suturing of aortic allograft valve into position. (Adapted from Hopkins, R. A. *Cardiac Reconstruction with Allograft Valves,* 1989, Springer-Verlag New York, Inc. New York, NY.)

Sutures for:
    Valve repair or replacement (with or without Teflon felt pledgets)
    Closure of the atrium

Valve sizers (Fig. 13-69)

Prosthetic valves and holder (assortment of sizes and types of valves are usually necessary)

Annuloplasty rings (see Fig. 13-73)

Suture holders (Fig. 13-70)

Single venous cannula (2) and Y connector

Suction tip with open end

Foley catheter for holding valve in open position

Rongeur

Echocardiogram machine with transesophageal probe

Procedure

Key steps

1. The usual sternotomy incision is done (left posterolateral incision can be used).

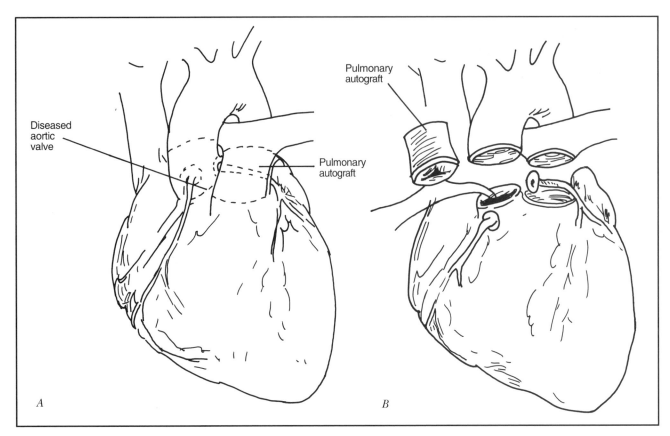

FIGURE 13-67 *A*, Pulmonary autograft prepared to suture into aortic root. *B*, Pulmonary allograft (with pulmonic valve) sutured into the pulmonary artery position. Pulmonary autograft sutured into aortic position. Adapted from Constancia, P. The Ross Procedure, *Critical Care Nursing Clinics of North America,* 1991, 3:4; 717. 721, W. B. Saunders Co., Philadelphia, PA.)

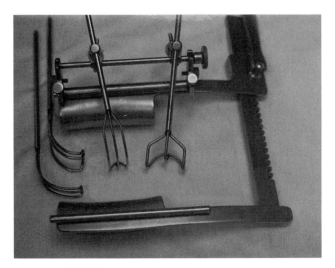

FIGURE 13-68 Cosgrove mitral retractor.

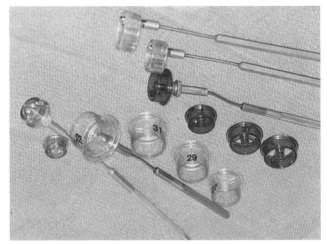

FIGURE 13-69 Valve sizers, used to measure the annulus after the patient's native valve has been removed. This instrument determines the size of the prosthetic valve needed.

2. CPB: two venous cannulae and tapes are placed around the inferior vena cava and the superior vena cava.

3. The aorta is cross-clamped.

4. Cardioplegia is accomplished.

5. A left atrial incision is carried out (Fig. 13-71,*A*).

6. A right atrial incision may be used, with access to the mitral valve through an incision in the atrial septum.

7. The atrial walls are retracted, taking care to avoid tearing or injuring the atrium and/or surrounding structures (Fig. 13-71,*B*)

8. Sutures may be placed through the valve leaflets for traction on the valve.

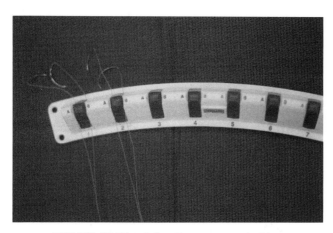

FIGURE 13-70 Gabey-Frater suture holder.

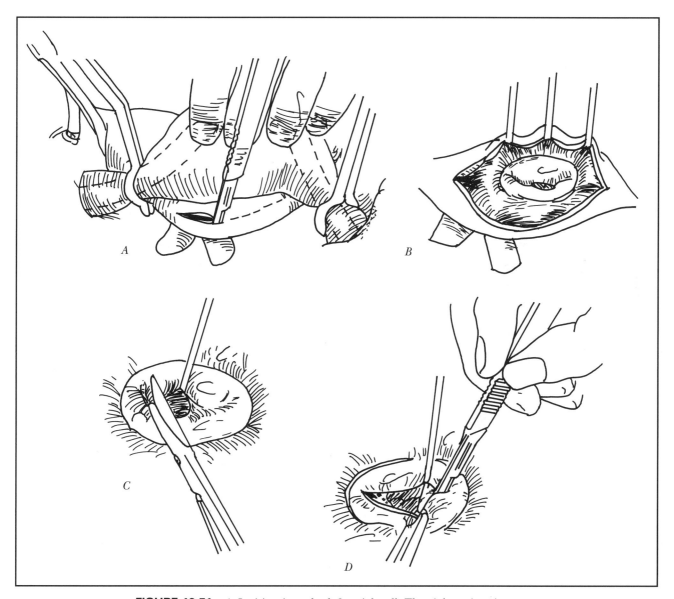

FIGURE 13-71 *A,* Incision into the left atrial wall. The right atrium is retracted by an assistant. *B,* Atrial retractor in position, exposing the mitral valve. *C,* Commissurotomy with scissors. *D,* Commissurotomy with knife.
(Adapted from Cooley, D. *Techniques in Cardiac Surgery, 2/e,* 1984, W. B. Saunders Co., Philadelphia, PA.)

Valve repair procedures

Commissurotomy of fused valve leaflets Commissures can be cut with scissors or a knife (Fig. 13-71,*C* and *D*).

Annuloplasty This is done to reduce the size of the annulus and prevent regurgitation.

1. Suture technique (Fig. 13-72)
2. Ring annuloplasty (Fig. 13-73). Rigid, semirigid, flexible, and adjustable styles of rings are available.

Chordae tendineae repair

1. Elongated chordae can be repaired by various chordoplasty procedures.
2. Ruptured chordae may be repaired by various techniques.
   a. Quadrangular resection of the prolapsed segment of the valve leaflet and reapproximation with suture (Fig. 13-74)
   b. Plication of valve leaflet (Fig. 13-74,*A*)
   c. Attachment of leaflet to papillary muscle with suture (Fig. 13-74)
   d. Replacement of ruptured chordae with expanded polytetrafluoroethylene suture (Gore-Tex)

Valve replacement

Key steps

1. The valve is retracted with sutures or an Allis clamp.
2. The leaflets are excised with a #15 knifeblade or scissors.
3. The chordae and a portion of the papillary muscle are excised with scissors. The posterior valve leaflet and chordal attachments and papillary muscle are left intact if possible (important for ventricular contractility). Excessive resection of papillary muscle may result in left ventricular wall rupture.

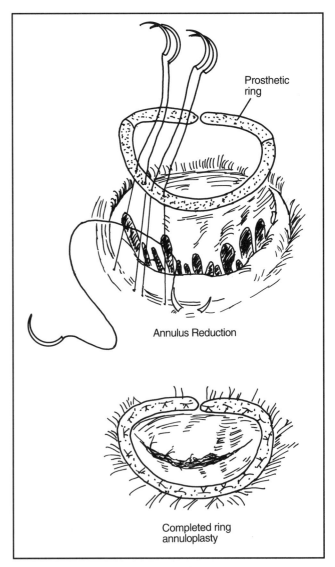

Prosthetic ring

Annulus Reduction

Completed ring annuloplasty

FIGURE 13-73 Mitral valve annuloplasty: ring technique. (Adapted with permission from the illustrator Joan Livermore, CMI, from Khonsari, *Cardiac Surgery Safeguards: Pitfalls in Operating Techniques,* 1988, Raven Press, New York, NY.)

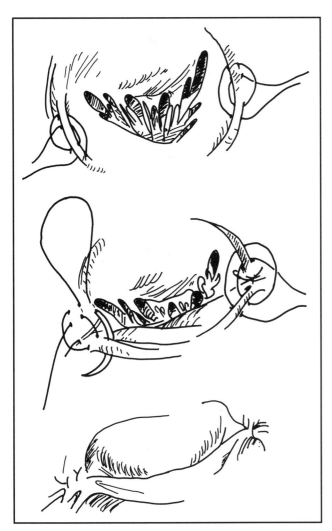

FIGURE 13-72 Mitral valve annuloplasty: suture technique.

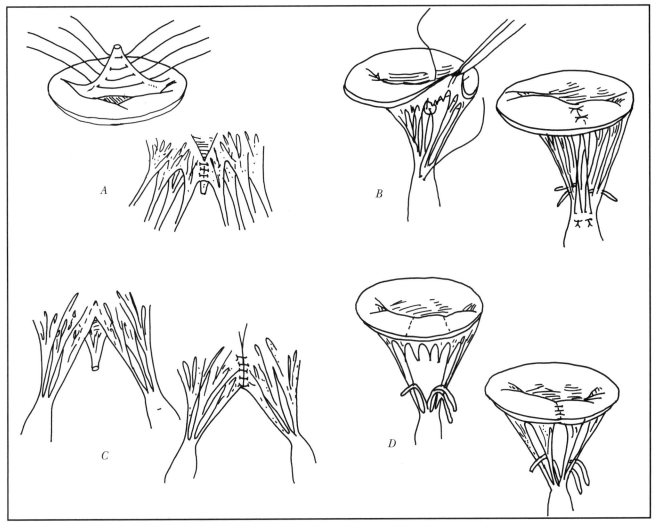

FIGURE 13-74 *A,* Plication of valve leaflet. *B* and *C,* Attachment of leaflet to papillary muscle with suture. *D,* Quadrangular resection of valve leaflet. (From McGoon, D. [1987]. *Cardiac surgery, Ed. 2.* Chap. 10, figure 2, page 133. With permission of F. A. Davis Company.)

4. Valve sizers are used to measure the annulus and determine the size of the prosthesis.
5. Valve sutures are placed into the valve annulus and kept in order with hemostat clamps or a special suture holder (see Fig. 13-70).
6. The valve prosthesis is obtained from the circulating nurse:
   - Verify the type, size, model (mitral versus aortic), and identification number.
   - Handle carefully to avoid damage.
   - Tissue valves:
     Do not touch the leaflets.
     Use care not to deform the cage.
     Follow rinsing instructions to remove glutaraldehyde.
     Do not use antibiotic solution because it will damage the leaflets.
     Keep the valve in the final rinse solution to prevent drying.

Keep the valve moist with saline while placing sutures in the sewing ring.
7. Valve holders are used to minimize chance of possible damage.
8. Sutures are placed through sewing ring and valve is slid into place (Fig. 13-75). Forceps with protected tips may be used to position valve as it is tied into place.
9. Sutures are cut.

Closure of left atrium

Key steps

1. A Foley catheter is placed across the valve into the left ventricle in order to keep the valve from closing and trapping air in the heart. The balloon is filled with saline, not air, in the event of rupture.
2. The atrial incision is closed, leaving space for the catheter.
3. Air is evacuated from the heart:
   The patient is placed in Trendelenburg's position.

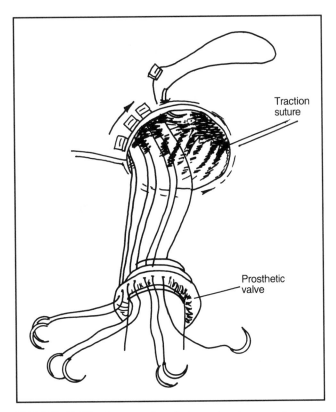

FIGURE 13-75 Sutures placed through valve annulus and through prosthetic valve sewing ring.

The vena caval tapes are released.

The venous return line is partially occluded and blood goes through the heart and fills it.

The aortic root is vented with a hypodermic needle to remove any air.

The aortic cross-clamp is removed.

4. The heart is defibrillated.
5. The Foley catheter balloon is deflated and removed from the heart.
6. Atrial sutures are tied and cut.
7. CPB is discontinued.
8. Standard closure is done.

Aortic valve surgery

Special instrumentation, equipment, and supplies

Valve leaflet retractors

Sutures for:
  Valve repair or replacement (with or without Teflon felt pledgets)
  Closure of aorta

Teflon felt strips

Valve sizers, holders, and prosthetic valves

Suture holders

A two-stage venous cannula

Discard suction tip with open end

Coronary cannula

Rongeur

Echocardiogram machine with transesophageal probe

Procedure

Key steps

1. A sternotomy incision is made.
2. CPB: use single two-stage venous cannula.
3. The aorta is cross-clamped.
4. Cardioplegia is accomplished:
   Retrograde (standard procedure)
   Antegrade: The initial dose is given through the aorta before the incision is made; subsequent doses are administered through a special coronary cannula.
5. Left ventricle venting is done.
6. Retraction sutures are placed in epicardial fat overlaying the aortic root; sutures are placed on the anterior aorta on each side of the incision site.
7. Aortic incision
   Low transverse incision is made 10 to 15 mm above the origin of the right coronary artery (most common).
   Oblique incision starts high on the lateral aspect of the aorta and descends diagonally to the noncoronary sinus.
   Valve leaflet retractors are used to retract the aorta and expose the valve.

Valve repair procedure

Key steps

1. A commissurotomy is done as in mitral valve surgery.
2. Plication or resection of a portion of the valve leaflet is done to restore competence to the valve.

Valve replacement procedure

Key steps

1. Leaflets are excised with scissors and/or a #15 knife blade.
2. Calcification in the valve annulus is removed with a rongeur.
3. The left ventricular cavity is inspected and irrigated to remove any debris from the valve resection.
4. Valve size is determined; a valve is obtained; sutures are inserted as in mitral valve surgery:
   If an allograft valve is used, thawing and handling instructions must be followed closely
5. Closure of the aorta is accomplished.
   Teflon felt strips may be used on each side of the aortic incision to bolster sutures and prevent tearing of the tissues.
   Sutures are placed, starting from each end of the incision and meeting in the center of the incision.
6. Prior to tying the sutures together:
   The patient is placed in Trendelenburg's position; the heart is filled with blood and air is evacuated.
   The cross-clamp is removed from the aorta and air escapes through the aortic opening; the sutures are then tied together.

7. Aortic root vented with hypodermic needle.
8. The left ventricle vent is removed.
9. Pacing wires are placed.
10. CPB is discontinued.
11. Standard closure is done.

Tricuspid valve surgery

Special instrumentation, equipment, and supplies

Retractors for the right atrium

Sutures for:
   Valve repair or replacement (with or without Teflon felt pledgets)
   Closure of right atrium

Valve sizers

Prosthetic valves and holders (assortment of sizes and types of valves that may be needed)

Annuloplasty rings

Suture holders

Single venous cannulae (2) and Y connector

Discard suction tip with open end

Echocardiogram machine with transesophageal probe

Procedure

Key steps

1. A sternotomy incision is made.
2. CPB is accomplished. Two venous cannulae are placed and tapes around the venae cavae are tightened prior to opening the atrium.
3. The aorta is cross-clamped.
4. Cardioplegia is accomplished.
5. Left ventricle venting is done.
6. A right atrial incision is made.
7. Atrial walls are retracted.
8. Sutures are placed through the valve leaflets for traction if necessary.

Valve repair procedures

Commissurotomy is done as in mitral valve surgery (rare).

Annuloplasty is accomplished as in mitral valve surgery.

Chordae tendineae repairs are not indicated.

Valve replacement procedure

This is the same as in mitral valve surgery, but is rarely done.

Closure of right atrium

The right ventricle and the atrium are allowed to fill with blood as the atrium is sutured (this removes any air).

The aortic cross-clamp is removed, the left ventricle vent is removed, and pacing wires are placed.

CPB is discontinued.

Standard closure is done.

Pulmonic valve surgery

Special instrumentation, equipment, and supplies

Valve leaflet retractors

Single venous cannulae (2)

Sutures for closure of pulmonary artery

Echocardiogram machine with transesophageal probe

Procedure

Key steps

1. A sternotomy is done.
2. CPB: two venous cannulae are placed as are the occlusion tapes around the venae cavae. Cardioplegia is optional.
3. The pulmonary artery incision is usually longitudinal above the valve, and leaflet retractors or sutures are used to provide exposure.
4. Commissurotomy is the most common procedure as valve replacement is rare.
5. As the PA is closed, the right heart is allowed to fill with blood and air is removed.
6. The vena caval tapes are released after the PA is closed.
7. CPB is discontinued.
8. Standard closure is done.

Surgery for Congenital Heart Defects (CHD)

Pediatric cardiac surgery is a highly challenging and demanding practice area for the perioperative nurse. Sophisticated team work and technical exactness are essential characteristics. Unique knowledge and skill are needed to provide surgical care for pediatric patients. Imagination, ingenuity, courage, and competence are needed to surgically manage the magnitude and complexity of congenital heart defects. Some heart teams may find it necessary to transport children to other cardiac surgery centers where the technology and personnel are available to surgically treat complex congenital defects.

Correction of cardiac defects is being done earlier because there is better recognition and understanding of the advantages in relation to cardiac, pulmonary, and cerebral function (Crupi et al., 1990). Advances in diagnostic technology, supportive care, and operative techniques are significant factors. Controversies and variations in surgical interventions will continue as we strive to determine what procedures provide the best outcomes for our patients.

The causes of CHD are related to environmental and genetic factors (Hurst & Schlant, 1990). The American Heart Association has identified 35 recognizable forms of CHD, and approximately 30,000 infants are born annually in the United States with such defects (American Heart Association, 1992).

The signs and symptoms of CHD will vary based on the type of defect and the degree of physiological alteration. The major complications, which can be severe and cause the patient to be critically ill, are congestive heart failure, cyanosis, pulmonary artery hypertension and pulmonary vascular obstructive disease (related to excessive pulmonary circulation), growth and developmental retardation, and exertional limitations.

Surgical insult is less tolerated in the pediatric patient with an immature heart because of structural, metabolic, and functional differences from the adult heart. The patient with a congenitally malformed heart is subject to preoperative stress that can affect recovery (Corno, 1990).

CPB techniques for the pediatric patient must consider the patient's size and blood volume (85 ml/kg for a neonate), as well as the complexity of the operative procedure. Hemodilution techniques decrease blood viscosity, vasoconstriction, and pulmonary and/or coagulation problems. For patients who weigh less than 12 kilograms there is increased risk of fluid retention. Blood is usually added to the CPB primer fluid because the fluid volume needed to prime (e.g., pump tubing, oxygenator) far exceeds the patient's blood volume.

Hypothermia techniques are used to protect the patient while on CPB. Moderate (24 to 26° C) hypothermia is commonly used, but deep hypothermia (18° C) and circulatory arrest may be necessary for adequate protection and operative exposure. A maximum of 30 to 40 minutes of circulatory arrest is ideal for preventing brain damage, although longer periods of circulatory arrest have been reported (Monro, 1990). Cold cardioplegia is used for myocardial protection and the desired myocardial temperature is <10° C. Cardioplegia is readministered every 20 to 25 minutes while the aorta is cross-clamped.

For most pediatric procedures, two venous cannulae are needed. Occlusive venal caval tapes are needed for preventing airlock in the venous line when the heart is opened.

Because of platelet destruction while the patient is on CPB, platelets are usually administered after the patient is rewarmed in order to prevent bleeding problems.

Special instrumentation, supplies, and equipment

Instrumentation

Chest retractors (sternal and rib spreaders), variety of sizes

Vascular clamps, various sizes and angles (small, delicate) (see Fig. 13-23)

Sternal saw

Tissue forceps, scissors, needle holders; designed for microscopic surgery (see Figs. 13-24, 13-25, and 13-28)

Malleable retractors, various small sizes

Hegar dilators for dilating aorta for cannulation and to measure vascular or valvular sizes or openings

Supplies

Specially designed cannulae (venous and arterial)

Small chest tubes, urinary catheters, arterial monitoring lines

Microvascular sutures, nonabsorbable and absorbable

Vessel loops, regular and fine sizes

Tourniquets, small sizes

Prosthetic graft material, Dacron and PTFE patch and tube grafts in variety of sizes

Conduits, Dacron prosthetic devices or allografts

Pediatric defibrillator and paddles (external and internal)

Equipment

Echocardiogram machine with transesophageal and/or epicardial probe

Modified positioning devices

Procedure

A median sternotomy incision is used for most cardiac procedures requiring CPB. Anterolateral and posterolateral thoracotomy incisions are indicated for selected procedures and will be identified.

The thymus gland is usually present in children and is resected to facilitate exposure.

The size of the heart varies with patient age and size. A neonate's heart is approximately 3 cm in length from the apex to the base. Surgical techniques must be precise to avoid injury.

Cardioplegia is usually administered antegrade through the aortic root. Retrograde cannulae are available for pediatric patients but rarely are needed.

The left ventricle can be vented as in an adult patient, but in situations where the heart chambers are opened, the venting can be done within the heart (i.e., across the septum).

Surgeons use extreme care not to damage the cardiac conduction system, but the potential of injury exists. Therefore, temporary pacing wires, especially ventricular, are frequently needed.

Echocardiography (epicardial or transesophageal) is used for many of the cardiac surgeries for repair of CHD to determine the effectiveness of the surgical correction or repair (Fig. 13-76). This is used after the patient is removed from CPB and before the chest is closed. If necessary, the patient can be returned to CPB for additional surgery.

Systemic–pulmonary artery shunts

The goal of a systemic to pulmonary artery shunt is to increase the blood flow through the pulmonary circula-

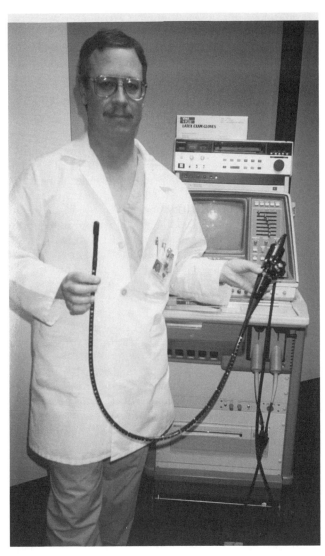

FIGURE 13-76 Echocardiography machine. The esophageal probe is held by the technician.

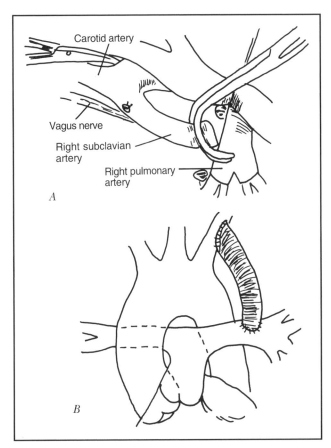

FIGURE 13-77 *A,* Classic Blalock Taussig shunt: right subclavian artery to right pulmonary artery. *B,* Modified Blalock Taussig shunt: PTFE tubular graft positioned between left subclavian and left pulmonary arteries.

tion and increase oxygenation of the blood. The shunt may also be needed to promote growth of hypoplastic pulmonary arteries (Pacifico & Sand, 1987).

Advances in corrective surgery for infants have decreased the indications for shunts. However, shunts may be needed for palliation or as a first-stage repair of a cardiac defect (Amato et al, 1988).

The modified Blalock-Taussig, the classic Blalock-Taussig, and central shunts are the most common shunts used today (Pacifico & Sand, 1987; Amato et al., 1988). The Waterston and Potts shunts have generally been abandoned because of increased incidence of congestive heart failure, pulmonary hypertension, or pulmonary vascular disease. Both are anatomically difficult to do and difficult to disconnect later. The Glenn shunt has limited application today (Pacifico & Sand, 1987; Doty, 1985).

These procedures do not require CPB, but the patient does need to be heparinized (1 mg/kg) prior to clamping any vessels. The heparin is usually reversed with protamine.

Classic Blalock-Taussig A lateral thoracotomy incision is used. The subclavian artery is clamped with a vascular clamp and divided. The distal end is ligated or sutured closed. The proximal end is mobilized and positioned so it can be anastomosed to the side of the pulmonary artery (right or left) (Fig. 13-77).

Modified Blalock-Taussig A lateral thoracotomy incision is used. The subclavian artery is isolated and clamped with a vascular clamp in a manner that permits incision into the side of the artery. The proximal end of a PTFE tube graft is sutured to the side of the subclavian artery. The distal end of the PTFE tube graft is sutured in a similar manner to the side of the pulmonary artery (see Fig. 13-77).

Central shunt A median sternotomy is used. A partial occlusion vascular clamp is used on the side of the ascending aorta and another similar clamp is used on the side of the main pulmonary artery. Incisions are made into both vessels and a short PTFE tube graft is sutured into place. Care is taken not to kink or curve the graft (Fig. 13-78).

Waterston shunt A right lateral thoracotomy incision is used. A partial occlusion vascular clamp is used to occlude the posterior segment of the ascending aorta. The right

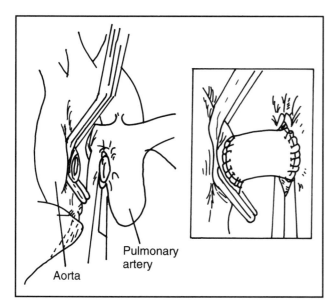

FIGURE 13-78 Central shunt: PTFE tubular graft placed between the aorta and the pulmonary artery.

pulmonary artery is occluded and incisions are made into the sides of both arteries. The two vessels are anastomosed together.

Potts shunt A left lateral thoracotomy incision is used. The left branch of the pulmonary artery is occluded with vessel loops or ligatures. The descending aorta is clamped with a partial occlusion vascular clamp. Incisions are made in both vessels and a side-to-side anastomosis is done.

Glenn shunt A median sternotomy or right anterolateral incision is used. The superior vena cava (SVC) is mobilized and the azygous vein is ligated. The right pulmonary artery is mobilized, ligated, and divided as close to the main pulmonary artery as possible. The proximal end of the pulmonary artery is sutured closed and the distal end is occluded with vessel loops or a vascular clamp. A partial occlusion vascular clamp is placed on the SVC at the site of the azygous vein. The azygous vein is divided and an incision is extended into the side of the SVC. The distal end of the divided pulmonary artery is anastomosed to the side of the SVC. The SVC is ligated below the anastomosis site (toward the heart). All of the flow from the SVC is then diverted into the right pulmonary artery.

Pulmonary artery banding

The purpose of banding the pulmonary artery is to decrease blood flow through the pulmonary circulation. There are limited indications for its use today.

A left anterolateral or median sternotomy incision is used. This procedure does not require CPB. The pulmonary artery is mobilized proximally and encircled with a band of cotton umbilical tape, PTFE graft, or Teflon felt. The pressures in the pulmonary artery and in the systemic system are measured simultaneously and the band

is tightened until the pulmonary artery pressure is one-half of the systemic pressure, or 40 mm Hg. The band is secured with sutures and sutured to the adventitia of the pulmonary artery to prevent migration. The band will be removed when more definitive surgery is done (Khonsari, 1988).

Patent ductus arteriosus (PDA) closure

The ductus arteriosus is the normal communication between the pulmonary artery and the aorta during fetal circulation. The ductus normally closes within 2 to 3 weeks after birth and the ligamentum arteriosum is formed. The ductus is located at the origin of the left pulmonary artery and connects to the lower aspect of the aortic arch beyond the origin of the left subclavian artery.

If the ductus does not close, the flow from the aorta into the pulmonary circulation can cause heart failure and/or pulmonary hypertension. The risk of infectious endarteritis is always present. Early surgical intervention is needed for the newborn with uncontrollable heart failure or for the premature infant in order to decrease pulmonary problems. Elective surgical intervention is done at from 6 months to 2 years of age (Hurst & Schlant, 1990).

The first successful surgical correction of a PDA was done in 1939 by Gross (Cooley, 1984). This procedure is done without CPB or heparinization. It is not uncommon to operate on premature infants right in the neonatal intensive care unit.

Procedure

Key steps

1. A left posterolateral thoracotomy incision is used. The ductus can be closed through a median sternotomy if other surgery is indicated.
2. The lung is retracted with a moist sponge and a malleable retractor.
3. The parietal pleura is opened and retracted with sutures.
4. The duct is dissected free, and heavy suture or an umbilical tape is passed around the duct.
5. The surgeon may dissect the aorta free, above and below the duct, and pass vessel loops or tapes around the aorta for control of any bleeding should the aorta tear at the ductal site. The duct may be ligated with a suture or metallic clip and may or may not be divided (Fig. 13-79).
6. When necessary (e.g., large ductus), vascular clamps may be placed across the duct. The duct can be divided between the clamps with a knife and the ductal ends can be closed by suturing, starting with the aortic side first (Fig. 13-79).

Coarctation of the aorta

This defect is a narrowing of the distal segment of the aortic arch. Approximately 50% of the infants born with this defect present with congestive heart failure within the

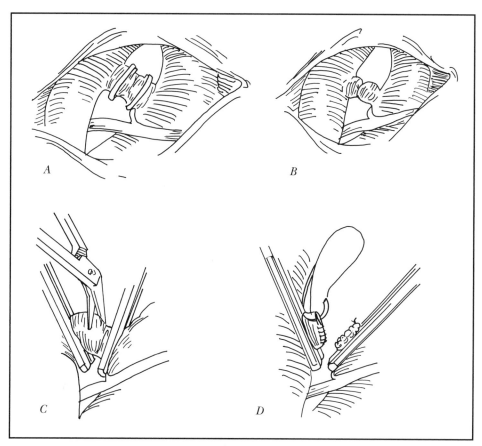

FIGURE 13-79   *A*, Use of a metallic clip to ligate a patent ductus arteriosus (PDA). *B*, Use of suture to ligate a PDA. *C*, Use of vascular clamp on a PDA and dividing with scissors. *D*, Suture closure of PDA sites on the aorta and pulmonary artery.

first month of life. A classic sign is a decrease in blood pressure in the lower extremities, with diminished or absent femoral pulses. Early surgical repair is indicated for infants not responding to medical therapy. Coarctations must be corrected to prevent cardiac and vascular complications (Hurst & Schlant, 1990).

When the defect has been repaired on an infant, recoarctation can occur as the aorta grows. Recoarctation is defined as a 20-mm Hg gradient between the blood pressure in the right arm and the legs (Amato et al., 1991).

Balloon dilation of the coarctation was introduced in the 1980s but is recommended for infants with complex intracardiac defects. This procedure has a high restenosis rate and aneurysm formation of the aorta (Messmer et al., 1991). The first repair of coarctation of the aorta was done in 1945 by Crawford in Sweden (Cooley, 1984).

Procedure

Key steps

1. A left posterolateral thoracotomy incision is used. Exposure is as for PDA.
2. The left subclavian artery and aorta are exposed and mobilized.
3. Vessel loops or tapes are passed around the aorta above and below the coarctation and around the subclavian artery.
4. If a PDA is present it is ligated and divided.
5. There are several repair techniques, and the choice usually depends on the length of the coarctation (Fig. 13-80).
   a. End-to-end anastomosis (this is the procedure of choice) (Jonas, 1991; Messmer et al., 1991)
   b. Patch enlargement of the aorta
   c. Subclavian flap aortoplasty
   d. Subclavian displacement aortoplasty
   e. Interposition graft insertion

Coarctation of the aorta with hypoplastic aortic arch

Hypoplasia can occur in various portions of the aortic arch in association with coarctation. The types of hypoplasia are:

Type I: distal arch (82%)

Type II: entire arch (13%)

Type III: absence of proximal arch (5%) (Lacour-Gayet, 1991)

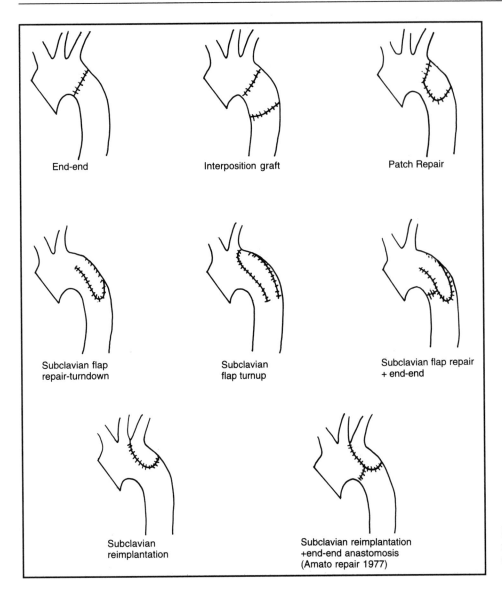

End-end

Interposition graft

Patch Repair

Subclavian flap
repair-turndown

Subclavian
flap turnup

Subclavian flap repair
+ end-end

Subclavian
reimplantation

Subclavian reimplantation
+end-end anastomosis
(Amato repair 1977)

FIGURE 13-80 Various methods of repairing coarctation of the aorta.

Approximately 24% to 50% of patients with coarctation have hypoplasia of the arch. Repair of this condition is limited to infants with extreme degrees of hypoplasia that restricts blood flow and strains the left ventricle (Siewers et al., 1991).

Procedure

Key steps

1. The incision is similar to that done for coarctation repair or median sternotomy.
2. The proximal and distal aorta are dissected free and encircled with vessel loops or tapes.
3. The left carotid and subclavian arteries are also dissected free and may be encircled with tapes or vessel loops.
4. The proximal aorta is cross-clamped with a vascular clamp.
5. The distal aorta and, if necessary, the other arteries are occluded with vascular clamps and/or vessel loops.
6. The PDA is ligated and divided.

7. The coarctation area of the aorta is excised and the underside of the hypoplastic arch is incised proximally to the normal area of the aorta.
8. The distal aorta is tailored to fit the proximal aorta incision, and the two portions of aorta are sutured together (Fig. 13-81).

Interruption of the aortic arch

In this defect there is a lack of continuity between the aortic arch and the descending aorta. Blood flow to the descending aorta comes from the PDA. Over 90% of these infants have a ventricular septal defect (VSD). These infants require surgery usually within the first few days of life because of congestive heart failure. Primary or staged repair may be done for patients with a VSD. The staged repair will include banding of the pulmonary artery with the surgery for the interruption. Primary repair would include closure of the VSD and surgery for the interruption. It has only been recently that these patients have been treated successfully with surgery (Irwin et al., 1991).

Types of interruptions to the aortic arch are:

Type A: distal to the left subclavian artery (42%)

Type B: distal to the left carotid artery (53%)

Type C: distal to the innominate or right carotid artery (5%) (Fig. 13-82) (Hurst & Schlant, 1990)

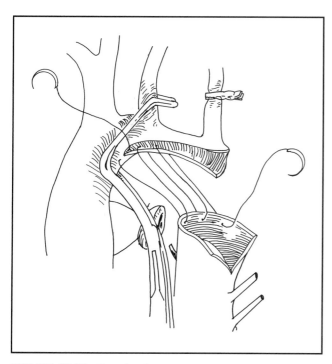

FIGURE 13-81 Repair of coarctation of the aorta with hypoplastic aortic arch. Incisions in the aortic arch and distal aorta are sutured together.

Procedure

Key steps

1. Incision is as for PDA.
2. A partial occlusion vascular clamp is applied to the side of the ascending aorta, and a vascular clamp is placed across the proximal end of the descending aorta.
3. The PDA is ligated and divided.
4. A PTFE tubular vascular graft is sutured end to side to the ascending aorta and to the proximal end of the descending aorta (Fig. 13-82).
5. CPB would be required if the VSD is closed.

Double aortic arch

This defect occurs when there is persistence of the right embryonic arch that results in two aortic arches. The right arch is usually larger and goes behind the esophagus and trachea and joins the left arch to form the descending aorta. Compression of the trachea and esophagus by this vascular ring can cause symptoms of respiratory distress and dysphagia. Infants are usually symptomatic within the first to second month of life, and surgery is necessary (Hurst & Schlant, 1990).

Procedure

Key steps

1. Incision is as for PDA.
2. Vascular clamps are placed across the left arch between the origin of the left carotid and left subclavian arteries. Two clamps may be used as with a PDA.
3. The left arch is divided and both ends are closed with suture. The PDA (if present) is ligated and divided.

Atrial septal defect (ASD)

When the atria communicate through an opening in the septum, the blood shunts from the left side to the

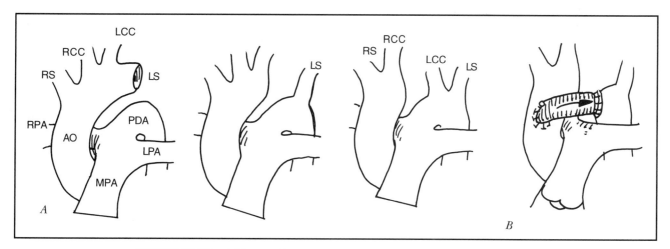

FIGURE 13-82 *A,* Types of interruptions of the aortic arch. *B,* Repair of interruption of the aortic arch with insertion of vascular graft and closure of PDA.

right side of the heart. This creates an increased workload for the right heart and increases the pulmonary circulation. Fatigue, dyspnea, arrhythmias, murmur, and congestive heart failure are common signs and symptoms. ASDs are classified according to their location on the septum:

1. Sinus venosus: this is located high on the septum and extends to the orifice of the superior vena cava.
2. Ostium secundum: this is located in the mid septum and is the most common type.
3. Ostium primum: this is located low in the septum and is associated with atrioventricular (AV) canal defect (Hurst & Schlant, 1990) (Fig. 13-83).

Procedure

Key steps

1. Median sternotomy incision is common, but a right anterolateral thoracotomy incision may be used for cosmetic purposes.
2. CPB is necessary with hypothermia.
3. Circulatory arrest is occasionally used for small hearts or if exposure is difficult.
4. Incision is made into the right atrium, which is then retracted.
5. A cardiotomy suction is placed across the septum to decompress the left ventricle.
6. Small defects might be closed directly with suture while larger defects may require patching. The patient's pericardium or synthetic vascular patch material may be used (Dacron; PTFE) (see Fig. 13-83).

7. Prior to completion of the defect repair, the left heart is allowed to fill with blood to remove any air.
8. As the atrial wall incision is closed, the right heart is allowed to fill with blood to remove air.
9. An aortic vent site for removal of air is established prior to releasing the aortic cross-clamp.

Ventricular septal defect (VSD)

This is an opening in the septum between the ventricles. The size of the defect varies and small defects may close spontaneously. Moderate to large defects permit an increased left-to-right shunt of blood and can cause congestive heart failure, pulmonary hypertension, and pulmonary vascular disease. Early closure is necessary for infants with congestive heart failure and for those infants with pulmonary hypertension. Elective repair is done within the first year of life.

VSDs are classified according to location (Fig. 13-84). About 75% are located in the outflow tract of the right ventricle and are perimembranous (Hurst & Schlant, 1990).

Procedure

Key steps

1. Median sternotomy incision is used.
2. CPB with hypothermia or circulatory arrest is used if necessary.

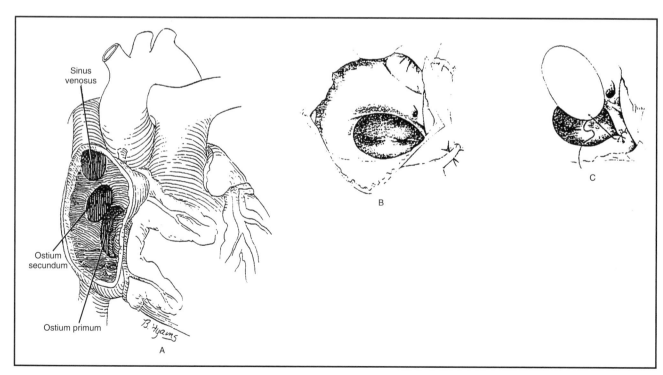

FIGURE 13-83 *A*, Location of various types of atrial septal defects. (Reprinted with permission from Cooley, D. *Techniques in Cardiac Surgery 2/e.* [1984] W. B. Saunders Co., Philadelphia, PA.) *B*, Exposure of atrial septal defect through right atrial incision. *C*, Closure of atrial septal defect with a patch. (Illustrated by Joan Livermore, CMI, from Khonsari, S. *Cardiac Surgery Safeguards: Pitfalls in Operating Techniques*, 1988, Raven Press, New York, NY.)

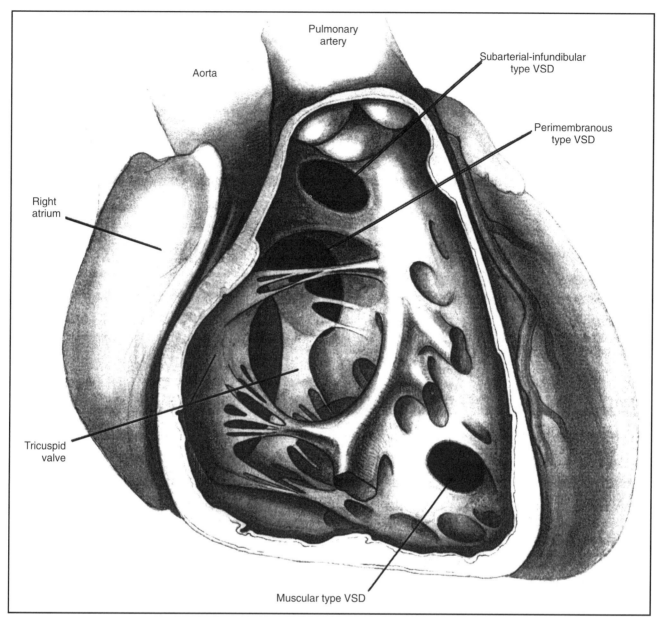

Aorta

Pulmonary artery

Subarterial-infundibular type VSD

Perimembranous type VSD

Right atrium

Tricuspid valve

Muscular type VSD

FIGURE 13-84 Location of various types of ventricular septal defects. (Illustrated by Joan Livermore, CMI, from Khonsari, S. *Cardiac Surgery Safeguards: Pitfalls in Operating Techniques,* 1988, Raven Press, New York, NY.)

3. The approach to the VSD will depend on its location and the surgeon's preference.
   a. Right atrial incision: The defect can be repaired through the tricuspid valve. This incision is usually used for the perimembranous type.
   b. Right ventricular or pulmonary artery incision: This incision is used for the subarterial-infundibular type.
   c. Left ventricular incision: This incision is used for the muscular type in the apex area of the septum.
4. It may be possible to directly close small defects with suture. Larger defects require a patch of Dacron or PTFE. A pericardial patch is not used for the ventricular septum because it cannot withstand the increased pressure.
5. Teflon felt bolsters may be needed for the sutures to prevent tearing of the septal tissues.

6. The left heart is allowed to fill with blood to remove air before repair is completed.
7. The right heart is filled with blood while the suturing of the heart incision site is completed.
8. The aortic root is vented to remove air.

Right ventricular outflow tract obstruction (RVOTO)

RVOTO results in decreased blood flow through the pulmonary circulation. Right ventricular obstruction is due to infundibular stenosis because of underdevelopment of the outflow tract (tubular hypoplasia) or hypertrophy of the infundibular septum. Obstruction can also result from pulmonary valve or artery stenosis or atresia. The best known RVOTO is tetralogy of Fallot. Surgical techniques used in repairing tetralogy of Fallot are applicable to other forms of RVOTO.

Characteristics of tetralogy of Fallot are:

1. VSD
2. Biventricular origin of the aorta
3. Obstruction to pulmonary flow
4. Varying degrees of right ventricular hypertrophy

Lillehai in 1954 and Kirklin in 1955 were the first to report successful surgical repair of this defect (Hurst & Schlant, 1990). Obstruction of pulmonary flow results in hypoxemia and produces a right-to-left shunt of blood through the VSD, causing cyanosis. Signs and symptoms include exertional dyspnea, polycythemia, systolic murmur, clubbing of the fingers and toes, and hypoxia "tet" spells. Hypoxia spells are sudden attacks of increasing cyanosis and hyperpnea that can result in syncope, seizures, or death. Squatting with exercise that occurs between $1\frac{1}{2}$ to 10 years of age is associated with this condition (Hurst & Schlant, 1990).

Elective primary surgical correction is recommended for infants over 6 months of age or earlier if the repair can be done by a transatrial and transpulmonary artery approach. Urgent surgery is indicated for the newborn with severe cyanosis, and prostaglandin can be administered to maintain patency of the PDA. When a palliative systemic shunt (e.g., modified Blalock-Taussig) is used, total repair may be delayed until 2 years of age. The experiences and judgment of the surgeon and cardiologist will determine the course of treatment (McGrath, 1992).

Occasionally, for infants with multiple extracardiac sources of pulmonary artery blood flow (i.e., collateral arteries from the thoracic aorta to the pulmonary circulatory system), a unifocalization procedure may be done. Multiple communications are eliminated, the pulmonary arteries are repaired if necessary, and a central shunt is created. This eliminates regional imbalances of pulmonary flow and promotes pulmonary arterial growth (Puga et al., 1989).

Procedure

Key steps

1. A median sternotomy incision is used. CPB with hypothermia and/or circulatory arrest is done.
2. Any systemic to pulmonary artery shunts must be ligated, including PDA if present.
3. A transatrial/transtricuspid valve approach is used when possible.
4. Incision is made in the right atrium.
5. A cardiotomy suction is used to vent the left ventricle via the foramen ovale. VSD is repaired.
6. Excision of hypertrophied infundibular septum is done as needed.
7. If necessary, a right ventricular incision is made over the infundibular area of the right ventricle and can be extended across the pulmonic valve annulus and onto the pulmonary artery. A Dacron or PTFE patch or gluteraldehyde-treated pericardial patch can be used to enlarge the outflow tract if needed. Simple

pulmonic valve stenosis can be relieved by commissurotomy. Transannular patching is controversial because of resultive pulmonic valve incompetence and potential for right ventricular failure.

8. If necessary, a Dacron valved conduit or pulmonary artery allograft conduit may be used to bypass annular pulmonic valve stenosis or valve atresia. The allograft conduit is preferred because it is more durable and superior to the Dacron conduit.
9. The size of the allograft conduit is based on the patient's size.
10. The distal pulmonary anastomosis is done based on anatomical findings. Modifications depend on the involvement of the pulmonary arteries.
11. The proximal anastomosis is made by suturing the allograft valve to the posterior segment of the pulmonary valve annulus.
12. A triangular shaped hood of allograft tissue or PTFE patch material is sutured to the anterior segment of the allograft and to the right ventricular incision (Maloney, 1980; Hopkins, 1989).
13. The left ventricular venting cardiotomy suction is removed, the heart is filled with blood to remove air, the atrial defect is closed, the right atrium is closed, and the aorta is vented to remove air.

Transposition of the great arteries (TGA)

With this congenital defect the aorta rises from the right side of the heart and the pulmonary artery arises from the left. A VSD is present in approximately one-third of the patients. If untreated, 30% of these infants will die within the first week of life and 90% will die within the first year. Severe, progressive cyanosis and congestive heart failure are the early signs and symptoms (Hurst & Schlant, 1990).

Palliative procedures such as the Rashkind balloon septostomy (ASD is created by tearing the septum with a balloon-tipped catheter) and pulmonary artery banding may not be needed if urgent surgical correction is undertaken.

Senning in 1959 and Mustard in 1975 introduced intracardiac corrective surgical procedures. Glutaraldehyde-treated pericardium is used to construct a baffle at the atrial level to reroute the venous and arterial blood.

Janeten in 1975 introduced the arterial switch procedure where the aorta and pulmonary artery are transected and reversed to correct the transposition (Hurst & Schlant, 1990; Mavroudis et al., 1992). This is an anatomical and physiological correction, and the surgery must be done within the first few days of life before there is a decrease in the left ventricular muscle (Mayer et al., 1986).

Procedure

Key steps

1. A median sternotomy incision is used.
2. CPB is accomplished, usually with profound hypothermia and circulatory arrest or low flow.

3. The PDA is ligated prior to placing the patient on bypass.

4. Arterial switch procedure:

   a. The ASD is closed through a right atrial incision.

   b. A left ventricular vent catheter can be inserted via the right superior pulmonary vein.

   c. If a VSD is present, it is closed.

   d. The aorta and pulmonary artery are transected, and the coronary artery ostial patches are excised for transfer to the neoaorta (Fig. 13-85). The Le Compte maneuver, placing the aorta behind the pulmonary artery, is performed to provide more length to the aorta (Fig. 13-85).

   e. The coronary artery ostial patches are sutured into the bases of the neoaorta (old pulmonary artery) after segments of the wall have been removed. The aorta is anastomosed to the old pulmonary artery (Fig. 13-85).

   f. To reconstruct the neopulmonary artery, a pericardial pantaloon patch or a PTFE patch is used to repair the area of the pulmonary artery where the coronary ostial patches were removed. By oversizing the patch, supravalvular stenosis can be avoided (Fig. 13-85) (Mavroudis et al., 1992).

5. The Senning procedure:

   a. An incision is made in the right atrium, and the atrial septum is incised to form a flap. The flap can be enlarged with a Dacron or PTFE patch.

   b. The interatrial grove is dissected in order to free the posterior atrial walls, and an incision is made into the left atrium.

   c. The flap is sutured to the left atrial wall in front of the left superior and inferior pulmonary veins.

   d. The anterior edge of the right atrial posterior aspect of the incised atrium is sutured to the anterior part of the septal defect between the mitral and tricuspid valves.

   e. The anterior segment of the right atrial wall is sutured to the left atrial incision around the caval channel.

   f. A patch of pericardium or Dacron/PTFE may be needed to enlarge the atrial wall.

6. Mustard procedure:

   a. A large segment of the anterior pericardium is removed and prepared for the baffle.

   b. Incision is made in the right atrium, and a portion of the atrial septum is removed.

   c. The baffle is sutured below the caval openings and inside the left atrium above the pulmonary vein orifices. It is then sutured to the anterior segment of the atrial septal opening.

   d. The right atrium is then closed.

Atrioventricular canal defect (cushion defect)

This anomaly involves the inferior atrial septum and the superior ventricular septum. The tricuspid and mitral valves are involved as a common valve with various deformities.

There are three forms of this defect:

1. Partial: 60% to 70% of patients have this form. This is an ostium primum ASD in which the valves are attached to the ventricular septum.

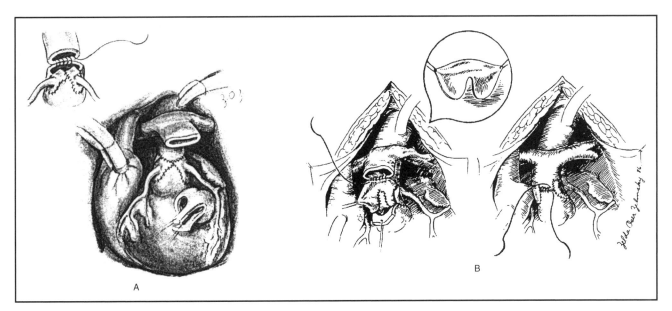

FIGURE 13-85   Arterial switch procedure for transposition of the great arteries (TGA). *A*, The aorta and pulmonary artery have been transected. The coronary arteries are sutured to the neoaorta and the neoaorta is reconstructed. (Reprinted with permission from Mavroudis, C. et al. Arterial switch for T.G.A. and associated malposition anomalies, *Advances in Cardiac Surgery*, pp. 214, 217 [1992]. Mosby-Year Book, Inc., St. Louis, MO.) *B*, The neopulmonary artery is constructed, using pericardial pantaloon patches. (Reprinted with permission from Idriss, FS et al. *J Thoracic Cardiovasc Surg*, 1988; 95:255–262. Mosby-Year Book, Inc., St. Louis, MO.)

2. Intermediate: This is the same as the partial except the valves are incompletely attached to the septum.
3. Complete: ASD and VSD are present and variations occur in the valve leaflet attachment. The Rastelli classification is based on the shape, size, location, and attachment of the left superior valve leaflet:
   Type A: Common. Chordal attachment is at the crest of the VSD and leaflet over the left ventricle.
   Type B: Rare. Chordal attachment is on the right ventricular side of the septum.
   Type C: Common. Leaflet bridges the VSD and the right ventricle. Chordal attachments vary (Khonsari, 1988; Hurst & Schlant, 1990).

Mitral valve regurgitation may be severe, causing congestive heart failure, cardiac enlargement, and murmur. Early, complete repair is indicated (within the first year of life) (Pacifico & Sand, 1987; Hurst & Schlant, 1990).

Procedure

Key steps

1. A median sternotomy incision is done.
2. CPB is accomplished with moderate hypothermia or profound hypothermia with circulatory arrest.
3. An incision is made in the right atrium.
4. Partial and intermediate defects are repaired as for an ASD. It may be necessary to suture edges of the mitral valve leaflets if a cleft is present. A patch of pericardium, Dacron, or PTFE may be needed to repair the ASD.
5. Complete defects require repair of the mitral cleft, VSD, tricuspid cleft, and ASD. The mitral valve is evaluated for competence prior to closing the ASD, the heart is filled with blood to remove air.
6. The aorta is vented.

Ebstein's anomaly

With this anomaly, there is downward displacement of the posterior and septal leaflets of the tricuspid valve into the right ventricle. The right ventricle is divided into two sections: the atrialized segment and the functional segment. An ASD is usually present. Symptoms are related to right ventricular obstruction and tricuspid regurgitation. Right heart failure, cyanosis, arrhythmias, murmurs, and cardiomegaly are common findings. Decisions regarding surgical intervention are based on progression of symptoms and their severity. Surgical results vary, but mortality decreases in older patients (Hurst & Schlant, 1990).

Procedure

Key steps

1. A median sternotomy incision is used.
2. CPB with moderate hypothermia is accomplished.
3. An incision is made in the right atrium.
4. The tricuspid valve is repaired by using buttressed sutures to bring the leaflets up into place with the tricus-

pid annulus into the right atrial level. Redundant atrial wall in the right ventricle is incorporated into the reconstruction of the valve.
5. If the abnormality cannot be repaired without leaving right ventricular obstruction, a tricuspid valve replacement may be needed.
6. The ASD is closed.
7. The heart is filled with blood to remove air, and the right atrial incision is closed.
8. The aorta is vented.

Truncus arteriosus and pseudotruncus

This defect occurs when the embryonic truncus arteriosus fails to undergo normal septation of the pulmonary artery and aorta, therefore leaving a single arterial trunk that arises from the left ventricle. A VSD is present. Surgery is indicated in infancy because of congestive heart failure and cyanosis.

This defect is classified according to the origin of the pulmonary artery or arteries (Fig. 13-86):

Type I: The common pulmonary artery arises from the proximal left side of the truncal artery.

Type II: The right and left pulmonary arteries originate together at the side or back of the truncal artery.

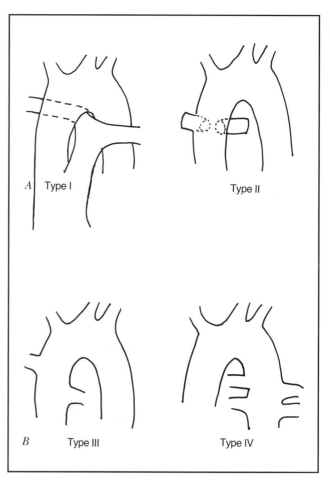

FIGURE 13-86 Types of truncus arteriosus.

Type III: The right and left pulmonary arteries arise at different areas of the truncal artery.

Type IV: The pulmonary arteries come from the descending aorta. This is considered a form of pulmonary atresia.

Pseudotruncus is an absence of any true pulmonary arteries, and the blood supply to the lungs is from bronchial collateral flow (Hurst & Schlant, 1990; Khonsari, 1988).

Procedure

Key steps

1. A median sternotomy incision is used.
2. CPB with moderate hypothermia is accomplished.
3. The VSD is repaired with a patch through a right ventricular incision.
4. The truncal valve (aortic) is inspected and repaired if necessary.
5. An allograft or Dacron valved graft conduit is placed from the right ventricle to the pulmonary artery (arteries).
6. The pulmonary arteries are detached from the truncal artery, and the artery is repaired.

Anomalous pulmonary venous return

The return of the pulmonary veins into the right atrium can occur. This can be partial or complete. An ASD is usually present. The anomaly is classified according to the location and type of venous (pulmonary) return:

Type I: Supracardiac is the most common. All the pulmonary veins enter a common vein behind the heart and connect to the innominate vein.

Type II: Intracardiac or paracardiac. The pulmonary veins enter into the right atrium itself or into the coronary sinus.

Type III: The pulmonary veins drain into a common vertical vein that goes down behind the heart and into the inferior vena cava.

Type IV: The pulmonary veins from the right lung enter the inferior vena cava. This is a scimitar deformity.

Congestive heart failure and cyanosis are the common signs and symptoms. Surgical repair in early infancy is indicated to prevent severe or irreversible deterioration (Yee et al., 1987; Cooley, 1984).

Procedure

Key steps

1. A median sternotomy incision or a thoracotomy incision may be used for Types I and III.
2. CPB is used.

3. Moderate hypothermia or profound hypothermia with circulatory arrest may be used.
4. Surgical repair is based on the type of deformity (see Fig. 13-86):
   a. Type I: A side-to-side anastomosis is made between the common vein behind the heart into the left atrium. The vertical vein that connects to the innominate vein is ligated and the ASD is closed.
   b. Type II: A right atrial incision is made and the septal wall is removed. A Dacron or PTFE patch is sutured over the vein openings and to the septal defect to shunt the blood to the left side of the heart. When the veins drain into the coronary sinus, the patch is placed posterior to the coronary sinus orifice.
   c. Type III: An incision is made into the side of the common vertical vein behind the heart and another incision is made into the left atrium. The vein is anastomosed to the left atrium and the distal common vein is ligated. The ASD is closed.
   d. Type IV: The vein is detached from the inferior vena cava and anastomosed to the right atrium. The cava is repaired where the vein has been removed. The ASD or foramen is enlarged, and a Dacron patch is sewn over the septal defect and over the vein anastomosis site. This forms a tunnel for draining the blood to the left side of the heart.

Left ventricular outflow tract obstruction (LVOTO)

Symptoms are based on the degree of obstruction of blood flow from the left ventricle. Dyspnea, growth retardation, fatigue with feeding, or congestive heart failure may be present. Timing of surgical intervention is based on the severity of symptoms (Hurst & Schlant, 1990). Surgical treatment in infancy is indicated for infants with cardiomegaly, congestive heart failure, and left ventricular hypertrophy with left ventricular strain on ECG (Stark & de Leval, 1983).

The location of the obstruction is based on the relationship to the aortic valve: subvalvular, valvular, or supravalvular. The types of obstructive deformities are membranous, fibromuscular, or asymmetric (Stark & de Leval, 1983).

Procedure

Key steps

1. A median sternotomy incision is used.
2. CPB with moderate hypothermia or profound hypothermia with circulatory arrest is accomplished.
3. A transaortic approach is used.
4. The type of incision in the aorta will depend on the intended repair.
4. **Subvalvular**
   a. Membranous: A diaphragm or crescent-shaped wedge occurs across the anterior two-thirds of the left ventricular outflow tract that is removed with a knife.
   b. Fibromuscular: Benign forms can be repaired by resecting the muscle or fibrotic tissue. Tunnel subaor-

tic stenosis is the most severe and may require insertion of a Dacron valved conduit from the apex of the left ventricle to the descending aorta. The sternotomy incision will need to be extended downward to provide access to the abdominal aorta. The conduit is placed through the diaphragm and into the aorta in such a manner as to prevent kinking.

   c. Asymmetric septal hypertrophy (idiopathic hypertrophic subaortic stenosis) can be excised with a knife.

5. Valvular: This defect usually can be repaired by an aortic valve commissurotomy or valve replacement if necessary.

6. Supravalvular: A narrowing in the aorta above the valve may be localized or diffuse and extend to the innominate artery. A partial resection may be needed if there is an annular ridge, and the aorta is enlarged by patching with a Dacron patch. Mixed lesions may require patch enlargement of the aorta and the left ventricular outflow tract across the annulus and include a valve replacement.

Single ventricle heart

CHD such as tricuspid atresia, double outlet right ventricle, and univentricular heart leave the patient with one functional ventricle. There is intracardiac mixing of pulmonary and systemic venous return, which results in cyanosis, polycythemia, and myocardial failure (Bartmus et al., 1990).

Palliation procedures may include (depending on the defect):

1. Systemic to pulmonary artery shunt in order to increase pulmonary blood flow
2. Pulmonary artery banding to decrease the pulmonary blood flow

In 1971 Fontan and Baudet reported the first successful surgery for tricuspid atresia where the systemic venous blood was diverted from the heart and into the pulmonary arterial system. This provided physiological correction of the pulmonary and systemic venous returns (Stein et al., 1991).

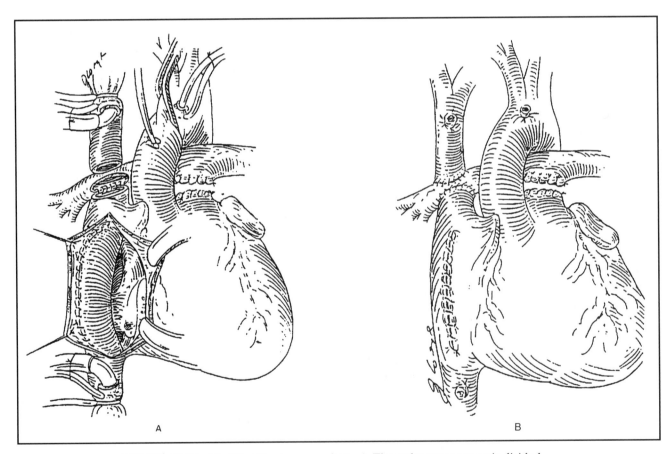

FIGURE 13-87 Modified Fontan procedure. *A,* The pulmonary artery is divided and oversewn. The superior vena cava is divided. Incision is made in the right atrium and a tunnel is constructed with atrial tissue or PTFE graft. The tunnel shunts the blood from the inferior vena cava to the pulmonary artery. *B,* Completed repair. The superior vena cava is sewn to the upper side of the right pulmonary artery. The upper end of the right atrium with the tunnel is sutured to the proximal side of the right pulmonary artery. (Reprinted with permission from Stein, D. G., et al. Results of total cavopulmonary connection in the treatment of patients with a functional single ventricle. *Journal of Thoracic and Cardiovascular Surgery* [1991]; 102:280–287. Mosby-Year Book, Inc., St. Louis, MO).

Modifications of the Fontan procedure have been made, and the one used today is the total cavopulmonary connection with an intraatrial baffle or tunnel (Stein et al., 1991; Bartmus et al., 1990; Chu et al., 1991; Jonas & Castaneda, 1988). The tunnel can be fenestrated to provide temporary communication between the systemic venous return and the cardiac chambers. This is done to prevent postoperative ventricular dysfunction or increased pulmonary vascular resistance from developing by decreasing the venous flow through the pulmonary circulation. This allows right-to-left shunting and helps maintain cardiac output. The fenestration can be closed later by using a transcatheter double umbrella "clamshell" device inserted through the opening (Bridges et al., 1990).

Procedure

Key steps

1. A median sternotomy incision is used.
2. CPB is used with profound hypothermia and circulatory arrest.
3. If a systemic to pulmonary artery shunt is present, it is ligated prior to placing the patient on the pump.
4. The right atrium is incised, and the atrial septum is excised.
5. An intraatrial tunnel of PTFE graft is anastomosed to the orifice of the inferior vena cava.
6. The superior vena cava is divided at the atrium, and the cardiac end is anastomosed to the upper end of the PTFE graft and sutured to the inferior side of the right pulmonary artery.
7. The main pulmonary artery is transected and oversewn.
8. The proximal end of the superior vena cava is sutured to the superior side of the right pulmonary artery.
9. The PTFE tunnel is fenestrated using an aortic punch 4 to 6 mm in diameter, depending on the desired shunt.
10. The right atrial incision is closed. Air has been removed from the heart by allowing it to fill with blood (Fig. 13-87).

Aortopulmonary window

With this relatively rare defect there is communication between the ascending aorta and the pulmonary artery. This communication can occur directly with the main pulmonary artery, at the level of the right pulmonary artery, or by an anomalous origin of the right pulmonary artery.

This defect can cause congestive heart failure and pulmonary hypertension, so it must be corrected. Closure of this defect under direct vision is the method of choice (Khonsari, 1988).

Procedure

Key steps

1. The pulmonary artery branches must be occluded at the beginning of CPB.

2. A longitudinal incision is made in the ascending aorta below the cross-clamp, and the defect is closed with a patch.
3. The aortotomy is closed.
4. If an anomalous origin of the right pulmonary artery is present, it is detached and anastomosed to the main pulmonary artery, and the aortic defect is repaired with a patch.

Cor triatriatum

With this defect there are two chambers for the left atrium that are divided by a membrane. A perforation in the membrane allows blood to flow through the mitral valve. There is usually a patent foramen ovale, and flow can be diverted to the right atrium. Symptoms depend on the obstruction to flow through the left atrium and the degree of shunting to the right atrium. Pulmonary venous congestion, dyspnea, right ventricular hypertension, and right heart failure can occur. Usually, the patient becomes symptomatic in early childhood and only occasionally as an infant (Hurst & Schlant, 1990).

Procedure

Key steps

1. A median sternotomy is done, and CPB is accomplished. A right atrial or left atrial incision is used.
2. If a right atrial incision is done, the membrane can be reached by incising the atrial septum.
3. The membrane separating the two chambers is excised, and the septum (if opened) and atrial incisions are closed.

Cardiac Tumors

The first successful surgical removal of an intracardiac tumor was in 1955 using CPB. Over 75% of the primary tumors of the heart are benign. Myxomas are the most common (approximately 50%) and arise from the endocardium in the left atrium, although they can occur in the other cardiac chambers (Fig. 13-88). Fragments of tumor can embolize into the systemic circulation and may be the first sign. Left atrial obstruction can cause symptoms of dyspnea, pulmonary edema, chest pain, pulmonary hypertension, right-sided heart failure, or death. Surgical removal is the only treatment.

The most frequent benign tumor seen in infants is the rhabdomyoma, and it usually involves the ventricular myocardium. Fibromas can occur in the ventricle or intramurally. Papillary fibroelastomas arise from the cardiac valves or ventricular endocardium. Lipomas can also be found in the heart tissues.

The most common malignant tumor is a sarcoma (angiosarcoma) that can originate in the right atrium or pericardium. Because of widespread metastasis, surgery is impractical. Rhabdomyosarcomas have a poor prognosis. Metastatic tumors to the heart occur through the lymphatic system or by direct growth from adjacent tumor. Radiation may provide symptomatic relief. Surgical resec-

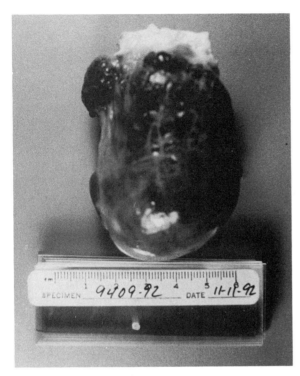

FIGURE 13-88 Left atrial myxoma.

tion for palliation is debatable (Hurst & Schlant, 1990; Carrel et al., 1992).

Procedure

Key steps

1. A median sternotomy incision is made.
2. CPB is used.
3. Left atrial myxomas are removed (usually), with a right atrial incision and across the septum.
4. Biatrial incisions can be used.
5. The area of the atrial septum where the tumor is attached is to be excised. Minimal manipulation of the heart and the tumor is done in order to prevent fragmentation of the tumor.
6. Tumors located in other chambers of the heart will require use of various incisions that provide access to the tumor.

Cardiac Trauma

Cardiac injury can result from penetrating and nonpenetrating wounds. Penetrating wounds from knives, sharp objects, bullets, or projectiles can injure various areas of the heart and surrounding tissues. Blunt or nonpenetrating injuries can occur from forces against the chest, from compression to the chest, or from indirect pressure caused by pressure on the abdomen, concussive forces against the chest, and deceleration forces. Septal, valvular, chordal, or papillary muscle rupture can occur. Myocardial contusion can cause ischemia or infarction. Cardiac

tamponade can occur if blood is trapped in the pericardium.

Ionizing radiation can cause pericarditis and electrical injuries can result in burns of the heart and/or great vessels. Arrhythmias can occur with electrical shocks (Hurst & Schlant, 1990).

Procedure

Key steps

1. The procedure will be related to the type of injury to the heart.
2. CPB may be necessary.
3. Direct closure of cardiac lacerations can usually be done without CPB.

Thoracic Aortic Diseases and Trauma

Diseases of the thoracic aorta can involve the ascending, arch, or descending aorta. Weakness in the medial wall of the aorta can cause aneurysm formation, dissection, rupture, or occlusion of the aorta.

The causes of aortic disease are:

1. Atherosclerosis
2. Medial degeneration, which causes the aorta to dilate and/or elongate. This can result in annuloaortic ectasia. Marfan's syndrome and medial necrosis are common causes.
3. Aortitis; bacterial, syphilitic, Takayasu's disease
4. Congenital abnormalities; coarctation, PDA, or aortic valve stenosis causing poststenotic dilation

Aneurysms are described as fusiform (circumferential dilatation; spindle-shaped) or saccular (balloon-like) or a combination of the two. The risk of aneurysmal rupture increases with age, aneurysms over 6 cm in diameter, and hypertension. Urgent surgery is recommended for large aneurysms or if signs and symptoms suggesting expansion or rupture of aneurysm occur, such as pain, cardiac murmur, shock, dyspnea, or absent pulses in the extremities.

Dissection of the aorta occurs when there is a tear in the intima that allows blood flow to separate the media and form a false lumen or channel in the aortic wall. The dissection plane is usually longitudinal but can be medial or spiral in direction.

Approximately 60% of dissections occur in the ascending aorta and can dissect proximally and distally. Proximal dissection can involve the aortic valve, annulus, and sinus of Valsalva. Aortic dissections are classified according to the location of the intimal tear and the area of the aorta involved (Fig. 13-89).

The DeBakey classification is as follows:

Type I: Ascending aorta, arch, and descending aorta involved

Type II: Only involves the ascending aorta and arch

Type III: Only involves the descending aorta distal to the origin of the left subclavian artery

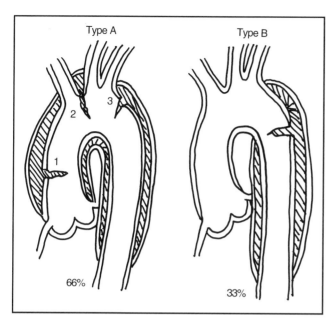

FIGURE 13-89 Classification of aortic dissection by location. Type A and B = Stanford classification. 1, 2, and 3 = the DeBakey classification.

The Stanford classification is:

Type A: Ascending and/or arch of aorta (60% of dissections)

Type B: Descending aorta

Aortography remains the most definitive method of diagnosing aortic problems. CT scans and MRI are useful but limited diagnostic tools (Hurst & Schlant, 1990; Fuster & Ip, 1991).

Trauma to the thoracic aorta can involve the ascending, arch, and/or descending aorta. The trauma can be due to penetrating or blunt injury. The most common location of aortic traumatic rupture is the descending aorta distal to the left subclavian artery or the ascending aorta proximal to the innominate artery (Hurst & Schlant, 1990). Of patients with blunt trauma due to deceleration injuries from vehicular accidents or falls, 85% die at the scene. Early recognition and treatment are essential for survival of those who reach the hospital. An abnormal chest X-ray and the type of accident will usually alert the physician to this type of aortic injury. Aortography is essential (Mattox, 1991).

Surgical techniques for treating thoracic aortic disease are continually being refined, such as:

1. Composite vascular grafts; Dacron vascular grafts with aortic valve.
2. Coating of grafts with 25% albumin and autoclaving for 5 minutes at 270° C to decrease bleeding through the graft. Collagen-impregnated grafts are available, eliminating this process (Svensson et al., 1992).
3. Various techniques for anastomosis of the coronary arteries to the prosthetic graft are:
   a. Direct reimplantation: Bentall technique. May be more prone to false aneurysm formation at the coronary anastomosis (Svensson et al., 1992).

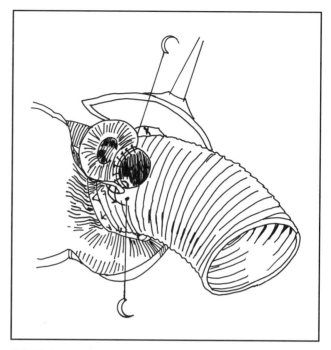

FIGURE 13-90 Aortic button resection of the coronary artery ostia and suturing to the aortic graft.

   b. Use of a separate Dacron tube graft: Cabrol's technique. Tension on the anastomosis and bleeding sites cannot be easily identified, but technical problems can result in occlusion of the right coronary artery (Svensson et al., 1992).
   c. Aortic button resection (Fig. 13-90) is more time-consuming but gives good long-term results (Svensson et al., 1992).
   d. Vein bypass grafts.
4. Graft inclusion techniques: The aortic wall is not totally removed, which decreases the amount of dissection and possible injury to surrounding tissues. The remaining wall is fashioned to fit around the vascular prosthetic graft and loosely sutured together. This provides support to the graft and decreases infection of the graft.

   If bleeding occurs when a graft has been placed in the aortic root and ascending aorta, bleeding into the space between the graft and the aortic wall can result in formation of a false aneurysm and dislodge coronary anastomosis. Creating an opening between this area and the right atrium shunts blood from this space and avoids this complication (Cabrol et al., 1991; Lewis et al., 1992).
5. Intraluminal grafts are easier to use, but there is concern regarding leaks, migration, aortic injury, thromboembolism, and/or technical problems (Lansman et al., 1991).
6. With bypass exclusion techniques there is graft bypass around the problem area of the aorta.
7. Cerebral protection techniques:
   a. Profound hypothermia with circulatory arrest can assist with making the surgical repair technically easier, but there are time limitations and CPB time is increased for cooling and rewarming the patient:

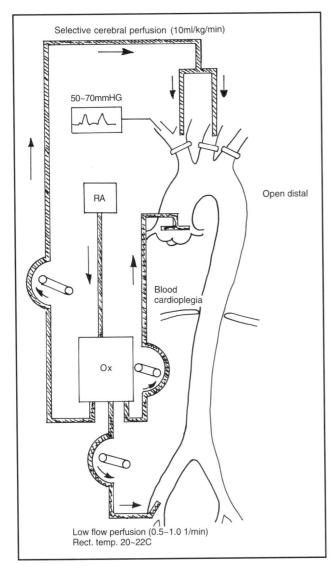

Selective cerebral perfusion (10ml/kg/min)

50~70mmHG

RA

Open distal

Blood cardioplegia

Ox

Low flow perfusion (0.5~1.0 1/min)
Rect. temp. 20~22C

FIGURE 13-91 Method of providing selective cerebral perfusion.

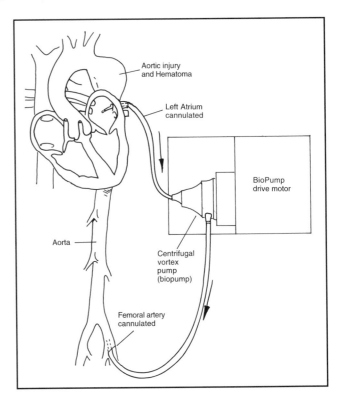

Aortic injury and Hematoma

Left Atrium cannulated

BioPump drive motor

Aorta

Centrifugal vortex pump (biopump)

Femoral artery cannulated

FIGURE 13-92 Partial pump bypass from the left atrium to the femoral artery using a centrifugal vortex pump.

Special supplies, instrumentation, and equipment

Vascular clamps: assortment of larger clamps and various shapes

Vascular grafts: assortment of various sizes of tubular Dacron grafts and composite grafts

Arterial and venous cannulae: assortment of those needed for cerebral perfusion or partial bypass

Sternal and thoracotomy instruments

Vascular sutures

Teflon felt

Positioning devices for thoracotomy

Procedure

Key steps

1. Ascending or aortic arch aortic repair:
   a. A median sternotomy incision is made. CPB is used.
   b. The arterial cannula may be inserted in the ascending or arch of the aorta if aortic repair can be done.
   c. Femoral arterial cannulation is needed if the aortic repair involves the arch.
   d. Single-, two-stage, or bicaval cannulation for venous return is done.
   e. Left ventricle vent is used.

15° C—60 minutes of arrest time; 20° C—30 minutes of arrest time.
   b. Selective cerebral perfusion can be done by cannulating the innominate and left carotid arteries and using a separate perfusion circuit (Fig. 13-91). Flows need to be 10 ml/kg/minute (Kazui et al., 1992). Retrograde perfusion via the SVC could be used as an alternative method of cerebral perfusion.
8. Pump bypass methods for distal perfusion when the descending aorta is cross-clamped are superior to passive shunts (e.g., Gott) and are the most frequently used. These techniques prevent hypertension proximally and provide adequate perfusion distally. Partial bypass from the left atrium or left ventricular apex to the femoral artery can be done using the roller pump or centrifugal pump without an oxygenator or reservoir. Systems that include an oxygenator and reservoir require the patient to have full-dose heparinization and femoral vein to femoral artery bypass (Fig. 13-92) (Ergin et al., 1991).

f. The aorta is cross-clamped and cardioplegia is given retrograde if possible; the antegrade method may require cannulation of the coronary ostia.

g. A longitudinal incision is made in the aorta and may require excision of the aortic valve. Excess aortic wall tissue is removed.

h. If the arch is involved, circulatory arrest may be used or cerebral protection provided by perfusing the arch vessels.

i. The distal anastomosis is done first for arch repairs. With ascending aortic repairs, the proximal repair is done first. When composite grafts are used, the coronary arteries are anastomosed as discussed earlier.

j. Teflon felt strips may be needed to reinforce cut edges of the aorta.

k. Dissection planes must be identified (if present), and the entry closed to prevent further dissection.

l. Air is removed from the heart and the aorta prior to releasing the aortic cross-clamp.

m. CPB is discontinued and a standard closure is done.

2. Descending aorta repairs:

a. A left thoracotomy incision is used.

b. Simple cross-clamping above and below the involved area with resection and end-to-end closure or graft insertion may be possible, providing the aorta is not cross-clamped longer than 20 to 25 minutes (Kouchoukos, 1991).

c. To prevent spinal cord ischemia, distal perfusion must be provided by active pump bypass techniques when the aortic repair will take longer than 20 to 25 minutes.

d. Total CPB with circulatory arrest may be indicated for complex aortic repairs.

e. Reimplantation of intercostal arteries may be necessary to prevent spinal cord ischemic injury.

Cardiac transplantation

The first heart transplant from one human to another was performed by Barnard in 1967. In 1980, the immunosuppressive drug cyclosporine was introduced, which resulted in prolonged survival for heart and heart–lung transplant patients. This accelerated the number of transplant procedures being done. By 1990, 16,355 heart transplants and 1025 heart–lung transplants has been done worldwide. Currently, there are 161 heart transplant centers and 41 heart–lung transplant centers worldwide (Muirhead, 1992; Young, 1992).

Survival for adult heart transplant patients is 81% at 1 year following transplant and 69% at 5 years. For pediatric patients, survival is 70% at 1 year after transplant and 60% at 5 years. There is an increase in transplants for infants under 1 year of age. Heart–lung transplantation survival is 59% at 1 year after transplant (Pennington & Swartz, 1991).

Scarcity of donor organs continues to be a problem, and 30% of patients approved for heart transplant die awaiting an organ. The lack of organ donation is primarily because the request may not have been made. Several international, national, and regional agencies facilitate the process of matching donors with recipients. The United Network for Organ Sharing (UNOS) provides a computerized service in the United States. The North American Transplant Coordinators Organization (NATCO) expedites the procurement, preservation, and distribution of donor organs. Careful, coordinated planning is essential if transplantation is to be successful (Cooper & Novitzky, 1990).

Heart transplant candidates have conditions that cannot be treated by other medical or surgical methods and have a prognosis of 6 to 12 months of survival. They are New York Heart Association Class III and IV and have a left ventricular ejection fraction of less than 20%. Cardiomyopathy; ischemic, valvular, and congenital heart disease; or life-threatening arrhythmias are the types of diseases that may result in transplantation.

Contraindications for heart transplant are the following:

Absolute contraindications
  Active infection
  Malignancy, untreated or uncontrolled
  Systemic disease, uncontrolled
  Irreversible dysfunction of other major organs
  Irreversible pulmonary hypertension

Relative contraindications
  Advanced age; no absolute age limit; physiologic age most important
  Pulmonary infarction, recent or unresolved
  Type I diabetes mellitus
  Significant peripheral or cerebrovascular disease
  Active peptic ulcer or diverticulitis
  Psychological instability or noncompliant behavior

Heart–lung transplantation candidates have conditions of isolated pulmonary hypertension, cardiac disease with severe pulmonary hypertension or underdeveloped pulmonary vasculature, or parenchymal lung disease. These patients have severe functional limitations with an estimated 6- to 12-month survival and cannot be treated by other medical or surgical methods.

Contraindications for heart–lung transplant are:

Major contraindications
  Active systemic infection
  Severe chest deformity
  Malignant disease
  Severe renal or hepatic disease
  Uncontrolled systemic disease
  Severe central nervous system disability
  Positive hepatitis or HIV serology
  Psychological instability or noncompliant behavior

Minor contraindications
  Advanced age, over 40 years
  Previous thoracic surgery
  Type I diabetes mellitus
  Active peptic ulcer
  Current corticosteroid therapy
  Major or numerous bronchial collaterals
  (Muirhead, 1992; Cooper & Novitzky, 1990)

Criteria have been established for donor selection for heart and heart–lung transplantation:

1. Donor–recipient matching of ABO blood group must be done.
2. Cytotoxicity of the recipient must be determined and further tests may be indicated.
3. Body size and weight of the donor must be comparable with the recipient's.
4. Normal cardiac function is determined by appropriate tests.
5. The donor must have no transferable disease.
6. The donor must be under 60 years of age.
7. A donor may be excluded if there is a history of diabetes mellitus or longstanding hypertension.
8. Thoracic cavity size and shape must be similar to recipient's.
9. There must be no history of lung disease.
10. The lungs must have good pulmonary function.
11. The donor must be a nonsmoker. (Cooper & Novitzky, 1990; Muirhead, 1992).

Complications can occur after transplantation. The most common are:

1. Infection, because of immunosuppression of the patient
2. Rejection of the organ
3. Myocardial and/or respiratory dysfunction
4. Accelerated form of atherosclerosis; requires retransplantation
5. Lymphoproliferative disease; most common is lymphoma, related to immunosuppression
6. Obliterative bronchiolitis; fibrosing, inflammatory process that causes small airway obstruction; related to rejection episode or viral pneumonia (Cooper & Novitzky, 1990; Muirhead, 1991)

There are two types of heart transplantation procedures. *Orthotopic:* The recipient's heart is excised and replaced with the donor heart in the correct anatomical position. *Heterotopic or "piggy-back":* The donor heart is placed in the right chest alongside the recipient's heart. It is anastomosed to allow blood to pass through either or both hearts. Heterotopic transplantation is used when the patient's own heart may recover, if the donor heart function will be inadequate to maintain circulation by itself, with severe angina that is unresponsive to therapy and the left ventricular function is good, or with fixed pulmonary vascular resistance.

Procedure

Key steps

1. The donor heart is excised; a median sternotomy incision is used.
2. The aorta, pulmonary artery, and venae cavae are mobilized.
3. The donor is heparinized and the cardioplegia needle is positioned in the aorta.

4. The cavae are cross-clamped and the heart is allowed to empty prior to cross-clamping the aorta and administering the cold cardioplegia solution (4° C).
5. An incision is made into the inferior vena cava and the right pulmonary vein to allow the cardioplegia solution to escape and not overdistend the heart.
6. At least 1000 ml of cardioplegia solution is administered and the heart is covered with iced saline or slush; 2 minutes is allowed for adequate cooling.
7. The cavae and aorta are divided, and the heart is lifted up in order to divide the pulmonary veins; the pulmonary artery is divided at the bifurcation with a cuff of both branches attached.
8. The heart is removed from the donor and placed in ice-cold solution in a plastic bag and sealed.
9. Additional plastic bags may be used and the heart is transported packed in ice to the recipient. Ischemic times of 4 to 6 hours may be safe (Hurst & Schlant, 1990).
10. For orthotopic transplantation, the recipient is taken to the operating room about 1½ hours prior to the arrival of the donor heart.
11. A median sternotomy incision is made, and the patient is prepared for CPB with bicaval cannulation.
12. The donor heart is prepared as the recipient is prepared for CPB by ligating the superior vena cava, incising the right atrium, interconnecting the pulmonary veins, and tailoring the aorta and pulmonary artery (Fig. 13-93).
13. The recipient is placed on CPB and cooled to 28° C, caval tapes are tightened, the aorta is cross-clamped, and the right atrium is incised across the septum and into the left atrium.
14. The aorta and pulmonary artery are divided and the heart is removed.
15. The donor heart is anastomosed, beginning with the left atrium and proceeding to the right atrium.
16. The heart is filled with iced saline or slush and topically cooled with iced saline.
17. The pulmonary artery is anastomosed end to end as is the aorta.
18. Air is evacuated from the heart and the aortic cross-clamp is removed.
19. Systemic rewarming of the patient was begun at the beginning of the aortic anastomosis.
20. Heterotopic transplantation can be done in two ways (Fig. 13-94): For left ventricular bypass the pulmonary artery of the donor is anastomosed to the recipient's right atrium, and the left atria are anastomosed together, as are the aortas. For total heart bypass, the superior vena cava, left atria, pulmonary arteries, and aortas are anastomosed together.

Cardiomyoplasty

This procedure provides assistance to the heart by wrapping it in the latissimus dorsi muscle and stimulating the muscle to contract. The procedure was introduced in the 1980s by Carpentier and Chachques, and by 1990 over 100 procedures had been done worldwide. The major in-

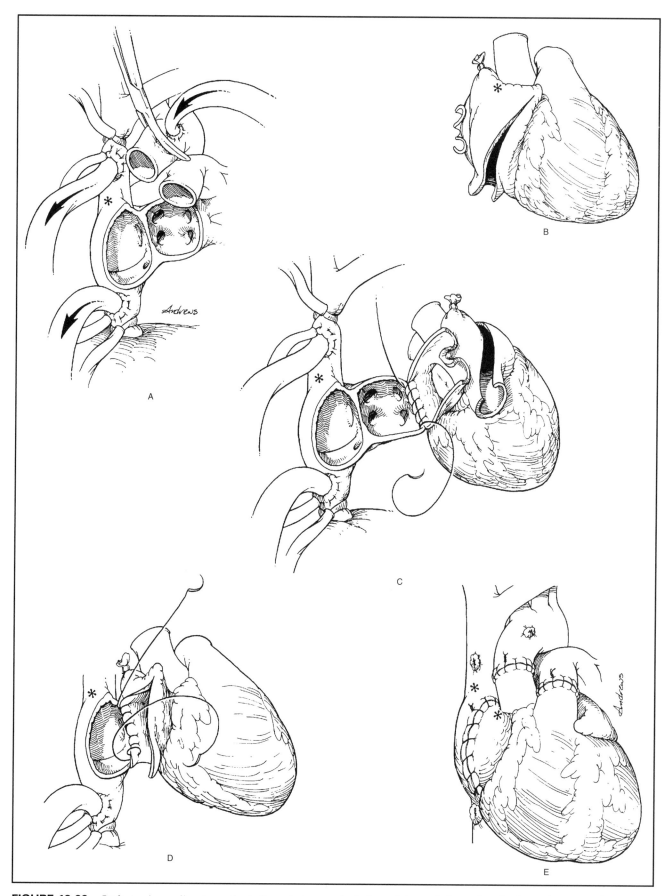

FIGURE 13-93 Orthotopic cardiac transplantation. *A,* Anatomical view of the recipient after the heart is removed. *B,* Incision in right atrium of the donor heart. *C,* Incision in left atrium of the donor heart is being sutured to the recipient's left atrium. *D,* Right atrium of the donor heart and right atrium of the recipient heart are sutured together. *E,* Procedure completed by suturing donor and recipient pulmonary arteries and aortas together. (Reprinted with permission from Cooley, D., *Techniques in Cardiac Surgery 2/e.* [1984] W. B. Saunders, Philadelphia, PA.)

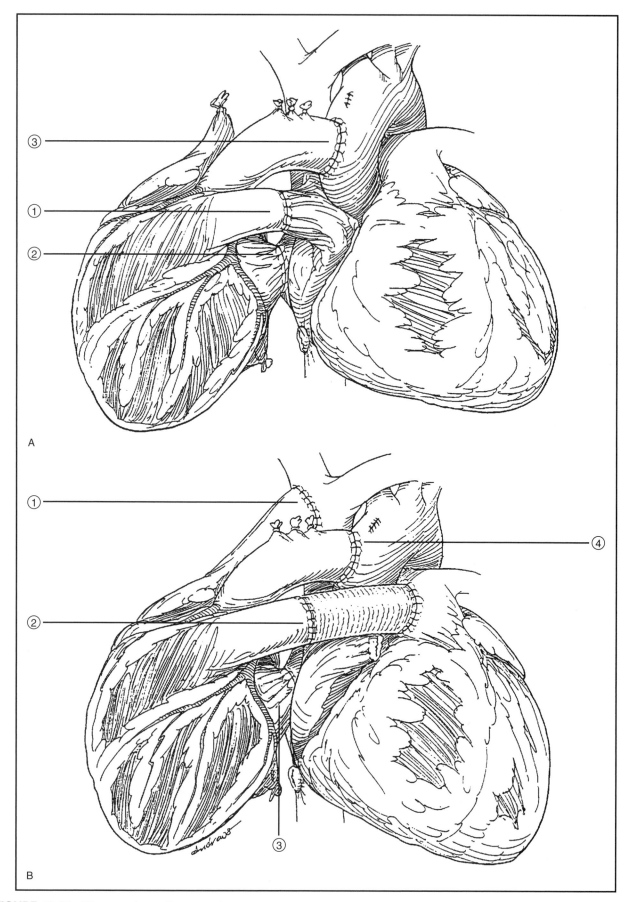

FIGURE 13-94 Heterotopic cardiac transplantation. *A,* Left ventricular bypass: (1) Donor pulmonary artery is anastomosed to the recipient's right atrium. (2) Donor and recipient's left atria are anastomosed together. (3) Donor's aorta is anastomosed to the recipient's aorta. *B,* Total heart bypass: (1) The superior venae cavae are anastomosed together. (2) The pulmonary arteries are anastomosed together. (3) The left atria are anastomosed together. (4) The aortas are anastomosed together. (Reprinted with permission from Cooley, D., *Techniques in Cardiac Surgery,* 2/e. [1984] W. B. Saunders Co., Philadelphia, PA.)

dications for this procedure are ischemic heart disease and cardiomyopathies. This technique assumes 25% to 50% of the cardiac workload.

Procedure

Key steps   This procedure is done in two stages:

1. Stage 1: The left latissimus dorsi muscle is mobilized from the chest wall and subcutaneous tissues, preserving the neurovascular pedicle. Stimulating leads are attached near the muscle body and the thoracodorsal nerve. A 5- to 6-cm portion of the anterior third of the second rib is removed and the muscle flap is positioned inside the chest (Fig. 13-95).
2. Stage 2: A median sternotomy incision is used, and CPB is usually not required. The muscle is positioned around the heart and sutured to the ventricular surfaces of the heart. An intramyocardial sensing electrode is attached to the heart for synchronization of the heart and muscle. All electrodes are attached to the cardio-myostimulator that is placed in an abdominal pocket beneath the rectus abdominis muscle. All incisions are closed (Carpentier & Chachques, 1991; Heckler & White, 1991).

Other Surgical Procedures

Circulatory assist devices

Indications for using circulatory assist devices include patients who cannot be "weaned" from CPB, those with acute myocardial infarction (MI) and cardiogenic shock, and candidates for heart transplant awaiting a donor organ (Ruzevich, 1991). Approximately 2% to 6% of those patients undergoing cardiac surgery experience postcardiotomy shock. Therefore, perioperative nurses practicing in cardiac surgery must be familiar with the use of these devices (Pae et al., 1992).

Intraaortic balloon pump (IABP)   This device was introduced in 1962 and has become widely used in the past 15 years. The IABP may be inserted preoperatively for unstable or high-risk patients; however, its most frequent use is intraoperatively when patients cannot be removed from CPB (Hazelrigg et al., 1992). The advantages are its low cost, ease of insertion, and relative low risk. Some left ventricular activity is necessary as the IABP only provides limited support (Wampler et al., 1991). The balloon is usually placed into the descending aorta retrograde via the femoral artery with a subcutaneous puncture or direct exposure with a cut-down. Transthoracic placement via the aortic arch may be necessary if peripheral vascular disease prevents the balloon from being inserted retrograde (Hazelrigg et al., 1992).

The balloon provides counterpulsation and increases the blood flow to the coronary arteries during cardiac diastole (Fig. 13-96). The balloon deflates with systole and does not obstruct blood flow from the heart. It then inflates with diastole and increases the blood pressure in the proximal aorta. Helium gas is used to inflate the balloon because of helium's rapidity of transport in and out of the balloon and because it is harmless if the balloon ruptures and allows the gas to escape into the bloodstream.

Care must be taken during patient transfer to prevent accidental dislodgement. Possible complications include dissection or injury of the femoral artery or aorta; throm-

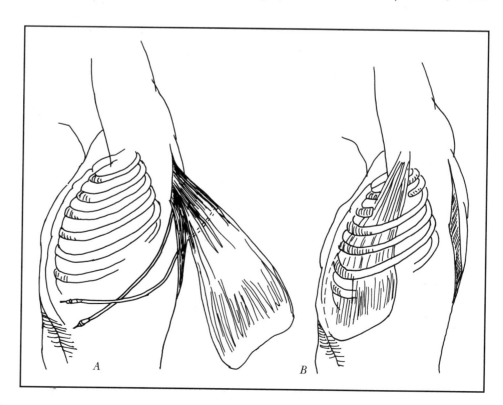

FIGURE 13-95 *A,* Mobilization of the latissimus dorsi muscle. Stimulating lead is attached. *B,* Positioning of the muscle flap inside the chest.

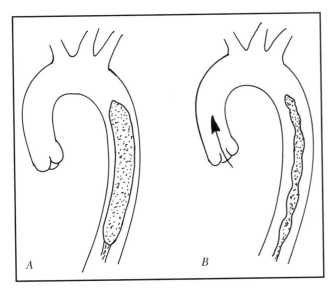

FIGURE 13-96 Position of the intraaortic balloon inside the aorta. *A,* Balloon inflated. *B,* Balloon deflated.

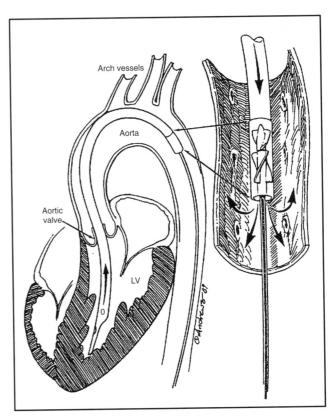

FIGURE 13-97 Hemopump Cardiac Assist. (Reprinted with permission from Duncan, J. M., et al. Implantation Techniques for the Hemopump. Society of Thoracic Surgeons [*The Annals of Thoracic Surgery,* 1989 48:733].)

boembolism; and ischemia of the involved leg if flow is obstructed.

Ventricular assist devices These devices can be used to provide cardiac support for cardiogenic shock that cannot be relieved by IABP and/or inotropic medications. Support can be provided to the right ventricle (RVAD), the left ventricle (LVAD), or both ventricles (BiVAD). The LVAD can provide 80% to 100% of the cardiac workload (Pennington & Swartz, 1990; Wampler et al., 1991).

There are three basic types of assist pumping devices: the roller, pneumatic, and centrifugal. The centrifugal pump is the most commonly used because it is less expensive and less complex, and causes less destruction to the blood elements. However, it does require the patient to be anticoagulated. The centrifugal pump consists of rotating cones that propel the blood (Curtis et al., 1992; Pae et al., 1992).

For RVAD, the right atrium and pulmonary artery are cannulated and the blood is drained from the right atrium and pumped into the pulmonary artery. For LVAD, the left atrium and aorta are cannulated and blood is drained from the left atrium and pumped into the aorta. Oxygenation is provided by the patient's lungs. BiVAD would require both the RVAD and LVAD systems.

The hemopump cardiac assist system This assist system is still an investigational device in the United States but is available in other countries. The pump is inserted retrograde through a Dacron graft sutured to the femoral artery, up the aorta, and into the left ventricle. It provides direct circulatory assistance by pumping the blood from the left ventricle into the aorta (Fig. 13-97). Possible complications include dislodgement of the cannula, ventricular ectopy, inflow obstruction of the cannula, intracardiac shunting, bleeding, thromboembolism, and lower extremity ischemia (Baldwin et al., 1992; Wampler et al., 1991).

Implantable left ventricle assist devices These devices are used to support patients awaiting cardiac transplantation

(bridge to transplant). This device is implanted intra-abdominally and the blood is pumped from the left ventricle apex to the ascending aorta. Two available systems are Heartmate 1000 1P (Thermocardio Systems, Inc.) and Novacor Model 1000 LVAS (Baxter Corp.). Anticoagulation is required, and possible complications include hemorrhage or thromboembolism (Ruzevich, 1991).

Direct mechanical ventricular assist Experimentation with this device is encouraging, and it has been used successfully as a "bridge to transplant." An anterior thoracotomy incision is needed in order to place the "cup" over the heart and the drive system is brought through the chest wall to the power source. The "cup" is held onto the ventricles by a vacuum. The cup has two layers, and with positive and negative pneumatic force the ventricles are compressed and released. There is no contact with blood, so anticoagulation is not necessary (Lowe et al., 1991).

Total artificial heart This device has been used as a "bridge to transplant" since 1985. The Symbion J-7 and the recent Vienna Heart have been used successfully, with the Symbion having been used over 170 times. This device is now restricted in the United States by the FDA. Extensive adhesion formation can increase the difficulty in removing the device and implanting the donor organ. Initial problems included bleeding, hemolysis, renal failure, need for reoperation, and thromboembolism. Although lifesaving, poor patient selection will result in increased complications and, perhaps, wasteful use of scarce resources (Emery et al., 1992).

Extracorporeal membrane oxygenation (ECMO) See Chapter 19, Pediatric Surgery, in this volume.

Cardiac pacemakers

The purpose of cardiac pacemakers is to electrically stimulate the heart to beat. The first permanent pacemaker was implanted in 1958 and since then over 1 million have been implanted worldwide (Hurst & Schlant, 1990). Perioperative nurses working in cardiac surgery must be familiar with pacemakers as temporary pacemakers are usually used for cardiac patients. The nurse may be involved with the implantation of permanent pacemakers or pulse generator change procedures.

Failure of pulse formation and failure of the cardiac conduction system are the major reasons for implanting pacemakers. The American College of Cardiology (ACC) and the American Heart Association's (AHA) "Guidelines for Implantation of Cardiac Pacemakers and Antiarrhythmic Devices" were approved in 1991 (ACC-AHA 1991). These guidelines outline the indications for implanting pacemakers in adults and children.

Pacemaker technology continues to advance, and changes have resulted in smaller devices, increased reliability and longevity of the devices, and multiprogrammability. Two basic varieties of pacemakers exist: single chamber, for use in the atrium or ventricle; and dual chamber, to be used in the atrium and the ventricle. Pacemaker modes are described in universal terminology: the first letter indicates the chamber paced; the second letter indicates the chamber sensed; the third letter indicates the pacemaker response to a sensed event; the fourth letter denotes the presence or absence of rate response; and the fifth letter indicates antitachycardia function (Table 13-7) (Shakespheare & Camm, 1992).

The pulse generator of the pacemaker system contains the power source (lithium anode battery) and the electronic circuits, which control timing, output, and sensing.

The electronics have mechanisms for programming, switches, telemetry, memory, and dual-chamber and rate-responsive features. Programmable pacemakers allow the rate, sensitivity, and output to be changed.

The pacemaker lead serves two purposes: sensing intracardiac activity and sending a message to the generator and conducting the electrical charge to the myocardium. Leads may be placed endocardially (transvenous), using fluoroscopy, or on the epicardium (requires a thoracotomy). Ninety percent are placed transvenously. The leads may be unipolar (one active pole) or bipolar. Some leads incorporate a fixation device to secure the lead to the inside of the heart. Two leads are usually needed for atrioventricular sequential pacing. Epicardial leads puncture or screw into the surface of the heart and are usually secured with a suture (Hurst & Schlant, 1990).

Temporary pacer leads can be inserted transvenously, but during cardiac surgery they are placed on the epicardium. Ventricular and atrial wires are usually placed so the patient can be atrially, ventricularly, or atrioventricularly sequentially paced. The circulating nurse will set the battery-powered external pacemaker according to the surgeon's directions. The nurse must know how to operate the pacemaker correctly.

Procedure

Key steps
Transvenous electrode placement is done under fluoroscopy in order to ensure accurate placement of the lead in the right ventricle. It can be done under local or general anesthesia and often is done in the cardiac catheterization department:

1. An incision is made in the subclavicular area of the anterior chest in order to provide access to the cephalic vein.
2. The vein is divided and the lead is threaded down the vein into the heart.
3. The vein is secured to the lead with a suture and attached to the generator after it has been tested for conduction.
4. The pulse generator is placed in a pocket in the subcutaneous tissue in the upper chest.

TABLE 13-7 Universal Terminology for Pacemaker 5-Letter Codes

Chamber Paced (First Letter)	Chamber Sensed (Second Letter)	Mode Response (Third Letter)	Rate Response* (Fourth Letter)	Tachycardia Function (Fifth Letter)
V = ventricle	V = ventricle	I = inhibited	R = rate response	P = pacing
A = atrium	A = atrium	T = triggered	O = none	N = normal rate competition
D = atrium and ventricle	D = atrium and ventricle	D = atrium and ventricle	P = programmability	S = shock
	O = none	O = none	M = multiprogram	O = none
			C = communicating	D = dual

*Includes programmability functions.

5. The incisions are closed (Fig. 13-98).

Epicardial leads are placed using an anterior thoracotomy or subxiphoid incision. The pulse generator can be placed in the subcutaneous abdominal tissue and the lead can be tunneled subcutaneously to the pacer pocket. All incisions are closed (see Fig. 13-98).

Implantable cardioverter–defibrillator (ICD)

Since the first implant of an ICD in 1980 by Mirowski, over 24,000 have been implanted worldwide (Damiano, 1992). This device has proved to be effective in preventing sudden death. The indications for use are patients with life-threatening arrhythmias that cannot be treated by conventional therapies. Criteria include:

1. One or more hemodynamically significant episodes of ventricular tachycardia or fibrillation
2. Continued ability to induce these arrhythmias with electrophysiological studies
3. Must have adequate left ventricular function

Contraindications include:

1. Ventricular tachyarrhythmias that cannot be terminated by antitachycardia pacing
2. Arrhythmias due to drug toxicity, acute MI, hypoxemia, sepsis, or electrolyte imbalance
3. Inability to induce tachyarrhythmias in patients with unexplained syncope (Damiano, 1992).

The self-contained ICD unit monitors the heart, identifies ventricular fibrillation or tachycardia, and delivers the corrective discharge. Some ICDs also provide pacer features. The unit is powered by lithium vanadium silver pentoxide batteries with a life expectancy of 5 years and the ability to deliver 100 discharges at a maximum output of 30 to 40 joules. The epicardial or transvenous electrode senses the heart rhythm and sends the message to the generator, and the defibrillation energy is sent to the heart via implanted electrode patches on the epicardium or pericardium, or transversely (Fig. 13-99). Possible postoperative complications include infection, bleeding, pulmonary problems, and/or generator erosion (Damiano, 1992; Hurst & Schlant, 1990).

Special electrophysiological testing equipment is needed for testing and programming the ICD. The defibrillation threshold is tested by inducing ventricular fibrillation. The testing process can be tedious and may require repositioning of the patches or sensing leads.

Procedure

Key steps

1. Median sternotomy, left anterolateral thoracotomy, bilateral thoracotomies, subxiphoid, or subcostal thoracotomy incisions can be used.
2. CPB is not usually required, but standby CPB may be indicated.
3. The pericardium is opened; the epicardial electrode is positioned on the heart, and the defibrillator patches are positioned in an anterior/posterior or lateral/lateral orientation.

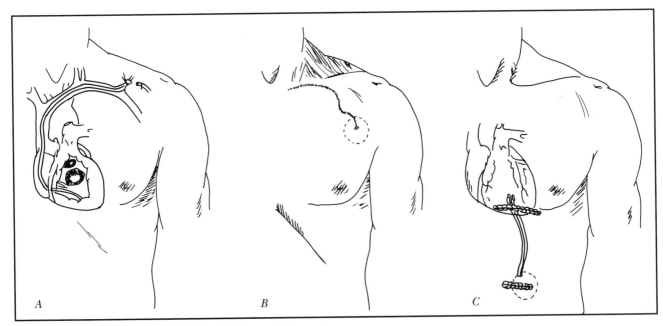

A *B* *C*

FIGURE 13-98 *A*, Transvenous pacemaker lead threaded into the right heart via the cephalic vein. *B*, Pacemaker implanted in a subcutaneous pocket in the upper chest. *C*, Transthoracic approach, with pacing leads placed on the epicardium and connected to the pacemaker. The pacemaker is implanted in a subcutaneous tissue pocket in the abdominal area (above the belt line).

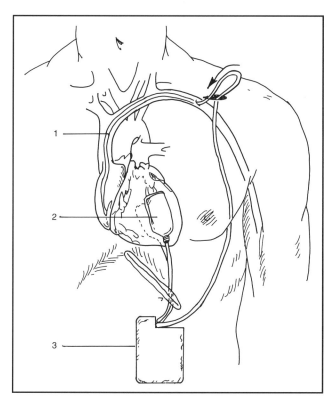

FIGURE 13-99 ICD implantation: (1) Transvenous lead inserted via the cephalic vein into the right ventricle. (2) Electrode patches placed over the ventricles. (3) Generator.

4. Transvenous leads (if used) are inserted via the left subclavian vein and tunneled subcutaneously to the generator placement site, usually the left upper quadrant of the abdomen in a subcutaneous pocket. A thoracotomy is not necessary if sensing and discharge leads are transvenous.

Interventional cardiology procedures

Percutaneous transluminal coronary angioplasty (PTCA) Introduced in 1977, this technique of reducing coronary artery obstruction by compressing atherosclerotic lesions with a balloon has become a common procedure (Fig. 13-100). Limitations include lesions longer than 2 cm in length, diffuse disease, possible abrupt closure of the target vessel, and biological problems related to elastic recoil, endovascular disruptions, and proliferative responses that can cause restenosis (National Heart, Lung, and Blood Institute, 1992).

Surgical standby for PTCA procedures is based on the possibility of acute occlusion and the risk based on the site of the lesion, collateral circulation, and myocardial function distal to the lesion (Meier et al., 1992). *The Guidelines for Percutaneous Transluminal Coronary Angioplasty* from the American College of Cardiology and the American Heart Association (1988) recommend that an experienced cardiovascular surgical team be available within the institution. Institutional policies for PTCA surgical standby will vary and include no standby (surgery

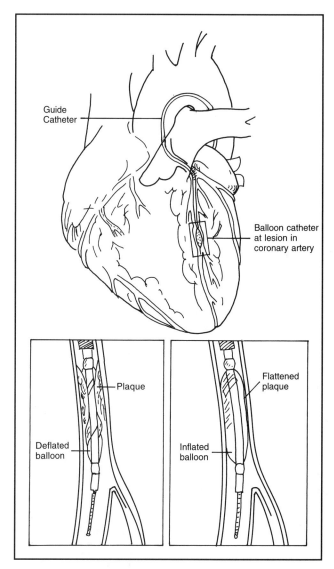

FIGURE 13-100 PTCA. *A,* Catheter inside the coronary artery. *B,* Catheter at plaque site. *C,* Catheter balloon inflated and plaque compressed.

would not be considered), next available room, or full standby. The choice of standby is based on the patient risk and/or condition during the PTCA (Cameron et al., 1990).

Directional coronary atherectomy This procedure uses a side-cutting device built into a coronary artery catheter that can be used to remove atheroma. Its use is limited to large arteries with noncalcified plaques. Technically this is a complex procedure. The FDA has approved its use in coronary arteries (Grab, 1992).

Transluminal extraction atherectomy This uses a forward-cutting device that cuts plaque from the artery and removes it with a suction. It is technically complex and can result in a substantial blood loss (Good & Gentzler, 1992).

Rotational atherectomy A conical burr with diamond chips is used to abrasively cut and pulverize plaque (National Heart, Lung, and Blood Institute, 1992).

Over the wire ablative lasers This is used for long stenoses and diffuse disease, but its limitations include its high cost and the small luminal diameter attained (National Heart, Lung, and Blood Institute, 1992).

Laser balloon angioplasty This involves heating the artery wall near the balloon with an Nd:YAG laser. There is a high rate of restenosis (Dougherty et al., 1991).

Direct laser angioplasty Experimental studies using the CO_2 and excimer laser intraoperatively for diffuse coronary artery disease are encouraging, but further research is needed (Dougherty et al., 1991).

Endovascular stents These expandable metal devices are placed inside of an artery to keep it open. The effectiveness of this technique is questionable, and anticoagulation is necessary to prevent thrombosis (National Heart, Lung, and Blood Institute, 1992).

Catheter ablative procedures This technique is used to control drug-resistant supraventricular tachyarrhythmias and was first introduced in 1981. Electrical current is used through a cardiac catheter to render selected conduction pathways inactive. Initially, direct current (DC) was used and general anesthesia was required because of the discomfort to the patient. DC caused significant tissue trauma, and often a permanent pacemaker was implanted owing to the atrioventricular node's becoming inactive.

Recently introduced radiofrequency ablation techniques have been successful without the adverse effects of DC ablation and are more precise.

Surgical division of accessory atrioventricular conduction pathways has been effective and continues to be the procedure of choice for certain ventricular tachycardias. Complex electrophysiological mapping equipment is necessary. Surgical intervention can be avoided for those arrhythmias treatable by catheter ablative technique (Seale, 1992; Scheinmann et al., 1991).

Percutaneous balloon valvuloplasty This procedure is done for stenotic heart valves. The valve is opened with the use of a balloon. Severe calcification and/or subvalvular disease or the presence of thrombus are major contraindications for this procedure. Patients who are not considered operative candidates or have severe noncardiac disease are candidates for this procedure. Long-term follow-up is limited (Hurst & Schlant, 1990).

SUMMARY

This chapter has covered various cardiac surgery procedures and their indications, and preparation of the patient and the operating room. The perioperative nurse is challenged by this specialty because patients already have compromising disease; because equipment and instrumentation are multifaceted and extensive; and because intense assessment, anticipation, and preparation are always required. Prevention of complications, especially postoperative infections, begins during the preoperative and intraoperative phases of care and is a significant part of perioperative nursing.

Progress in cardiac surgery has resulted from the determination to develop methods of helping patients with cardiac problems. Careful review and evaluation of patient outcomes are essential for continued progress in this exciting area of surgical treatment.

REFERENCES

Abramowicz, M. (1992). Antimicrobial prophylaxis in surgery. *The Medical Letter on Drugs & Therapeutics, 34,* 862.

Akins, J. (1991). Mechanical cardiac valvular prostheses. *Annals of Thoracic Surgery, 52,* 161–172.

Amato, J., Cotroneo, J., Galdieri, R., Heldman, E., Stark, F., Bushong, J., & Lepeniotis, C. (1990). Perfusion primes, flow rates, and perfusion pressures for CPB in pediatric practice. In *Perspectives in Pediatric Cardiology* (Vol. 2, pp. 192–195). Mt. Kisco, NY: Futura Publishing Co.

Amato, J., Galdieri, R., & Cotroneo, J. (1991). Role of extended aortoplasty related to the definition of coarctation of the aorta. *Annals of Thoracic Surgery, 52,* 615–620.

Amato, J., Marbey, M., Bush, C., Galdieri, R., Cotroneo, J., & Bushong, J. (1988). Sytemic-pulmonary polytetrafluoroethylene shunts in palliative operations for congenital heart disease. *Journal of Thoracic and Cardiovascular Surgery, 95,* 62–69.

American College of Cardiology and American Heart Association Task Force Report (1991a). Guidelines and indications for coronary artery bypass graft surgery. *Journal of the American College of Cardiology, 17,* 543–589.

American College of Cardiology and American Heart Association (1991b). Guidelines for implantation of cardiac pacemakers and antiarrhythmia devices. *Circulation, 84,* 455–465.

American College of Cardiology and American Heart Association (1988). Guidelines for percutaneous transluminal coronary angioplasty. *Circulation, 78,* 486–502.

American College of Surgeons (1991a). Guidelines for minimal standards in cardiac surgery. *Bulletin of the American College of Surgeons,* August, 27–29.

American College of Surgeons (1991b). *Socio-economic factbook for surgery 1991–1992,* Chicago: American College of Surgeons.

American Heart Association (1992). Statistics. *Circulation, 85,* A104.

American Heart Association (1991). *Heart and stroke facts.* Dallas: American Heart Association.

American Hospital Association (1991). *Hospital statistics,* Chicago: American Hospital Association.

Anderson, R., & Ho, S. (1989). The surgical anatomy of the Fontan procedure. In *Perspectives in pediatric cardiology* (Vol. 2): *Pediatric cardiac surgery, Part II* (pp. 162–166.). Mt. Kisco, NY: Futura Publishing Co.

Anderson, R., Necheo, W., Park, S., & Zuberbuhler, J. (1988). *Perspectives in pediatric cardiology* (Vol. 1). Mt. Kisco, NY: Futura Publishing Co.

Anderson, S. (1990). ABGs: Six easy steps to interpreting blood gases. *American Journal of Nursing, 90,* 42–45.

Andreoli, K., Zipes, D., Wallace, A., Kinney, M., & Fowkes, V. (1987). *Comprehensive cardiac care* (6th ed.). St. Louis: C. V. Mosby.

Aren, C. (1990). Heparin and protamine therapy. *Seminars in Thoracic and Cardiovascular Surgery, 2,* 364–372.

Arom, K., & Emery, R. (1992). Coronary sinus cardioplegia: Clinical trial with only retrograde approach. *Annals of Thoracic Surgery, 53,* 967–971.

Association of Operating Room Nurses (1994). *Standards and recommended practices.* Denver: Author.

Baldwin, R., Radovanceviro, B., Duncan, J., Wampler, R., & Frazier, O. (1992). Management of patients supported on the hemopump cardiac assist system. *Texas Heart Institute Journal, 19,* 81–86.

Barner, H. (1991). Blood cardioplegia: A review and comparison with crystalloid cardioplegia. *Annals of Thoracic Surgery, 52,* 1354–1367.

Bartmus, D., Driscoll, D., Offord, K., Humes, R., Mair, D., Schaff, H., Puga, J., & Danielson, G. (1990). The modified Fontan operation for children less than four years of age. *Journal of the American College of Cardiology, 15,* 429–435.

Behrendt, D., & Austen, W. G. (1985). *Patient care in cardiac surgery* (4th ed.). Boston: Little, Brown & Co.

Bell, P., & Diffee, G. (1991). Cardiopulmonary bypass principles: Nursing implications. *AORN Journal, 53,* 1480–1496.

Bonchek, T. (1987). Basis for selecting a valve prosthesis. In *Cardiac Surgery* (2nd ed., pp. 103–125). Philadelphia: F. A. Davis.

Bridges, N., Jonus, R., Mayer, J., Flanagan, M., Keane, J., & Castaneda, A. (1990a). Bidirectional cavopulmonary anastomosis as interim palliation for high-risk Fontan candidates. *Circulation, 82* (Suppl. IV), 170–176.

Bridges, N., Lock, J., & Castaneda, A. (1990b). Baffle fenestration with subsequent transcatheter closure: Modification of the Fontan operation for patients at increased risk. *Circulation, 82,* 1681–1689.

Buckberg, G. (1987). Recent progress in myocardial protection during cardiac operations. In *Cardiac Surgery* (2nd ed., pp. 291–319.). Philadelphia: F. A. Davis.

Cabrol, C., Gandjbahch, I., & Pavie, A. (1987). Techniques of ascending aorta reconstruction. In *Heart Valve Replacement and Reconstruction.* Chicago: Year Book Medical Publishers.

Cabrol, C., Gandjbakhch, I., Pavie, A., & Bors, V. (1991). Total replacement of the ascending aorta: La Pitie experience. *Seminars in Thoracic and Cardiovascular Surgery, 3,* 177–179.

Calderon, M., & Ott, D. (1991). Surgical treatment of post infarction rupture of interventricular septum. *Texas Heart Institute Journal, 18,* 282–285.

Cameron, D., Stinson, S., Greene, P., & Gardner, T. (1990). Surgical standby for PTCA: A survey of patterns of practice. *Annals of Thoracic Surgery, 51,* 35–39.

Carpentier, A., & Chachques, J. (1991). Clinical dynamic cardiomyoplasty: Method and outcome. *Seminars in Thoracic and Cardiovascular Surgery, 3,* 136–139.

Carrel, T., Linka, A., & Turnia, M. (1992). Tricuspid valve obstruction caused by plasmacytoma metastasis. *Annals of Thoracic Surgery, 54,* 352–354.

Carrier, M., Gregoire, J., Tronc, F., Cartier, R., Leclerc, Y., & Pelletier, L. C. (1992). Effect of internal mammary artery dissection on sternal vascularization. *Annals of Thoracic Surgery, 53,* 115–119.

Chitwood, W. (1992). Retrograde cardioplegia: Current methods. *Annals of Thoracic Surgery, 53,* 352–355.

Chu, S., Leu, M., Chang, C., & Wang, J. (1991). Total cavopulmonary connection: A modified technique without prosthetic material. *Journal of Cardiac Surgery, 6,* 294–298.

Cohen, A., Cleveland, D., Dyck, J., Poppe, D., Smallhorn, J., Freedom, R., Trusler, G., Coles, J., Moes, C., Rebeyka, I., & Williams, W. (1991). Results of the Fontan procedure for patients with univentricular heart. *Annals of Thoracic Surgery, 52,* 1266–1271.

Constancia, P. E. (1991). The Ross procedure: Aortic valve replacement using autologous pulmonary valve. *Critical Care Nursing Clinics of North America, 3,* 717–721.

Cooley, D. (1991). Experience with hypothermic circulatory arrest and treatment of aneurysms of the ascending aorta. *Seminars in Thoracic and Cardiovascular Surgery, 3,* 166–170.

Cooley, D. (1984). *Techniques in cardiac surgery* (2nd ed.). Philadelphia: W. B. Saunders.

Cooper, D., & Novitzky, D. (1990). *The transplantation and replacement of thoracic organs.* Boston: Kluwer Academic Publishers.

Corno, A. (1990). Myocardial protection in immature hearts. *Perspectives in Pediatric Cardiology* (Vol. 2.). Mt. Kisco. NY: Futura Publishing Co.

Crawford, E. S., & Coselli, J. (1991a). Replacement of the aortic arch. *Seminars in Thoracic and Cardiovascular Surgery, 3,* 194–212.

Crawford, E. S., & Coselli, J. (1991b). Thoracoabdominal aneurysm surgery. *Seminars in Thoracic and Cardiovascular Surgery, 3,* 300–322.

Crawford, E. S., & Crawford, J. L. (1984). *Diseases of the aorta.* Baltimore: Williams & Wilkins.

Crawford, F. A. (1987). *Cardiac surgery current heart valve prostheses* (Vol. 1, No. 2.). Philadelphia: Hanley and Belfus.

Crupi, G, Parenzan, L., & Anderson, R. (1990). *Perspectives in pediatric cardiology* (Vol. 2): Pediatric Cardiac Surgery (Vol. 1). Mt. Kisco, NY: Futura Publishing Co.

Curtis, J., Walls, J., Schmaltz, R., Boley, T., Nawarawong, W., & Landreneau, R. (1992). Experience with the Sarns centrifugal pump in postcardiotomy ventricular failure. *Journal of Thoracic and Cardiovascular Surgery, 104,* 554–560.

Damiano, R. (1992). Implantable cardioverter defibrillators: Current status and future directions. *Journal of Cardiac Surgery, 7,* 36–57.

David, T. (1990). A rational approach to surgical treatment of mitral valve disease. In *Advances in Cardiac Surgery* (Vol. 2, pp. 63–73). St. Louis: C. V. Mosby.

David, T. (1989). Replacement of chordae tendineae with expanded polytetrafluoroethylene sutures. *Journal of Cardiac Surgery, 4,* 286–290.

Docker, C., Muthusamy, R., Balasundaram, M., & Duran, C. (1992). Intraoperative echocardiography: An essential tool in cardiac surgery. *AORN Journal, 55,* 167–176.

Doty, D. (1985: updated 1991). *Cardiac Surgery.* Chicago: Year Book Medical Publishers.

Dougherty, K., Marsh, J., Lambert, B., Schulz, D., Reece, B., & Nangle, M. (1991). Laser ablation of coronary arteries. *AORN Journal, 54,* 244–261.

Dugan, L. (1991). Pacemakers. *Nursing '91, 21* (6), 47–52.

Elliott, M. (1990). Perfusion for pediatric open heart surgery. *Seminars in Thoracic and Cardiovascular Surgery, 2,* 332–340.

Emery, R., Joyce, L., Prietro, M., Johnson, K., Goldenberg, J., & Pritzker, M. (1992). Experience with the Symbion total artificial heart as a bridge to transplantation. *Annals of Thoracic Surgery, 53,* 282–288.

Ergin, M., Galla, J., Lansman, S., Taylor, M., & Griepp, R. (1991). Distal perfusion methods for surgery of the descending aorta. *Seminars in Thoracic and Cardiovascular Surgery, 3,* 293–299.

Ferguson, T., & Cox, J. (1991). Temporary external DDD pacing after cardiac operations. *Annals of Thoracic Surgery, 51,* 723–732.

Frater, R., Salomon, N., Rainer, W., Cosgrove, D., & Wickham, E. (1992). Carpentier Edwards pericardial aortic valve intermediate results. *Annals of Thoracic Surgery, 53,* 764–771.

Fuster, V., & Ip, J. (1991). Medical aspects of acute aortic dissection. *Seminars in Thoracic and Cardiovascular Surgery, 3,* 219–224.

Glick, D., Liddicoat, J., & Karp, R. (1990). Alternative conduits for coronary artery bypass grafting. In *Advances in Cardiac Surgery* (Vol. 2, pp. 191–201). St. Louis: Mosby–Year Book.

Good, L., & Gentzler, R. (1992). Coronary atherectomy: An alternative to balloon angioplasty. *AORN Journal, 53,* 32–39.

Gore, J., Alpert, J., Benotti, J., Kotilainen, P., & Haffajee, C. (1985). *Handbook of hemodynamic monitoring.* Boston: Little, Brown & Co.

Grab, C. (1992). The cutting alternative to PTCA. *RN, 55,* 22–26.

Hammon, J. W. (1989). The role of the automatic implantable cardioverter defibrillator in the treatment of ventricular tachycardia. *Seminars in Thoracic and Cardiovascular Surgery, 1,* 88–96.

Hazelrigg, S., Auer, J., & Seifert, P. (1992). Experience in 100 transthoracic balloon pumps. *Annals of Thoracic Surgery, 54,* 528–532.

Heckler, F., & White, M. (1991). Isolation of skeletal muscle for biomechanical circulatory assist. *Seminars in Thoracic and Cardiovascular Surgery, 3,* 128–131.

Hopkins, R. (1989). *Cardiac reconstructions with allograft valves.* New York: Springer-Verlag.

Hurray, J., & Saver, C. (1992). Arterial blood gas interpretation. *AORN Journal, 55,* 180–185.

Hurst, J. W., & Schlant, R. C. (1990). *The heart* (7th ed.). San Francisco: McGraw-Hill.

Irwin, E., Braunlin, E., & Foker, J. (1991). Staged repair of interrupted aortic arch and ventricular septal defect in infancy. *Annals of Thoracic Surgery, 52,* 632–639.

Jonas, R. (1991). Coarctation: Do we need to resect ductal tissue? *Annals of Thoracic Surgery, 52,* 604–607.

Jonas, R., & Castaneda, A. (1988). A modified Fontan atrial baffle and systemic venous to pulmonary artery anastomotic techniques. *Journal of Cardiac Surgery, 3,* 91–96.

Jones, E., Weintraub, W., Craver, J., Guyton, R., & Cohen, C. (1991). Coronary bypass surgery: Is the operation different today? *Journal of Thoracic and Cardiovascular Surgery, 101,* 108–115.

Karp, R., Lak, H., & Wechsler, A. (1992). *Advances in cardiac surgery.* St. Louis: Mosby–Year Book.

Kazui, T., Inoue, N., Yamada, O., & Komatsu, S. (1992). Selective cerebral perfusion during operations for aneurysms of the aortic arch: A reassessment. *Annals of Thoracic Surgery, 53,* 109–114.

Khonsari, S. (1988). *Cardiac surgery: Safeguards and pitfalls of operative technique.* Rockville, MD: Aspen Publishers.

Kirklin, J., & Barratt-Boyes, B. (1993). *Cardiac Surgery* (2nd ed.). New York: Churchill Livingstone.

Kloner, R. (1990). *Cardiology reference book,* New York: CoMedical.

Komeda, M., David, T., Malik, A., Ivanov, J., & Sun, Z. (1992). Operative risks and long term results of operations for left ventricular aneurysms. *Annals of Thoracic Surgery, 53,* 22–29.

Kouchoukos, N. (1991). Spinal cord ischemic injury: Is it preventable? *Seminars in Thoracic and Cardiovascular Surgery, 3,* 323–328.

Kumar, A., Kumar, R., Schrivastava, S., Venugopal, P., Sood, A., & Gopinath, N. (1992). Mitral valve reconstruction. *Texas Heart Institute Journal, 19,* 107–111.

Lacour-Gayet, F. (1991). Commentary: Indications for extended aortic arch reconstruction. *Annals of Thoracic Surgery, 52,* 613–614.

Lansman, S., Ergin, A., Galla, J., Taylor, M., & Griepp, R. (1991). Intraluminal graft repair of ascending, arch, descending, and thoracoabdominal aortic segments for dissecting and aneurysmal disease: Long term follow-up. *Seminars in Thoracic and Cardiovascular Surgery, 3,* 180–182.

Lewis, C., Cooley, D., Murphy, M., Talledo, O., & Vega, D. (1992). Surgical repair of aortic root aneurysms in 280 patients. *Annals of Thoracic Surgery, 53,* 38–46.

Lichtenstein, S., & Abel, J. (1992). Warm heart surgery: Theory and current practice. In *Advances in Cardiac Surgery* (Vol. 3, pp. 135–154). St. Louis: Mosby–Year Book.

Lowe, J., Anstadt, M., Vantrigt, P., Smith, P., Hendry, P., Plunkett, M., & Anstadt, G. (1991). First successful bridge to cardiac transplantation using direct mechanical ventricular actuation. *Annals of Thoracic Surgery, 52,* 1237–1245.

Lundy, E., Gassmann, C., Bonchek, L., Smith, R., Burlingame, M., & Vazales, B. (1992). A simple and safe technique of left ventricular venting. *Annals of Thoracic Surgery, 53,* 1127–1129.

Magovern, G. (1991). Introduction to the history and development of skeletal muscle plasticity and its clinical application to cardiomyoplasty and skeletal muscle ventricle. *Seminars in Thoracic and Cardiovascular Surgery, 3,* 95–97.

Maloney, S. (1989). Tetralogy of Fallot using pulmonary allograft conduits to reconstruct the right ventricular outflow tract. *AORN Journal, 50,* 554–562.

Mattox, K. (1991). Contemporary issues in thoracic aortic trauma. *Seminars in Thoracic and Cardiovascular Surgery, 3,* 281–285.

Mavroudis, C., Backer, C., & Idriss, F. (1992). Arterial switch for transposition of great arteries and associated malposition anomalies. *Advances in Cardiac Surgery* (Vol. 3, pp. 175–242). St. Louis: Mosby–Year Book.

Mayer, J., Jonas, R., & Castaneda, A. (1986). Arterial switch operation for transposition of the great arteries with intact ventricular septum. *Journal of Cardiac Surgery, 1,* 97–104.

McGoon, D. (1987). *Cardiac Surgery* (2nd ed.). Philadelphia: F. A. Davis.

McGrath, L. (1992). Tetralogy of Fallot with pulmonic stenosis. In *Advances in Cardiac Surgery* (Vol. 3, pp. 175–203). St. Louis: Mosby–Year Book.

Meier, B., Urgan, P., Dorsaz, P., & Favre, J. (1992). Surgical standby for coronary balloon angioplasty. *Journal of the American Medical Association, 268,* 741–745.

Menasche, P., & Piwnia, A. (1991). Cardioplegia by way of the coronary sinus for valvular and coronary artery surgery. *Journal of the American College of Cardiology, 18,* 628–636.

Messmer, B., Minale, C., Muhler, E., & Bernuth, G. (1991). Surgical correction of coarctation in early infancy: Does surgical technique influence the result? *Annals of Thoracic Surgery, 52,* 594–603.

Monro, J. (1990). Circulatory arrest versus cardiopulmonary bypass. *Perspectives in Pediatric Cardiology* (Vol. 2, pp 203–207). Mt. Kosco, NY: Futura Publishing Co.

Moriera, L., Stolf, N., & Jatene, A. (1991). Benefits of cardiomyoplasty for dilated cardiomyopathy. *Seminars in Thoracic and Cardiovascular Surgery, 3,* 140–144.

Moulton, A. (1984). *Congenital heart surgery current techniques and controversies.* Pasadena, CA: Appleton Davies.

Muirhead, J. (1992). Heart and heart–lung transplantation. *Critical Care Nursing Clinics of North America, 4,* 97–109.

National Heart, Lung, and Blood Institute (1992). Evaluation of emerging technologies for coronary revascularization. *Circulation, 85,* 357–361.

Nichols, G. M., Eiriksson, C., Olsen, C., Mellinger, C., Harritt, P., & Leary, P. (1991). Transesophageal echocardiography: A new tool in the diagnostic tool box. *IATROS, 2,* 1–6.

Nurse's Clinical Library (1984). *Cardiovascular disorders,* Springhouse, PA: Springhouse Corp.

O'Brien, M., & Griffin, D. (1990). Aortic and pulmonic allografts in contemporary cardiac surgery. In *Advances of Cardiac Surgery* (Vol. 1, pp. 1–25). Chicago: Year Book Medical Publishers.

Pacifico, A., & Sand, M. (1987). Advances in surgical management of congenital heart disease in infants and children. In *Cardiac Surgery* (2nd ed., pp. 177–219). Philadelphia: F. A. Davis.

Pae, W., Miller, C., Matthews, Y., & Pierce, W. (1992). Ventricular assist devices for postcardiotomy shock. *Journal of Thoracic and Cardiovascular Surgery, 104,* 541–543.

Parenteau, G., Van Anderson, R., Siegman, M., Vastia, S., & Clark, R. (1992). New concepts in cardiopulmonary bypass. In *Advances in Cardiac Surgery (Vol. 3,* pp. 9–56). St. Louis: Mosby–Year Book.

Pearson, D. (1990). Gas exchange: Bubble and membrane oxygenators. *Seminars in Thoracic and Cardiovascular Surgery, 2,* 313–319.

Pennington, D., & Swartz, M. (1990). Current status of temporary circulatory support. *Advances in Cardiology I* (pp. 177–198). Chicago: Year Book Medical Publishers.

Pennington, D., Noedel, N., McBride, L., Naunheim, K., & Ring, W. (1991). Heart transplantation in children: An international survey. *Annals of Thoracic Surgery, 52,* 710–715.

Perez, J., Villagra, F., Leon, J., Gomez, R., Diaz, P., Diez, J., Checa, S., Sanchez, P., Alonso, A., & Villibre, D. (1990). Total hemodilution in children during open heart surgery. In *Perspectives in pediatric cardiology (Vol. 2): Pediatric cardiac surgery (Part 3,* pp. 196–202). Mt. Kisco, NY: Futura Publishing.

Pluth, J. (1987). Mitral valve reconstruction versus prosthetic valve replacement. In *Cardiac Surgery* (2nd ed., pp. 122–139). Philadelphia: F. A. Davis.

Powell, M., & Costanzo, J. (1990). Tricuspid atresia: Surgical treatment, pediatric nursing care. *AORN Journal, 52,* 567–574.

Puga, F., Leoni, F., Julsrud, P., & Mair, D. (1989). Complete repair of pulmonary atresia, ventricular septal defect, and severe peripheral arborization abnormalities of the central pulmonary arteries. *Journal of Thoracic and Cardiovascular Surgery, 98,* 1018–1029.

Reed, C. (1985). *Cardiopulmonary bypass* (2nd ed.). Houston: Texas Medical Press.

Ruzevich, S. (1991). Heart assist devices: State of the art. *Critical Care Nursing Clinics of North America, 3,* 723–732.

Sabiston, D. (1986). *Textbook of Surgery (13th ed.).* Philadelphia: W. B. Saunders.

Saver, C., & Hurray, J. (1990a). Electrocardiogram monitoring: Interpreting normal cardiac rhythms. *AORN Journal, 52,* 264–271.

Saver, C., & Hurray, J. (1990b). Electrocardiogram monitoring: Interpreting abnormal cardiac rhythms. *AORN Journal, 52,* 273–283.

Sawatari, K., Imai, Y., Kurosawa, H., Isomatsu, Y., & Momma, K. (1989). Staged operation for pulmonary atresia and ventricular septal defect with major aortopulmonary collateral arteries. *Journal of Thoracic and Cardiovascular Surgery, 98,* 738–750.

Scheinmann, M., Laks, M., DiMarco, J., & Plumb, J. (1991). Current role of catheter ablative procedures in patients with cardiac arrhythmias. *Circulation, 83,* 2146–2151.

Seale, W. (1992). Radiofrequency catheter ablation for cardiac arrhythmias. *IATROS, 3,* 1–6.

Shakespheare, C., & Camm, A. (1992). Benefits of advances in cardiac pacemaker technology. *Clinical Cardiology, 15,* 601–606.

Siewers, R., Ettedgui, J., Pahl, E., Tallman, T., & del Nido, P. (1991). Coarctation and hypoplasia of the aortic arch: Will the arch grow? *Annals of Thoracic Surgery, 52,* 608–614.

Society of Thoracic Surgeons (1992). Practice guidelines in cardiothoracic surgery. *Annals of Thoracic Surgery, 53,* 1138–1146.

Starek, P. (1987). *Heart valve replacement and reconstruction.* Chicago: Year Book Medical Publishers.

Stark, J., & de Leval, M. (1983). *Surgery for congenital heart defects.* New York: Grune & Stratton.

Stark, J., & Kostelka, M. (1991). The use of right atrial flap in total cavopulmonary connection. *Journal of Cardiac Surgery, 6,* 362–366.

Stein, D., Laks, H., & Drinkwater, D. (1992). Myocardial protection in children. In *Advances in Cardiac Surgery (Vol. 3,* pp. 113–133). St. Louis: Mosby–Year Book.

Stein, D., Laks, H., Drinkwater, D., Permut, L., Louie, H., Pearl, J., George, B., & Williams, R. (1991). Results of total cavopulmonary connection in treatment of patients with a functional single ventricle. *Journal of Thoracic and Cardiovascular Surgery, 102,* 280–287.

Svensson, L., Crawford, E. S., Hess, K., Coselli, J., & Safi, H. (1992). Composite valve graft replacement of the proximal aorta: Comparison of techniques in 348 patients. *Annals of Thoracic Surgery, 54,* 427–439.

Tavilla, G., van Son, J., Verhagen, A., & Smedts, F. (1992). Retrogastric versus antigastric routing and histology of right gastroepiploic artery. *Annals of Thoracic Surgery, 53,* 1057–1061.

Thurer, R., Luceri, R., & Bolooki, H. (1986). A.I.C.D.: Techniques of implantation and results. *Annals of Thoracic Surgery, 42,* 143–147.

Utley, J. (1990). Historical perspectives and basic pathophysiology of cardiopulmonary bypass. *Seminars in Thoracic and Cardiovascular Surgery, 2,* 292–299.

Vouche, P., & Neveux, J. (1991). Surgical management of diffuse subaortic stenosis: An integrated approach. *Annals of Thoracic Surgery, 52,* 654–662.

Wampler, R., Frazier, O., Lansing, A., Smalling, R., Nicklas, J., Phillips, S., Guyton, R., & Golding, A. (1991). Treatment of cardiogenic shock with the hemopump left ventricular assist device. *Annals of Thoracic Surgery, 52,* 506–513.

Wells, F., & Milstein, B. (1990). *Thoracic surgical techniques.* Philadelphia: Bailliere Tindall.

Yee, E., Turley, K., Wen-Ren, H., & Ebert, P. (1987). Infant total anomalous pulmonary venous connection: Factors influencing timing of presentation and operative outcome. *Circulation, 76* (Suppl. III), III83–87.

Young, J. (1992). Heart transplantation: Where we stand at 25 years. *The Newspaper of Cardiology,* May, 7.

Zwischenberger, J., & Bartlett, R. (1990). Extracorporeal circulation for respiratory or cardiac failure. *Seminars in Thoracic and Cardiovascular Surgery, 2,* 320–331.

Chapter 14

Thoracic Surgery

Key Concepts

- Thoracic surgery involves body structures and functioning that are critical to life and sustenance. Enclosed within the thorax are the major organs of respiration and circulation.

- Pertinent patient information that is gathered by the perioperative nurse includes physical status and physiological responses; understanding, perceptions, and expectations regarding the surgical procedure; previous responses to illness, surgery, and hospitalization; and results of diagnostic studies.

- Diagnosis of thoracic diseases and disorders usually requires a variety of tests, including X-rays, computed tomography (CT scan), magnetic resonance imaging (MRI), nuclear techniques, arteriograms, pulmonary function tests, arterial blood gases, esophagrams, electrocardiogram (ECG), and other laboratory tests.

- Procedures integral to thoracic surgery and sometimes helpful in establishing diagnoses include bronchoscopy, esophagoscopy, mediastinoscopy, thoracoscopy, video-assisted thoracic surgery (VATS), and needle biopsies.

- Incisional sites for thoracic surgery are posterolateral, anterolateral, median sternotomy, anterior, axillary, and thoracoabdominal.

- Because many thoracic surgery patients have coexisting diseases, especially cardiac, and numerous risk factors are present, the importance of intraoperative monitoring becomes evident: ECG, blood pressure, pulse oximetry, arterial pressure, temperature, urinary output, and ventilation parameters (e.g., peak airway pressure, tidal volume, expiratory time, and minute ventilation).

INTRODUCTION

This chapter discusses a myriad of thoracic surgical procedures, some diagnostic, some curative, and some palliative. The perioperative nurse understands that impaired gas exchange, ineffective breathing patterns, and ineffective airway clearance are potential problems/nursing diagnoses related to thoracic surgery. These patients are also at high risk for infection.

The perioperative nurse plays an important role in preparing the patient and operating room for surgery and assists with positioning (sometimes of a complex nature), knows and anticipates needed instrumentation and equipment, and understands and works toward desired patient outcomes.

Historical Perspective

By performing thoracic surgery in a negative pressure chamber, Sauerbruch in 1904 was able to open the thoracic cavity without collapsing the lung (Meade, 1961). With the introduction of intratracheal anesthesia by Elsberg in 1911, thoracic surgery became feasible as a treatment modality. Traumatic injuries and infections were the primary reasons for thoracic surgery prior to 1925 (Hurwitz & Degenshein, 1958). By the 1930s and 1940s, pulmonary and esophageal surgical procedures were being done successfully (Meade, 1961).

ANATOMY

The thorax is a "cage-like cone" that is composed of bones, muscles, cartilage, and other tissues. Enclosed within the thorax are the major organs of respiration and circulation, as well as other important anatomical structures.

The major functions of the thorax are to provide:

1. Movement needed for respiration
2. Structural support for the upper body
3. Protection to the heart, lungs, trachea, esophagus, and major blood vessels (Shields, 1989).

External landmarks of the thorax are used to identify the location of underlying structures (Fig. 14-1).

Structures of the Thorax

Chest wall muscles

Those muscles primarily responsible for movement and control of the arms, shoulders, and scapulae include the anterior and posterior chest wall muscles (Fig. 14-2).

1. Anterior:
   Pectoralis major
   Pectoralis minor
   Latissimus dorsi
   Sternocleidomastoid
   Serratus anterior
2. Posterior:
   Trapezius
   Rhomboideus major and minor
   Levator scapulae
   Serratus posterior (superior and inferior)
   Latissimus dorsi

Diaphragm

The diaphragm is a dome-shaped muscle that separates the thoracic and abdominal cavities. Stimulation of the phrenic nerve causes the diaphragm to contract and provide a respiratory function (Fig. 14-3).

Intercostal muscles

The intercostal muscles are located in the spaces between the ribs and are accompanied by neurovascular structures. The muscle layers include:

1. The external intercostal muscles are diagonally located from one rib to the next and assist with inspiration by contracting and elevating the rib cage (Fig. 14-4).
2. The internal intercostal muscles are located in a downward and backward direction between the ribs and assist with expiration. With contraction these muscles pull the ribs downward (Fig. 14-4).

Neurovascular structures

The neurovascular structures in the intercostal spaces are located in the upper area of each space along the lower side of the rib. Incisions are made along the top edge of the rib in order to avoid injury to these structures.

Bony structures

The bony structures include the sternum, 12 thoracic vertebrae, 12 pairs of ribs (10 ribs have costal cartilages), 2 clavicles, and 2 scapulae.

The sternum The sternum (Fig. 14-5) is 15 to 20 cm in length and consists of three sections:

1. The manubrium is the upper section. It articulates with the clavicles and forms the suprasternal notch.
2. The body is the longest section of the sternum; the upper portion articulates with the manubrium to form the sternal angle.
3. The xiphoid process is the cartilaginous tip of the sternum.

Ribs and costal cartilages

1. The upper seven pairs of ribs are vertebrosternal ribs (Fig. 14-5). They are attached posteriorly to the verte-

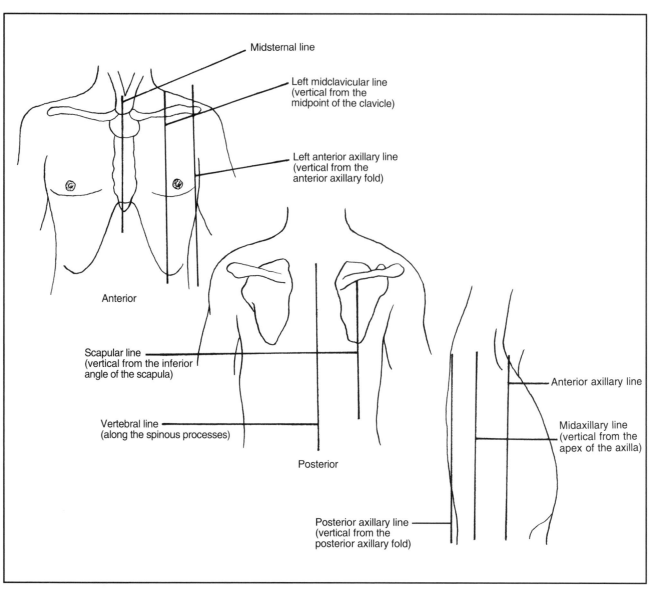

FIGURE 14-1 Location of external landmarks.

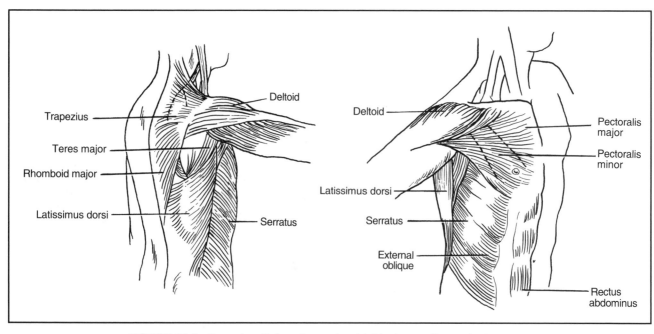

FIGURE 14-2 Posterior (*left*) and anterior (*right*) chest wall muscles.

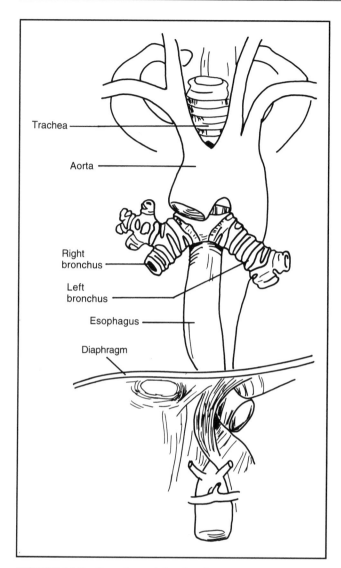

FIGURE 14-3   Location of the diaphragm in relation to mediastinal structures.

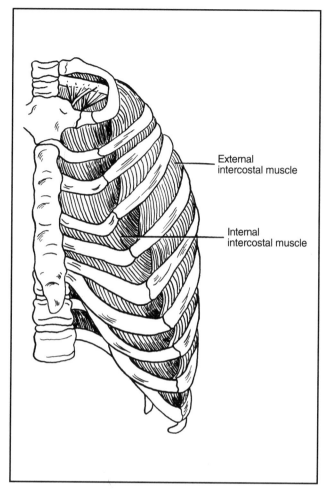

FIGURE 14-4   Intercostal muscles.

brae and anteriorly to the sternum by the costal cartilages.

2. Vertebrocostal ribs are the eighth, ninth, and tenth pairs of ribs. They do not articulate with the sternum but with the suprajacent cartilages.

3. Vertebral ribs are the eleventh and twelfth pairs of ribs. They do not have an anterior attachment and form a cartilaginous tip that ends in the muscles of the abdominal wall.

Pleura

The pleura is a delicate serous membrane that covers the lung surfaces (visceral layer) and reflects to cover the inside of the chest wall (parietal layer). The space between the layers creates a slight suction that holds the lungs against the thoracic wall. The pleural fluid provides lubrication that allows the lungs to move during respiration (Fig. 14-6).

Lungs

The lungs are the organs of respiration. They are normally pink and feel "spongey." They are composed of tissue, air, and blood. The airways are hollow and flexible tubes that branch from the trachea into the bronchi, bronchioles, alveolar ducts, and sacs, and terminate into small pouches called alveoli. The alveoli are honeycombed structures in which gas exchange occurs between the air and the blood. The alveolar surface area in the adult is 97 to 194 m^2 (Shields, 1989). Surfactant is the fluid substance that prevents collapse and adherence of the alveolar walls (Sabiston & Spencer, 1990). The pulmonary circulatory system comes from the heart via the pulmonary arteries, with the capillary beds occurring at the alveolar structures of the lung. Gas transfer occurs (carbon dioxide is eliminated and oxygen is absorbed by the blood) through the alveolocapillary membrane, and the blood returns to the heart via the pulmonary veins (Shields, 1989).

The right and left lungs are separated by the mediastinal structures. The lungs are divided into lobes: three in the right lung and two in the left lung. The lobes are separated by fissures and are further divided into segments, usually ten in the right lung and eight in the left lung. Bronchial vessels arise from the aorta, intercostal

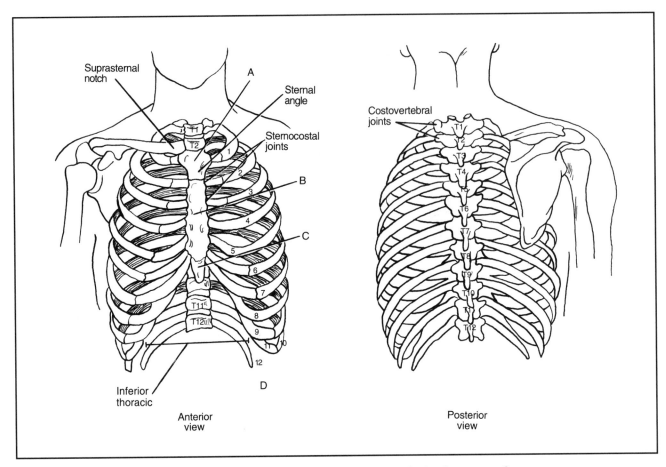

FIGURE 14-5 Sternum and ribs. *A*, manubrium; *B*, body of sternum; *C*, xiphoid process; *D*, ribs 1 to 12.

arteries, and occasionally from the subclavian or innominate arteries (Shields, 1989; Guyton, 1991; Gray, 1977) (Fig. 14-7).

Mediastinum

The mediastinum is the space in the middle of the thorax that contains all viscera except the lungs. Structures in the mediastinum include the following:

1. The thoracic duct, which drains the majority of the lymphatic vessels and empties into the left subclavian vein (posterior)
2. The esophagus, which goes from the pharynx to the stomach and is located in the posterior mediastinum behind the trachea and to the right side of the aorta (see Fig. 14-3)
3. The trachea, which is located behind the heart and major vessels and bifurcates at the level of the fourth dorsal vertebra into the right and left main stem bronchi (see Fig. 14-3)
4. Major vascular structures: the ascending aorta, aortic arch, and descending aorta and branches; the vena cavae; and the pulmonary circulatory system (see Fig. 14-3).
5. Nerve structures, which include the vagus, recurrent laryngeal, and phrenic nerves and their branches

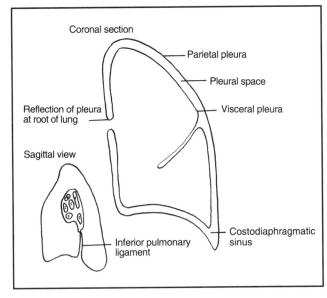

FIGURE 14-6 Pleural components.

6. The heart, which is located in the middle of the mediastinum and is separated from the other structures by the pericardial sac

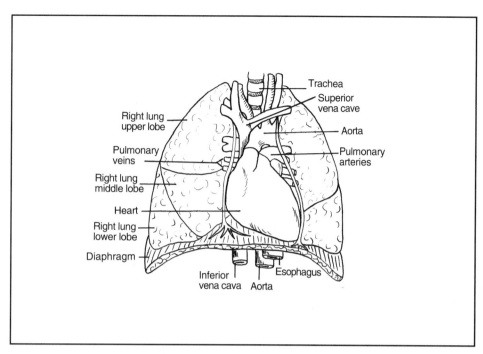

FIGURE 14-7   Intrathoracic organs.

7. The thymus, which is located in the upper anterior mediastinum. After childhood this gland shrinks but remnants remain.

The Respiratory Cycle

The two phases of the respiratory cycle are inspiration and expiration.

Inspiration

Inspiration occurs when the intrathoracic space is enlarged and increases the negative pressure within the thoracic cavity. The anteroposterior dimensions increase with the contraction of the external intercostals with assistance from the sternocleidomastoid, anterior serratus, and scalenus muscles. The vertical dimensions increase as the diaphragm contracts.

Expiration

Expiration is primarily a passive action that occurs when the muscles of respiration relax and the chest walls recoil. The elastic recoil of the lungs also forces the air out of the lungs. The abdominal recti and internal intercostal muscles assist in expiration by pulling the rib cage downward and compressing the abdominal organs against the diaphragm (Guyton, 1991; Shields, 1989).

The respiratory center is located in the medulla oblongata and pons areas of the brain. Increased carbon dioxide levels in the blood stimulate the center. Other factors that affect respirations include airway irritants, brain edema, anesthesia, decreased oxygen levels in the

blood (via peripheral chemoreceptors), and voluntary control of respirations (Guyton, 1991).

NURSING CONSIDERATIONS

Care Planning

The perioperative nurse implements the nursing process in providing care for the surgical patient. The priority of data collection is determined by the patient's immediate condition or needs, and by the relationship to the proposed intervention. Information about the patient is collected (Standard I: The perioperative nurse collects patient health data: *Standards of Perioperative Clinical Practice* [AORN, 1994]), related to:

1. The medical diagnoses and therapies
2. Physical status and physiological responses
3. Psychosocial status of the patient
4. Cultural, spiritual, and lifestyle information
5. Understanding, perceptions, and expectations regarding the surgical procedure
6. Previous responses to illness, hospitalization, and surgical, therapeutic, or diagnostic procedures
7. Results of diagnostic studies

In addition to the assessment of the patient, the perioperative nurse plans the intraoperative care based on the intended surgical procedure.

Patient teaching related to the perioperative care is provided by the perioperative nurse if the patient's condition and the time frame permit.

Expected Outcomes

Patients undergo thoracic surgical procedures for various reasons. The intent of the procedure may be to improve, cure, or palliate a certain condition. Many patients are at increased risk for intraoperative complications because of the underlying and/or associated disease processes. Increased technical difficulty for certain procedures must be considered when anticipating potential problems. Pulmonary function is always compromised when the thoracic cavity is entered.

Perioperative nurses facilitate these surgical procedures by understanding the procedure and preparing the needed instruments, supplies, and equipment. The intraoperative plan of care is individualized and designed to provide supportive, therapeutic, and safe care for the patient. The *Patient Outcomes: Standards of Perioperative Care,* published by the Association of Operating Room Nurses, Inc. (1994), addresses the anticipated effects of care provided by perioperative nurses and other members of the health care team.

Indications for Thoracic Surgery

Pulmonary and tracheal disorders

A. Congenital
  1. Tracheal agenesis or atresia
  2. Bronchial abnormalities
    a. Tracheal bronchus and diverticulum
    b. Tracheal atresia
    c. Anomalous bronchus (tracheoesophageal fistula is the most common)
    d. Bronchial stenosis
    e. Bronchobiliary fistula
  3. Lobar emphysema
  4. Diaphragmatic hernia
  5. Sequestration
  6. Bronchogenic cysts
  7. Cystic adenomatoid malformation
  8. Vascular lesions of the lung
  9. Vascular rings
B. Bullous emphysema (blebs, cysts, bullae)
C. Bacterial lung disease (bronchiectasis, abscess)
D. Hydatid cyst
E. Bronchial adenoma
  1. Carcinoid (85%–90%)
  2. Adenoid cystic cancer (10%)
  3. Mucoepidermoid tumor (less than 1%)
  4. Bronchial mucous gland adenoma (rare)
F. Carcinoma
  1. Non–small-cell carcinoma
    a. Epidermoid carcinoma (35%)
    b. Adenocarcinoma (25%–50%)
    c. Undifferentiated large-cell carcinoma
    d. Mixed-cell types (4%–15%)
  2. Small-cell tumors
    a. Typical small-cell tumors
    b. Intermediate-cell tumors
    c. Combined-cell types

  3. Less common malignant tumors
    a. Soft tissue sarcomas
    b. Carcinosarcoma
    c. Pulmonary blastoma embryoma
    d. Lymphoma
    e. Malignant melanoma
    f. Malignant teratoma
  4. Secondary tumors (metastatic from elsewhere in the body)
G. Tracheal conditions
  1. Primary neoplasms
  2. Secondary neoplasms (invasion by tumors of the esophagus, lung, thyroid, or larynx)
  3. Compression lesions
    a. Goiter
    b. Vascular ring
    c. Aneurysm
  4. Inflammatory disease
    a. Post-infection strictures
    b. Post-trauma stenosis
    c. Post-intubation damage

Pleural disorders

A. Empyema thoracis
  1. Exudative (acute) fluid in pleural pace
  2. Fibrinopurulent or transitional (fibrin traps lung)
  3. Organizing (chronic) pleural peel formation
B. Tumors
  1. Mesothelioma (asbestos exposure)
    a. Diffuse or localized
    b. Benign or malignant
  2. Metastatic tumors

Mediastinal disorders

A. Infection (mediastinitis)
B. Hemorrhage
C. Emphysema
D. Tumors
E. Cysts
F. Inflammatory disorders

Esophageal disorders

A. Congenital anomalies (see Chap. 18, this volume)
  1. Esophageal atresia and tracheoesophageal fistula
  2. Esophageal atresia without tracheoesophageal fistula
  3. Esophageal stenosis
  4. Laryngotracheoesophageal cleft
B. Motor disturbances
  1. Achalasia
  2. Chalasia
C. Diverticula
D. Hiatal hernia and esophageal reflux (Barrett's esophagus)
E. Benign strictures
F. Benign tumors and cysts
G. Carcinoma
H. Trauma

Diaphragmatic disorders

A. Hernias due to congenital defects, trauma, stress
B. Eventration
C. Tumors
D. Trauma

Skeletal disorders

A. Deformities
1. Pectus excavatum
2. Pectus carinatum
3. Poland's syndrome
4. Sternal clefts
B. Infections
C. Tumors
D. Radiation necrosis
E. Thoracic outlet syndrome
F. Trauma

Cardiovascular disorders

See Chapter 13, Cardiac Surgery, in this volume.

Foreign bodies (aerodigestive tract)

1. Laryngeal
2. Tracheal
3. Bronchial
4. Esophageal

Trauma

A. Fractures
B. Open wounds
C. Hemothorax
D. Air embolism (due to laceration of lung)
E. Tracheobronchial lacerations
F. Cardiac/major vessel injury

Diagnostic Procedures

Diagnosis of thoracic diseases and disorders often requires a variety of testing modalities, described in this section.

Radiology (chest X-ray)

A chest X-ray is a necessity for any patient undergoing a thoracic surgical procedure. The standard views are a posteroanterior (PA) and a left lateral. Other views that may be used are the oblique, lateral decubitus, lordotic, and kyphotic. Skeletal structures, tracheal position, areas above and below the diaphragm, mediastinal borders, hilar shadows, rib interspaces, vascular structures, cardiac size and contour, and abnormal densities or lucencies can be seen and evaluated (LoCicero, 1992; Hurst & Schlant, 1990).

Computed tomography (CT scan)

This technique provides cross-sectional imaging, which eliminates the problem of superimposition of anatomical structures. It provides higher contrast resolution, which makes lesions and abnormalities more visible.
CT is used for:

1. Staging lung cancer, nodal involvement, and metastases
2. Viewing vascular pathology
3. Confirming the presence of disease
4. Guiding biopsies
5. Differentiating between pleural and lung disease
6. Characterizing diffuse lung disease (Naidich et al., 1991; LoCicero, 1992)

Magnetic resonance imaging (MRI)

MRI is useful because of its ability to image blood vessels, distinguish between various tissues, and provide images in multiplane views. The longitudinal views are coronal (front to back) or sagittal (from the side). Transaxial views are cross-sectional. This technique is used for more detailed evaluation of lung cancer or chest wall and/or mediastinal invasion, and to demonstrate adenopathies or masses (Shields, 1989; Naidich et al., 1991; LoCicero, 1992).

Nuclear techniques

Ventilation perfusion scintigraphy (V/Q scan) The most frequent use of this technique is for diagnosis of pulmonary embolus. It is useful for assessment of pulmonary neoplasms, obstructive airway disease, inhalation injuries, and the effects of pulmonary treatments.
The ventilation imaging is done by having the patient inhale a radioactive gas (xenon 133 is most commonly used). The perfusion imaging is done by injecting technetium-99m. The gamma scintillation camera is used and at least 6 views are imaged. Defects in ventilation or perfusion in the lungs can be seen (LoCicero, 1992; Shields, 1989).

Gallium imaging This technique is used for evaluation of inflammatory and neoplastic diseases of the lung. Gallium-67 citrate is injected and is taken up by tissues where these types of pathology exist. Imaging is done 48 to 72 hours after the injection (LoCicero, 1992).

Arteriograms

This technique is used for more definitive visualization of vascular structures. It continues to be the most definitive test for pulmonary embolus (LoCicero, 1992).

Pulmonary function tests (PFT)

Preoperative evaluation of pulmonary function is essential for patients needing pulmonary resection procedures. Thoracotomy incisions and pulmonary resections always cause pulmonary dysfunction postoperatively. Age, smoking history, obesity, length of anesthesia, and intra-operative positioning are other factors that can increase pulmonary dysfunction.

The degree of preoperative pulmonary functional impairment and response to treatment assist the surgeon in determining the resectability of lung lesions and the anticipation of survival. The mortality from thoracotomies is estimated at 5% to 50%, and the morbidity is estimated at 25% to 75% (LoCicero, 1992).

PFTs determine lung volumes, lung mechanics, flow rates, and diffusing capacity. The perioperative nurse caring for patients undergoing thoracic procedures needs an understanding of the PFT results in order to anticipate patient responses (Hen, 1992) (Table 14-1).

Arterial blood gases (ABGs)

Measuring the ABGs provides an indirect method for determining pulmonary gas exchange (see Chapter 13 in this volume).

Upper gastrointestinal series

This test would be indicated for patients with diseases involving the esophagus.

Esophagrams

Esophagrams are fluoroscopic studies of swallowing mechanisms.

Esophageal manometry

This test assesses the motility with pressure measurements of the esophagus.

Electrocardiogram (ECG)

All male patients over 40 years of age and females over 55 years of age need a preoperative ECG (American College of Surgeons, 1989) in order to evaluate cardiac status. Additional testing of the cardiovascular system may be indicated prior to surgery.

Standard laboratory tests

According to the American College of Surgeon's publication, *Care of the Surgical Patient* (1989), the purpose of perioperative patient evaluation is to:

1. Evaluate the patient's presenting complaint
2. Screen for related problems
3. Assess the risk factors for surgical intervention

Based on the patient evaluation findings, the surgical procedure may be delayed, modified, or cancelled. Preoperative stability of cardiac, pulmonary, vascular, endocrine, and metabolic conditions is desired (American College of Surgeons, 1989).

The Practice Guidelines for Cardiothoracic Surgery from the Society of Thoracic Surgeons (1992) recom-

TABLE 14-1 Pulmonary Function Tests: Normal Values

Test	Normal Values Male	Female
VC = vital capacity (slowly exhaled volume)	4–5 L	3–4 L
FVC = forced vital capacity (forced maximum exhaled volume)	>4.0 L	>3.0 L
FRC = functional residual volume (volume remaining in lungs after normal exhalation)	2–3 L	1–2 L
RV = residual volume	1–2 L	1–2 L
ERV = expiratory reserve volume	1–2 L	1–2L
TLC = total lung capacity (volume after full inhalation or VC + RV)	6–7 L	5–6 L
FEV_1 = maximum volume of air exhaled in first second during forced exhalation	>3 L	>2 L
FEV_1/FVC	>60%	>70%
FEF = Forced expiratory flow	>2 L/sec	>1.6 L/sec
Lung mechanics		
R_{aw} = airway resistance (pressure drop along airways per unit of airflow)	<2.5 cm H_2O/sec/L	
Compliance (the volume change per unit of pressure change; reflects elasticity or stiffness of lung)	0.2 L/cm H_2O	
MIP = maximum inspiratory pressure (forcibly inhale)	>90 cm H_2O	>50 cm/H_2O
MEP = maximum expiratory pressure (forcibly exhale)	>150 cm H_2O	>120 cm H_2O
DL_{cosb} = diffusing capacity (efficiency of gas exchange in lungs)	20 ml CO_2/min/mm Hg	

mend the following preoperative evaluation for all patients undergoing major thoracic procedures:

1. Thorough history and physical examination
2. Chest X-ray
3. Urinalysis
4. Electrocardiogram
5. Blood sample for typing in all patients and a type and crossmatch for blood products in cases having a risk of significant blood loss. Patients who have previously provided blood via autologous donation may be excused from this requirement.
6. Blood analysis to include complete blood count, platelet count, prothrombin time, partial thromboplastin time, and SMA-18.

7. Room air arterial blood gas determination, including pCO_2, O_2, and pH, in patients with suspected pulmonary compromise
8. Appropriate medical consultation
9. Assessment of nutritional status

Culturing of the sputum or cytological examination may be indicated for certain pulmonary conditions.

Intraoperative Considerations

The perioperative nurse may assist in the intraoperative processes of monitoring and laboratory testing, and must be familiar with thoracic instrumentation and equipment, all discussed in the following section.

Monitoring

Electrocardiogram The ECG must be monitored because many patients undergoing thoracic surgical procedures have coexisting cardiac disease. Numerous risk factors may be present. Surgical intervention in the thoracic cavity has the potential of causing cardiac arrhythmias and instability (Sabiston & Spencer, 1990).

Blood pressure This is routinely monitored.

Pulse oximetry All patients undergoing thoracic surgery are to be monitored continuously with the SaO_2 monitor. Pulse oximetry is a noninvasive method of monitoring the hemoglobin saturation and pulse rate (see Chapter 13 in this volume).

Arterial pressure line This provides a continuous measurement of the arterial blood pressure and access to arterial blood samples intraoperatively (see Chapter 13 in this volume).

Temperature Continuous monitoring of the patient's temperature can alert the team to any untoward changes. Thoracic cavity procedures can cause heat loss and may lead to hypothermia.

Urinary output Measurement of urinary output may not be necessary for procedures of less than 2 hours' duration. If there is concern regarding renal function and/or perfusion, a urinary catheter should be inserted and urine output measured every 30 minutes. Measuring urinary output is helpful in determining fluid volume replacement. It is important not to overload patients undergoing any lung resection procedures because of reduced venous capacitance (Shields, 1989).

Blood loss Blood loss in sponges and suction canisters must be measured. Major blood loss can occur during thoracic surgery.

Ventilation During thoracic procedures, the anesthesia provider monitors the peak airway pressure, tidal volume, expiratory time, and minute ventilation. Early

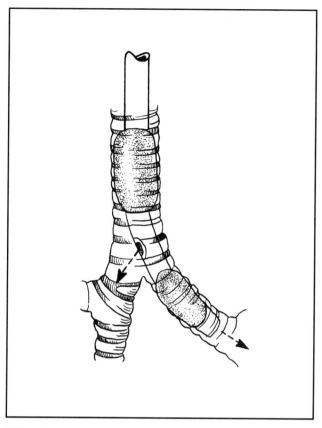

FIGURE 14-8 Double-lumen endotracheal tube positioned in the trachea and left main bronchus.

detection of physiological changes can facilitate prompt interventions.

One-lung ventilation using a double-lumen endotracheal tube is indicated to:

1. Prevent spillage or cross-contamination from one lung to the other
2. Provide adequate ventilation in the presence of large bronchopleural fistula or for pulmonary lavage
3. Provide better exposure and less trauma to the lung on the operative side by collapsing the lung (Sabiston & Spencer, 1990) (Fig. 14-8).

Laboratory tests

Arterial blood gases (ABGs) This test is done during thoracic surgery to determine if ventilation is adequate. ABGs are done after the induction of anesthesia and positioning. ABGs need to be done if the patient is on one-lung anesthesia and at any other time there is a question regarding ventilation.

Cultures There are multiple cultures that may be requested on fluids or tissues. These may include tests for bacterial (aerobic, anaerobic, mycobacteria), fungal, parasitic, or viral infections.

Smears Exudative or fluid material may be sent for a smear to determine the type of bacteria present (Gram stain) or other tests as requested.

Tissue specimens All tissue specimens must be handled carefully in order to have accurate test results. Careful labeling regarding the type of tissue and its location (in the patient) is essential. Multiple specimens are common. Frozen sections are used for determination of adequacy of the operative procedure, for diagnostic purposes, or to determine if surgery is possible. Clarification with the surgeon regarding specimens and tests is essential.

Special Equipment

1. Electrosurgical unit
2. Positioning devices
   a. Pillows; sandbags; heel, elbow, and head protectors
   b. "Bean bag" device, used for supporting the patient in lateral positions. Air is suctioned from the device and the bag conforms to the patient, providing firm support.
   c. Towels
3. Suction lines
   a. 1 for the operative field
   b. 1 for the "bean bag" positioning device, if used
   c. 1 for anesthesia
4. Temperature probe and control box
5. Headlights and power source

Special Instrumentation and Supplies

Thoracic

1. Retractors (appropriate for patient size)
   a. Rib spreaders: different sizes and blade depths (Fig. 14-9)
   b. Sternal retractor (if sternotomy incision is made)
   c. Abdominal retractor for esophageal or hiatal hernia

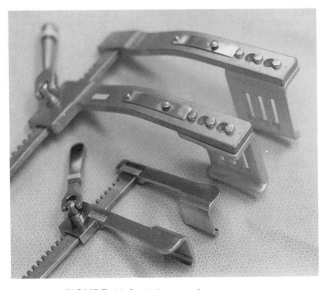

FIGURE 14-9 Rib spreader retractors.

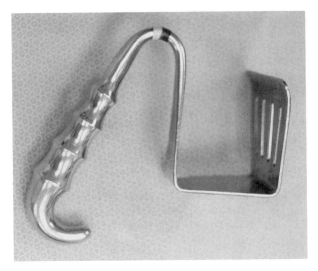

FIGURE 14-10 Scapula retractor.

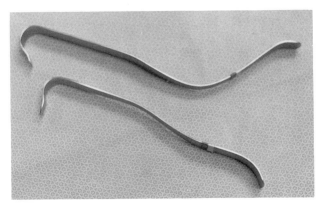

FIGURE 14-11 Esophageal retractors.

   d. Assorted sizes of Deaver, malleable, Richardson, and double-ended retractors
   e. Scapula retractor (Fig. 14-10)
   f. Esophageal retractors (Fig. 14-11)
2. Rib instruments (Figs. 14-12 to 14-14)
   a. Shears
   b. Periosteal elevators
   c. Rib raspatories
   d. Rongeurs
   e. Approximater
   f. Punch
3. Lung clamps (Fig. 14-15)
4. Hemostatic clamps of adequate length
   a. Tonsil clamps
   b. Mixter right-angled clamps
   c. Pean clamps
5. Scissors and tissue forceps of adequate length
6. Babcock clamps
7. Sponge sticks with folded 4 × 4s
8. Dissecting sponges ("pills," "peanuts")
9. Vascular clips (assorted sizes)
10. Stapling devices (Fig. 14-16)
    a. Vascular (Fig. 14-16,*A*)
    b. Bronchus (Fig. 14-16,*B*)

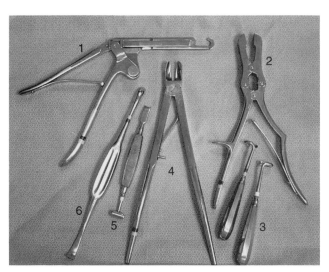

FIGURE 14-12 Rib instruments. Clockwise from top left: *1*, Sauerbruch-Frey rib shears; *2*, Sauerbruch Conyllos (box end) rib rongeurs; *3*, Doyen costal elevators (rib raspatories); *4*, Bethune rib shears; *5*, Alexander periosteotome; *6*, Cameron Haight periosteal elevator.

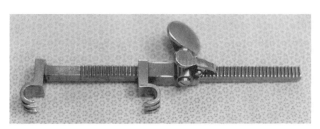

FIGURE 14-13 Bailey rib approximator.

c. Tissue (Fig. 14-16,*C*)
11. Vascular clamps (for management of inadvertent bleeding from major vessels, e.g., pulmonary artery or vein)
12. Vessel loops or umbilical tapes
13. Long knife handle
14. Extension for cautery tip
15. Warm irrigation fluids
16. Sutures (adequate length) according to surgeon's preference
17. Chest tubes, connectors, and drainage sets
18. 2″ adhesive tape for positioning

Endoscopic

See specific procedure.

SPECIAL PROCEDURES

Procedures complementary to or integral with thoracic surgery are discussed in this section.

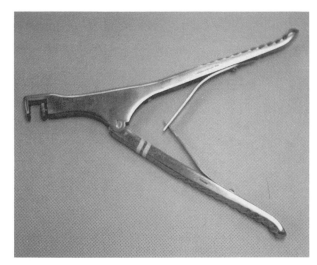

FIGURE 14-14 Sternal and/or rib punch used for making suture holes in the sternum and/or ribs.

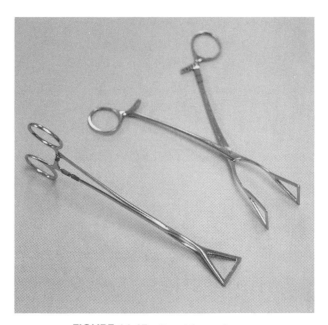

FIGURE 14-15 Duval lung clamps.

Endoscopy

Bronchoscopy

Endoscopic visualization of the tracheobronchial tree may be done for diagnostic or therapeutic reasons. Direct inspection and obtainment of tissue samples, secretions, brushings, and washings may be done. Therapeutic interventions to remove secretions or foreign bodies, control bleeding, or open a narrowed airway may be indicated (Sabiston & Spencer, 1990).

Diagnostic bronchoscopy is indicated for chronic cough, hemoptysis, wheezing, frequent pulmonary infections, bronchial obstructions, suspicion of pulmonary tumor, or staging of lung cancer (Sabiston & Spencer, 1990; Shields, 1989) (Table 14-2).

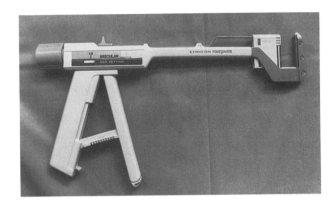

A

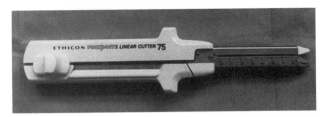

C

FIGURE 14-16 *A*, Vascular stapling device. *B*, Bronchus stapling device. *C*, Linear Cutter (Proximate). (*A*, *B*, and *C*, courtesy of ETHICON ENDO-SURGERY, Cincinnati, OH.)

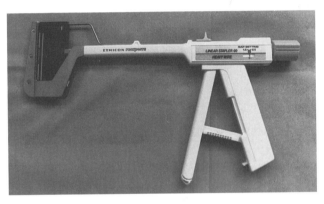

B

Complications may include pneumothorax, bleeding, hypoxia, bronchospasm, respiratory depression, fever, lacerations of oral or pharyngeal mucosa, laceration or rupture of the bronchus, breaking of teeth, and pulmonary or systemic infections. Deaths are usually related to advanced cardiopulmonary disease, end-stage lung disease, pneumonia, or cancer (Sabiston & Spencer, 1990; LoCicero, 1992).

Anesthesia Anesthesia can be local or general. General anesthesia is generally used for rigid, open-ended bronchoscopy, to increase comfort and safety. Rigid scopes have a side arm for anesthesia administration, and a lens cap is used to cover the end of the scope. The lens cap can be removed for biopsies or aspiration. Flexible scopes can be passed through the endotracheal tube. Topical application or spray of 2% lidocaine (flexible scope) or 3% to 10% cocaine (rigid scope) provides local anesthesia (Shields, 1989; Sabiston & Spencer, 1990).

Monitoring Patients undergoing bronchoscopy are at increased risk for cardiac arrhythmias and hypoxia and must be monitored with an ECG, pulse oximetry, and blood pressure. Supplemental oxygen is administered to minimize hypoxia (LoCicero, 1992; Shields, 1989; Sabiston & Spencer, 1990).

The perioperative nurse provides supportive care (comfort and reassurance) and observes for adverse changes in the patient's condition. Appropriate nursing interventions must be initiated.

Position Supine or sitting positions can be used.

Instrumentation Scopes may be either the rigid, open-ended type or of flexible fiber. Rigid scopes are preferred for removal of foreign bodies or aspiration of thick or copious secretions, and are safer for biopsy of vascular tumors and/or control of bleeding because they provide a larger working area. Flexible scopes allow deeper penetration into the bronchial tree, provide a wider angle of vision, and are easier to insert. A variety of sizes for adult and pediatric patients must be available. Light carriers, cords, light sources, telescopic attachments, forceps for biopsies or foreign body retrieval, suction tips and tubing, collection traps and specimen containers, lubricant, and camera equipment (if used) must be prepared (Shields, 1989; Wells & Milstein, 1990).

Procedure

Key steps

1. The patient is positioned comfortably and securely.
2. Draping is minimal; the patient's hair and eyes are covered and a sheet or towel is placed across the patient's chest.
3. Rigid scope (Fig. 14-17)
   a. The scope is introduced through the right side of the patient's mouth.
   b. The patient's head is lowered and extended or the scope is angled backward as it is advanced.
   c. Telescopic attachments and instrumentation are used as requested by the surgeon.
   d. The patient's head is moved to the left or right as necessary for visualization.
   e. Secretions are aspirated and collected for specimens.
   f. All specimens are handled appropriately, labeled, and sent to pathology.
4. Flexible scope (Fig. 14-18)
   a. The scope is inserted through the nose or mouth or may be inserted through an endotracheal tube. The tubing should not be bent or kinked.
   b. Flexible forceps, brushes, or curettes are used as needed.
   c. Secretions are aspirated and collected for specimens.

TABLE 14-2 Staging System for Lung Cancer

Summary of Staging Definitions (cont.)	
TX	Tumor proved by the presence of malignant cells in bronchopulmonary secretions but not visualized roentgenographically or bronchoscopically, or any tumor that cannot be assessed as in a retreatment staging
T0	No evidence of primary tumor
T_{is}	Carcinoma in situ
T1	A tumor that is 3.0 cm or less in greatest dimension, surrounded by lung or visceral pleura, and without evidence of invasion proximal to a lobar bronchus at bronchoscopy
T2	A tumor more than 3.0 cm in greatest dimension, or a tumor of any size that either invades the visceral pleura or has associated atelectasis or obstructive pneumonitis extending to the hilar region. At bronchoscopy, the proximal extent of demonstrable tumor must be within a lobar bronchus or at least 2.0 cm distal to the carina. Any associated atelectasis or obstructive pneumonitis must involve less than an entire lung.
T3	A tumor of any size with direct extension into the chest wall (including superior sulcus tumors), diaphragm, or the mediastinal pleura or pericardium without involving the heart, great vessels, trachea, esophagus or vertebral body, or a tumor in the main bronchus within 2.0 cm of the carina without involving the carina
T4	A tumor of any size with invasion of the mediastinum or involving heart, great vessels, trachea, esophagus, vertebral body, or carina, or presence of malignant pleural effusion

Nodal Involvement (N)

NX	Minimum requirements to access the regional nodes cannot be met
N0	No demonstrable metastasis to regional lymph nodes
N1	Metastasis to lymph nodes in the peribronchial or the ipsilateral hilar region, or both, including direct extension
N2	Metastasis to ipsilateral mediastinal lymph nodes and subcarinal lymph nodes
N3	Metastasis to contralateral mediastinal lymph nodes, contralateral hilar lymph nodes, ipsilateral or contralateral scalene, or supraclavicular lymph nodes

Distant Metastasis (M)

MX	Minimum requirements to assess the presence of distant metastasis cannot be met
M0	No (known) distant metastasis
M1	Distant metastasis present

Stage grouping

Occult stage	TX	N0	M0
Stage 0	T_{is}	N0	M0 (in situ)
Stage I	T1	N0	M0
	T2	N0	M0
Stage II	T1	N1	M0
	T2	N1	M0
Stage IIIa	T3	N0	M0
	T3	N1	M0
	T1-3	N2	M0
Stage IIIb	Any T	N3	M0
	T4	Any N	M0
Stage IV	Any T	Any N	M1

Summary of Staging Definitions

Occult stage	Microscopically identified cancer cells in lung secretions on multiple occasions (or multiple daily collections); no discernible primary cancer in the lung
Stage 0	Carcinoma in situ
Stage I	Tumor surrounded by lung or visceral pleura arising more than 2 cm distal to the carina (T1-2, N0)
Stage II	Tumor not extending to adjacent organs, pleura, or chest wall, with hilar lymph-node involvement (T1-2, N1)
Stage IIIa	Tumor invading chest wall, pleura, or pericardium or within 2 cm but not involving carina; nodes in hilum or ipsilateral mediastinum (T3, N0-1; T1, N2)

(continued)

TABLE 14-2 Staging System for Lung Cancer *(continued)*

Summary of Staging Definitions (cont.)	
Stage IIIb	Direct extension to adjacent organs (pleura, heart, chest wall, diaphragm, or mediastinum); or associated with contralateral mediastinal or supraclavicular lymph-node involvement (T4 or N3)
Stage IV	Any tumor with distant metastases (M1)

(From Schwartz, S., Shires, G., Spencer, F., & Husser, W. [1994] *Principles of Surgery* (6th ed.) Reprinted with permission of McGraw-Hill, New York.)

d. All specimens are handled appropriately, labeled, and sent to pathology.
5. Inspection is done for bleeding and providing appropriate intervention.
6. The scope is removed.
7. Instrumentation is cleaned, and high-level disinfection or sterilization is done.

Postoperative care The patient is taken to the recovery room for close observation of pulmonary and cardiac status. Discharge from the recovery room to home or to a patient care area occurs when established protocols have been met.

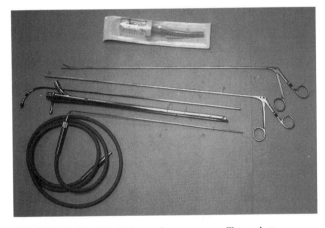

FIGURE 14-17 Rigid bronchoscopy set. *Top to bottom:* specimen collection set, grasping, biopsy forceps, suction tip, bronchoscope, light carrier and cord.

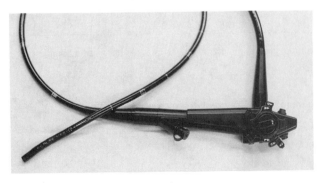

FIGURE 14-18 Flexible bronchoscope.

Esophagoscopy

Endoscopic examination of the esophagus is indicated for dysphagia, hematemesis, regurgitation, and retrosternal pain and to determine the effects of caustic agent ingestion and/or trauma. Treatments such as removal of foreign bodies, placement of stents, laser therapy, or dilation of strictures may be done through the esophagoscope. The scope is not necessary for certain types of dilation procedures.

The esophagus is thin and flexible, which increases the risk of complications. Perforation, subcutaneous emphysema, sepsis, shock, bleeding, and pulmonary aspiration may occur. Patients with large thoracic aneurysms, Zenker's diverticulum, bony jaw abnormalities, advanced cervical spinal hypertrophy, and major cardiac and/or pulmonary disorders are usually not candidates for this procedure (Shields, 1989; Sabiston & Spencer, 1990).

Anesthesia Anesthesia is the same as in bronchoscopy procedures, both local and general. General is usually used for the rigid, open-ended scope because of discomfort.

Monitoring Monitoring is the same as for bronchoscopy procedures.

Position Positioning is left lateral decubitus for flexible esophagoscopy under local anesthesia. Supine positioning is with the head extended if general anesthesia is used.

Instrumentation Flexible or rigid scopes may be used. The rigid, open-ended scope allows for direct vision during insertion and provides a larger working space (Figs. 14-19 and 14-20). It can be used for removing foreign bodies or for dilating strictures (Fig. 14-21). The flexible scope provides more patient comfort, permits examination of the entire upper gastrointestinal tract, and may allow examination on patients with jaw or spinal deformities. The flexible scope is introduced "blindly," which may increase perforation risks. Only small biopsies may be obtained through the flexible scope (Sabiston & Spencer, 1990). Various sizes of scopes must be available for adult and pediatric patients. Light carriers, cords, light sources, biopsy and grasping forceps, suction tips and tubing, collection traps, specimen containers, esophageal bougies and dilators, lubricant, and camera equipment are prepared as needed.

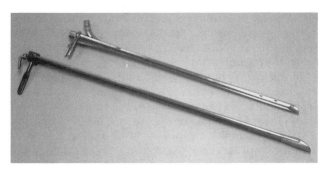

FIGURE 14-19 *Top,* rigid bronchoscope; *bottom,* rigid esophagoscope (esophagoscope is longer, flatter, and wider than bronchoscope).

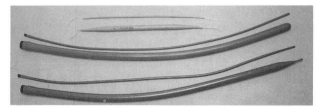

FIGURE 14-21 Esophageal bougies and dilators, small and large sizes. *Top,* Tucker; *middle,* Hurst (16 & 60 Fr); *bottom,* Maloney (20 & 60 Fr).

9. Instruments are cleaned and high level disinfected or sterilized.

Postoperative care Postoperative care is the same as in bronchoscopy procedures.

Mediastinoscopy

This procedure is done to evaluate mediastinal lymphadenopathy as determined by computed tomography examination. Nodes greater than 1 cm in diameter need to be biopsied. If the nodes are positive for cancer, pulmonary resection for lung cancer is usually not indicated (Pearson, 1993).

Paratracheal, supratracheobronchial, and anterior subcarinal nodes can be biopsied through the mediastinoscope. Transpleural inspection and aspiration of pleural fluid are possible.

Injury to the left recurrent laryngeal nerve, pneumothorax, and esophageal and vascular injuries have been reported. A thoracotomy may be required to control major bleeding (Shields, 1989).

Anesthesia General anesthesia is usually used to prevent patient coughing or movement (Ravitch & Steichen, 1988).

Monitoring Monitoring is the same as in bronchoscopy.

Position The patient is supine.

Instrumentation Instruments include a mediastinoscope, light carrier, cord, light source, suction tips and tubing, biopsy and grasping forceps, cautery, specimen containers, and vascular clips. Emergency thoracotomy instruments should be immediately available.

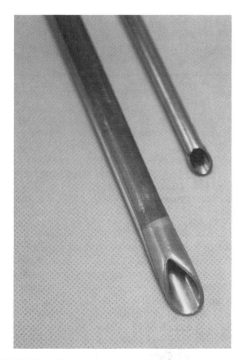

FIGURE 14-20 Close-up of tips of esophagoscope (*left*) and bronchoscope (*right*). Esophagoscope tip is broader and more blunt.

Procedure

Key steps

1. The patient is positioned comfortably and securely.
2. Draping (as in bronchoscopy) is done.
3. Scopes are introduced through the patient's mouth, with the head extended.
4. Care is taken to protect the flexible scope from kinking or bending.
5. Instrumentation is used as needed for the procedure.
6. Specimens are handled appropriately, labeled, and sent to pathology.
7. Secretions are aspirated from the mouth and upper airway, if needed.
8. The scope is removed.

Procedure

Key steps

1. The patient is positioned comfortably and securely.
2. Draping provides exposure of the upper anterior chest and neck.
3. A small, transverse 2- to 3-cm incision is made above the sternal notch.
4. Finger dissection is done along the anterior and lateral trachea into the mediastinum.

5. The scope is inserted.
6. Biopsies are obtained, properly handled, labeled, and sent to pathology. Frozen sections are usually needed.
7. The surgical area is inspected for bleeding.
8. The incision is closed.
9. Instrumentation is cleaned and high level disinfected or sterilized.

Postoperative care Postoperative care is the same as in bronchoscopy procedures.

Mediastinotomy

When mediastinal nodes cannot be reached with a mediastinoscope, it may be necessary to do a mediastinotomy. Bleeding, pneumothorax, and phrenic nerve injury are potential complications.

Anesthesia General anesthesia is used.

Monitoring Monitoring is the same as in bronchoscopy.

Instrumentation Soft tissue dissection instruments are needed, as well as a periosteal elevator and heavy scissors.

Procedure

Key steps

1. The patient is positioned comfortably and securely.
2. Draping provides exposure of the anterior chest.
3. An incision is made over the second or third costal cartilage.
4. The costal cartilage is removed.
5. The pleura and the internal mammary artery are retracted laterally.
6. Blunt dissection is used to enter the mediastinum.
7. Nodes are removed, properly handled, labeled, and sent to pathology. Frozen sections are usually needed.
8. The area is inspected for bleeding.
9. A small tube is used to evacuate air if the pleura has been opened.
10. The incisions are closed.
11. Instruments are cleaned and terminally sterilized. (Ravitch & Steichen, 1988)

Postoperative care Postoperative care is the same as in bronchoscopy.

Thoracoscopy and video-assisted thoracic surgery (VATS)

Thoracoscopy was first described in 1910 as a method of diagnosing and treating pleural disease (Mack et al., 1992). This technique is limited to simple diagnostic and therapeutic procedures because of the small visual field and minimal access and has been replaced by VATS in many instances (Lewis et al., 1992; Oakes, 1993).

In the 1980s, advances in instrumentation, telescopes, microcameras, and video display expanded the scope of thoracoscopy procedures. Complex intrathoracic surgical procedures are possible with VATS, and traditional thoracotomies are often avoided (Lewis et al., 1992; Tampinco-Golos, 1992; Coltharp, 1992).

Thoracic surgeons doing VATS must have successfully completed educational courses designed to acquire the technical and judgmental skills needed for these procedures (Table 14-3) (McKneally, 1993).

VATS procedures are for diagnostic and/or therapeutic purposes of various types of pathology, including:

1. Pleural conditions: cysts, blebs, effusions, pleurodesis, biopsies, pleurectomy
2. Pulmonary resections: wedge resection, stapling of blebs, biopsies

TABLE 14-3 Statement of the AATS/STS Joint Committee on Thoracoscopy and Video Assisted Thoracic Surgery

The Councils of The American Association for Thoracic Surgery and The Society of Thoracic Surgeons have formed a Joint Committee on Thoracoscopy and Video Assisted Thoracic Surgery. The purpose of this Committee is to facilitate the education of thoracic surgeons in this new technology and to provide guidelines for appropriate training in and performance of thoracoscopy and video assisted, minimally invasive thoracic surgery.

The following guidelines are recommended by the Joint Committee:

1. In order to ensure optimal quality patient care, thoracoscopy and video assisted thoracic surgery (TVATS) should be performed only by thoracic surgeons who are qualified, through documented training and experience, to perform open thoracic surgical procedures and manage their potential complications. The surgeon must have the judgment, training, and capability to proceed immediately to a standard open thoracic procedure if necessary.

    The preoperative and postoperative care of patients treated by TVATS should be the responsibility of the operating surgeon.

2. It is recommended that TVATS techniques be learned through appropriate instruction:
    a. As part of a formal approved thoracic surgical residency or fellowship program that includes structured and documented experience in these procedures.
    b. For the practicing thoracic surgeon, completion of a course that follows the guidelines approved by the Joint Committee, with hands-on laboratory experience, plus observation of these techniques performed by thoracic surgeons experienced in such procedures.

3. The granting of privileges to perform TVATS remains the responsibility of the credentialing body of individual hospitals.

© 1992 by The Society of Thoracic Surgeons. From *The Annals of Thoracic Surgery* (1992), *54*, 1. For the AATS/STS Joint Committee on Thoracoscopy and Video Assisted Thoracic Surgery: Martin F. McKneally, MD, and Ralph J. Lewis, MD, Co-Chairmen; Richard P. Anderson, MD, Richard G. Fosburg, MD, William A. Gay, Jr., MD, Robert H. Jones, MD, and Mark B. Orringer, MD

3. Pericardial biopsies, pericardiectomy
4. Lymph node biopsies
5. Sympathectomy, vagotomy
6. Esophageal biopsies
7. Evacuation of empyema, decortication
8. Drainage of spinal abscesses
9. Lysis of adhesions
10. Ligation of thoracic duct for chylothorax
11. Exploration of thoracic cavity
    (Mack et al., 1992, 1993; Lewis et al., 1992; Tampinco-Golos, 1992; Caccavale & Arzouman, 1993; LoCicero, 1992)

Other possible procedures:

1. Esophageal myotomy
2. Spinal discectomy and/or fusion
3. Lobectomy/pneumonectomy
4. Esophagogastrectomy
5. ICD (implantable cardioverter defibrillator) implantation

Possible complications include perforation of the diaphragm, air embolus, tension pneumothorax, hemorrhage, and infection. Contraindications include obliteration of the pleural space, dense adhesions, inability to tolerate one-lung anesthesia, lesions located near major vessels, and coagulopathies (Lewis et al., 1992; Tampinco-Golos, 1992)

Anesthesia General anesthesia with one-lung ventilation is used.

Monitoring Monitoring is standard.

Positioning The patient is positioned supine, semi-lateral, or lateral, depending on the location of the surgical pathology (Fig. 14-22).

Instrumentation and special equipment

Video equipment, electrosurgical unit, suction

Soft tissue instrument set

Graspers, dissectors, ligators, scissors, suction/coagulater, stapling devices, trocars, clip appliers, thoracoscope (Fig. 14-23)

Chest instrumentation is present in the operating room in the event a thoracotomy is necessary.

Procedure

Key steps

1. The patient is draped, providing adequate exposure of the chest for all puncture sites and emergency thoracotomy if necessary.
2. The incisions are made. The first incision is for the trocar, and then the lens is inserted. Additional incisions are made, trocars are inserted, and instrumentation is inserted.
3. The surgical procedure is undertaken.

4. A chest tube is inserted.
5. The instruments are removed, the incisions are closed, and dressings are applied.
   (Coltharp, 1992; Tampinco-Golos, 1992)

Postoperative care The patient is transported to the recovery area and is discharged from the recovery area to a nursing care unit or home, according to protocol.

Needle Biopsies

Transbronchial needle aspirations

Needle aspiration biopsies can be done through the rigid or flexible bronchoscope. Three samples from each area should be obtained. Fluoroscopic guidance may be needed for peripheral lesion aspiration. Bleeding complications are rare and usually minimal (LoCicero, 1992).

Transthoracic percutaneous fine needle aspiration biopsy (PFNAB)

This procedure is usually done in the radiology department under fluoroscopic or computed tomography guidance. Ultrasound guidance is possible for masses in contact with the chest wall. Local anesthesia is used and the patient is supine or prone, depending on the location of the area to be biopsied. Contraindications include an uncooperative patient, emphysema, pulmonary hypertension, coagulation disorders, and/or suspected hydatid cyst. Possible complications are pneumothorax, hemorrhage, hemoptysis, air embolus, or hemopericardium with tamponade (Pan et al., 1993; LoCicero, 1992).

Thoracentesis

Fluid and/or air can be removed from the thoracic cavity by inserting a needle through the chest wall. The needle is inserted into the posterior thorax at the sixth or seventh interspace, with the patient in a sitting or lateral position. Local anesthesia is used. Fluid removal should not exceed 1000 ml at a time. Possible complications include pneumothorax, hemothorax, vasovagal reactions, lacerations of the spleen or liver, subcutaneous emphysema, air embolus, pulmonary edema, and/or pain (LoCicero, 1992; Hood, 1986; Ravitch & Steichen, 1988).

Pericardiocentesis

Blood and/or fluid can be removed from the pericardial space with a long needle and aspirating syringe. This may be done to relieve cardiac tamponade or to diagnose pericarditis or effusion. The needle is inserted to the left of the sternum at the fourth or fifth interspace or subxiphoid. Possible complications include laceration of the heart, coronary arteries, or internal mammary artery; penetration of the pleural cavity; laceration or puncture of a lung; perforation of abdominal organs; pneumothorax; or bleeding (Sabiston & Spencer, 1990).

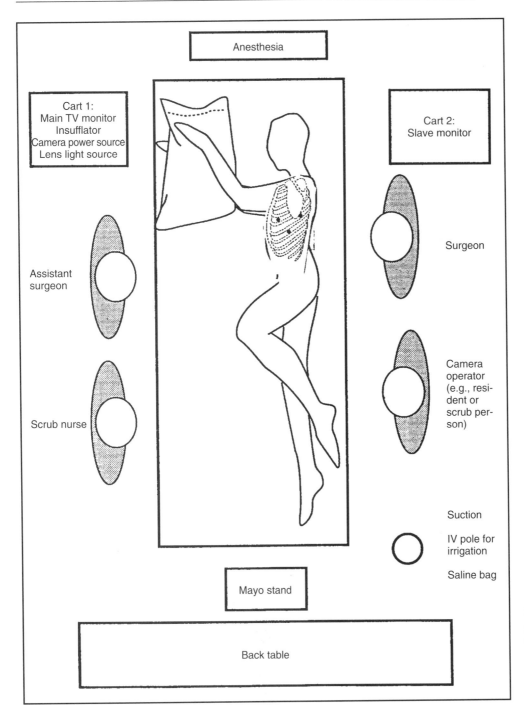

FIGURE 14-22 Positioning for VATS. Reprinted with permission from the Association of Operating Room Nurses, Inc., Denver, CO; *AORN Journal,* May 1992, p. 1171.

Chest Tube Insertion

A chest tube (thoracostomy tube) may be inserted to remove air and/or fluid from the thoracic cavity. After thoracotomy there is usually some degree of pneumothorax. After a pulmonary resection, 2 tubes are usually inserted: 1 for air that goes to the apex, and 1 for fluid located posteriorly and inferiorly. A chest tube is usually not inserted after a pneumonectomy as air is aspirated from the chest after the procedure. This creates a slightly negative pressure in the chest and helps maintain the mediastinum in the midline (Shields, 1989).

Procedure

Key steps

1. Chest tube incisions are made inferiorly to the chest incision.
2. An incision is made along the upper border of the rib to avoid bleeding from intercostal vessels.
3. Hemostasis of the tube incision is obtained.
4. A long hemostatic clamp is inserted through the skin incision and tunneled through tissues until the thoracic cavity is entered. The surgeon palpates the inside of the chest for the entry site (Fig. 14-24,*A*).

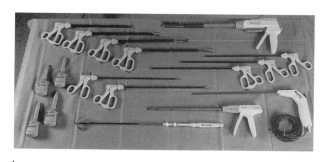

A

FIGURE 14-23   VATS instrumentation. *A, Clockwise from top left:* *1*, 10-mm thoracic instruments; *2*, 60-mm endoscopic linear cutter; *3*, 5-mm hand instruments; *4*, probe plus suction, cautery, and irrigation; *5*, 10-mm endoscopic multiple clip applier; *6*, 5-mm tissue manipulator; *7*, thoracic trocars. *B, Left to right:* *1*, thoracic curved Kelly forceps; *2*, Glassman clamp; *3*, right-angle clamp; *4*, Debakey tissue forceps; *5*, lung forceps; *6*, Metzenbaum scissors; *7*, dissector; *8*, "cherry." (Courtesy ETHICON ENDO-SURGERY, Cincinnati, OH.)

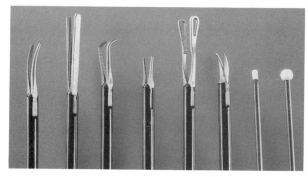

B

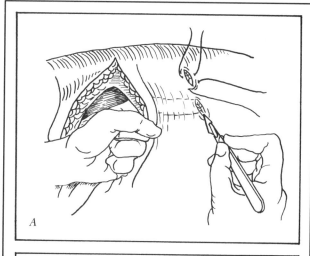

A

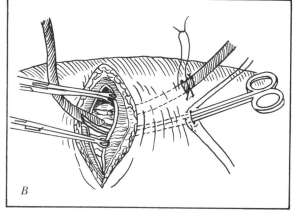

B

FIGURE 14-24   Insertion of a chest tube. *A*, Making incisions for the chest tubes. *B*, A long hemostat clamp is inserted through the incision into the chest cavity, and the chest tube is grasped and will be pulled through the chest wall.

5. The chest tube is grasped inside the chest and pulled through the tunnel to the skin level. The tube is positioned inside the chest and secured to the skin with a suture (Fig. 14-24,*B*).
6. A connector is used to attach the chest tube to the chest drainage set tube. The connection is secured with tape.
7. The chest drainage set (if sterile) can be prepared by the scrub nurse or the circulating nurse. A three-chamber system is usually used, and disposable units are widely available (Fig. 14-25). The chambers are for collection, water seal (prevents air from entering the chest cavity), and suction control for maintaining continuous negative pressure in the chest (25 cm of water).

Precautions

1. Do not clamp the tubes unless accidental separation occurs.
2. Do not elevate the drainage set above the patient's chest since water could be siphoned into the chest.

3. Maintain appropriate fluid levels in the chest drainage set.
4. If suction is inadequate, chest drainage flow will reverse during inspiration or there will be intermittent bubbling of the water seal.

Possible complications include bleeding from the intercostal vessels or lung trauma; pneumothorax from air leak around the tube site or from lacerated lung; pain; infection; and/or tube obstruction and inadequate drainage of pleural space (Wells & Milstein, 1990; Shields, 1989).

Tracheostomy

The development of low-pressure, cuffed endotracheal tubes and fiberoptic intubation technique has resulted in a decreased need for tracheostomy procedures. Tracheostomy is usually indicated for patients with:

1. Need for mechanical ventilation longer than 2 weeks
2. Severe head injury

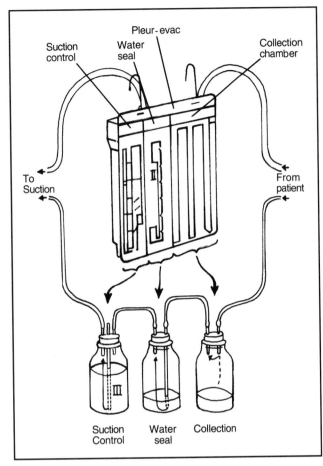

FIGURE 14-25 Single-use chest drainage set as compared to the standard 3-bottle (chamber) set.

3. Chest trauma resulting in a large flail segment of the chest wall and decreased lung compliance
4. Need for management of pulmonary secretions
5. Airway obstruction that cannot be managed with endotracheal intubation
6. Glottic edema or poor oral hygiene (potential infection) from endotracheal tube
7. Diaphragmatic pacing
(Shields, 1989; Wells & Milstein, 1990; Sabiston & Spencer 1990)

The operating room environment is preferred for this procedure, but it may be necessary to do the procedure in the intensive care unit or emergency room because of the patient's condition and because of difficulty in transporting the patient to the operating room.

Possible complications during the procedure include hypoxia; cardiac arrest; injury to nerves, esophagus, or vascular structures; hemorrhage; and/or pneumothorax. Late complications may include erosion of the tracheal wall (cuff site) into the innominate artery, tracheoesophageal fistula, circumferential tracheal damage, and persistance of the stoma (3 to 6 months after the tube is removed).

Anesthesia General or local anesthesia can be used. An endotracheal tube is usually in place and respirations are controlled.

Monitoring Monitoring is standard.

Positioning The patient is supine, with shoulders elevated so the neck is moderately extended. The head is stabilized with a positioning device.

Instrumentation and special equipment Equipment includes a soft tissue dissection set, appropriate assortment of tracheostomy tubes, and a tracheal hook and spreader.

Procedure

Key steps

1. The patient is draped to expose the anterior neck from the chin to the sternal notch.
2. A transverse incision (4 to 5 cm) is made over the trachea midway between the sternal notch and the cricoid cartilage and between the borders of the sternocleidomastoid muscles.
3. The dissection is continued through the platysma muscle, fascial layers, and the strap muscles. The thyroid isthmus is retracted or divided if necessary.
4. Hemostasis is obtained with electrosurgery or suture ligatures.
5. A tracheal hook is inserted into the trachea at the level of the second tracheal ring.
6. The endotracheal tube cuff is deflated and the tube is withdrawn to a level in the trachea above where the incision will be made.
7. The trachea is incised vertically at the second, third, and fourth tracheal rings if necessary, or a portion of the trachea is excised and removed, except in children. Hemostasis is attained.
8. A suction catheter is used to suction secretions from the trachea and bronchus.
9. A tracheostomy tube is inserted. The cuff should be checked prior to insertion. The obturator is removed. The cuff is inflated until an adequate seal exists; caution is needed to ensure the cuff is not overinflated, causing pressure inside the trachea. The endotracheal tube is removed and ventilation tubing is connected to the tracheostomy tube.
10. Skin edges may be closed.
11. Dressings are applied, and the tube is secured with a tie around the neck that is attached to the tube flanges.

Postoperative care The patient must be monitored for adequate ventilation. Suctioning may be needed to remove bronchial and tracheal secretions. The obturator and tracheal spreader should be kept at the bedside in the event of accidental dislodgement of the tracheostomy tube.

SURGICAL PROCEDURES

Incisions

Common incisional sites are illustrated in Chapter 13 in this volume. This section includes the basic steps in thoracic surgery (openings and closings) according to incisional sites.

Posterolateral incision

The posterolateral incision offers the most exposure and versatility. The disadvantages include increased muscle and soft tissue dissection, increased time to access the thoracic cavity, and increased postoperative discomfort (Shields, 1989; Sabiston & Spencer, 1990).

Position

1. The patient is placed in lateral decubitus position with appropriate positioning devices. Sandbags, pillows, and a "bean bag" should be available. Ensure patient stability and protect neurovascular structures from injury.
2. The patient's arms are forward and flexed at the elbows. The upper arm may be positioned on an overhead armboard or pillows and the lower arm on the bed or armboard.
3. An axillary roll is carefully placed beneath the lower axilla to decrease pressure on the brachial plexus (a small "fluid bag" may be used).
4. Pillows are placed between the patient's legs to decrease pressure, and the lower leg is flexed at the hip and knee while the upper leg is straight.
5. Pelvic support is provided by positioning devices and secured with a strap across the hips.

Procedure

Key steps

1. The incision is from midway between the spinous processes and the medial border of the scapula (posteriorly) and at a level halfway between the inferior angle of the scapula and the spine at the level of the fifth thoracic vertebra. The incision curves down 1 inch below the inferior angle of the scapula and forward to the midaxillary line.
2. Electrocautery is used to divide the subcutaneous tissues and muscle layer. Retraction of wound edges is necessary to provide exposure, and the retractor size will be adjusted as necessary.
   a. The trapezius and latissimus dorsi muscles are divided.
   b. The rhomboid and serratus anterior muscles are divided. The serratus may be retracted if exposure is adequate.
3. The surgeon identifies the interspace desired by slipping his or her hand up under the scapula and counting the ribs. A scapula retractor is used.

4. Entry into the thoracic cavity is done as follows:
   a. Without rib resection, by:
      (1) Separating the intercostal muscle from the upper border of the lower rib or
      (2) Stripping the periosteum with a periosteal elevator from the upper border of the lower rib and underneath the rib. The chest is entered through the rib bed (Fig. 14-26).
   b. With rib resection:
      Removal of the rib is only occasionally done. The indications are patients with rigid chests, the need for maximum exposure, repeat thoracotomy with adhesions, and anytime there is a risk of causing rib fractures (Shields, 1989; Sabiston & Spencer, 1990).
      (1) Partial resection of a rib or ribs may be done anteriorly or posteriorly to increase exposure, decrease trauma, and decrease postoperative pain.
      (2) Rib resection is done by:
         • Stripping the periosteum from the rib with a periosteal elevator and rib raspatories (Fig. 14-26)

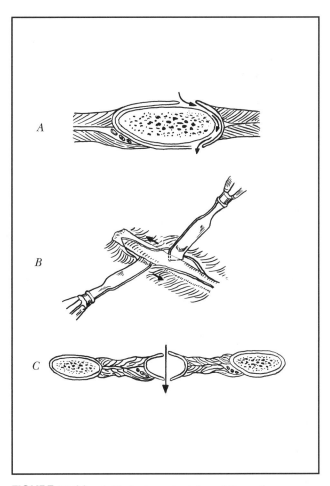

FIGURE 14-26 *A,* Periosteum is stripped from the upper half of the rib and the chest is entered through the rib bed. *B,* Periosteum being stripped from the rib prior to its removal. *C,* Entrance into the chest cavity after the rib is removed.

- Using the rib cutter and removing the rib (Fig. 14-26)
  - A rongeur is used to smooth the cut rib edges.
  (3) The rib regenerates if the periosteum is left intact.
5. Pleural incision
   a. The surgeon observes for lung motion prior to incising the pleura. Absence of motion could indicate adhesions.
   b. Single-lung anesthesia is instituted, and the lung on the operative side collapses.
   c. The pleura is incised with scissors and/or cautery. The lung is protected by retracting it with a sponge stick. The ends of the incision are retracted to increase exposure.
6. Rib spreader retractor is inserted and opened gently.
7. The surgical procedure is done.
8. An intercostal nerve block in the posterior aspect of the second to the seventh ribs will decrease postoperative pain. Marcaine 0.5% with epinephrine is usually used.
9. Chest tubes are inserted prior to closing the chest (see Fig. 14-24).
10. Chest closure
    a. Pericostal sutures of heavy absorbable suture (6 to 8) are placed around the upper rib and through a punch hole in the lower rib. A rib punch is used. This increases postoperative comfort and decreases the chance of vascular injury when placing the suture around the lower rib (Fig. 14-27).
    b. The rib approximator may be used to hold the chest incision closed while tying the sutures.
    c. If pericostal sutures are not used, the intercostal muscles are approximated and closed with an absorbable suture.
    d. Chest muscle layers are approximated and closed in layers with absorbable suture.
    e. Subcutaneous and skin layers are closed and dressings are applied.

Anterolateral incision

This incision is being used more frequently because it causes a minimum of circulatory and ventilatory disturbances. There is rapid access to the thoracic cavity, and fewer muscles need to be divided. There is limited exposure with this incision, especially the lower lobes and vertebral area (Sabiston & Spencer, 1990; Shields, 1989).

Position

1. The patient is supine, with the operative side elevated 30 degrees. Positioning devices are used to support the chest, shoulders, and pelvis.
2. The patient's lower arm is straight at the side or flexed on the bed. The upper arm is elevated above the head, flexed and supported.
3. Pillows are placed between the legs, and the lower leg is straight while the upper leg is flexed at the hip and knee.

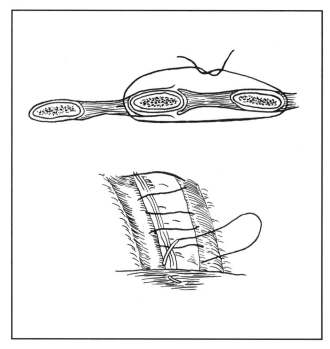

FIGURE 14-27 Pericostal suturing technique.

4. An axillary roll may be used.

Procedure

1. An incision is made from the inferior edge of the scapula to the sternal border (if necessary) (submammary for women and following the fifth rib for men).
2. The pectoralis major and serratus anterior muscles are divided as needed. The latissimus dorsi muscle may be retracted if there is adequate exposure.
3. Usually there is no rib resection.
4. The costal cartilages may be divided to increase exposure.
5. Closure is done as for a posterolateral incision (modified).

Anterior incision

This incision provides access to the anterior mediastinum and pericardium; however, exposure is limited. It is frequently used for lung biopsy. Circulation and ventilation are improved because of position (Sabiston & Spencer, 1990; Shields, 1989).

Position The patient is supine, with the arm on the operative side flexed and secured to the anesthesia screen.

Procedure

1. An inframammary incision is made from midline to midaxilla.
2. The pectoralis major and minor muscles are divided.
3. The intercostal muscle incision extends to the posterior axillary line.

4. Closure is done as for the posterolateral incision (modified).

Axillary incision (Fig. 14-28, A)

This incision has the advantages of the anterolateral incision but with less trauma to the muscle layers. It provides good access to the upper chest and upper lobes.

Position The patient is positioned as for the anterolateral incision except the operative side is positioned at a 45-degree angle.

Procedure

1. The incision starts high in the midaxilla, between the pectoralis major and latissimus dorsi muscle roots.
2. The incision can be extended anteriorly along the fourth rib to the midline if necessary.

Median sternotomy

This incision is used for most cardiac and mediastinal surgical procedures. Access to both lungs is possible, but lobectomy of the lower lobes is difficult.

Refer to Chapter 13 in this volume for information regarding positioning and the procedure.

Thoracoabdominal incision (Fig. 14-28, B)

It is rare to use this type of incision. It provides increased exposure in the upper abdominal area and allows simultaneous upper abdominal and lower chest exposure. The major disadvantages are the increased time needed to open and close this incision and that patients have increased postoperative pain (Sabiston & Spencer, 1990).

Position The patient is positioned with the shoulders and upper chest in a lateral position, with hips rotated back.

Procedure

1. The incision starts in the abdominal midline midway between the tip of the xiphoid process and the umbilicus.
2. The incision goes up and across the costal margin to the seventh or eighth intercostal space to the posterior axillary line.
3. The serratus anterior and external oblique muscle fibers are split in the incisional line, the intercostal muscles are divided, and the pleural cavity is entered.
4. The anterior rectus sheath, the rectus muscle, and the posterior rectus sheath are divided and the peritoneal cavity is entered.
5. The costal margin is divided, and the diaphragm is incised as needed.
6. Appropriate abdominal and chest retractors are used to provide exposure.
7. Closure of this incision involves reapproximation of the incised layers. The diaphragm is repaired with interrupted nonabsorbable sutures.

Lung and Pleural Procedures

Pneumonectomy

Bronchial cancer is the most common reason for total removal of the lung. Other reasons include extensive infections, other types of malignant tumors, and metastatic lesions (Sabiston & Spencer, 1990).

Position The patient is usually positioned as for a posterolateral chest incision.

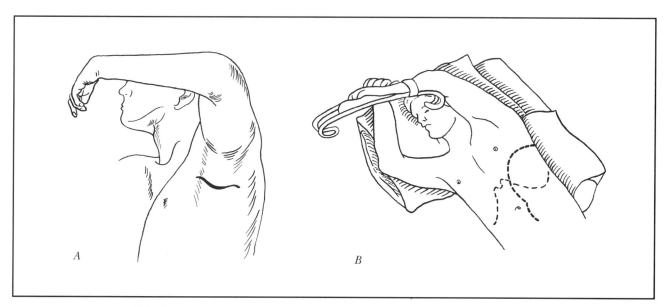

FIGURE 14-28 *A,* Axillary incision location. *B,* Thoracoabdominal incision location.

Instrumentation and special equipment Thoracic instruments, mechanical stapling devices (if used), and positioning devices are needed. Chest tubes and drainage sets are usually not used.

Procedure

1. The chest incision and positioning of the rib-spreading retractor are carried out.
2. The lung is deflated and retracted by using Duval lung clamps, stick sponges, and/or lap sponges as needed.
3. The pulmonary ligament is divided.
4. The pleura is incised along the hilus, and vascular structures are identified, mobilized, and divided. The main pulmonary artery, superior and inferior pulmonary veins, and the azygos vein on the right side are the major vascular structures.
   a. Suture ligation and transfixation suture technique are done (Fig. 14-29); or
   b. Mechanical stapling devices are used (Fig. 14-30).
5. The main stem bronchus is divided at the tracheal junction by:
   a. Clamping with bronchial clamps, dividing, and suturing the proximal end of the bronchial stump; or
   b. Mechanically stapling the bronchus (Fig. 14-31), incising with a knife.
6. Tracheal sleeve technique may be necessary if the cancer involves the trachea, carina, or opposite bronchus.
   a. The involved area of the trachea is excised and removed with the lung.
   b. Remaining bronchus is anastomosed to the tracheal stump.
7. The bronchial stump may be covered with adjacent pleural tissue to prevent an air leak.
8. Warm irrigation fluids are poured into the chest cavity covering the bronchial stump. The anesthesia provider uses increased ventilation pressure while the surgeon observes for air bubbles, indicating an air leak.

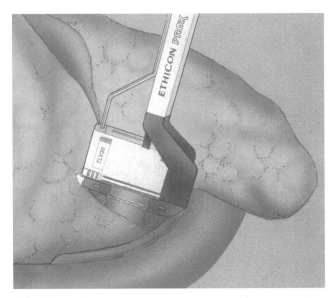

FIGURE 14-30 Vascular stapling device used to staple the left pulmonary artery. (Courtesy of ETHICON ENDO-SURGERY, Cincinnati, OH.)

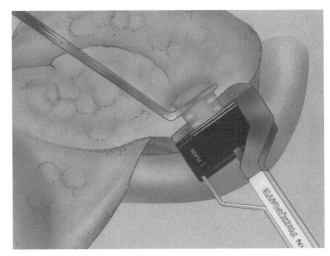

FIGURE 14-31 Bronchus stapling device used to staple the left main stem bronchus. (Courtesy of ETHICON ENDO-SURGERY, Cincinnati, OH.)

9. Biopsies of lymph nodes are done to determine metastases of the cancer.
10. The chest incision is closed. No chest tubes are inserted.
11. Pleural space pressure is adjusted after the incision is closed by aspirating air from the chest cavity until the trachea is midline.

Postoperative care Major postoperative complications are development of a bronchopleural fistula, causing massive air leak and respiratory distress; bleeding; empyema; and/or cardiac arrhythmias. Mortality of 3% to 30% can occur, and common causes are sepsis, pulmonary insuffi-

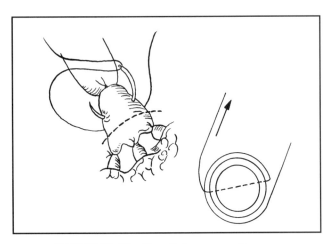

FIGURE 14-29 Transfixion suture ligature.

ciency, heart failure, and myocardial infarction (Shields, 1989).

Pleuropneumonectomy

This is a technically difficult and hazardous procedure and is indicated for patients with total lung destruction associated with chronic empyema and bronchopleural fistula (Hood, 1986).

Position The patient is usually positioned as for a posterolateral chest incision.

Instrumentation and special equipment This is as for pneumonectomy.

Procedure

Key steps

1. The chest incision is made, usually with rib resection. A retractor is inserted.
2. The empyema cavity and lung are resected as a unit.
3. Dissection is begun at the extrapleural plane and carried out to the mediastinum.
4. Hilar dissection of vascular structures and bronchus is carried out as in pneumonectomy. Intrapericardial dissection of vascular structures may be necessary.
5. The pleural space is irrigated with antibiotic solution.
6. A chest tube may be needed for drainage of the pleural space if gross contamination occurred during the surgical procedure.
7. The chest incision is closed.

Postoperative care
The postoperative complications that may occur are the same as with pneumonectomy. The mortality rate is 20% to 40% (Hood, 1986).

Lobectomy

The primary reason for removing a lobe of the lung is bronchogenic cancer. Other indications include extensive infectious processes, metastatic lesions, and solitary benign lesions (Shields, 1989).

Position The patient is positioned as for posterolateral or anterolateral incisions.

Instrumentation and special equipment As in pneumonectomy. Chest tubes and a drainage set are needed.

Procedure

Key steps

1. The chest incision is made and the rib-spreading retractor is placed.
2. The lung is deflated and retracted.
3. Hilar dissection, mobilization, and division of lobar branches of the pulmonary artery and pulmonary vein are done.

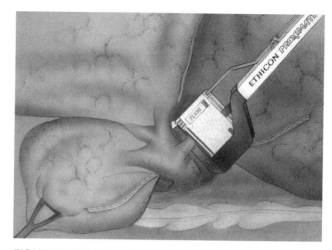

FIGURE 14-32 Vascular stapling device used to staple intralobar arteries. Note the staple lines where the fissure has been divided. (Courtesy of ETHICON ENDO-SURGERY, Cincinnati, OH.)

4. For division of the fissure between lobes, a linear stapler or cutter may be used (Fig. 14-32).
5. The interlobar vascular branches are divided.
6. The lobar bronchus is identified. Temporary occlusion of the bronchus while the anesthesia provider inflates the lung provides assurance that the correct bronchus is being divided.
7. The lobar bronchus is divided with a stapling or clamp technique.
8. Sleeve resection of the bronchus (Fig. 14-33):
   a. A portion of the adjacent bronchus is removed if there is tumor involvement.
   b. The bronchus is anastomosed end to end and the suture line is covered with a parietal pleural flap.
   c. Intraoperative fiberoptic bronchoscopic examination may be done to check the anastomosis site for stenosis or kinking.
9. Check for air leaks with irrigation fluid.
10. Two chest tubes are inserted: one in the apex, the other at the base.
11. The chest is closed.

Postoperative care Chest tubes remain in place until there is no air leak and less than 50 ml drainage in 24 hours. Complications are similar to those encountered in pneumonectomy patients. Mortality is 1% to 3% (Shields, 1989).

Segmental resection

The minimal amount of lung tissue is resected to remove the involved area. A segment or segments of the lung lobe may be removed.

Position The position is as for posterolateral, anterolateral, or anterior chest incision.

Instrumentation and special equipment This is the same as in pneumonectomy and lobectomy procedures.

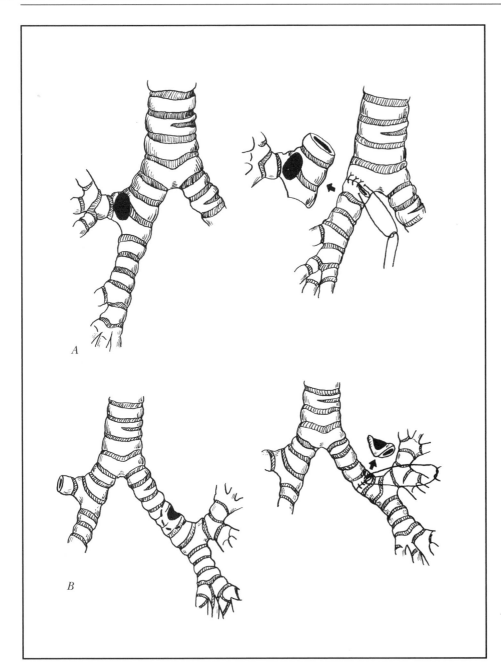

FIGURE 14-33 *A*, Bronchial sleeve resection. *B*, Partial bronchial sleeve resection. (Adapted from Lowe, J. E. et al. "The role of bronchoplastic procedures in the surgical management of benign and malignant pulmonary lesions," *Journal of Thoracic and Cardiovascular Surgery*, 83:227, 1082, Mosby-Year Book, Inc., St. Louis, MO).

Procedure

Key steps

1. The chest incision is made and a rib-spreading retractor is placed.
2. The lung is deflated and retracted.
3. The involved area of lung is identified.
   a. Simple removal of a segmental area can be done with a mechanical stapling device, or
   b. The segment is divided and vascular and bronchial structures are identified and divided. The segment is separated from the lobe by using blunt dissection. Hemostasis is obtained.
4. Checking for air leaks is done with irrigation fluid.
5. A chest tube is inserted.

6. The incision is closed.

Postoperative care Postoperative care is as in lobectomy. The mortality is 1% or less (Shields, 1989).

Wedge resection

The wedge resection is used for peripheral lesions that are usually benign, such as blebs, granulomas, tumors, or biopsy specimens.

Position The position is the same as for anterolateral or anterior chest incision.

Instrumentation and special equipment This is as in lobectomy procedures.

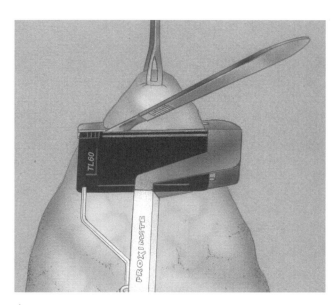

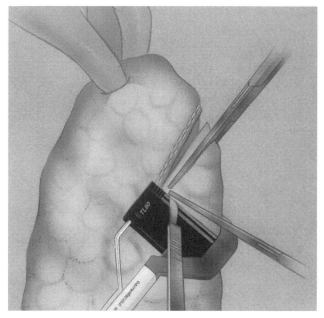

A

FIGURE 14-34   *A*, Apical biopsy using vascular stapling device. *B*, Wedge resection.   (Courtesy of ETHICON ENDO-SURGERY, Cincinnati, OH.)

B

Procedure

Key steps

1. The chest incision is made, and a rib-spreading retractor is placed.
2. The involved area of lung is identified and grasped with a Duval lung clamp.
3. The area to be resected can be removed by using a mechanical stapling device or by clamping, incising, and suturing technique (Fig. 14-34,*A*, *B*).
4. Air leaks are checked with irrigation fluid. A chest tube is inserted.
5. The incision is closed.

Postoperative care   As in lobectomy. The mortality rate is low, 0.5% (Shields, 1989).

Decortication

The collection of pus in the pleural cavity, empyema, is usually a secondary complication of pneumonia. Trauma, spontaneous pneumothorax, abscesses of the lung, or subphrenic, postoperative complications, and/or foreign bodies in the bronchial tree are other causes. Decortication is indicated in the chronic stage of empyema, when the lung is trapped and unable to expand. The fibrotic "peel" that forms in the pleural space is removed so the lung can reexpand (Sabiston & Spencer, 1990).

Position   Usually the positioning is for a posterolateral incision.

Instrumentation and special equipment   This is as in lobectomy, except materials needed for lung resection. Cultures are taken.

Procedure

Key steps

1. The chest incision is made, and a rib-spreading retractor is placed.
2. The visceral pleural peel is incised with a knife, and the peel is bluntly dissected. Sharp dissection with the scissors or knife may be necessary.
3. Removal of the parietal pleural peel depends on the surgeon's preference.
4. The empyema collection may be entered, cultured, and evacuated.
5. The anesthesia provider periodically expands the lung so the surgeon can identify adhesed areas.
6. The chest cavity is irrigated with an antibiotic solution.
7. Chest tubes are inserted.
8. The chest incision is closed.

Postoperative care   Persistent air leak, hemorrhage, and sepsis are the major postoperative complications. Mortality is 1% to 8% and is usually related to the patient's septic condition and/or hemorrhage (Shields, 1989).

Thoracoplasty/thoracomyopleuroplasty

This rare procedure is used to treat chronic empyema when the lung tissue is insufficient to obliterate the pleural space. Unresolved empyema has a mortality of 10% to 50%.

If the empyema space is small enough, muscle flaps can be positioned to obliterate the space (Hammond et al., 1993).

Thoracoplasty is the removal of several ribs or portions of ribs in order to allow the chest wall to collapse.

The Andrews thoracomyopleuroplasty involves removal of ribs, or a portion of the ribs, over the space; entering and curetting the space; and suturing the chest wall to the mediastinal and visceral pleura. This obliterates the space (Fig. 14-35) (Deslauriers & Lacquet, 1990; Sabiston & Spencer, 1990; Shields, 1989).

Position Positioning is as for anterior, anterolateral, or posterolateral chest incision.

Instrumentation and special equipment Rib resection instruments are needed, and retractors (i.e., Richardsons) are needed for exposing ribs. Curettes are also needed.

Procedure

Key steps

1. An incision over the area of the ribs to be removed is done.
2. Ribs to be removed are identified and removed.
3. Muscle layers are closed over the site of rib removal.
4. Note: no chest tube is used because the purpose of this surgery is to obliterate the pleural space.

Postoperative care Complications are related to nerve or vascular injury, respiratory distress, sepsis, and/or chylothorax. Scoliosis of varying degrees can occur with the resulting chest wall deformity. Mortality is approximately 5%, usually due to the underlying disease (Deslauriers & Lacquet, 1990; Shields, 1989; Sabiston & Spencer, 1990).

Pleurodesis

This procedure is used to treat recurring spontaneous pneumothorax. Patients at risk for repeat pneumothorax are those with chronic obstructive pulmonary disease (COPD), air leak for more than 48 hours, large air cysts of the lung, and more than one episode of these. Recurrence is 20% after the first episode and 60% to 80% if there is more than one episode.

Pleurodesis is the creation of an inflammatory process within the pleural space. Adhesions form with the inflammation, and the lung surface adheres to the inside of the chest wall, thereby preventing further air leaks. The three methods used are chemical pleurodesis (instilling foreign substances, such as talc), which can be toxic and may not create uniform adhesions; removal of parietal pleura in the area of the air leak, which creates an inflammatory surface and adhesions between the lung and the thoracic fascia, making future thoracotomies difficult; and mechanical pleurodesis, where a dry sponge is used to abrade the parietal pleura until bleeding occurs. Adhesion formation will occur between the lung and the parietal pleura. Any blebs or bullae of the lung are stapled or sutured (Deslauriers & Lacquet, 1990). Chemical pleurodesis is usually done through a chest tube. The other two procedures require a thoracotomy.

Position The positioning is as for an anterior or anterolateral incision.

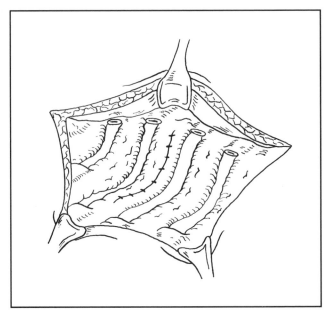

FIGURE 14-35 Andrews thoracomyopleuroplasty. Note areas where ribs have been removed.

Instrumentation and special equipment Thoracotomy instruments, chest tube(s), and a drainage set are needed. Stapling devices must be available.

Procedure

Key steps

1. The chest incision and positioning of the retractor are accomplished.
2. The lung is inspected. Resection of blebs/bullae, if present, is done, using the stapling device or suture. Any area of the lung where air leak is occurring is closed.
3. The pleurodesis procedure is done.
4. A chest tube is inserted.
5. The chest incision is closed.

Postoperative care Postoperative care is as for other pulmonary surgical procedures.

Tracheal procedures

Tracheal resection

Tracheal resection may be indicated for tracheal problems that obstruct the airway. The primary causes are neoplasms, congenital deformities, infections, and/or injuries. Prolonged endotracheal intubation may cause tracheal injury because of the pressure from the tube's cuff.

The development of surgical mobilization techniques and the use of cervical flexion postoperatively are major factors in facilitating tracheal resection procedures. Up to 6 cm of trachea can be removed by using these techniques (Shields, 1989; Mathison & Grillo, 1991).

The use of tracheal prosthetic devices frequently results in strictures, sepsis, and/or erosion of the device into major vessels, with resultant hemorrhage (Shields, 1989). Neville reports using the Neville silicone prosthesis in 65 patients since 1970. Selected patient outcomes have been encouraging with the use of this device (Neville et al., 1991).

The surgical approach is determined by the location of the tracheal lesion. Those occurring in the upper third of the trachea can be repaired through a cervical incision. Exposure can be increased by splitting the upper sternum if necessary. A right posterolateral thoracotomy incision is used for lesions in the lower two-thirds of the trachea. A combination of cervical, sternal, and/or thoracotomy incisions may be needed for complex resections and repair. Cardiopulmonary bypass is rarely needed (Shields, 1989).

Position   The patient is supine for cervical and sternal incisions and in the lateral decubitus position for posterolateral incisions.

Instrumentation and special equipment   A soft tissue set is needed for the cervical incisions. A sternal saw and sternal sutures are used for the sternal approach. Thoracotomy instruments, appropriate retractors, and umbilical tapes are needed.

Procedure

Key steps

1. Incision and retraction are accomplished.
2. Mobilization of the trachea is done by dissecting adjoining tissues. Umbilical tapes are placed around the trachea above and below the area to be resected.
3. Continuing anesthesia while the trachea is being resected and reconstructed may be accomplished by using a longer endotracheal tube (thoracic approach) or by attaching sterile anesthesia tubing to a tube that is inserted into the distal trachea.
4. Traction sutures are placed in the lateral aspects of the trachea above and below the area to be resected. Once the trachea has been resected, the traction sutures are used to align and support the trachea while it is being anastomosed.
5. The trachea is incised and resected. Margin edges are checked by frozen section for malignant cells.
6. Cervical flexion (tilting the patient's head forward) facilitates the anastomosing. Hilar mobilization is done by incising the pericardium. Suprahyoid laryngeal release will add 1 to 2 cm in tracheal length.
7. The thoracic tracheal anastomosis site is wrapped with a segment of pleura to protect the suture line and decrease possible air leak.
8. Carinal resection and reconstruction can be complex (Fig. 14-36).
9. A drain or chest tube (or several tubes) is positioned.
10. The incision is closed.

Postoperative care   The cervical flexion can be maintained by placing a suture from the chin to the upper chest and supporting the head with pillows. The suture can be released 7 days postoperatively. The majority of postoperative complications are related to anastomotic problems (infection, disruption of suture line, air leak, delayed healing). Long-term followup is important, with bronchoscopic procedures done periodically to evaluate the suture line.

Esophageal Procedures

Esophageal resection

Cancer is the most common reason for resecting the esophagus. Other reasons include strictures, tumors, or extensive injury. Fifteen percent of esophageal cancer occurs in the upper one-third, 50% in the middle one-third, and 35% in the lower one-third of the esophagus. The majority are squamous cell, with adenocarcinoma being the most common in the esophagogastric junction. Although uncommon, esophageal cancer is a highly lethal disease, and wide resection is necessary. Possible causes include cigarette smoking, excessive alcohol consumption, caustic injuries, achalasia, gastroesophageal reflux, irradiation, chronic inflammation, and nutritional deficiencies. Symptoms include progressive dysphagia, rapid weight loss, weakness, and odynophagia (Mayer, 1993; Sabiston & Spencer, 1990).

The decision regarding the type of surgical approach is determined by the location of the tumor, the intent of the procedure (curative or palliative), the organ to be used for the esophageal replacement (stomach, colon, or jejunum), the planned treatment program (chemotherapy and/or radiotherapy), and the surgeon's preference (Delarue et al., 1988; Sugarbaker & DeCamp, 1993).

The surgical approaches are:

1. Transhiatal or orthotopic (via the posterior mediastinum) (retrosternal or subcutaneous are alternate routes) (Fig. 14-37). Abdominal and cervical incisions are required.
2. Transthoracic requires right thoracotomy and abdominal incisions (a left thoracoabdominal incision is occasionally used) (Fig. 14-38).
3. Transthoracic–abdominal–cervical approach requires incisions in all three areas (Sugarbaker & DeCamp, 1993; Sabiston & Spencer, 1990; Orringer, 1993).

Position   Supine positioning is used for cervical and abdominal incisions. The thoracotomy position is used for a posterolateral or anterolateral incision.

Instrumentation and special equipment   Instrumentation is based on the incision. The transthoracic/abdominal approach may be done in two stages: the abdominal incision is closed and the patient repositioned and redraped for the thoracic incision. Stapling devices, Penrose drains, chest tubes, jejunostomy feeding tube, and vascular clips are needed.

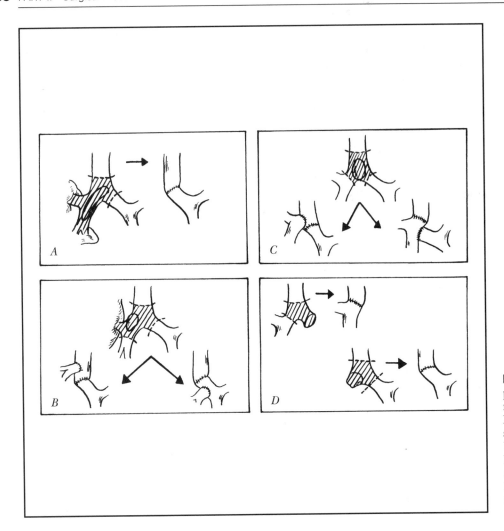

FIGURE 14-36 *A*, Right pneumonectomy with carina resected and reconstructed. *B*, Resection of the carina segment and reconstruction. *C*, Upper and/or middle lobectomy, resection of carina, and reconstruction. *D*, Resection of carina after prior right or left pneumonectomy.

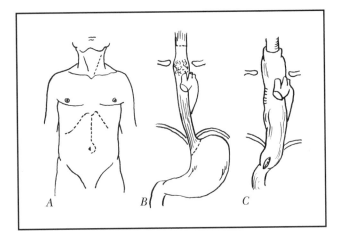

FIGURE 14-37 *A*, Location of incisions for transhiatal esophageal resection. *B*, Location of the portion of the esophagus to be excised is shown by dotted lines. *C*, Location of the stomach tube in the chest cavity and sutured to the proximal end of esophagus.

Procedure

Key steps

Transhiatal

1. An upper midline abdominal incision is done. Exposure is enhanced with the use of a table-mounted, self-retaining retractor (i.e., Gomez, Upper Hand).
2. Inspection is done for tumor invasion, and the stomach is evaluated for use as an esophageal substitute.
3. The stomach, along the greater curvature, is mobilized.
4. Pyloromyotomy is done to prevent delayed gastric emptying.
5. A Penrose drain is placed around the esophagus, and the esophagus is bluntly dissected through the hiatus 5 to 10 cm.
6. Cervical incision is carried out along the border of the left sternocleidomastoid.
7. The cervical esophagus is mobilized and encircled with a Penrose drain (for traction).
8. Simultaneous blunt dissection of the posterior transhiatal and anterior transhiatal areas is done from the abdominal and the cervical incisions (Fig. 14-39).
9. The cervical esophagus is stapled and divided using a linear stapler/cutter.

10. A long Penrose drain is sewn to the distal end of the cervical esophagus.
11. The esophagus is then pulled into the abdominal incision and each end of the drain is secured with a hemostat.
12. The esophagogastric esophagus is divided using a linear stapler cutter device; the cardia portion of the stomach is oversewn, and the abdominal end of the Penrose drain is sewn to the fundus of the stomach (Fig. 14-40).
13. The stomach is guided through the transhiatal space while pulling on the upper end of the Penrose drain (Fig. 14-41). A sterile plastic bag may be placed

around the stomach to decrease the friction as it is pulled through the chest.
14. A feeding jejunostomy tube is positioned and secured with a suture to the inside abdominal wall. The abdominal incision is closed.
15. The proximal end of the cervical esophagus is anastomosed to an opening made in the fundus of the stomach.
16. The nasogastric tube is inserted, drains are placed, and the cervical incision is closed.

Transthoracic (esophagogastrectomy)

1. Abdominal procedure is followed, as in the transhiatal approach. The esophagus is not divided.
2. The abdominal incision is closed, and the patient is repositioned, reprepped, and redraped for the thoracotomy.
3. A posterolateral or an anterolateral thoracotomy incision is made and the chest retractor is positioned.
4. The lung is collapsed and retracted.
5. The mediastinal pleura is opened and the esophagus is exposed and mobilized. A Penrose drain is placed around the esophagus for traction.
6. The distal esophagus and stomach are pulled into the chest through the hiatus.
7. A linear stapler cutter device is used across the upper stomach, and the staple line is oversewn (Fig. 14-42). This frees the distal end of the esophagus.
8. The esophagus is transected proximally, and the specimen is removed.
9. The proximal end of the esophagus is anastomosed to the opening made in the stomach tube.

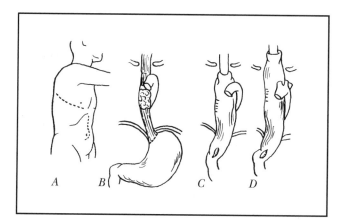

FIGURE 14-38 *A*, Location of the incisions for transthoracic esophageal resection. *B*, Location of the portion of esophagus to be excised. *C*, Location of the stomach in the chest cavity. *D*, Location of the stomach after it is passed through the chest into the neck incision.

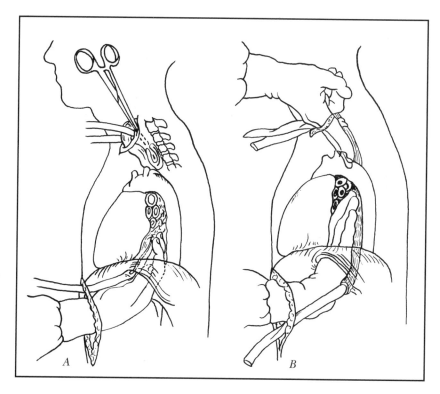

FIGURE 14-39 Blunt dissection of transhiatal area through abdominal and cervical incisions. *A*, posterior area. (Reprinted with permission from Orringer, M. B., and Sloan, H. J. *Thoracic Cardiovascular Surgery* 76:643, 1978, Mosby-Year Book, Inc., St. Louis, MO.) *B*, anterior area. (Reprinted with permission from Orringer, M. B.: Transhiatal blunt esophagectomy without thoracotomy. In Cohn, L. H. editor: *Modern technics in surgery: Cardiothoracic surgery*, New York, 1983, Futura Publishing Co.)

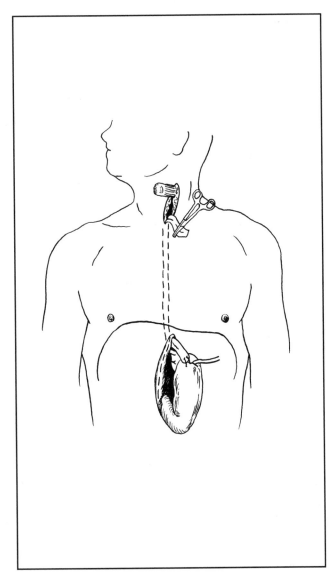

FIGURE 14-40 Location of Penrose drain after it is sutured to the stomach. (Adapted from Nyhus and Baker, *Mastery of Surgery*, 1984, Little, Brown and Company, Boston, MA).

10. The nasogastric tube is positioned, chest tubes are placed, and the chest incision is closed.

Transthoracic–abdominal–cervical

1. Abdominal, thoracic (right side), and cervical incisions are made, as in the other two approaches.
2. The abdominal incision is usually done first; the thoracic incision is needed to free the esophagus when the lesion is high in the esophagus intrathoracicly. The stomach can be easily positioned through the hiatus, into the chest, and into the neck. The cervical incision is made on the right side of the neck.
3. Incisions are closed in the usual manner.

Postoperative care A 5-year survival rate of approximately 15% is reported for patients undergoing esopha-

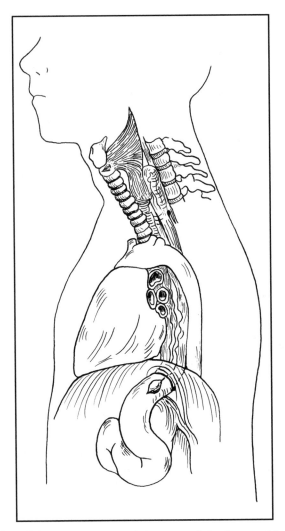

FIGURE 14-41 Location of the stomach in the transhiatal space. (Adapted from Orringer, M. B. and Sloan, H. J. *Thoracic Cardiovascular Surgery*, 76:643, 1978, Mosby-Year Book, Inc., St. Louis, MO).

geal resection procedures (Orringer, 1993). Hospital mortality is 3% to 5%. Possible complications include respiratory problems, injury to the recurrent laryngeal nerve, and anastomotic leak and/or stricture. Mortality is related to infections, other organ failure, and intraoperative complications (i.e., hemorrhage) (Sabiston & Spencer, 1990).

Esophageal perforation or rupture

The most common causes of esophageal perforation or rupture are instrumentation, foreign bodies, spontaneous rupture (Boerhaave's syndrome with prolonged emesis), postoperative leak or separation of esophageal anastomosis, or thoracic trauma (usually penetrating).

Symptoms include dysphagia, pain, fever, dyspnea, and/or cervical crepitation. Surgical exploration, repair, and drainage are the methods of treatment. The incisional site depends on the location of the esophageal problem. The type of repair depends on the extent of the tear or rupture. Pleural or muscle tissue may be used to

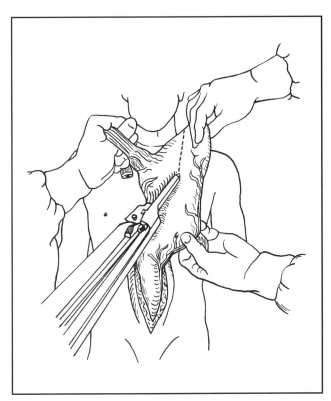

FIGURE 14-42 Use of a linear cutter to prepare the stomach for esophagogastrectomy. (Adapted from Nyhus and Baker, *Master of Surgery*, 1984, Little, Brown and Company, Boston, MA).

wrap the suture line to decrease possible leaking at the repair site. Delay in treatment beyond 24 hours has a mortality rate of over 25%. Antibiotics, nutritional support, and gastric decompression are indicated during the postoperative period. Sepsis is the leading cause of death (Sabiston & Spencer, 1990; Guth & Gouge, 1992).

Antireflux repair

The thoracic approach may be selected for some patients with gastroesophageal reflux and secondary esophagitis associated with hiatal hernia. Indications for the thoracic approach include previous repair, need for esophageal resection or esophagomyotomy, extensive esophagitis, presence of pulmonary or mediastinal disease, need to expose the esophagus, and obesity. Both the Nissen and Belsey Mark IV fundoplication procedures can be done thoracicly (see Chapter 7 in this volume) (Sabiston & Spencer, 1990).

Esophageal myotomy (Heller myotomy)

Achalasia, which results in a lack of peristalsis in the body of the esophagus, and diffuse esophageal spasm are the usual problems treated by esophageal myotomy. Symptoms include obstruction to swallowing, regurgitation, and pain.

A left thoracotomy incision is used. The esophagus is exposed and an incision (5 to 7 cm) is made on the left anterolateral surface of the esophagus through the mus-

cle layer to the mucosal layer. The muscle is dissected free of the mucosa laterally for half the circumference of the esophagus (Sabiston & Spencer, 1990).

Esophageal diverticula

Esophageal diverticula are blind pouches or pockets in the main esophageal lumen. The three common types are pharyngoesophageal (Zenker's), epiphrenic or supradiaphragmatic, and parabronchial. Symptoms are related to esophageal obstruction, retention, regurgitation, secondary respiratory aspiration, choking, foul breath, strangling, and noisy deglutition.

Zenker's diverticulum

The Zenker's diverticulum is the most common and occurs frequently in elderly patients. Surgical treatment may be a cricopharyngeal myotomy for a small sac and diverticulectomy for larger sacs.

Position The patient is supine, with the head toward the right side.

Instrumentation and special equipment A soft tissue dissection set, a stapler, and a drain are needed.

Procedure

Key steps

1. An incision is made along the anterior border of the left sternocleidomastoid muscle.
2. Underlying structures are retracted, and the esophagus is exposed.
3. Esophageal muscle fibers are incised inferior to the diverticulum (myotomy for a small diverticulum).
4. Resection of a larger diverticulum at the neck of the sac can be done with a stapler or by resecting and closing the esophagus.
5. A drain is placed.
6. The incision is closed.

Epiphrenic diverticulum

Epiphrenic diverticula usually occur in the lower 10 cm of the esophagus. The usual cause is esophageal obstruction.

Position The patient is positioned as for a right posterolateral thoracotomy.

Instrumentation and special equipment Thoracotomy instruments and a chest drainage tube and set-up are needed.

Procedure

Key steps

1. A posterolateral incision is made at the level of the eighth rib.

2. The esophagus is mobilized, and tapes are placed around the esophagus above and below the diverticulum.
3. The neck of the diverticulum is dissected free, and the diverticulum is removed; the esophagus is closed.
4. An esophagomyotomy is done on the side opposite the repair.
5. A chest tube is placed.
6. The incision is closed.

Parabronchial diverticulum

Parabronchial diverticula are usually asymptomatic unless a fistula with the tracheobronchial tree occurs. Surgery is indicated and is done through a right posterolateral incision.

1. The diverticulum is excised.
2. The esophagus is closed in layers over a 40 to 50 French catheter or esophageal dilator to ensure an adequate lumen.
3. Fistulas are closed and the suture line is covered with pleura, muscle, or connective tissue to prevent recurrence.

(Shields, 1989; Ravitch & Steichen, 1988)

Chest Wall Procedures

Congenital deformities of the chest wall primarily involve the sternum, costal cartilages, and ribs. Chest wall deformities may result from infections, trauma, radiation therapy, and/or surgical excision of tumors. Surgery is indicated if pulmonary or cardiac function is impaired but frequently is done for cosmetic reasons.

Position Patient positioning depends on the location of the deformity and the need to access other body areas.

Instrumentation and special equipment Equipment needed includes a soft tissue set; bone instruments—periosteal elevators, rongeurs, curettes, bone cutters, drills, saws, wires, and pins; reconstruction materials—polypropylene mesh, polytetrafluoroethylene sheets, and methylmethacrylate glue; and special sutures.

Pectus excavatum

This is the most common congenital deformity of the sternum. The sternum is depressed due to the concave deformity of the costal cartilages.

Ravitch technique
Key steps (Fig. 14-43)

1. A midline sternal or transverse submammary incision is made.
2. The pectoral muscles are dissected and retracted to expose the deformed cartilages.

3. The perichondrium flaps are reflected, and a periosteal elevator is used to dissect the cartilages free. Cartilages are cut and removed.
4. The xiphoid is divided from the sternum, and the underlying tissues are bluntly dissected from under the sternum.
5. The sternum is dissected free from the cartilages and tissue on both sides and is lifted up. A posterior osteotomy is done at the sternomanubrium joint. A wedge of bone or cartilage is placed in the osteotomy, thus elevating the sternum. A Steinmann pin or Kirschner wire may be placed under the sternum to provide support.
6. A mediastinal drain is placed, and chest tubes are inserted if the pleural space is entered.
7. The pectoral muscles are sutured together over the sternum.
8. Subcutaneous tissue and skin are closed.

Sternal eversion ("turnover")
Key steps (Fig. 14-44)

1. An incision is made as in the Ravitch technique.
2. The deformed portions of the sternum, cartilages, and ribs are resected en bloc with the intercostal muscles.
3. The resected bloc is turned over and sutured into place.
4. Optional vascular supply may be provided by the internal mammary vessels from the rectus muscle.

Pectus carinatum ("pigeon breast") (Fig. 14-45) Upward curve of the lower costal cartilages causes the sternum to protrude.

Key steps

1. A midline sternal or transverse submammary incision is made.
2. The pectoral muscles are dissected free and retracted; the rectus and external oblique muscles are dissected free from the lower cartilages and xiphoid.
3. Deformed cartilages are removed, and sutures through the perichondrial beds are used to "reef" the tissues together and remove redundant space.
4. The pectoral muscles are sutured together; the rectus and external oblique muscles are sutured to the pectoral muscles.
5. Usually no drain is required. The subcutaneous tissue layer and the skin are closed.

Sternal cleft or fissure

This congenital defect results in the incomplete joining of the sternum. The defect may involve the upper, lower, or complete sternum. The pericardial and peritoneal cavities may be joined, and other congenital anomalies may exist (Sabiston & Spencer, 1990; Ravitch & Steichen, 1988).

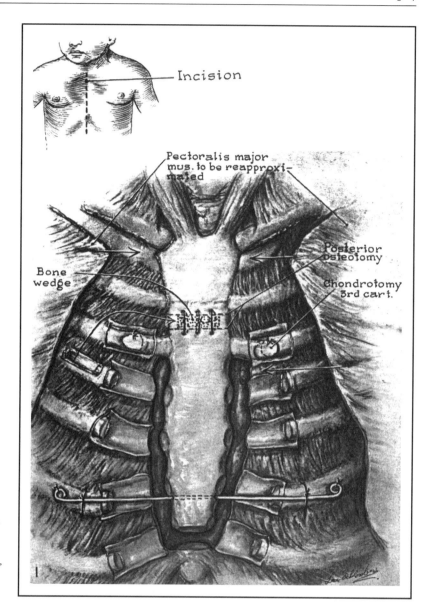

FIGURE 14-43 Repair of pectus excavatum using the Ravitch technique. (Reprinted with permission from Ravitch & Steichen: *Atlas of General Thoracic Surgery* [1988] W. B. Saunders Co., Philadelphia, PA.)

Procedure

Key steps

1. U- and V-shaped defects of the upper sternum can be closed in infancy.
   a. Sternal edges are notched.
   b. A bone wedge is removed from the lower end of the defect.
   c. The sternum is held together with peristernal sutures.
2. Older children (3 to 4 years of age) have the costal cartilages released in order to pull the sternal edges together.
3. Adolescent/adult patients need prosthetic devices.
4. Defects of the lower or complete sternum require procedures that separate the peritoneal and pericardial cavities.

Poland's syndrome

Absence of the pectoralis major muscle and other nearby musculoskeletal components on one side of the chest results in asymmetry. The defect is surgically repaired for cosmetic reasons or when substantial chondral or costochondral defects exist. Surgical repair may involve chest wall reconstruction and the use of latissimus dorsi muscle transfer (Ravitch & Steichen, 1988; Sabiston & Spencer, 1990; Seyfer et al., 1988).

Procedure

Key steps (Fig. 14-46)

1. A submammary incision is made well below the defect.
2. Rib ends are freshened, and rib grafts are inserted.
3. The medial ends of the rib graft are sharpened and pressed into holes made in the sternum.

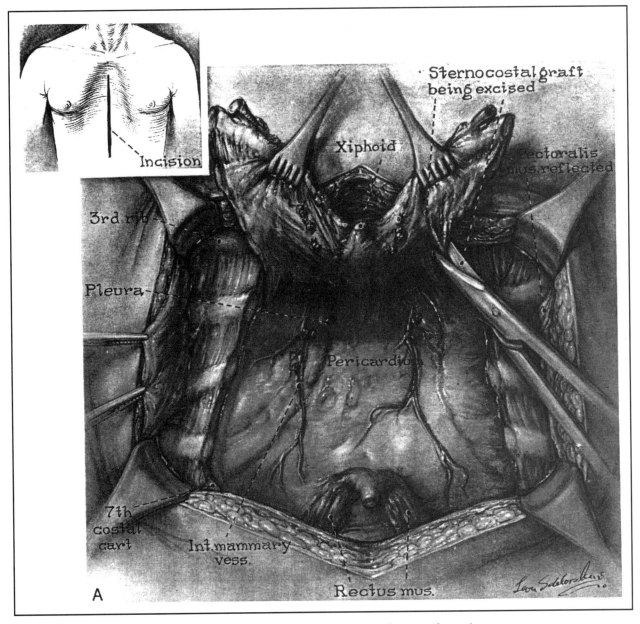

FIGURE 14-44 Repair of pectus excavatum using the sternal eversion (turnover) technique. (Reprinted with permission from Ravitch & Steichen: *Atlas of General Thoracic Surgery* [1988] W. B. Saunders Co., Philadelphia, PA.)

4. A sheet of prosthetic graft material is sutured into place over the rib grafts.
5. A latissimus dorsi muscle transfer is used to replace the absent pectoralis major muscle.
6. A drain is placed.
7. The incision is closed.

Resection of chest wall neoplasms

Chest wall neoplasms involve various bone and/or soft tissues. Benign tumors are excised at biopsy, whereas malignant tumors require wide resection. Removal of the entire involved bony structure is necessary for high-grade malignancies.

The development of chest wall reconstructive procedures has increased the use of surgical treatment for chest wall neoplasms. The size, location, and depth of the tumor, as well as the patient's general condition, prognosis, and local skin condition, are factors that must be considered.

Large skeletal defects need to be supported in order to stabilize the chest. Prosthetic materials, such as polypropylene mesh, polytetrafluorethylene patch material, and meshes impregnated with methyl methacrylate, can be used. Smaller defects may be repaired with a rib graft covered with a mesh.

Muscle or omentum is used to reconstruct soft tissue defects. Muscle flaps alone or musculocutaneous flaps are

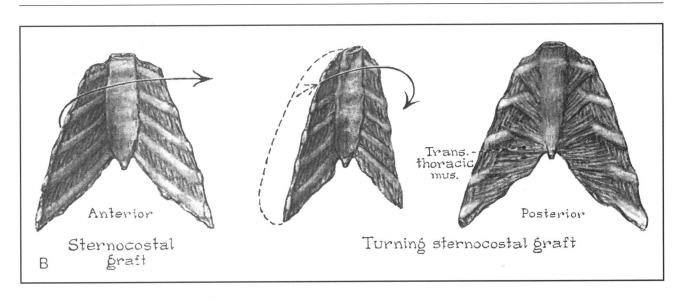

B   Sternocostal
graft

Anterior

Turning sternocostal graft

Trans.-
thoracic
mus.

Posterior

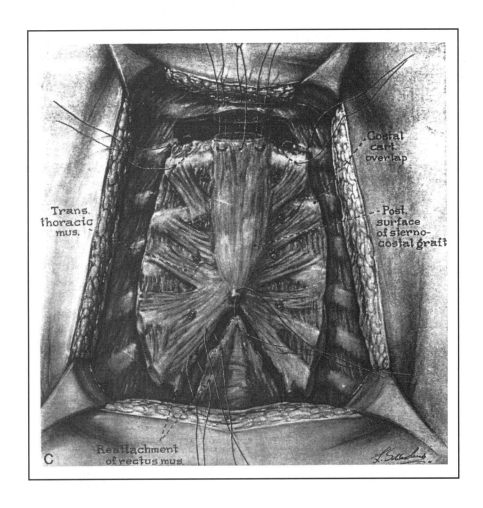

Trans.
thoracic
mus.

Costal
cart.
overlap

Post.
surface
of sterno-
costal graft

Reattachment
of rectus mus.

C

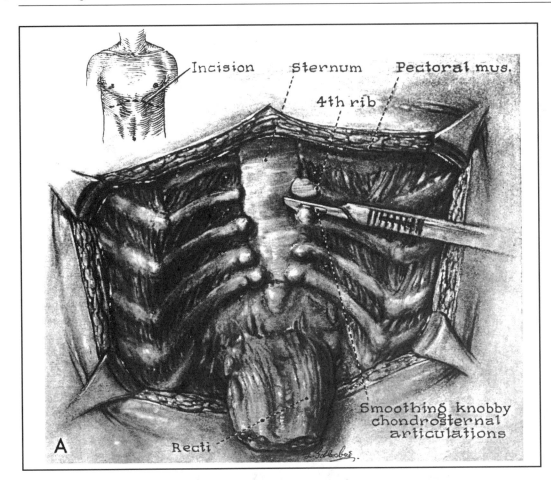

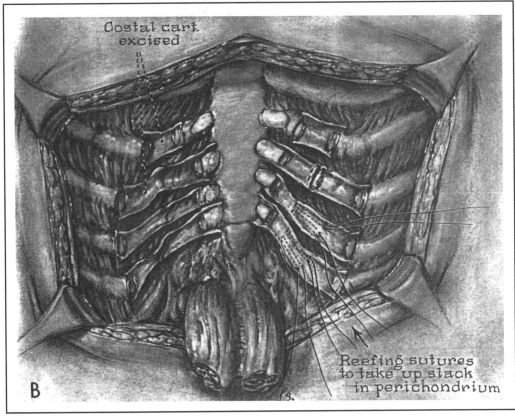

FIGURE 14-45
Repair of pectus carinatum. (Reprinted with permission from Ravitch & Steichen: *Atlas of General Thoracic Surgery* [1988] W. B. Saunders Co., Philadelphia, PA.)

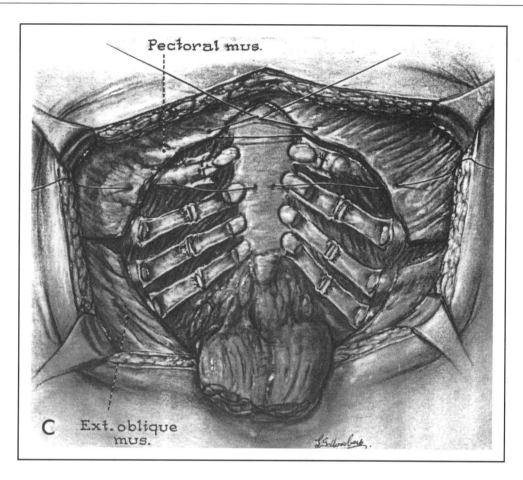

used. The muscles commonly used are the pectoralis major, latissimus dorsi, rectus abdominis, serratus anterior, external oblique, and trapezius (Sabiston & Spencer, 1990; Ravitch & Steichen, 1988).

Procedure

Key steps

1. An incision is made to provide access to the involved area.
2. The tumor and surrounding tissue and bone are excised.
3. The prosthetic device or rib graft is prepared and placed (Fig. 14-47).
4. Muscle or omentum transfer requires incision(s) that provide access to the muscle or omentum (Fig. 14-48). The transfer is completed.
5. Drains are placed.
6. The incisions are closed. A skin graft may be needed.

Sternal resection and reconstruction

When indicated, the sternum can be partially or totally removed. The most common indication is sternal infection. This occurs in approximately 2% of the patients who have had a median sternotomy. Risk factors for postoperative sternal infection include diabetes mellitus, obesity, malnutrition, COPD, uremia, prolonged operating room time, excessive use of electrosurgery on surrounding tissues, use of bone wax for hemostasis, bilateral internal mammary artery grafts, and prolonged postoperative ventilatory support (Ulicny & Hiratzka, 1991; Mansour et al., 1993).

Since 1980, sternal debridement with muscle or omental flap reconstruction has reduced the mortality rate for sternal infections from over 50% to near 0% (Pairolero et al., 1991). The wound is debrided of all infected and necrotic tissue and bone. If large areas of sternum and costal cartilages are removed, prosthetic materials may be used for reconstruction and to support the bony thorax. Pectoralis major muscle flaps are usually used for reconstruction of sternal defects. Omental transposition can be used, especially to obliterate mediastinal space and cover the heart. Staged procedures may be necessary for adequate debridement and cleaning of the wound (Houston et al., 1992; Mansour et al., 1993; Pairolero et al., 1991).

Procedure

Key steps

1. An incision is made over the involved area.
2. Debridement of the wound may include curetting sternal edges or removal of the sternum and costal cartilages. All infected and necrotic tissue is removed.

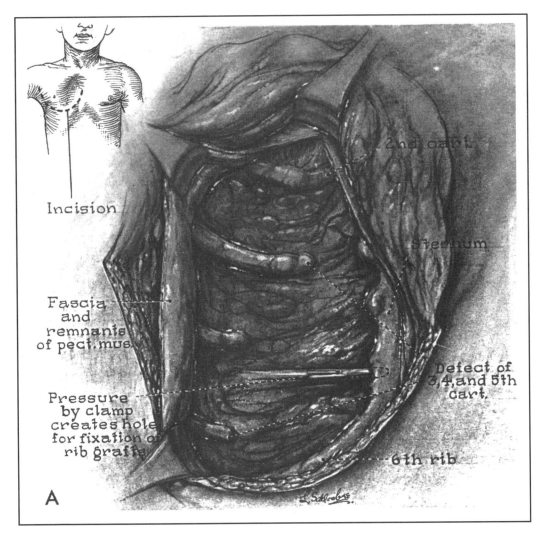

Incision

Fascia
and
remnants
of pect. mus.

Pressure
by clamp
creates hole
for fixation of
rib graft

A

2nd cart.

Sternum

Defect of
3, 4, and 5th
cart.

6th rib

FIGURE 14-46
Repair of Poland's syndrome anomaly. (Reprinted with permission from Ravitch & Steichen: *Atlas of General Thoracic Surgery* [1988] W. B. Saunders Co., Philadelphia, PA.)

3. The pectoralis muscle flap is prepared and positioned (Fig. 14-49).
4. Drains are placed.
5. The wound is closed.

Postoperative care Total parenteral nutrition (TPN) may be needed to promote healing. Adequate oxygenation is necessary, and ventilatory support may be indicated. Reoperation for debridement, drainage, and repeat reconstruction is necessary if infection recurs. Up to 17% of these patients will have a recurrence of their wound infection. Mortality is related primarily to multisystem organ failure (Ulicny & Hiratzka, 1991; Pairolero et al., 1991).

Mediastinal Procedures

The mediastinum lies between the two pleural cavities and is divided into the anterior, visceral, and paravertebral sulcus compartments (Fig. 14-50). The anterior compartment contains the thymus gland, internal mammary arteries, and lymph nodes. The visceral compartment contains the heart, pericardium, great vessels, trachea, portions of the left and right main stem bronchi, esophagus, thoracic duct, lymph nodes, and vagus and phrenic nerves. The paravertebral compartment contains proximal portions of the intercostal arteries and veins and numerous neurological structures. Certain primary tumors and cysts are located in these compartments (Table 14-4). Infections, trauma, vascular abnormalities, and congenital anomalies can be other causative factors for surgery involving the mediastinum.

Most mediastinal tumors and cysts are benign and asymptomatic. These are usually found by radiological examination. Symptoms are usually related to the location and type of tumor or cyst. Cough, chest pain, fever, chills, weight loss, fatigue, dysphagia, superior vena caval syndrome, and respiratory distress are the most common symptoms and are usually related to the compression of surrounding anatomical structures by the mass.

Diagnostic evaluation of a mediastinal mass is frequently done by mediastinoscopy or mediastinotomy. Surgical removal of the mass is usually done through a sternotomy or posterolateral or anterolateral incision. A partial sternotomy limited to the manubrium is used when exposure will be adequate. Positioning and instru-

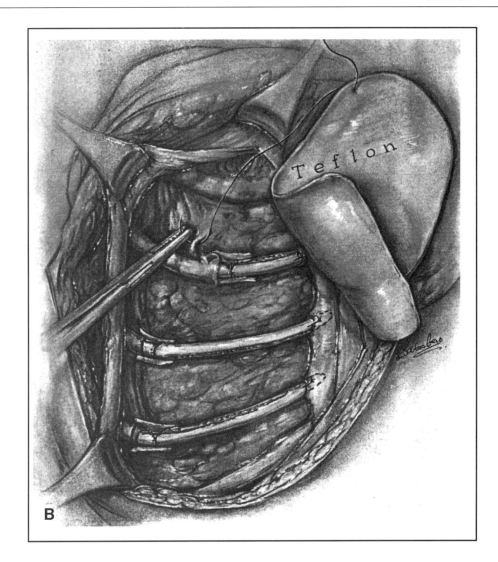

B

mentation are specific to the operative approach (Shields, 1991; Shields, 1989; Sabiston & Spencer, 1990).

Thymectomy

Removal of the thymus gland is indicated for treatment of myasthenia gravis or for thymic tumors (i.e., thymomas).

Procedure

Key steps

1. A sternotomy incision, partial or complete, is made.
2. A sternal retractor is placed.
3. The thymus is dissected from the pericardium and adjacent pleura. Resection of other tissues may be indicated to ensure complete removal of the thymic tissue. Frozen sections are done to ensure adequate tissue margins if malignancy is present.
4. Hemostasis is ensured, and a mediastinal drain is placed. Pleural drain tubes may be needed if the pleural spaces were entered.

5. Closure of the incision is completed.

Postoperative care   Myasthenia gravis patients must be monitored very closely for respiratory distress. Major complications include respiratory failure, bleeding, and infection.

Resection of "hourglass" tumors

These neurogenic tumors have an intraspinal and intrathoracic component that is joined by a narrow "waist" through the intervertebral foramen of the spine (Shields, 1991).

Procedure

Key steps

1. A vertical incision is made midline over the spinal processes and extended laterally along the rib at the appropriate level in relation to the location of the tumor.
2. The intrathoracic portion of the tumor is mobilized.

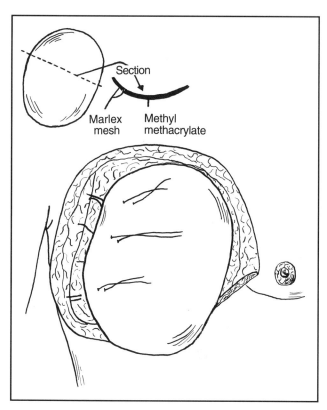

FIGURE 14-47 Use of prosthetic material to repair chest wall defect.

3. Bilateral laminectomy is done above and below the involved foramen.
4. The tumor is removed from the intravertebral foramen. If necessary the dura is opened to remove the tumor from around the spinal cord. The dura is then closed. The foramen is sealed with muscle or Gelfoam to prevent spinal fluid leak.
5. A chest drainage tube is placed.
6. The incision is closed.

Pericardiectomy

A chronic inflammatory process can result in constrictive pericarditis, which can compress the heart. The heart's diastolic filling and systolic ejection are both affected, which results in decreased cardiac output, lowered systemic blood pressure, and increased venous pressure. Weakness, pain, shortness of breath, and ascites are other signs and symptoms.

Removal of the thickened, dense, and scarred pericardium relieves the compression of the heart. Immediate improvement in cardiac function occurs. The amount of pericardium removed depends on the findings at surgery. Cardiopulmonary bypass may be needed for difficult adhesions where there is increased risk of hemorrhage or excessive manipulation of the heart (Sabiston & Spencer, 1990).

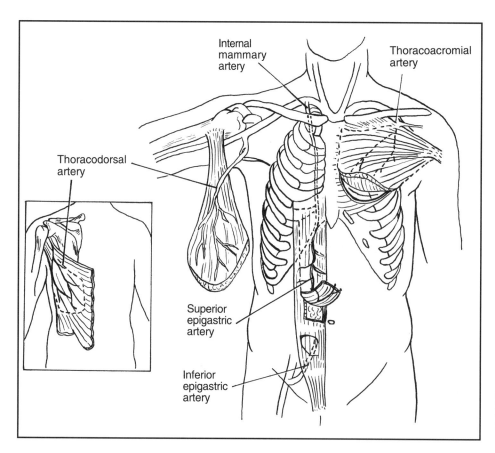

FIGURE 14-48 Anatomical location of various muscle flaps.

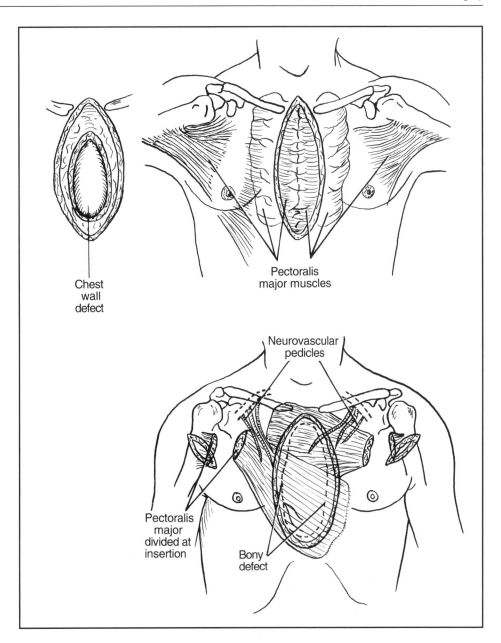

FIGURE 14-49 Use of pectoralis major muscle for sternal defect reconstruction.

Procedure

Key steps

1. A median sternotomy or left anterior or anterolateral thoracotomy incision is made.
2. A retractor is inserted.
3. The pericardium is incised and dissected free from the epicardium. The pericardium is removed from over both ventricles, the apex, and the right atrium. Injury to the phrenic nerves is avoided. Tissue and pericardial fluid samples are sent for culture.
4. Hemostasis is ensured.
5. Chest drains are placed.
6. Incisions are closed.

Pericardial window

Chronic pericardial effusion secondary to pericarditis may be better relieved with a pericardial window procedure. By creating an opening through the pericardium, the pericardial fluid can drain into the pleural space, where it will be absorbed.

Procedure

Key steps

1. A left anterior anterolateral thoracotomy incision is made.
2. A retractor is placed.
3. The pericardium is incised and a portion is removed. Cultures are taken.
4. A chest drain is placed.
5. The incision is closed.

Diaphragmatic Procedures

The diaphragm is the major muscle of inspiration and anatomically separates the abdominal and thoracic cavities. Abnormalities that may require surgical intervention include tumors, hernias, eventration and traumatic perforation.

Primary tumors

Although primary tumors of the diaphragm are rare, surgical resection is recommended whenever possible. Surrounding tissues that are involved (ribs, lung) will need to be included in the resection.

Repair of a Bochdalek diaphragmatic hernia

Diaphragmatic hernias are usually considered congenital defects and occur primarily in three areas of the diaphragm.

Bochdalek hernia (posterolateral) usually occurs on the left side. Herniation of the abdominal contents into the thoracic cavity causes acute respiratory distress in newborns.

Procedure

Key steps

1. An abdominal incision is made on the side of hernia.
2. The abdominal contents are moved from the chest to the abdominal cavity.
3. The hernia in the diaphragm is closed directly with suture, or a synthetic patch material is used for large defects.
4. Chest drain insertion depends on the surgeon's preference.
5. The incision is closed.

Postoperative care Because of hypoplastic lung and increased pulmonary vascular resistance, the patient's respiratory status may be compromised. Extracorporeal membrane oxygenation (ECMO) may be used. Even with immediate surgical repair, the mortality rate is 30% to 50% (Sabiston & Spencer, 1990; Shields, 1989).

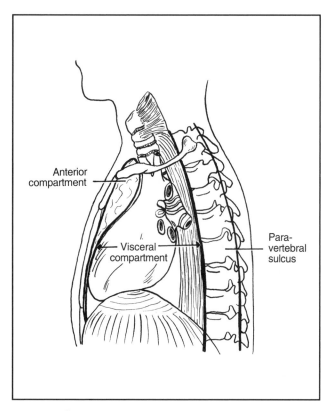

FIGURE 14-50 Mediastinal compartments.

TABLE 14-4 Usual Location of the Common Primary Tumors and Cysts of the Mediastinum

Anterior Compartment	Visceral Compartment	Paravertebral Sulci
Thymoma	Enterogenous cyst	Neurilemoma—schwannoma
Germ cell tumor	Lymphoma	Neurofibroma
Lymphoma	Pleuropericardial cyst	Malignant schwannoma
Lymphangioma	Mediastinal granuloma	Ganglioneuroma
Hemangioma	Lymphoid hamartoma	Ganglioneuroblastoma
Lipoma	Mesothelial cyst	Neuroblastoma
Fibroma	Neuroenteric cyst	Paraganglioma
Fibrosarcoma	Paraganglioma	Pheochromocytoma
Thymic cyst	Pheochromocytoma	Fibrosarcoma
Parathyroid adenoma	Thoracic duct cyst	Lymphoma
Aberrant thyroid		

(From Shields, T.W.: [1991] *Mediastinal Surgery,* Waverly-Lea & Febiger, Philadelphia, PA.)

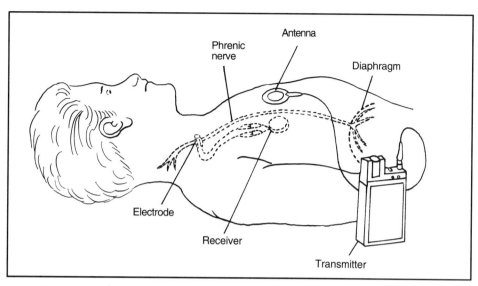

FIGURE 14-51 Location of diaphragmatic pacing components. The receiver and electrode are implanted. The antenna and transmitter are used externally.

Repair of a Morgagni diaphragmatic hernia

Morgagni hernia (subcostosternal) usually does not become symptomatic until the affected person is of an adult age.

Procedure

Key steps

1. An upper midline abdominal incision is made.
2. The defect is directly closed with suture.
3. The incision is closed.

Repair of an esophageal hiatal hernia

See antireflux surgery.

Repair of eventration

In eventration, part or all of the diaphragm on one side assumes an abnormally high position in the thoracic cavity. This may be due to paralysis, aplasia, or atrophy of muscle fibers (Sabiston & Spencer, 1990).

Procedure

Key steps

1. A thoracotomy incision (posterolateral) is made.
2. Plication sutures are placed in the diaphragm to remove the redundancy.
3. A chest drain is inserted.
4. The incision is closed.

Traumatic perforation

Traumatic perforation can be due to blunt or penetrating trauma to the chest or abdomen. Surgical repair is required, and usually a thoracotomy incision is used (Sabiston & Spencer, 1990).

Diaphragmatic pacing

Since 1969, over 10,000 patients worldwide have been treated with diaphragmatic pacing (McEwen, 1993). Electrical stimulation of the phrenic nerve causes the diaphragm to contract. This technique can be used for patients with chronic ventilatory insufficiency only if the lungs, diaphragm, and phrenic nerves are adequate to sustain ventilation. The receiver and electrode for the pacer are surgically implanted. The transmitter and antenna are used externally (Fig. 14-51) (Sabiston & Spencer, 1990).

Procedure

Thoracic approach: Key steps

1. The anterior thoracotomy incision is made over the second intercostal space. The incision for the receiver is usually made in the upper abdominal area.
2. The phrenic nerve is identified and exposed at the junction of the azygos vein and superior vena cava on the right side or between the aortic arch and left pulmonary artery on the left side.
3. The electrode is placed around the phrenic nerve and tunneled subcutaneously to the pocket containing the receiver.
4. The incisions are closed.

Cervical approach: Key steps

1. The transverse incision is made above the clavicle.
2. The sternocleidomastoid muscle and internal jugular vein are retracted and the phrenic nerve is identified by using a nerve stimulator. Fluoroscopy may be used to observe the contraction of the diaphragm.

3. The electrode is placed around the phrenic nerve.
4. A subcutaneous pocket is made below the clavicle through the same incision. The receiver is implanted and the electrode connected.
5. The incision is closed.

Postoperative care It is 12 to 14 days postoperatively before the pacer is used. This allows wound healing and recovery of the phrenic nerve from the surgical manipulation. Close monitoring and follow-up are needed (McEwen, 1993; Sabiston & Spencer, 1990).

Traumatic Injury Procedures

Pneumothorax

This is the most common result of chest injury requiring treatment (Hood, 1986). Air in the thoracic cavity can cause the lung to collapse and result in mediastinal shift, which interferes with the expansion of the good lung and impairs cardiac function. Life-threatening respiratory and hemodynamic problems can occur. Blunt trauma can cause injury to the lung, bronchus, trachea, or esophagus, which can lead to pneumothorax. Penetrating wounds allow air into the chest and may cause injury to other structures. Signs and symptoms include dyspnea, absent or decreased breath sounds, hyperresonance with percussion, tracheal shift, and respiratory distress. Aspiration of air from the thoracic cavity and chest X-ray are diagnostic (Blaisdell & Trunkey, 1986).

1. *Open pneumothorax* is an open wound that allows air to move in and out of the chest. Immediate tamponade and surgical closure are indicated. Large defects may require chest wall reconstruction (Hood et al., 1989) (Fig. 14-52).
2. *Tension pneumothorax* results when injury to the lung allows a continual leak of air into the thoracic cavity. This is an emergency situation treated by inserting a chest tube. Large leaks from the lung or bronchial or tracheal tears will need surgical closure (Hood et al., 1989) (Fig. 14-52).
3. *Partial pneumothorax* is when the lung is only partially collapsed; a chest tube should still be inserted as the air leak could increase or continue (Hood et al., 1989).

Subcutaneous emphysema

Air in the subcutaneous tissues can result from thoracic trauma. The most common ways for air to enter the tissues is by trauma that:

1. Penetrates the skin and allows air into the tissues
2. Causes a pneumothorax with a defect in the parietal pleura that allows air to escape into the tissues
3. Causes injury to mediastinal structures and air dissects to the cervical region, face, and anterior chest (Fig. 14-53).

The cause of the subcutaneous emphysema is treated. Decompression by skin incision or aspiration of air is rarely indicated (Hood et al., 1989).

Flail chest (Fig. 14-54)

An unstable chest wall occurs when there are multiple fractures of three or more ribs or costal cartilages. The sternum may or may not be fractured. The fractured segments move inward with inspiration and outward with expiration. This paradoxical motion causes pain and interferes with ventilation and coughing. Atelectasis and hypoxia can occur.

Treatment includes attention to pulmonary injuries, intubation, and mechanical ventilation if necessary and surgical stabilization of fractures when indicated. Intercostal nerve block or epidural injections are used to relieve pain, which results in improved ventilation and clearing of secretions. Rib and sternal fractures can be repaired surgically with wire sutures, staples, or steel plates (Fig. 14-55) (Hood et al., 1989; Blaisdell & Trunkey, 1986).

Hemothorax

Bleeding into the thoracic cavity can occur with penetrating and blunt trauma. Shock, respiratory distress, decreased or absent breath sounds, dullness to percussion, and tracheal shift can be seen with massive hemothorax. Emergency surgery is indicated when the chest X-ray shows complete opacification of the hemithorax, if 1000 ml or more of blood is obtained when the chest tube is inserted, or if unable to stabilize the patient with volume replacement. Surgery is indicated if there is a blood loss through the chest tube of 200 ml per hour for 3 to 4 hours, 500 ml per hour for more than 1 hour, or 1500 ml in 24 hours and still bleeding. Aortic and cardiac injuries are discussed in Chapter 13 in this volume (Blaisdell & Trunkey, 1986; Hood et al., 1989) (see Fig. 14-52).

Cardiac tamponode

Blunt or penetrating trauma to the chest, upper abdomen, or neck can result in blood accumulation within the pericardium. Cardiac compression begins to occur when over 100 to 150 ml of blood is present.

The classic signs of the triad of Beck are increased central venous pressure, muffled heart sounds, and hypotension. Increased venous pressure over 15 cm H_2O can be measured by inserting a central venous pressure line. Distended, pulsating neck veins, cyanosis of the head and face, and Kussmaul's sign (filling of neck veins on inspiration) may be seen with increased venous pressure. Decreased filling of the heart results in decreased cardiac output and hypotension. Tachycardia, agitation, restlessness, narrow pulse pressure, and paradoxical pulse may be present. The blood around the heart muffles the heart sounds and make them sound distant. Hypotension is seen without other evidence of blood loss and does not improve with the administration of intravenous fluid volume.

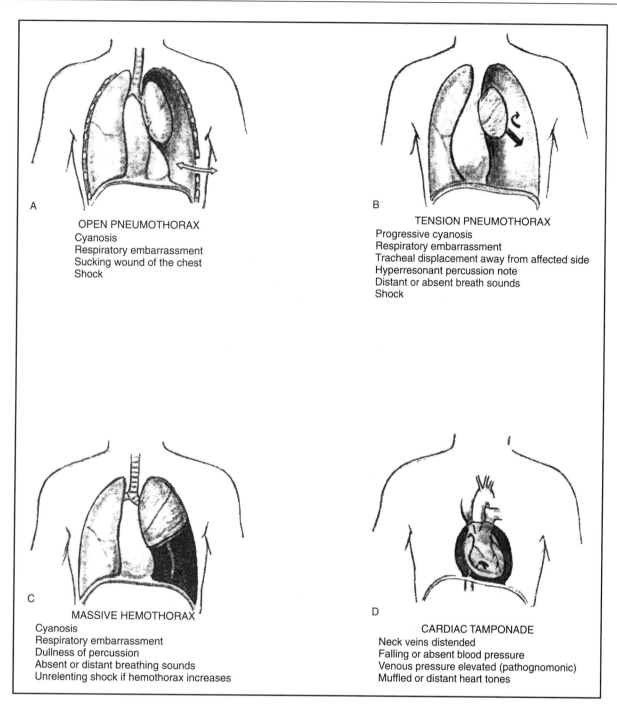

FIGURE 14-52 *A,* Open pneumothorax. Air can move in and out of the thoracic cavity. *B,* Tension pneumothorax. Air leaking from the lung into the thoracic cavity causes the lung to collapse. *C,* Hemothorax. *D,* Cardiac tamponade. (From Hood, R. M. [1989] *Thoracic trauma.* Philadelphia, W. B. Saunders. Reprinted with permission.)

The two-dimensional echocardiogram is useful for making the diagnosis. Pericardiocentesis is done to confirm the diagnosis and relieve the pressure. Emergency thoracotomy is done to determine and repair the source of the bleeding and to evacuate the blood from the pericardial space (Hood et al., 1989; Blaisdell & Trunkey, 1986) (see Fig. 14-52).

Airway obstruction

Trauma to the head, face, neck, or chest can result in compromise to the airway. Airway obstruction can occur with accumulation of blood, secretions, vomitus, or foreign bodies in the airway passages. Drug overdose or concussion can interfere with respiratory drive.

"Air hunger," cough, dysphonia or aphonia, stridor,

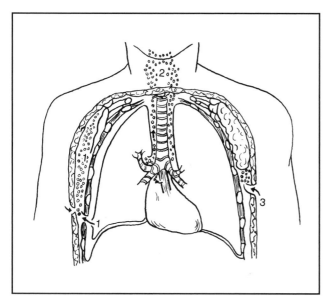

FIGURE 14-53 Locations of sources of subcutaneous emphysema. *1*, From air leak in lung. *2*, Air in mediastinal area moving up into cervical area. *3*, External penetration.

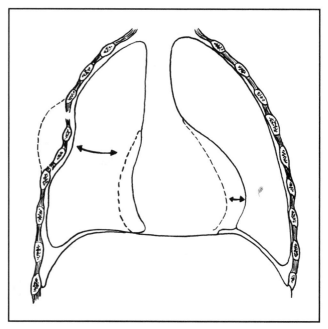

FIGURE 14-54 Flail chest. Note the concave deformity of the chest wall that occurs with inspiration.

hoarseness, hemoptysis, cyanosis, dyspnea, tachypnea, intercostal and supraclavicular retractions, and neck deformity (swelling, hematoma, subcutaneous emphysema) are signs and symptoms that may be present.

Endotracheal intubation (when possible and not hazardous), tracheostomy, or cricothyroidotomy may be needed. Laryngotracheal injuries may result in lacerations, fractures, or disruption to those structures. Direct laryngoscopy, X-rays, and computed tomography (CT) examinations are diagnostic tools. Surgical intervention may be needed to repair airway injuries (Hood et al., 1989).

Lung Transplantation Procedures

Lung transplantation surgery was first attempted in 1963 and became successful in the early 1980s. Advances in infection control, organ preservation, surgical techniques, and immunosuppressive drugs are the major contributors to this success.

There is an increasing demand for donor lungs but their supply is limited. The average patient wait for a donor lung is 270 days, and 30% of patients die while awaiting a donor lung. From 1983 to 1992, the St. Louis International Lung Transplant Registry entered 1,519 lung transplantation patients.

COPD, antitrypsin deficiency emphysema, cystic fibrosis, idiopathic pulmonary fibrosis, primary pulmonary hypertension, Eisenmenger's syndrome, and retransplantation are the major indications for lung transplantation.

Guidelines for recipient selection include:

1. Severe pulmonary disease
2. Ineffective or unavailable medical treatment
3. Significant physical limitations
4. Life expectancy of less than 18 to 24 months

5. Adequate cardiac function, no significant coronary artery disease, and right ventricular ejection fraction of over 24%
6. Ambulatory with rehabilitation potential
7. Satisfactory psychosocial profile and emotional support system
8. Meets maximum age limits: 50–55 years for double-lung transplantation, 60 to 65 years for single-lung transplantation.

Contraindications to lung transplantation:

1. Steroid dependence
2. Cancer of the lung
3. Other cancer that is uncured
4. Pulmonary sepsis
5. Active infection
6. Systemic disease with vital organ involvement (non-lung)
7. Vital organ dysfunction (non-lung)
8. Psychosocial problems: drug/alcohol abuse; history of noncompliance with medical management
9. Smoking cigarettes

Possible contraindications include:

1. Ventilator dependence
2. Prior cardiothoracic surgery (increased technical difficulty and increased hemorrhage)

Candidates for single-lung transplant include:

1. Higher-risk patients
2. Older patients
3. Previous thoracic surgery

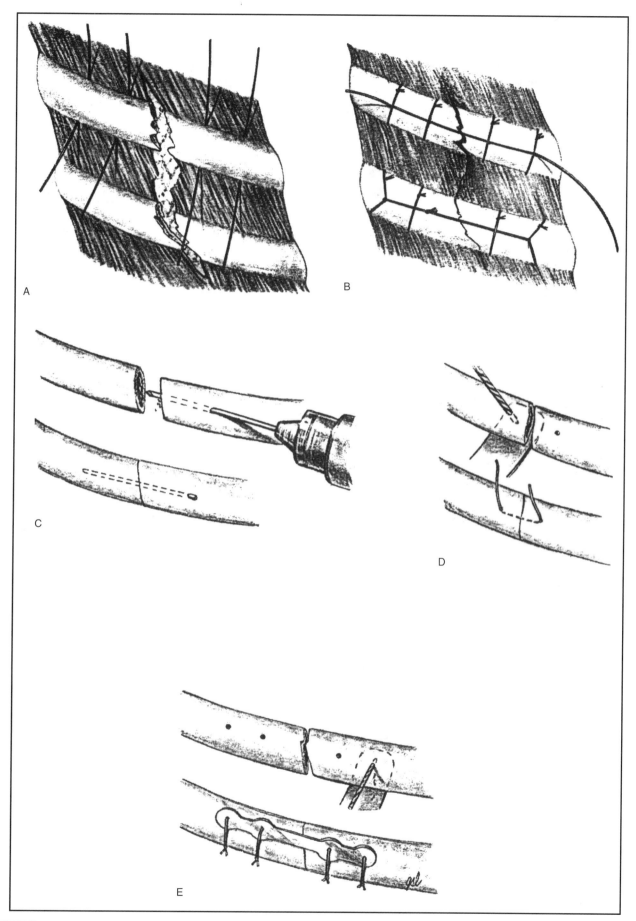

FIGURE 14-55 Methods of stabilizing fractured ribs. *A & B,* Use of wire to align fracture. *C & D,* Use of wire to connect ends of fractured rib. *E,* Use of bone plate to stabilize fracture site. (From Hood, R. M. [1989]. *Thoracic trauma.* Philadelphia, W. B. Saunders. Reprinted with permission.)

4. Significant difference in lung function between lungs
5. Pulmonary fibrosis disease

Candidates for double-lung transplant include:

1. Younger patients
2. Extensive bullae in both lungs
3. Severe bronchitic component to disease
4. Highly compliant lungs (COPD)
5. Infected lungs
6. If the donor lung is inadequate for a single lung

Guidelines for lung donor are the following:

1. Documentation of brain death
2. History of injury with no possibility of aspiration
3. Compatible ABO blood type
4. Adequate-size lung
5. Adequate oxygenation has been maintained
6. Serologic data negative

Contraindications for lung donor include:

1. Extremes in age
2. History of smoking
3. History of IV drug use
4. Previous pulmonary surgery
5. Thoracic trauma with pulmonary contusion
6. Intubation (endotracheal) for longer than 3 days
7. History of aspiration or possible aspiration
8. Fluid overload
9. Infection of lung
   (Patterson & Cooper, 1993; Cooper & Novitzky, 1990)

Lung procurement procedure

Position The donor is positioned for a median sternotomy incision.

Special equipment Equipment includes infusion systems and solutions, iced slush, and transportation supplies.

Procedure

Key steps

1. A median sternotomy incision is made.
2. Umbilical tapes are placed around the aorta and cavae.
3. The pleura is opened longitudinally and the pericardium is excised.
4. The pulmonary ligaments are incised; the right and left pulmonary arteries are dissected from the main pulmonary artery bifurcation to the hilum.
5. The donor patient is heparinized; prostaglandins (PGE$_1$) are infused intravenously.
6. After the donor becomes hypotensive, the superior vena cava is double ligated and divided; the inferior vena cava is transected; and the tip of the left atrium is removed. This allows venting of the heart once the

cardioplegia is administered and prevents overdistention.

7. Cardioplegia is administered through the aortic root, with the aorta cross-clamped. At the same time, 2 liters of Euro Collins solution (at 4° C) is infused into the main pulmonary artery as the lungs are being ventilated, which prevents vasospasm and more evenly distributes the solution. Euro Collins solution is high in potassium, low in sodium; it is an intracellular type of solution without the colloid used for organ presevation.
8. Iced slush solution is placed over the heart and lungs and removed after the solutions have been administered.
9. The heart is elevated and a part of the left atrium is removed with the pulmonary veins for a single-lung transplant or a larger cuff of atrium with all four of the pulmonary veins is removed for a double-lung transplant.
10. The pulmonary artery is stapled and divided at the bifurcation for one lung transplant or proximal to the bifurcation for a double-lung transplant.
11. The heart is removed.
12. The trachea or main stem bronchus is stapled, with the lung inflated and transected. The lung or lungs are removed.
13. The lung or lungs are triple bagged in plastic and packed in ice for transport and can be ischemic for up to 6 hours.
14. Lymph nodes have been removed for tissue typing.

Lung transplantation procedure

Position The patient is positioned for a posterolateral thoracotomy for a single-lung transplant. A bilateral anterior thoracotomy is done across the sternum to the anterior axillary line. The patient is supine with arms positioned above the head (Fig. 14-56). If an omental pedicle is used to wrap the tracheal anastomosis, a midline abdominal incision is made.

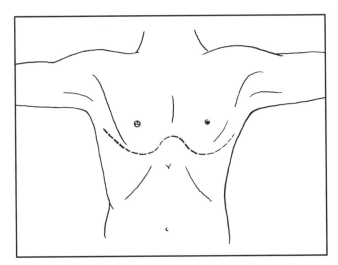

FIGURE 14-56 Bilateral anterior thoracotomy incisions.

Instrumentation and special equipment Instrumentation is as for a thoracotomy and for abdominal incisions. Supplies for a cardiopulmonary bypass may be necessary.

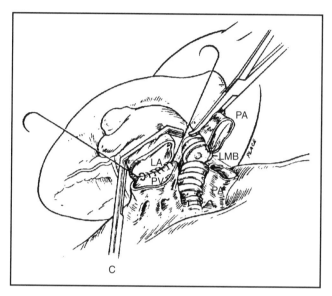

FIGURE 14-57 Donor lung pulmonary veins being sutured to recipient's left atrium. (From Calhoon, J., et al. [1991] Single Lung Transplantation, *Journal of Thoracic and Cardiovascular Surgery* 101:816–25, Mosby-Year Book, Inc., St. Louis, MO.)

Procedure

Key steps

1. The chest incision is made and a retractor is placed.
2. The lung on the operative side is deflated. If the patient becomes hypoxic, cardiopulmonary bypass may be necessary.
3. A pneumonectomy is done and the patient's lung is removed. A cuff of pulmonary artery is contained in a vascular clamp, as is a segment of the left atrium where the pulmonary veins have been transected (Fig. 14-57). The bronchus is transected below the bifurcation.
4. The donor lung is prepared by removing it from the ice bath, deflating it, and preparing the bronchus for anastomosis.
5. The donor lung is positioned in the chest, and the bronchial, pulmonary artery, and left atrial anastomoses are done. If the bronchus is anastomosed using the telescoping technique, an omental pedicle is not necessary (Fig. 14-58).
6. Prior to securing the pulmonary artery suture line, the pulmonary artery clamp is removed and the pulmonary vascular system is "flushed" of the preservation solution out through the suture line. The left atrial anastomosis site is filled with blood by releasing the left atrial vascular clamp, and the suture is tied.
7. Hemostasis is ensured, and the new lung is inflated.
8. If a double-lung transplant is being done, the same procedure is done on the other side. By doing sequential lung transplants, the use of cardiopulmonary bypass can usually be avoided.
9. Chest tubes are placed, and the incisions are closed.

FIGURE 14-58 Bronchial anastomosis. *A*, 4-0 Prolene traction sutures are placed at each end of the membranous portion of the bronchus. The first traction suture is tied and a continuous posterior suture line is placed before the second traction suture is tied. *B*, The posterior suture line has been completed and the bronchial blocker, a No. 7 Fogarty catheter 80 cm long with a 2.5 ml liquid balloon, is shown in place. *C*, The anterior bronchial anastomosis is completed by placing figure-of-eight 4-0 Prolene sutures around the cartilages. *D*, After the anterior sutures are tied, the bronchus naturally telescopes to a depth of one cartilage. (From Calhoon, J., et al. [1991] Single Lung Transplantation, *Journal of Thoracic and Cardiovascular Surgery* 101:816–25, Mosby-Year Book, Inc., St. Louis, MO.)

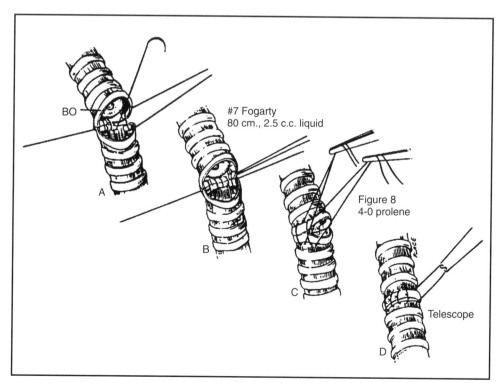

Postoperative care Early survival rates are now near 80% to 90% for patients receiving lung transplants. Postoperative care is related to the thoracic surgery and to pulmonary function. The use of immunosuppressive drugs increases the risk of postoperative infection, and appropriate precautions must be taken. Long-term follow-up with frequent evaluation for potential rejection of the lung is essential (Patterson & Cooper, 1993; Calhoon et al., 1991; Todd et al., 1988).

Chylothorax

Lymphatic fluid (chyle) accumulation in the chest cavity is caused by a leak in the thoracic duct or one of its major divisions. The causes include congenital abnormalities, trauma, and nontraumatic conditions (i.e., tumors, infections). Intraoperative injury can occur with surgery involving the aortic arch, left subclavian artery, or the esophagus.

Signs and symptoms are related to the chyle effusion causing pressure on the lung and resulting in respiratory problems. Examination of the fluid aspirated during thoracentesis confirms the diagnosis. Serious metabolic, nutritional, and immunologic problems can occur with chyle loss.

A 2-week period of conservative therapy may include multiple thoracentesis procedures and/or insertion of a chest tube. The patient is given nothing by mouth (NPO) and receives intravenous hyperalimentation. If the chyle drainage continues to be over 500 ml per day at the end of 14 days, surgery is usually indicated. A thoracotomy provides access for ligating the thoracic duct or for direct closure of the leak. For patients with less chyle drainage or those at risk with surgical intervention, a pleuroperitoneal shunt may be inserted (Shields, 1989; Milsom et al., 1985).

Insertion of a pleuroperitoneal shunt

The pleuroperitoneal shunt consists of two silicone catheters joined by a one-way valve. The unit is fused together, and the catheter length can be adjusted by cutting the tube or tubes. The Denver shunt is available from Denver Biomaterials, Inc.

Position The patient is supine.

Instrumentation and special supplies Soft tissue dissection instruments and the Denver shunt must be available.

Procedure

Key steps

1. A small inframammary incision is made on the appropriate side.
2. A subcutaneous "pocket" is developed for the "pump."
3. The shunt is prepared by filling the tubings and pump completely with normal saline solution.

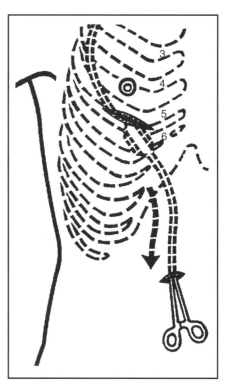

FIGURE 14-59 Position of pleuroperitoneal shunt. (Reprinted with permission of Denver Biomaterials, Inc., Evergreen, CO.)

4. The pleural arm of the shunt is placed into the chest through an introducer-type sheath, and the sheath is removed.
5. A subcostal abdominal incision is made on the same side.
6. A purse-string suture is placed in the peritoneum.
7. A long clamp is used to create a tunnel between the two incisions, and the peritoneal arm of the shunt is pulled through the tunnel to the abdominal incision (Fig. 14-59).
8. A small incision is made in the peritoneum, and the tubing is inserted into the peritoneal cavity and secured by tying the purse-string suture.
9. The pump is positioned and secured with sutures.
10. Both incisions are closed.

Postoperative care The pump is primed several times every hour for the first 24 to 48 hours. Each time the pump is compressed, 1.5 ml of fluid is pumped and 500 to 1000 pump compressions are needed every 24 hours. The patient and/or family are taught how to use the pump. Complications may include infection, fever, or shunt malfunction.

Thoracic Outlet Syndrome

Compression of the subclavian vessels and the brachial plexus against the first rib causes neurological and/or vascular signs and symptoms.

Congenital, traumatic, and atherosclerotic factors can contribute to this problem. Pain, paresthesias, arm weakness, arm coolness, and easy fatigue of the arm and/or hand are the usual symptoms. Absent radial pulse, venous distention, edema, muscle weakness, venous thrombosis, and trophic changes may be seen.

Delays in ulnar nerve conduction velocity, vascular impairment demonstrated by arteriograms, and reproduction of signs and symptoms with certain physical maneuvers are diagnostic for this condition.

Treatment may include physical therapy designed to strengthen shoulder muscles and improve posture, which may relieve the patient's symptoms. When necessary, resection of the first rib is done (Sabiston & Spencer, 1990; Shields, 1989).

Resection of the first rib

Position The patient is positioned in a lateral position with the arm abducted 90 degrees and attached to an overhead pulley with traction (2 to 3 lb). The incision is transaxillary.

Instrumentation and special supplies and equipment Equipment includes soft tissue dissection instruments, instruments for removing the rib, and an overhead pulley and traction device.

Procedure

Key steps

1. A transverse incision is made in the axilla between the pectoralis major and latissimus dorsi muscles.
2. Dissection is carried out along the thoracic fascia plane to the level of the first rib.
3. The scalenus anticus muscles are divided.
4. The first rib is dissected subperiosteally with a periosteal elevator.
5. The middle segment of the rib is removed, followed by the removal of the anterior and posterior segments.
6. If a cervical rib is present, it is removed.
7. A drain is placed.
8. The incision is closed.

Postoperative care A graduated exercise and physical therapy program is implemented, and the patient must avoid heavy lifting for 3 months.

SUMMARY

This chapter has outlined various lung, tracheal, esophageal, chest wall, mediastinal, diaphragmatic, traumatic, lung transplantation, and chylothorax procedures, including perioperative considerations, positioning, equipment and instrumentation, and key procedural steps.

The information bank for the perioperative nurse must include this knowledge and information. Expected patient outcomes usually relate to respiratory and circulatory functions, quality of life, absence of infection, and the ability to function in activities of daily living.

REFERENCES

American Association for Thoracic Surgery and the Society of Thoracic Surgeons. (1992). Statement of the A.A.T.S./S.T.S. Joint Committee on Thoracoscopy and Video Assisted Thoracic Surgery. *Annals of Thoracic Surgery, 54,* 1.

American College of Surgeons. (1989). *Care of the surgical patient, Vol. 2: Elective care,* New York: Scientific American, Inc.

Association of Operating Room Nurses, Inc. (1994). *Standards and recommended practices.* Denver: Author.

Blaisdell, F., & Trunkey, D. (1986). *Trauma management, Vol. III: Cervicothoracic trauma.* New York: Thieme.

Caccavale, R., & Arzouman, D. (1993). Video assisted thoracic surgery for pleural disease. *Chest Surgery Clinics of North America, 3,* 263–269.

Calhoon, J., Grover, F., Gibbons, W., Bryan, C., Levine, S., Baily, S., Nichols, L., Lum, C., & Trinkle, J. (1991). Single lung transplant alternative indications and technique. *Journal of Thoracic and Cardiovascular Surgery, 101,* 816–825.

Coltharp, W., Arnold, J., Alford, W., Burrus, G., Glassford, D., Lea, J., Petracek, M., Starkey, T., Stoney, W., Thomas, C., & Stadler, R. (1992). Videothoracoscopy: Improved technique and expanded indications. *Annals of Thoracic Surgery, 53,* 766–779.

Cooper, D., & Novitzky, D. (1990). *The transplantation and replacement of thoracic organs.* Boston: Kluwer Academic Publishers.

Delarue, N., Wilkins, E., & Wong, J. (1988). *International trends in general thoracic surgery, Vol. 4: Esophageal cancer.* St. Louis: C.V. Mosby.

Deslauriers, J., & Lacquet, L. (1990). *Thoracic surgery: Surgical management of pleural diseases: Vol. 6.* St. Louis: C.V. Mosby.

Gray, H. (1977). *Anatomy: Descriptive and surgical.* New York: Bounty Books.

Guth, A., & Gouge, T. (March, 1992). Recognition and treatment of thoracic esophageal perforations. *Surgical Rounds,* 269–272.

Guyton, A. (1991). *Textbook of medical physiology* (8th ed.). Philadelphia: W.B. Saunders.

Hammond, D., Fisher, J., & Meland, N. (1993). Intrathoracic free flaps. *Plastic and Reconstructive Surgery, 9,* 1259–1264.

Hen, J. (1992). Pulmonary function tests: Understanding and interpreting results. *Clinical Nurse Practitioner, 10*(1), 11–13.

Hood, R. (1986). *Surgical disease of the pleura and chest wall.* Philadelphia: W.B. Saunders.

Hood, R., Boyd, A., & Culliford, A. (1989). *Thoracic trauma.* Philadelphia: W.B. Saunders.

Houston, S., Luquire, F., & Jewell, M. (1992). Crafting postoperative care for sternal wound omentopexy. *American Journal of Nursing, 92,* 56–60.

Hurst, J. W., & Schlant, R. (1990). *The heart* (7th ed.). San Francisco: McGraw-Hill.

Hurwitz, A., & Degenshein, G. (1958). *Milestones in modern surgery.* New York: Hoeber-Harper Books.

Lewis, R., Caccavale, R., Sisler, G., & Mackenzie, J. (1992). One hundred consecutive patients undergoing video-assisted thoracic operations. *Annals of Thoracic Surgery, 54,* 421–426.

LoCicero, J. III (1992). Diagnostic procedures for thoracic surgery. *Chest Surgery Clinics of North America, 2* (3).

Mack, M. J., Aronoff, R. J., Acuff, T. E., Douthit, M. B., Bowman, R. T., & Ryan, W. H. (1992). Present role of thoracoscopy in the diagnosis and treatment of diseases of the chest. *Annals of Thoracic Surgery, 54,* 403–409.

Mack, M. J., Landreneau, R., Hazelrigg, S., & Acuff, T. (1993). Video thoracoscopic management of benign and malignant pericardial effusions. *Chest, 103,* 390S–393S.

Mansour, K., Anderson, T., & Hester, T. (1993). Sternal resection and reconstruction. *Annals of Thoracic Surgery, 55,* 834–843.

Mathisen, D., & Grillo, H. (1991). Carinal resection for bronchogenic CA. *Journal of Thoracic and Cardiovascular Surgery, 102,* 16–23.

Mayer, R. (1993). Overview: The changing nature of esophageal cancer. *Chest, 103,* 404S–405S.

McEwen, D. (1993). Diaphragmatic pacing: An option for patients with quadriplegic respiratory paralysis. *AORN Journal, 58,* 547–558.

McKneally, M. (1993). Video-assisted thoracic surgery standards and guidelines. *Chest Surgery Clinics of North America, 3,* 345–351.

Meade, R. (1961). *A history of thoracic surgery.* Springfield, IL: Charles C Thomas.

Milsom, J., Kron, I., Rheuban, K., & Rodgers, B. (1985). Chylothorax: An assessment of current surgical management. *Journal of Thoracic and Cardiovascular Surgery, 89,* 221–227.

Naidich, D., Zerhouni, E., & Siegelman, S. (1991). *Computed tomography and magnetic resonance of the thorax* (2nd ed.). New York: Raven Press.

Neville, W., Bolanowski, P., & Bentley, D. (1991). Tracheal reconstruction: Success with a silicone tracheal prosthesis. *AORN Journal, 54,* 470–482.

Nohl-Oser, H., Nissen, R., & Schreiber, H. (1981). *Surgery of the lung.* New York: Thieme-Stratton.

Oakes, D. (1993). Traditional therapeutic thoracoscopy. *Chest Surgery Clinics of North America, 3,* 183–199.

Orringer, M. (1993). Multimodality therapy for esophageal carcinoma: Update. *Chest, 103,* 406S–409S.

Pairolero, P., Arnold, P., & Harris, J. (June, 1991). Long term results of pectoralis major muscle transposition for infected sternotomy wounds. *Annals of Surgery,* 583–590.

Pan, J., Yang, P., Chang, D., Lee, Y., Kuo, S., & Luh, K. (1993). Needle aspiration biopsy of malignant lung masses with necrotic centers: Improved sensitivity with ultrasonic guidance. *Chest, 103,* 1452–1456.

Patterson, G., & Cooper, J. (1993). Lung transplantation. *Chest Surgery Clinics of North America, 3,* 1.

Pearson, F. G. (1993). Staging of the mediastinum: Role of mediastinoscopy and computed tomography. *Chest, 103,* 346S–348S.

Ravitch, M., & Steichen, F. (1988). *Atlas of general thoracic surgery.* Philadelphia: W.B. Saunders.

Sabiston, D., & Spencer, F. (1990). *Surgery of the Chest* (5th ed.). Philadelphia: W.B. Saunders.

Schwartz, S., Shires, G., Spencer, T., & Husser, W. (1994). *Principles of surgery* (6th ed.), New York: McGraw-Hill.

Seyfer, A., Icochea, R., & Graeber, G. (December, 1988). Poland's anomaly. *Annals of Surgery,* 776–782.

Shields, T. (1989). *General thoracic surgery* (3rd ed.). Philadelphia: Lea & Febiger.

Shields, T. (1991). *Mediastinal surgery,* Philadelphia: Lea & Febiger.

Sisler, G. (1993). Malignant tumors of the lung: Role of V.A.T.S. *Chest Surgery Clinics of North America, 3,* 307–317.

Society of Thoracic Surgeons (1992). Practice guidelines for cardiothoracic surgery. *Annals of Thoracic Surgery, 53,* 1138–1146.

Sugarbaker, D., & DeCamp, M. (1993). Selecting the surgical approach to cancer of the esophagus. *Chest, 103,* 410S–414S.

Tampinco-Golos, I. (1992). Endoscopic thoracotomy: A new approach to thoracic surgery. *AORN Journal, 55,* 1167–1180.

Todd, T., Goldberg, M., Koshal, A., Menkis, A., Boychuk, J., Patterson, G., & Cooper, J. (1988). Separate extraction of cardiac and pulmonary grafts from a single organ donor. *Annals of Thoracic Surgery, 46,* 356–359.

Ulicny, K., & Hiratzka, L. (1991). The risk factors of median sternotomy infection. *Journal of Cardiac Surgery, 6,* 338–351.

Wells, F., & Milstein, B. (1990). *Thoracic surgical techniques.* Philadelphia: Bailliere Tindall.

Chapter 15

Vascular Surgery

Key Concepts

- Patient positioning is critical for patients undergoing vascular surgery because of the length of many of the procedures and the often concomitant systemic vascular disease.

- The incidence of pressure ulcers and thrombus formation is greatly increased in a patient who has poor tissue perfusion.

- Poor tissue perfusion in vascular surgery patients greatly increases the risk of infection and poor wound healing, leading to prolonged recovery time, longer hospitalization, and increased morbidity.

- Careful asepsis is a prime infection preventative for all vascular patients, especially those receiving implants or free autografts.

- The potential for patient blood loss and the hemodynamic shifts caused by anesthesia, shifts in temperature, and immobility mandate that patient fluid balance be monitored and maintained. Irrigation fluid, urine output, and blood loss to suction and sponges must all be carefully measured.

- Physiologic monitoring is a standard for patients with conditions in which fluid volume shift is common.

- Vascular surgery patients face loss of limb and loss of life and generally are especially fearful on arrival in the operating room.

INTRODUCTION

Arterial diseases are a major cause of death in the United States and many other countries. The morbidity associated with vascular disease is as important as the mortality. Stroke with its subsequent permanent neurological deficit, angina pectoris, leg claudication, and ischemic foot lesions are all associated with long-term disability. Often the morbidity is associated with the progression of peripheral vascular disease concomitant with diabetes mellitus.

The goal of all arterial surgery is to revascularize previously compromised areas of the body. When that cannot be accomplished, amputation is necessary to prevent septicemia that results from gangrenous tissue.

Venous disorders range from varicose veins with a low morbidity and mortality to deep venous thrombosis, which debilitates or kills thousands each year. Pulmonary embolism is the most common lethal pulmonary disease in the United States (Hallett, Brewster, and Darling, 1987).

Patients undergoing vascular surgery provide a challenge to the perioperative nurse who must protect poorly perfused tissue from injury and infection.

This chapter presents anatomy related to vascular surgical procedures. The diagnostic procedures to determine disruption of blood flow through the vessels are also discussed. Common surgical procedures, instruments and supplies, and patient interventions are described to assist the perioperative nurse in planning and implementing care for the patient undergoing vascular surgery.

ANATOMY

Arteries and Veins

All blood vessels in the body have three layers: an intima, a media, and an adventitia. The intima, or inner layer, is composed of endothelial cells that line the luminal surface. If disrupted, this layer gives rise to thrombus formation; it must be smooth and contiguous throughout the vascular tree. The media, the middle layer, is formed of muscle tissue and is thinner and less developed in veins. Veins subjected to arterial pressures will become thickened and hypertrophic. The adventitia is an outermost layer of connective tissue (see Fig. 15-1).

Sympathetic nerve fibers distributed within the media of both arteries and veins allow the nervous system responses of contraction and dilatation to satisfy body requirements. The media itself is supplied by minute arteries in a system called the *vasa vasorum*. Veins additionally have a series of semilunar valves that promote one-way blood flow back toward the heart.

Vessels Associated with Carotid Surgery

The innominate, left common carotid, and left subclavian arteries all arise from the aortic arch (Fig. 15-2). The innominate artery then divides into right subclavian and right common carotid arteries. The common carotid bifurcates into internal and external carotid arteries at the carotid bulb, just below the mandible. The vagus nerve runs between the internal jugular vein and common ca-

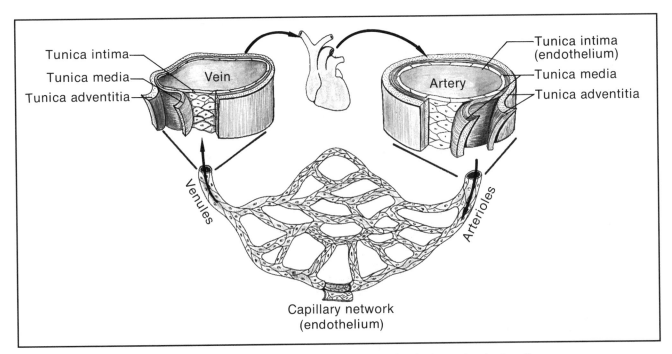

FIGURE 15-1 Blood vessels. This diagrammatic sketch shows the single-cell endothelium of all vessels and the layered muscular coats of arteries and veins. (From Anderson [1984]. *Basic human anatomy and physiology.* Monterey, CA: Wadsworth Health Sciences Division. Reprinted with permission of copyright owner.)

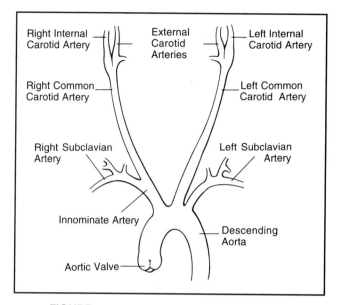

FIGURE 15-2 Arteries of the head and neck.

rotid artery and behind the internal carotid artery. The external carotid arteries supply blood to the face; the internal carotid arteries supply the brain. The ophthalmic artery is ultimately a branch of the circle of Willis and of the internal carotid supply. This artery is used in testing for carotid artery disease.

The Aorta

The abdominal aorta begins at the diaphragm and descends slightly to the left of the spine before bifurcating into right and left common iliac arteries approximately at the level of the umbilicus (Fig. 15-3). The celiac axis, superior mesenteric artery, renal arteries, and inferior mesenteric arteries are major branches of the aorta as it descends. The vena cava lies to the right of the aorta.

The thoracic aorta

The descending thoracic aorta lies to the left of the spine at its origin and gradually runs toward the midline anterior to the spine in the mediastinum. The intercostal arteries originate from the posterior thoracic aorta, and branches form the spinal arteries supplying the spinal cord and its membranes (Williams, 1989). The artery becomes the abdominal aorta at the level of the diaphragm (see Fig. 15-3).

Vessels of the Leg

The common femoral artery begins at the inguinal ligament and is an extension of the external iliac artery. The common femoral artery soon divides into superficial and deep, or profunda, femoral arteries. The profunda, as its name implies, runs deep into the thigh. The superficial femoral continues down the anteromedial thigh until it becomes the popliteal artery near the knee. The same

artery, now called popliteal, continues down the leg and ultimately becomes the anterior and posterior tibial arteries in the calf (Fig. 15-4).

The saphenous vein begins at the anterior surface of the medial malleolus in the ankle and continues up the medial aspect of the leg. A sensory nerve runs alongside the vein and is the source of the numbness or pain that sometimes occurs after dissection of this vein for cardiac or vascular grafting. The saphenous vein communicates with the femoral vein in one or more branches.

NURSING CONSIDERATIONS

General Information

Patients undergoing vascular surgery often have complex medical problems that require extensive planning and interventions during surgery in order to prevent further complications. The progression of vascular disease, often due to diabetes and a long history of smoking, leaves patients vulnerable to skin breakdown and ischemia. A pressure-relieving mattress and pads for heels and elbows should be used when positioning the patient on the operating room bed. Patients may be in pain due to ischemic changes, ulcers, gangrene, or neuropathy. If the sensation of touch is diminished due to neuropathy, the patient may not be aware of pressure, sharp objects, or temperature extremes. The nurse must monitor for items that could injure the patient without his or her knowledge. Peripheral pulses may be weak or absent, and a bruit may be heard over areas of obstruction. A patient with an abdominal aortic aneurysm (AAA) may have a pulsating abdominal mass.

Patients either arrive in the operating room with invasive monitoring lines in place or these lines will be inserted prior to surgery.

Nursing Diagnoses

Nursing diagnoses commonly seen in patients undergoing vascular surgery are impaired skin integrity (actual or high risk), altered tissue perfusion due to inadequate cellular nutrition and oxygenation, high risk for fluid volume deficit due to blood loss during surgery, pain due to ischemia or neuropathy, and anxiety or fear over the outcomes of surgery and prognosis.

Diagnostic Studies

Doppler ultrasound

Doppler ultrasound is an instrument that gives a direction-specific magnification of pulses that may not be felt by palpation. The Doppler probe is used at an angle to the vessel, most efficiently 30 to 60 degrees, and senses motion of fluid waves coming toward or away from it by detecting the motion of red blood cells within the plasma. Turbulent

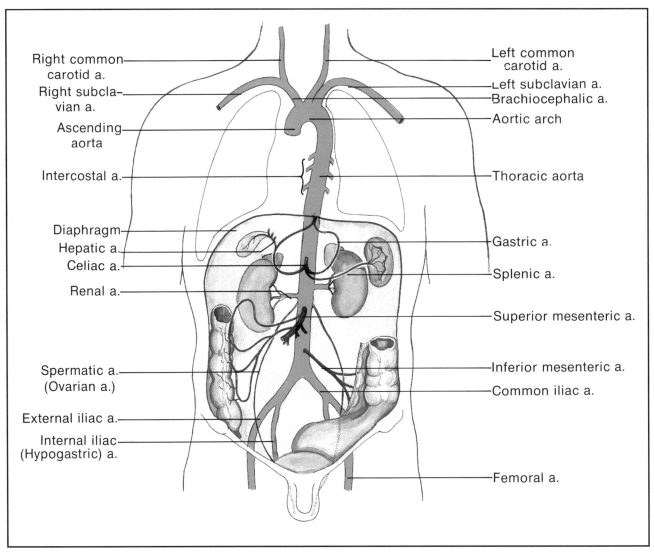

FIGURE 15-3 The aorta and its branches. (From Anderson [1984]. *Basic human anatomy and physiology.* Monterey, CA: Wadsworth Health Sciences Division. Reprinted with permission of copyright owner.)

flow will be heard as a muffled sound and is used to diagnose partial occlusion or obstruction within the vessel such as that caused by retained thrombus, plaque, or an obstructed suture line. The Doppler probe may be coupled with the skin using a gel, or it can be sterilized and used on the operative field on a moist surface.

Angiograms

Angiograms are radiographs of blood vessels visualized by injecting a radiopaque contrast medium into the bloodstream. Angiograms provide a luminal view of the vessel. The outer dimensions of a thickened arterial wall or the outline of an aneurysm sac filled with thrombus, for example, will not be seen on an angiogram. The contrast medium may be injected at the operative site or from remote locations, usually the femoral artery. Preoperative angiograms are frequently used as a reference in the operating room during surgery. Intraoperative angiograms

may be taken to study the immediate results of a surgical bypass before the patient is moved to the post-anesthesia care unit (PACU). The amount and dilution of contrast medium used will be determined by the size of the vessel, depth of tissue to be penetrated by X-rays, and the patient's renal tolerance to the contrast medium. Contrast medium can cause allergic reactions. A careful allergic history must be taken prior to use.

Angioscopy

An angioscope is a thin, flexible, fiberoptic scope used to directly view the lumen of arteries and veins. It uses a light source and foot-operated irrigation pump, and the image may be projected onto a video monitor for teaching or for documentation purposes. The vessel to be studied is clamped or manually occluded, and the scope is introduced via an arteriotomy. Irrigation is used to flush blood from the visual field. The angioscope may be used as a diagnostic instrument, as an aid to identify or retrieve

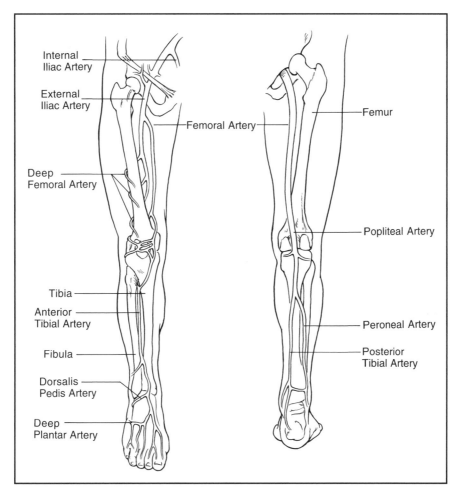

FIGURE 15-4 Major arteries of the right lower extremity. (From Anderson [1984]. *Basic human anatomy and physiology.* Monterey: CA: Wadsworth Health Sciences Division. Redrawn with permission of copyright owner.)

thrombus, or as an adjunct to a surgical technique (see Angioscopy-Assisted In Situ Femoropopliteal Bypass, later in this chapter) (Fig. 15-5).

Special Supplies and Equipment

Fine instruments (Fig. 15-6), synthetic prosthetic grafts (Fig. 15-7), and specially designed catheters for embolectomy are used in vascular surgery. The Doppler ultrasound and angioscope, used for diagnosis, may also be used during surgical procedures. Autotransfusion is used to salvage blood and to limit the amount of banked blood required.

Instrumentation

There are few instruments used only for vascular surgery. The atraumatic properties of forceps and the fine tips of scissors and needle holders have made the "vascular" instruments tools of many specialties. The few instruments that are unique to the vascular specialty are peripheral vascular clamps, aortic occlusion clamps, Satin-

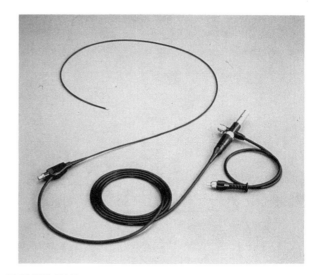

FIGURE 15-5 Angiofiberscope. (Photo courtesy of Olympus America, Inc. Medical Instrument Division.)

sky clamps, various bulldog clamps, and Fogarty occlusion clamps.

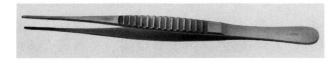

A

FIGURE 15-6 Instruments used in vascular surgery. (*A*) Debakey vascular forceps. (*B*) Senning bulldog clamp. (*C*) Curved cross-section bulldog clamp. (*D*) Straight Cooley bulldog clamp. (*E*) Potts scissors, 45 degree. (*F*) Crafoord coarctation clamp. (*G*) Satinsky vena cava clamp. (Instruments courtesy of Baxter Healthcare Corporation, V. Mueller Division.)

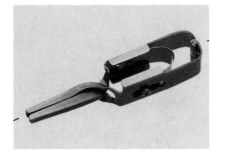

B

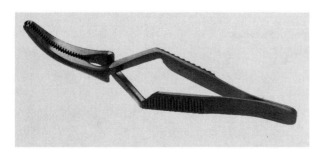

C

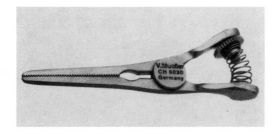

D

Vascular dilators, microvascular scissors, and a valvulotome are used for in situ procedures. Dacron tape or vessel loops are used for gentle retraction of vessels.

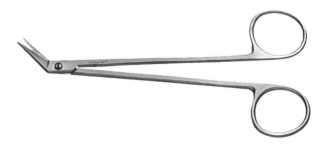

E

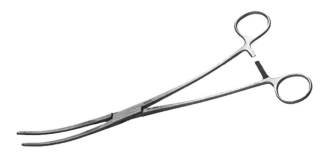

F

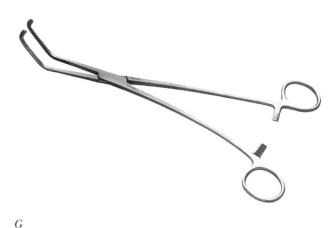

G

Prosthetic grafts

Prosthetic grafts may be knitted, woven, or made of Velour, Dacron, or Teflon material. Knitted grafts require preclotting to prevent leakage of blood. A small volume of the patient's blood is drawn off before heparinization and repeatedly drawn through the graft with syringes before the graft is sutured into the resected artery. Recent developments in graft technology include collagen- and albumen-impregnated knitted grafts requiring no preclotting (see Figs. 15-7 to 15-10). These were developed in response to the alternate technique of soaking a knitted graft in a small volume of the patient's albumen and then autoclaving the graft. The denatured protein filled the interstices of the graft and prevented bleeding. This time-consuming method also required the meticulous removal

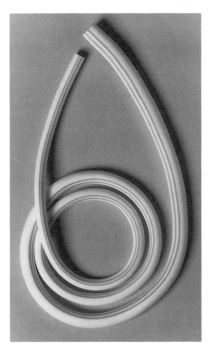

FIGURE 15-7   PTFE tapered graft.   (Courtesy of IMPRA, Tempe, AZ.)

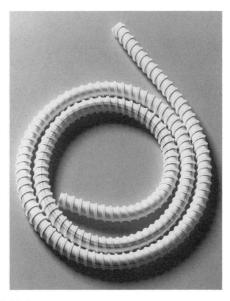

FIGURE 15-8   Externally supported PTFE graft.   (Courtesy of IMPRA, Tempe, AZ.)

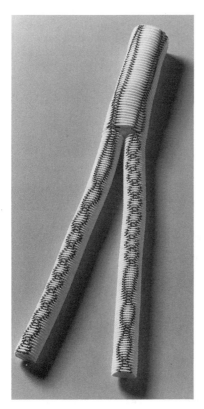

FIGURE 15-9   Vascutek Triaxial knitted Dacron bifurcated graft.   (Courtesy of IMPRA, Tempe, AZ.)

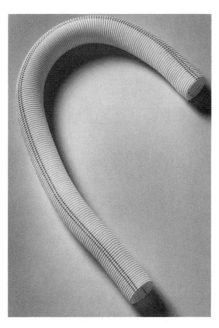

FIGURE 15-10   Vascutek extra soft woven straight Dacron tube graft.   (Courtesy of IMPRA, Tempe, AZ.)

of any remaining fragments of albumen to prevent embolization.

Woven grafts require no preclotting but are more diffi-cult to suture due to the tighter weave. They may be used in situations where nonheparinized blood is not immedi-ately available as in emergency situations, prehepariniza-tion, or cardiopulmonary bypass.

Fogarty embolectomy catheters

The Fogarty embolectomy catheter, which comes in various sizes, is an arterial catheter with a balloon tip. The catheter is inserted into the artery beyond the point of clot attachment. The balloon is inflated and then with-drawn, bringing the detached clot with it.

Autotransfusion

Autotransfusion allows shed blood from the operative field to be collected in a sterile fashion, filtered, washed, and reinfused into the patient as packed red cells. Platelets and clotting factors are lost in the supernatant, and crystalloid must be added for volume replacement. The autotransfusion apparatus may be set up in the operating room, or the blood may be collected in the operating room in a sterile fashion and sent to the blood bank to be spun.

Policies vary with institutions, but some antibiotics and iodophor solutions must not be used on the operative field if autotransfusion is to be employed. Contraindications to autotransfusion include presence of amniotic fluid, cancer, and fecal contamination of the wound.

SURGICAL PROCEDURES

Carotid Surgery

Carotid artery disease is a stenosis or narrowing of the internal, external, or common carotid arteries in the neck, usually at or above the common carotid bifurcation. The etiology is most commonly atheroma, beginning as a fatty streak and evolving into fibrous plaque. The damaged intimal surface often generates thrombus and contributes the added risk of embolism to the brain, resulting in stroke. Acute occlusion has been associated with hemorrhage into or behind this fibrous plaque (Baker, 1985). In rare instances, occlusion may occur from aneurysm or trauma to the neck, leading to embolization of the carotid arteries.

Endarterectomy is a procedure to remove atheromatous plaque, thrombi, and debris through an incision in the artery. Patients who benefit most from carotid endarterectomy are those with cerebral symptoms (Chassin, 1989). The obstructed blood flow can cause any of the warning signs or symptoms of brain ischemia, including syncope, visual disturbances, dizziness, weakness, or transient ischemic attacks (TIAs), and a bruit may be heard over the artery in the neck. The presence or severity of these symptoms depends on the degree of collateral circulation present. In the absence of these warning signs the presenting sign may be stroke. The goal of surgery in a symptomatic patient is the prevention of stroke.

Perioperative nursing considerations

Although carotid endarterectomy is sometimes performed under local anesthesia (Baker, 1985), it most often requires a general anesthetic both for patient comfort and hemodynamic control. The patient's blood pressure must be maintained at a level high enough to ensure perfusion of the brain via collateral circulation while the carotid artery is clamped. Anesthetic agents can cause unstable blood pressure and hypotension, and the anesthetist may use intravenous vasopressor agents to maintain an adequately high systolic pressure. An insufficient level of anesthesia may result in hypertension and can lead to intraoperative stroke. Preoperative medication may eliminate hypotension caused by cardiac arrhythmias.

With the patient in the supine position and shoulders elevated, a small firm pillow, inflatable pillow, or folded towel is placed between the scapulae to hyperextend the neck. The patient's head is turned to the nonoperative side and the arms are tucked alongside the torso to allow the surgeon easier access to the neck. The surgeon and assistant stand at either side of the patient's head, the scrub nurse stands at the level of the patient's waist on the operative side, and the anesthesia provider stands on the nonoperative side with a tent of surgical drapes to allow access to the endotracheal tube and the patient's face. Care is taken to ensure that no metal of the operating room bed comes into contact with the patient's hands and that the patient's hands are protected with padding from inadvertent leaning of the operating room team.

Carotid artery endarterectomy

Key steps

1. An incision is made over the carotid artery in the neck.
2. The soft tissue is dissected free of the artery. Retraction tapes are passed around the internal, external, and common carotid arteries with a right-angle clamp (Fig. 15-11). Manipulation of the vessels is avoided as much as possible to prevent disruption and embolization of the plaque or thrombus.

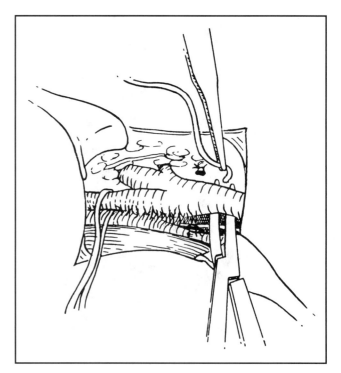

FIGURE 15-11 The internal, external, and common carotid arteries are isolated, and retraction tapes are placed around them.

3. After heparinization, the internal, external, and common carotid arteries are clamped with noncrushing vascular clamps or bulldog clamps. Electroencephalographic monitoring is used to detect any decrease in brain wave activity, which indicates cerebral ischemia. If ischemia is present, the procedure will be expedited to progress quickly to shunting of blood around the blocked vessel.

4. An arteriotomy is made with a knife and extended with Potts scissors (Fig. 15-12). Pooled blood is removed with suction. If shunting is to be used, the shunt is now passed between the internal and common carotid arteries.

5. The atheroma is excised using a blunt dissector (Fig. 15-13). Any remaining fragments on the luminal surface are removed with a soft peanut dissector (Fig. 15-14). Small fragments of plaque left behind may embolize to the brain once flow is reestablished in the artery. The artery is irrigated with heparinized saline solution to prevent formation of clots.

6. The arteriotomy is closed with running nonabsorbable sutures (Fig. 15-15). If used, the shunt is clamped and removed at the last moment. Before the last few sutures are tied down, the artery is "back-bled" to remove air. If necessary, a patch of Gore-Tex fabric or saphenous vein graft removed from the leg is used to maintain adequate size of the vessel lumen.

7. Clamps are removed last from the internal carotid artery to prevent air emboli or debris remaining in the

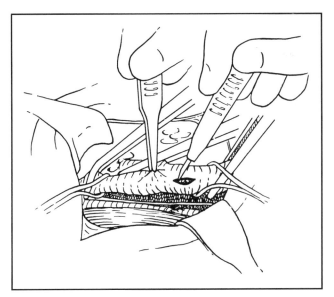

FIGURE 15-12   An arteriotomy is made with a knife, followed by Potts scissors.

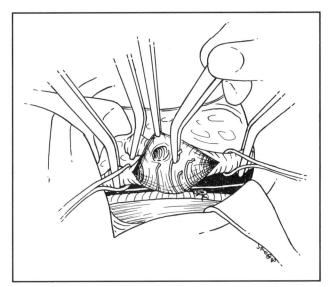

FIGURE 15-14   Any remaining fragments of atheroma are carefully removed to prevent embolization.

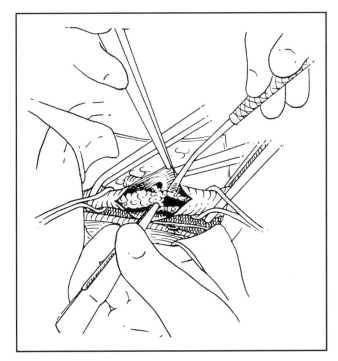

FIGURE 15-13   Atheromatous plaque is excised, using a blunt dissector.

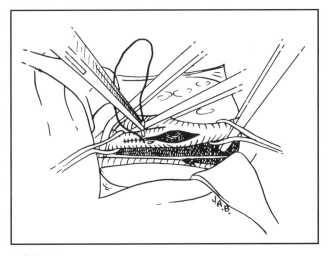

FIGURE 15-15   The arteriotomy is closed with a running suture line of monofilament.

vessel from being washed up toward the brain. A Doppler ultrasound is used to study the patency of the vessel.

8. The wound is closed with interrupted nonabsorbable sutures, and a loose-fitting dressing is applied.

9. The patient is monitored in the post-anesthesia care unit (PACU) or intensive care unit (ICU) for a minimum of 4 hours (O'Brien & Ricotta, 1991). Incisional bleeding in a heparinized patient can cause pressure on internal neck structures.

Surgery of the Aorta

Aortic resections may be performed for either aneurysmal or occlusive disease. In occlusive disease, atheromatous plaque built up within the walls of the aorta and the thrombus and debris it generates obstruct blood flow to the limbs and internal organs. The symptoms of ischemia vary with the tissue affected. Absence or lessening of pulses can occur, along with pain or cramping of the limbs or abdominal viscera. The diseased segment of aorta with its contents is transected and replaced with a prosthetic graft.

Aneurysmal disease is a weakening in the wall of the artery, with herniation into the surrounding area. Symptoms, if present, usually result from the pressure of this space-occupying mass on internal organs or the adjacent tissue. An uncomfortable pulsating mass may be found on abdominal examination or the patient may complain of abdominal or back pain. Thrombus formed within the aneurysm sac can embolize, causing pulselessness in the limbs or infarction of the abdominal viscera, with resulting pain or dysfunction. Often there are no symptoms, and the first presentation is one of acute pain, bleeding, or acute occlusion as the aneurysm ruptures. Although blood loss may be significant, if tamponaded by adjacent structures, the patient may survive until surgery. Elective surgery for a known aneurysm is done as it becomes symptomatic or enlarges. The diseased segment of aorta is transected and replaced with a prosthetic graft via either a transperitoneal or a retroperitoneal approach.

Perioperative nursing considerations

The transperitoneal approach to aortic resection is historically the most common. A retroperitoneal approach may be used when the patient is obese or has had multiple previous abdominal surgeries where the tedious lysis of adhesions will greatly prolong surgery time. In either case, a preoperative epidural catheter may be placed to supplement the general anesthesia, thus reducing the amount of inhalational agents needed and affording better hemodynamic control during surgery.

The patient is positioned supine with arms abducted on armboards for a *transperitoneal* approach to resection and replacement of a segment of the abdominal aorta. The knees may be flexed and abducted if access to the groins is anticipated as for bifemoral grafting.

Transperitoneal aortic resection

Key steps

1. A midline incision is made from the xiphoid process to the symphysis pubis.

2. The peritoneal cavity is opened and internal organs are examined for undetected disease before proceeding. The discovery of an inflamed appendix, infected gallbladder, or other acute disease processes may delay the elective repair of aortic disease. The severity of the vascular disease must be weighed against the risk of infection from intestinal surgery in a setting of implanted graft material.

3. The abdominal organs are retracted to one side and protected by a moist towel or plastic bag, and the retroperitoneum is opened.

4. The aorta is dissected free from surrounding tissues above and below the aneurysm site or segment to be resected, and retraction tapes are placed around the artery for control. Minimal handling of the aneurysm site prevents rupture.

5. Using a needle and syringe, 50 ml of blood is drawn for preclotting of the Dacron graft. The patient is heparinized.

6. The aorta is cross-clamped above and below the resection site with noncrushing vascular clamps of sufficient size to encompass the artery. The distal site is clamped first to prevent embolization of plaque material to the limbs, and then the proximal aorta is clamped. During the cross-clamp time, efforts are made to expedite the surgery so as to minimize the ischemia time. Urine output is closely monitored.

7. An incision is made into the aorta using a knife and is extended with Potts scissors to open the aneurysm sac (Fig. 15-16). The renal arteries or other aortic branches of significant size may be occluded from within the arterial lumen, using balloon catheters.

8. Gross atheromatous plaque, thrombus, and debris are removed, and bleeding lumbar arteries are suture-ligated with absorbable sutures (Fig. 15-17). The area is irrigated with heparinized saline solution.

9. After preclotting, a synthetic graft of knitted Dacron is sewn end-to-end into the proximal aorta, using 2-0 or 3-0 nonabsorbable suture material (Fig. 15-18). A running or interrupted suture technique may be used, and the sutures are double armed to allow stitching in either direction. Pledgets or strips of Teflon felt may be used for reinforcement of a thin aortic wall and are sewn directly into the suture line.

10. The first suture line is tested by clamping the open end(s) of the graft and removing the proximal aortic clamp. Blood fills the graft, and any additional sutures needed to stop bleeding are placed at this time. Placement of posterior aortic wall sutures for bleeding sites is more difficult once the distal anastomoses are completed.

11. The distal site is selected, the graft is trimmed to the correct length, and an end-to-end anastomosis is done in a fashion similar to that used for the distal aorta (tube graft) or common iliac or femoral arteries (bifurcated graft) (Fig. 15-19). Before tying down the

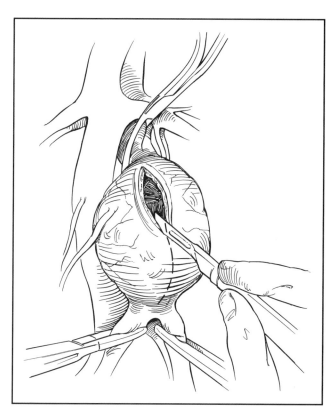

FIGURE 15-16 The aneurysm sac is opened with a knife, followed by Potts scissors.

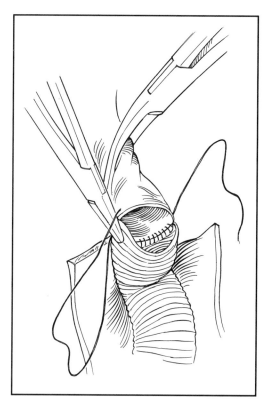

FIGURE 15-18 The proximal anastomosis is completed first.

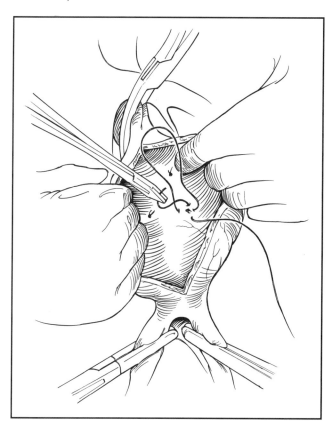

FIGURE 15-17 Lumbar arteries are suture-ligated as they are encountered.

last suture of each limb, the vascular clamps are partially opened to allow back-bleeding to fill the graft. Air is evacuated and debris flushed out of the artery. After the suture line is completed, the clamps are removed.

12. It may be necessary to replant visceral arteries into the graft, depending on the extent and location of the aneurysm. If done, a side-biting vascular clamp is applied to the side wall of the graft while allowing blood flow around it through the new conduit. A small incision is made with a knife or scissor in the isolated segment of graft wall of matching diameter to the artery to be side-grafted. The visceral artery is cut free of aortic wall, allowing sufficient cuff for suturing, and is sewn into the new graft with a running 4-0 or 5-0 nonabsorbable suture. On occasion, a prosthetic graft of 8-mm Dacron will be used for side-grafting. After air is evacuated, the side-biting clamp is removed.

13. The aneurysm wall is sewn over the graft for protection (Fig. 15-20). The retroperitoneum is closed, using interrupted fine silk or other nonabsorbable suture, and a sponge count is done.

14. The abdominal organs are returned to the peritoneal cavity, and the peritoneum is closed. Another sponge count is done.

15. The abdominal wall, subcutaneous tissue, and skin are closed, and a final sponge count is done. Generally, the patient is extubated before leaving the operating room.

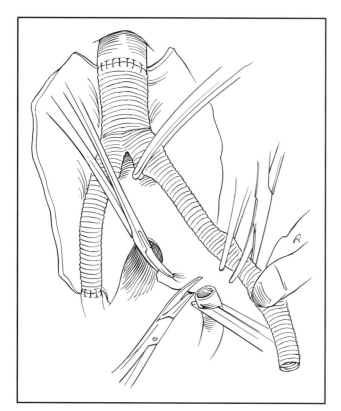

FIGURE 15-19 A bifurcated graft is trimmed to the correct length before each distal anastomosis is completed.

Retroperitoneal aortic resection

If the *retroperitoneal* approach is used, the patient is positioned in the right lateral position (right side down) with hips rotated back toward supine 45 degrees to allow access to both groins. The right arm is extended on an armboard, with the left arm over the right, supported by positioning devices and secured. The anesthesia provider may request an axillary roll to allow full expansion of the chest wall. A small support is placed at the level of the scapula to prevent the torso from rolling as the hips are rotated back toward supine. Pillows are placed between the knees and padding under the heels before the legs are secured with a padded safety strap. Pneumatic boots may be used on the lower legs to prevent thrombus formation in the venous circulation.

Key steps

1. The incision extends from the left lateral border of the rectus muscle 4 to 5 cm below the umbilicus, out to the posterior aspect of the eleventh or twelfth rib (Moore, 1991). The flank muscles are divided in this incision.
2. A retroperitoneal plane is created by blunt dissection, and the peritoneum with its contents and the left kidney are retracted anteriorly. The aorta is exposed from the side.
3. The aorta is dissected free of the surrounding tissues down to the bifurcation, and the left common iliac artery is exposed. An aneurysm affecting the right common iliac artery is more difficult to repair using this

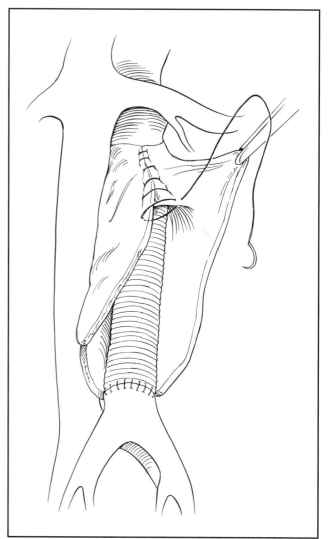

FIGURE 15-20 The aortic wall/aneurysm sac is closed over the tube graft.

approach (Greenhalgh & Mannick, 1990), and bleeding from the right iliac artery may necessitate the use of a balloon catheter in the artery lumen.

4. After heparinization, the aorta is clamped above and below the segment of resection and replaced as described above for transperitoneal resection. The aneurysm wall is closed over the graft.
5. Wound closure is somewhat more prolonged because of the muscle repair of the flank incision, which is done with layers of interrupted absorbable suture. Speed gained by not opening the peritoneal cavity and examining abdominal organs may be lost by the longer wound closure time, with the net result being the same (Cambria, 1990).

Thoracic aortic resection

A thoracic aneurysm may cause the patient to experience chest pain or shortness of breath from stretching of the pleura or displacement of the lung. Pressure on the left main bronchus may cause cough or dysphagia. Left recurrent laryngeal nerve pressure may cause voice changes or hoarseness. Hemoptysis may indicate erosion of the aneurysm into the bronchus with rupture, or a silent bleed may occur into the pleural space.

Thoracic aortic resection, usually for aneurysm repair, may or may not include extracorporeal circulatory bypass. In any case, autotransfusion apparatus may be employed for retrieval of blood loss.

All efforts will be made to keep the cross-clamp time as short as possible to minimize spinal cord ischemia. Intercostal arteries arising from the posterior thoracic aorta are preserved or replanted when possible, and the systemic blood pressure is maintained by vasopressors to ensure adequate perfusion of the spinal cord.

A thoracic resection will involve clamping the renal arteries, and an iced solution of lactated Ringer's, heparin, and a steroid is irrigated through the kidneys to preserve function. After the aortic cross-clamps are removed, urine output is closely monitored.

A double-lumen endotracheal tube may be used to allow deflation of one lung during thoracotomy, facilitating exposure.

The patient is placed in a right lateral position (right side down) with the hips rotated back toward supine 45 degrees, similar to positioning for retroperitoneal abdominal aortic resection.

Key steps

1. An incision is made in the sixth or seventh intercostal space, depending on the location of the proximal resection margin, and extending toward the midline of the abdomen to below the umbilicus (Cooley, 1986) (Fig. 15-21).
2. A self-retaining retractor is placed in the thoracic incision, and the diaphragm is incised to prevent injury to the phrenic nerve (Moore, 1991).
3. The left kidney is retracted forward, and the aorta is exposed from the side.
4. The site of proximal aortic anastomosis is dissected free of the surrounding tissues, and a retraction tape is passed around it for control. The renal vein may be divided (Moore, 1991).
5. Abdominal organs are retracted to one side, and the site of distal aortic anastomosis is identified and dissected free.
6. After heparinization, aortic cross-clamps are applied above and below the area of resection, and graft replacement is carried out as described above. The distal site of anastomosis may be the abdominal aorta (tube graft) or the iliac arteries (bifurcated graft).
7. Two teams of surgeons may be employed to facilitate the closure of this large wound. Pleural catheters with underwater seal are placed, and possibly a wound drain.

Femoral Vessel Surgery

Atherosclerotic plaque in the arteries of the leg and the thrombus and debris generated by the plaque cause obstruction to blood flow similar to the occlusive disease of

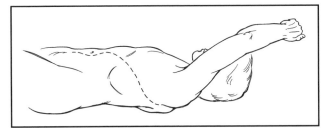

FIGURE 15-21 Thoracoabdominal incision and exposure.

the aorta. Diminishing or absent pulses in the leg, cramping or pain on walking, or ulcers that resist healing are indications for bypass of the popliteal, tibial, or pedal arteries. In some cases, blunt trauma, dislocation of the knee, or aneurysm of the popliteal artery will cause a defect that cannot be primarily repaired and requires a bypass procedure.

Perioperative nursing considerations

The saphenous vein in the leg, if present and free of varicosities, is the most commonly used conduit for arterial bypasses in similar-sized arteries. The vein may be dissected free of the leg and reversed to allow blood flow through unidirectional vein valves. Or it may be left in place (in situ) and anastomosed proximally and distally to the artery after lysis of the valve leaflets. In above-the-knee bypasses, synthetic material such as polytetrafluoroethylene (PTFE) may be used.

The patient is positioned supine on the operating room bed, with both legs circumferentially prepped and draped into the sterile field. Vein for grafting may be taken from either the operative or nonoperative leg. Having both legs prepped greatly reduces the preparation time if later it is decided more vein is necessary.

Femoropopliteal bypass using reversed vein or synthetic graft

Key steps

1. An incision is made over the femoral artery in the groin below the inguinal ligament. Lymphatic tissue over the femoral artery is divided and ligated with absorbable suture.
2. The femoral artery is dissected from the surrounding tissues at the site of the proximal anastomosis, and retraction tapes are placed around it. An incision is made in the lower leg at the site of the distal arterial anastomosis, and tapes are placed around the artery.
3. The proximal saphenous vein, located in the groin, is dissected free of soft tissues. It is transected at the saphenofemoral junction. The proximal skin incision is extended down the leg to follow the path of the saphenous vein. As the saphenous vein is dissected free of the leg, branches are divided and ligated with silk ties or polypropylene sutures. A Marks needle is tied to the proximal end, and the vein is irrigated with a solution of heparinized saline to prevent thrombus formation. When a vein of sufficient length has been freed

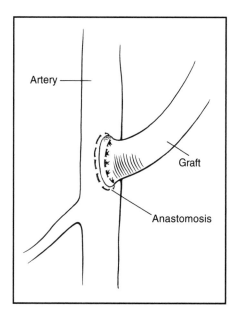

FIGURE 15-22 An end-to-end anastomosis.

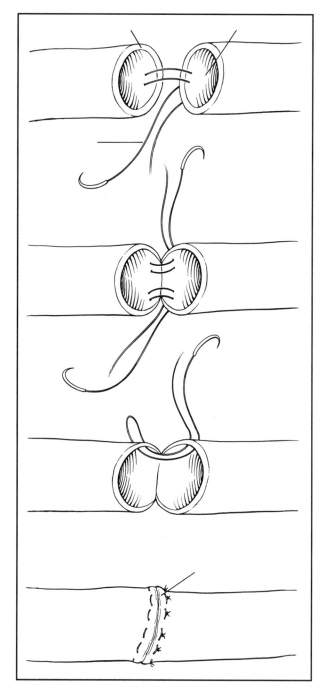

FIGURE 15-23 An end-to-end anastomosis using interrupted sutures.

from the leg, the distal end is ligated and the vein is removed and placed on the instrument table.

4. The femoral artery is clamped with a noncrushing vascular clamp, and an arteriotomy incision is made with a knife, followed by a Potts scissors. Heparinized saline is used to flush the artery. Using a running suture line of nonabsorbable suture, the *distal* end of the saphenous vein is anastomosed to the *proximal* arterial anastomotic site, the femoral artery.

5. An arteriotomy is made at the site of the distal anastomosis. Using a running suture line of nonabsorbable suture material, the *proximal* end of the saphenous vein is anastomosed to the *distal* popliteal or tibial artery in an end-to-side anastomosis (Fig. 15-22).

6. At times it may be necessary to splice segments of vein graft together. This is done using end-to-end anastomoses (Fig. 15-23). The vascular clamps are removed, and air is evacuated before the last suture is "tied down."

7. An arteriogram is done from the surgical field to examine the patency of the new graft and the suture line. The leg incision is closed, using interrupted layers of absorbable suture material.

In situ femoropopliteal bypass graft

The in situ saphenous vein bypass has the added advantage of close proximity in size of the graft with the artery to be bypassed. Leaving the vein in its anatomical bed may lessen the risk of trauma and injury during dissection and surgical manipulation. However, side branches of the vein may be missed when the vein is not fully dissected free and may later become arteriovenous fistulae when the vein is arterialized, and it is important to avoid this.

The patient is placed supine on the operating room bed. Only the operative leg is prepped.

Key steps

1. An incision is made over the femoral artery in the groin below the inguinal ligament. Lymphatic tissue is divided, and the femoral artery anastomotic site is identified as described above. The saphenous vein is located through the same incision. A second skin incision is made at the location of the distal arterial anastomosis, and retraction tapes are placed around the distal artery.

2. The proximal skin incision is extended the length of the leg to follow the saphenous vein. Side branches of

the vein are ligated with silk sutures, but the vein is not dissected free from the leg.

3. After heparin is administered, the vein is transected once at the saphenofemoral junction and again slightly below the level of the distal anastomosis. The distal artery is clamped with a noncrushing vascular clamp, usually of a bulldog variety, and an arteriotomy is made with a knife, followed by a Potts or angled microscissor. The distal vein is anastomosed to the artery, end to side, using a running nonabsorbable monofilament suture.

4. A valvulotome is passed into the proximal end of the vein and threaded to the level of the distal anastomosis. As the valvulotome is withdrawn, the vein valve leaflets are cut. The vein will distend with blood under arterial pressure.

5. An arteriotomy is made in the femoral artery with a knife, followed by a Potts scissors. The proximal saphenous vein is anastomosed, end to side, to the artery, using a running monofilament suture. The vascular clamps and bulldog clamps are removed from the artery, and air is evacuated before the last suture is "tied down."

6. A Doppler probe is used to study the patency of the graft at several locations. The graft is once again checked for patent vein side branches, which may become arteriovenous fistulae and, if found, are ligated. The leg wound is closed as described above.

Angioscopy-assisted in situ femoropopliteal bypass

An angioscope is a thin, flexible, fiberoptic scope used to view the lumen of blood vessels. When used in the femoropopliteal bypass, the angioscope has the potential of altering the surgical procedure to a significant degree. The angioscope follows the valvulotome through the in situ saphenous vein as valve leaflets are cut and gives a luminal view, in some cases eliminating the need for a full-length leg incision (Fogarty, 1991). The patient is placed in supine position.

Key steps

1. The femoral artery and saphenous vein are exposed in the groin as described above, but the skin incision is not extended down the leg. A second small skin incision is made at the site of the distal anastomosis, and the artery to be bypassed and the distal saphenous vein are exposed.

2. After heparinization, the saphenous vein is transected once at the saphenofemoral junction and again at the site of the distal anastomosis. A valvulotome is passed into the proximal saphenous vein and threaded through the length of the vein. The angioscope is passed into the distal end of the vein. As the valvulotome is withdrawn, the angioscope follows, allowing a visual inspection of the vein valve leaflets as they are cut (Fig. 15-24).

3. A foot-operated irrigation pump, primed with lactated Ringer's solution, is used to clear blood from view. By lessening the irrigation flow, vein side branches are

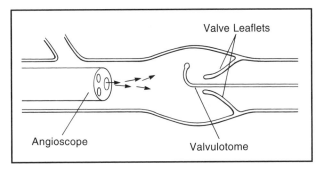

FIGURE 15-24 Valvulotome-obliteration of vein valve under angioscopic guidance.

identified by back-bleeding into the lumen. A mark is made on the skin surface at the location of each branch, and a small incision is later made to ligate each branch.

4. The image may be projected onto a video monitor. This helps to eliminate inadvertent contamination with a cap, mask, or eyeglasses while trying to look directly into the eyepiece of the scope.

5. After satisfactory examination of the lumen of the vein graft and assurance that all leaflets are obliterated, the distal anastomosis is done and the procedure completed as described above.

Laser-assisted femoropopliteal bypass using balloon angioplasty

Balloon angioplasty may be used in arteries of the lower limbs, using techniques similar to those used in coronary angioplasty. Lasers are used in combination with balloon angioplasty for the totally occluded blood vessel. The laser recannulates an opening through atheromatous plaque that can be followed by ballooning. If unsuccessful, the procedure can be immediately followed by a surgical bypass. The patient must be able to tolerate both a lengthy procedure and relatively large amounts of contrast medium excreted through the renal system.

The procedure is done in the operating room and is guided by fluoroscopy. All personnel need to wear protective lead garments, and warning signs should be displayed at all entrances to the operating room to prevent inadvertent entry of unprotected personnel.

Several laser systems have been developed for use with laser-assisted balloon angioplasty (Cull et al., 1991), including the neodymium-yttrium-aluminum-garnet (Nd:YAG) laser. This laser uses sterile, disposable fibers to recannulate the artery.

The patient is placed supine on the operating room bed, with the operative leg circumferentially prepped into the sterile field.

Key steps

1. The preoperative angiogram is used to measure the widest diameter of patent vessel lumen and the length of the atherosclerotic lesion.

2. An incision is made in the groin over the femoral vessels. The femoral artery is identified and isolated with retraction tapes.

3. After heparinization, an introducer sheath is passed into the femoral artery. Under fluoroscopic visualization and using half-strength contrast medium, a guidewire is passed to the site of the arterial lesion. Inability to pass the guidewire beyond the lesion, as in a total occlusion, is an indication for use of the laser.

4. The guidewire is removed and the laser fiber passed to the same site. The laser is activated and, under fluoroscopy, is advanced through the fibrous plaque, creating a narrow channel.

5. The guidewire is passed into this new channel through the plaque. An angioplasty balloon is threaded over the guidewire and inflated, compressing the plaque and recannulating the vessel. Half-strength contrast medium is used to inflate the angioplasty balloon so that it may be viewed fluoroscopically.

6. The balloon and guidewire are removed, and contrast medium is again injected to study the vessel. A patent or satisfactory result will end the procedure.

7. The wound is closed with interrupted absorbable suture material. A Doppler probe may be used on the skin to locate distal pulses. The patient is maintained on heparin anticoagulation overnight.

Femoral pseudoaneurysm repair

Pseudoaneurysm, or false aneurysm, of the femoral artery may occur as a complication of venipuncture, from angiographic studies, cardiac catheterization, or after percutaneous placement of an intra-aortic balloon pump (McCann et al., 1991). Puncture of the femoral vessels and the sheaths used to introduce diagnostic catheters may leave a communication between the femoral artery and vein. A thrill may be audible with Doppler, or a pulsatile hematoma may be felt at the groin. Repair may be done under local anesthesia. The patient is placed in supine position.

Key steps

1. An incision is made over the femoral vessels in the groin, and the vessels are identified.

2. The dissection is carefully carried out around the hematoma with as little disruption of the surrounding tissues as possible. The hematoma is frequently the result of bleeding into the soft tissue and tamponades the vessel puncture site in these heparinized patients.

3. Vascular clamps or bulldog clamps are applied above and below the puncture site. Frequently, vigorous bleeding will occur as the dissection nears the puncture site, and pressure is used to control bleeding until a clamp can be placed on the vessel.

4. The vessel is repaired with interrupted nonabsorbable sutures. A Doppler may be used to locate distal pulses if they are not palpable. An embolectomy may be required (see embolectomy below) to retrieve thrombi from the vessel lumen.

5. The wound is closed with interrupted layers of absorbable sutures.

Surgery for Vascular Complications

Embolectomy

Occlusion caused by thrombi or trapped emboli can cause acute ischemia. Emboli may be retrieved by the use of Fogarty embolectomy balloon catheters. The procedure for femoral embolectomy is similar in kind to an embolectomy of any vessel.

Key steps

1. An incision is made in the skin over the artery. The vessels are identified and retraction tapes placed around them.

2. The artery is clamped with noncrushing vascular clamps or bulldog clamps or occluded with pressure on the retraction tapes. An arteriotomy is made with a knife, followed by Potts scissor.

3. A Fogarty embolectomy catheter, with an inflatable balloon near the tip, is passed into the artery and beyond the point of occlusion.

4. The balloon is inflated with saline solution, and the catheter is withdrawn from the artery. If successful, the inflated balloon will have pulled thrombus, debris, or other obstructing material from the artery (Fig. 15-25). Vigorous back-bleeding and the increased strength of distal pulses indicate clearing of the artery.

5. The artery may be flushed with heparinized saline solution from the instrument table, delivered by syringe and soft catheter.

6. The arteriotomy is closed with a running suture line of nonabsorbable monofilament. A Doppler may be used to verify unobstructed blood flow.

7. The wound is closed with layers of interrupted absorbable suture.

Insertion of vena cava filter

Vena cava filters are placed to prevent the often fatal complication of pulmonary embolism that may result from deep vein thrombosis (DVT). Thrombus in large veins of the leg and pelvis can fragment, sending emboli into the flow of blood toward the heart and becoming trapped in the pulmonary vasculature. *Virchow's triad* of venous stasis, hypercoagulability, and injury to the venous endothelium (Fernsebner et al., 1984) contribute to the formation of venous thrombosis.

A filter such as the cone-shaped Greenfield filter can intercept clot before it reaches the lungs. The trapped embolus can then be treated with anticoagulation and fibrinolysis agents such as tissue plasminogen activator (TPN), streptokinase, and urokinase. The filter allows some blood flow through it even with clot trapped within. As a result, the filter does not completely occlude venous return to the heart (see Figs. 15-26 and 15-27).

The filters can be inserted operatively or percutaneously through either the femoral or jugular veins. Semi-

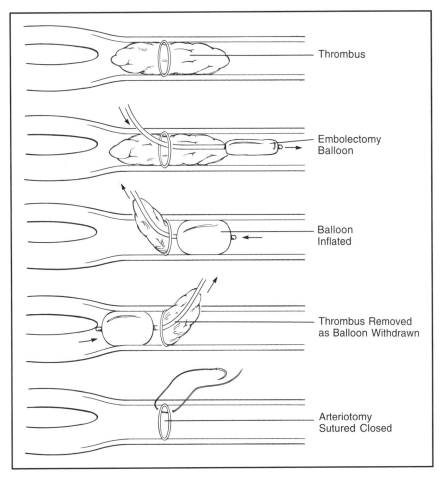

—— Thrombus

—— Embolectomy
Balloon

—— Balloon
Inflated

—— Thrombus Removed
as Balloon Withdrawn

—— Arteriotomy
Sutured Closed

FIGURE 15-25 Embolectomy facilitated by inflatable balloon catheter.

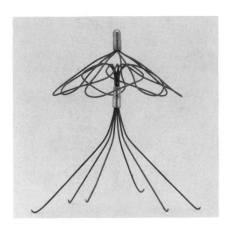

FIGURE 15-26 Simon Nitinol vena cava filter. (Photo courtesy of Nitinol Medical Technologies, Inc.)

Fowler's position is used, with the patient's head turned to the left for a transjugular approach. (Figure 15-28 illustrates deployment of a vena cava filter.)

Key steps

1. Under local anesthesia, an incision is made in the neck parallel to the clavicle.

2. The jugular vein is isolated, and a retraction tape is placed around it for control.
3. After heparinization, an incision is made in the vein with a knife. An intraoperative angiogram, including the renal veins, is taken with half-strength contrast medium.
4. The Greenfield filter is inserted through a No. 14 French sheath (Moore, 1991) and positioned below the renal veins. The placement is verified with angiography.
5. The venotomy is closed with interrupted 5-0 or 6-0 nonabsorbable sutures, and the wound is closed.

Venous Surgery

Varicose vein excision

A primary varicose vein occurs when the superficial branches of the saphenous vein in the leg become overdistended with blood. The distention causes unidirectional valves within the vein to become incompetent, and blood to pool within the leg. The veins dilate and become tortuous, resulting in a burning sensation, aching, and disfigurement in the leg that increase with standing. Varicose veins may be associated with dermatitis or ulcerations.

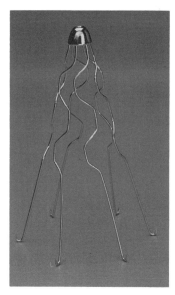

FIGURE 15-27 Titanium Greenfield vena cava filter. (Photo courtesy of Medi-tech, division of Boston Scientific Corp., Watertown, MA.)

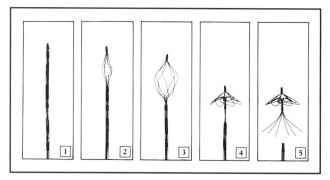

FIGURE 15-28 Nitinol filter as it is deployed in the vena cava. (Photo courtesy of Nitinol Medical Technologies, Inc.)

Varicose vein excision is performed when the patient is symptomatic and the more conservative treatments of elastic support stockings or injections of sclerosing agents have not provided substantive relief. Concerns about the salvage of these veins for potential use in vascular grafting are irrelevant because the diseased veins are unacceptable for grafting. The patient is positioned supine with the operative leg circumferentially prepped.

Key steps

1. Preoperatively, the skin over the veins to be excised is outlined using an indelible ink marker. The patient is standing when this is done. The markings must remain after the surgical prep.
2. A small incision is made in the skin over the site of the varicosity, and the vein is isolated.
3. The vein is transected, and the proximal end is ligated with nonabsorbable suture. A long, thin, flexible vein "stripper" is passed into the vein and threaded the length of the varicosed segment, or as far as possible.
4. A second skin incision is made over the end of the stripper at the distal site, and the end of the stripper is passed out through the skin.
5. A cap is placed over the end of the stripper and secured, and the stripper is pulled back into the wound and through the leg, withdrawing the vein. Pressure is applied to the leg with a rolled sponge or towel as the stripper is withdrawn.
6. Multiple skin incisions are usually necessary. After all affected veins have been excised, the skin incisions are closed, and compression dressings are applied.

Trauma

Traumatic injuries to blood vessels cause complications that vary with the area of the body affected. Acute arterial occlusions generally exhibit a characteristic progression of vasoconstriction, vasodilatation, and the establishment of collateral circulation (Burke et al., 1988). The injury may be obvious, presenting as frank hemorrhage, or it may be obscured in the shocky condition of the multiple injury patient. The surgical repair may involve a simple suture ligation or patch grafting, or may be more complicated as with interposition grafting using vein or synthetic conduit.

Carotid artery injuries

Blunt injuries to the neck caused by direct blow or stretching may cause intimal tears to the carotid arteries. Although not immediately symptomatic, the disrupted endothelium may serve as a source for thrombus formation with later occlusion. The injured carotid artery segment may be replaced with a reversed saphenous vein interposition graft.

Penetrating wounds to the neck can cause lacerations to the arteries that may be closed primarily; however, the entire neck and upper chest are generally prepped, as is a segment of leg for possible saphenous vein harvest. Depending on the path of a missile low in the neck, the thorax may have been entered, requiring the placement of thoracic catheters (Brewster, 1989).

Brachial artery injuries

Brachial artery injuries can occur in conjunction with orthopaedic fractures of the arm or dislocation of the elbow. An embolectomy using Fogarty balloon catheters and primary suturing of the artery may be adequate. More extensive injuries may require resection of a segment of artery with or without a saphenous vein interposition graft.

Intimal injury can occur from abrasion of angioscopic catheters during cardiac catheterization, causing thrombus formation. Embolectomy can be carried out under local anesthesia, or a more extensive repair may be necessary.

Popliteal artery injuries

Orthopaedic fractures of the knee and blunt injuries caused by dislocation can cause obstruction and injury to the popliteal artery. This artery is particularly vulnerable because of its anatomic location behind the knee and the lack of protection afforded it.

In the case of orthopaedic injury, amputation may be required because of combined orthopaedic and vascular injury. The vascular injury should be repaired first (Burke et al., 1989), followed by the bone fixation.

Arteriovenous Fistula

Indications

An arteriovenous fistula may be formed in the wrist to create hemodialysis access in patients with chronic renal failure. An end-to-side anastomosis is formed between the cephalic vein and radial artery in the wrist, usually on the ventral surface, and the remaining end of the cephalic vein is tied off. In small children and the elderly in whom fragile veins are a concern, a side-to-side anastomosis may be substituted.

Position

The patient is supine during the procedure.

Key steps

1. Under local anesthesia, a transverse incision is made over the cephalic vein and radial artery in the wrist, and the vessels are identified. The nondominant hand is selected if the vein is suitable.
2. Retraction tapes are placed around the vessels for control of bleeding, and the blood vessels are dissected free of the surrounding tissues.
3. The cephalic vein is transected, and the nonoperative end is tied off with a silk tie.
4. With pressure on the retraction tapes to prevent back-bleeding, an incision is made in the radial artery with a pointed microknife and extended with Potts scissors. The retraction tapes may be clipped to the drapes with bulldog clamps or snaps to maintain pressure while the vessels are sutured.
5. The free end of the cephalic vein is anastomosed to the side of the radial artery using two running suture lines of 7-0 nonabsorbable suture.
6. After the anastomosis is complete and the retraction tapes removed, patency of the fistula is confirmed by the presence of a vibration over the vessels, called a "thrill." The thrill is caused by turbulent blood flow beneath the vessel wall as higher-pressure arterial blood flow and lower-pressure venous blood flow mix. If a thrill is not felt, a bruit may be heard if a sterile stethoscope is held directly over the blood vessel.
7. The wound is closed with interrupted absorbable sutures.
8. The patient is instructed that he or she should feel a thrill similar to a cat "purring" over the fistula site.

SUMMARY

The progression and ravages of vascular disease can be devastating and life threatening for patients. The perioperative nurse caring for these patients must provide supportive care at a stressful and emotional moment during their surgical experience. Information has been provided in this chapter to assist the nurse in planning care for patients undergoing vascular surgical procedures.

REFERENCES

Baker, W.H. (Ed.) (1985). *Diagnosis and treatment of carotid artery disease* (2nd ed.). New York: Futura Publishing Co.

Brewster, D.C. (Ed.) (1989). *Common problems in vascular surgery*. Chicago: Year Book.

Burke, J.F., Boyd, R.J., & McCabe, C.J. (1988). *Trauma management: Early management of visceral, nervous system and musculoskeletal injuries*. Chicago: Year Book.

Cambria, R.P., Brewster, D.C., Abbott, W.M., Freehan, M., Megerman, J., LaMuraglia, G., Wilson, R., Wilson, D., Teplick, R., & Davison, J.K. (1990). Transperitoneal versus retroperitoneal approach for aortic reconstruction: A randomized prospective study. *Journal of Vascular Surgery, 11,* 314–324.

Chassin, M.R. (1989). *The appropriateness of selected medical and surgical procedures*. New York: Association for Health Services Research and Health Administration Press.

Cooley, D.A. (1986). *Surgical treatment of aortic aneurysms*. Philadelphia: W.B. Saunders.

Cull, D.L., Feinberg, R.L., Wheeler, J.R., Snyder Jr., S.O., Gregory, R.T., Gayle, R.G., & Parent III, F.N. (1991). Experience with laser-assisted balloon angioplasty and a rotary angioplasty instrument: Lessons learned. *Journal of Vascular Surgery, 14,* 332–339.

Fernsebner, B., Baum, P.L., & Bartlett, C. (1984). Surgical prevention of pulmonary emboli, vena cava interruption. *AORN Journal, 39,* 56–64.

Fogarty, A.M. (1991). Angioscopy, new developments in vascular surgery. *AORN Journal, 53,* 725–728.

Greenhalgh, R.M., & Mannick, J.A. (Eds.) (1990). *The cause and management of aneurysms*. Philadelphia: W.B. Saunders.

McCann, R.L., Schwartz, L.B., & Pieper, K.S. (1991). Vascular complications of cardiac catheterization. *Journal of Vascular Surgery, 14,* 375–381.

Moore, W.S. (Ed.). (1991). *Vascular surgery: A comprehensive review* (3rd ed.). Philadelphia: W.B. Saunders.

O'Brien, M.S., & Rocotta, J.J. (1991). Conserving resources after carotid endarterectomy: Selective use of the intensive care unit. *Journal of Vascular Surgery, 14,* 796–802.

Williams, P.L. (Ed.) (1989). *Gray's Anatomy*. New York: Churchill Livingstone.

Zweibel, W.J. (1982). *Introduction to vascular ultrasonography*. New York: Grune & Stratton.

Chapter 16

Plastic Surgery

Key Concepts

- Successful plastic surgery depends on meeting the patient's perception of success as well as achieving a positive clinical outcome. This means that patient preparation, patient education, and realistic expectations are imperative for a successful outcome. The successful outcome in other surgical disciplines is dependent on more objective criteria.

- Body image is a significant motivator for patients seeking plastic surgical procedures.

- Plastic surgical procedures are loosely categorized as *cosmetic,* when the primary objective is to improve the appearance of a body part, and *reconstructive,* when improving function is the most important goal. All procedures fall, to some extent, into both categories.

- It is essential that health care professionals maintain a nonjudgmental approach to plastic surgery patients. Patients undergoing cosmetic procedures require and deserve the same support and quality of care that reconstructive surgery patients enjoy.

- Many plastic surgical procedures are performed with local anesthesia and/or intravenous conscious sedation. The perioperative nurse must possess the knowledge and skill to monitor these patients effectively.

- An increasing number of plastic surgical procedures are being performed on an outpatient basis. Preoperative preparation and effective postoperative teaching are essential as these patients or family members must be prepared to assume a large portion of the responsibility for their postoperative care.

- Many plastic surgical procedures involve grafts or flaps—the advancement, rotation, or transfer of skin and underlying tissues.

- Advancement in microscope and instrument technology has driven the subspecialty of microvascular surgery to new heights of achievement. With this advanced technology, plastic surgeons can either address defects that they were previously unable to repair, or they can achieve results far superior to those using less sophisticated techniques.

INTRODUCTION

Plastic surgery is a broad term used in connection with surgical procedures performed for cosmetic or reconstructive purposes. The term *plastic* is derived from the Greek word *plastikos*, meaning to mold, form, or give shape. The goal of a plastic surgical procedure is to achieve the most normal form of appearance and the highest degree of function possible for the patient. Plastic surgery addresses congenital deformities as well as those caused by disease, trauma, and the aging process.

This chapter discusses general principles related to plastic surgery, such as factors affecting the healing process, anatomy of the skin, and closure for minimal scarring. The most common cosmetic and reconstructive surgical procedures will be described, as well as the supplies, equipment, and instruments used for each.

The scope of plastic surgery is broad, and few operating room suites will provide perioperative nurses the opportunity to participate in the full range of procedures. For example, many cosmetic procedures are performed in a physician's office in order to control cost to the patient, as most procedures are not covered by health insurance. Procedures such as cleft palate and lip repair will be done only in settings where pediatric surgery is performed, and reconstructive surgery is done primarily at facilities that are trauma centers and where there is a physician trained in microvascular surgery.

This chapter will be most helpful for the perioperative nurse who will be caring for patients undergoing plastic surgery procedures, but all perioperative nurses can benefit from the chapter as principles of plastic surgery are often incorporated into general surgery. For example, the surgeon who removes a lesion from the face of a patient will close the wound with what is referred to as a "plastic closure." The incision will be made in a natural crease, when possible, and closure will be done using a fine suture and needle. The reader will find many other examples and principles that can be incorporated into daily perioperative practice.

Historical Perspectives

Plastic surgery is one of the oldest surgical specialties. Ancient records verify attempts to change and improve the appearance of people. The Egyptians grafted skin as early as 3500 BC. Accounts of surgical reconstruction of the amputated nose appear as early as 600 BC in the *Ayurdeva*, the sacred Hindu medical record. Reconstruction of congenital anomalies was documented in Greek literature, and the early Roman, Celcius, documented the use of living tissue for facial reconstruction. Galen, in the second century A.D., described reconstruction of lips, ears, and nostrils.

Tagliocozzi, in sixteenth century Italy, used a delayed flap to reconstruct the nose, ear, and lip. Surgeons continued to use this technique until the development of microvascular surgery in this century. The concept of asepsis and the refinement of anesthesia techniques decreased surgical mortality and distress and made surgery a more feasible option for patients.

Skin transplants, or skin grafts, met with limited success before World War I. The types of injuries that occurred in the succession of modern wars presented new challenges that resulted in the rapid development of successful techniques in skin grafting and flap reconstruction. This advancement established plastic surgery as a recognized surgical specialty. The development of microvascular surgery provided the specialty with even more sophisticated techniques, enabling plastic surgeons to address defects previously impossible to repair.

NURSING CONSIDERATIONS

General Information

The plastic surgery patient and body image

It is said that plastic surgery is not only surgery of the body, but also of the mind. Body image is the way the individual *thinks* he looks. That perception has a significant impact on self-concept and self-esteem and affects the way the individual interacts with others. Individuals with a healthy body image acknowledge both their strong and weak attributes and accept them. Body image involves both appearance and function. Individuals with a healthy self-concept are more secure and comfortable with themselves and with others. Conversely, individuals who *think* their appearance or ability to function is less than acceptable can be insecure and uncomfortable with others. Body image plays an important role in a patient's motivation to seek both cosmetic and reconstructive surgical procedures. Surgery that enhances an individual's outward appearance may also foster a new feeling of confidence and inner satisfaction.

For the patient who perceives that some feature or body function is unacceptable, correcting or improving the defect can facilitate an improvement in self-image and increase the patient's mental and psychological well-being. A desire to feel better about oneself and to be able to function more effectively are both valid motives for seeking plastic surgery.

Expectations

The success of a plastic surgical procedure is largely dependent on the degree to which the patient's expectations are realized. A clinically successful procedure may be considered a failure if the patient is disappointed. It is imperative that the plastic surgeon and nurse assess the patient's expectations and reality orientation carefully during the initial assessment. A patient with inappropriate expectations is a poor surgical candidate. During the preoperative assessment, the perioperative nurse might identify difficulties with the patient's realistic expectations of surgery. These should be communicated to the surgeon so that he can address the issues with the patient prior to surgery.

It is essential that health care professionals be nonjudgmental and supportive. This is particularly pertinent to patients having elective, cosmetic surgery. When health care professionals judge cosmetic surgery to be less or less worthy than other procedures, they communicate these feelings nonverbally. Each patient, regardless of the severity of the deficit being corrected, needs acceptance and support. Nurses must remember that a patient who feels alienated from others because drooping eyelids and facial wrinkles make him look tired and old needs as much support for his surgery as the patient who has lost a thumb in an accident.

Categories of Plastic Surgery

Several general principles apply to plastic surgery regardless of whether the surgery is classified as cosmetic or reconstructive. The categorization of procedures is often arbitrary and based on whether insurance coverage will pay for the procedure, although many cosmetic procedures are also reconstructive in nature. Factors affecting the healing process are important in all surgical procedures, but especially so when microvascular procedures, such as grafts, have been performed. Anatomy of skin and wound closure for minimal scarring apply to all surgical procedures, but achieve a different level of importance in plastic surgery.

Plastic surgical procedures are very loosely categorized as aesthetic (cosmetic) and reconstructive. Cosmetic procedures strive primarily to improve the appearance of a body part, whereas reconstructive procedures are concerned more with function. All plastic surgical procedures fall, to a certain extent, into both categories. For example, a facelift, primarily done for cosmetic reasons, involves reconstruction of the facial tissues using the same principles of tissue handling and transfer as the reconstruction of a post-traumatic soft tissue facial defect. And, when reconstructing a deformity of any kind, the plastic surgeon strives for an acceptable appearance as well as optimal function.

Common cosmetic surgical procedures include rhytidectomy (facelift) and blepharoplasty (eye lift). Brow lift, mentoplasty (chin reshaping), dermabrasion (sanding of the skin), and chemical peels are also cosmetic procedures of the face that can be done in various combinations to achieve optimal results. Other cosmetic procedures of the face include rhinoplasty (reshaping of the nose) and otoplasty (ear pinning).

Elective procedures of the breast include augmentation, reduction, and mastopexy (breast lift involving only the skin). Abdominoplasty, brachioplasty (arm recontouring), and natoplasty (reshaping of the buttocks) are all procedures that help to achieve a more pleasing body contour. Liposuction can be used in conjunction with many surgical procedures to "fine tune" contouring.

Cosmetic procedures, considered elective surgery, are not covered by third party payers. However, a cosmetic procedure may have a significant functional component and, under those circumstances, might be covered by a third party payer. For example, a septorhinoplasty may correct an obstructed airway in addition to improving the appearance of a nose. Reduction mammaplasty can relieve neck and back pain as well as improve body proportion and appearance.

The goal of reconstructive surgery is to repair or replace a damaged or absent part of the body. Deformity of a body part can be congenital, such as cleft lip, craniofacial anomalies, or the absence of digits. Deformity can also be the result of trauma, such as burns and accidents. Disease processes such as cancer can result in the removal of a body part such as a breast or a skin tumor. Reconstructive surgery replaces missing tissue and repairs deformities using a variety of tissue transfer techniques involving flaps and grafts.

Factors Affecting the Healing Process

Healing is a slow process that occurs over a significant period of time. Both the health care professional and the patient assume responsibility for managing the environment in which healing takes place. For outpatients, preoperative and postoperative teaching is essential to prepare the patient to assume this responsibility. Hospitalized patients and the health care professional share the responsibility in the early postoperative period, but the patient must be prepared to continue to manage his environment and promote wound healing once he leaves the health care facility.

Plastic surgery is heavily dependent on grafts and flaps, which must have good vascularity to survive. Factors that affect blood flow to the operative site are critical to wound healing.

Nicotine is a potent vasoconstrictor that inhibits blood flow. Smokers should refrain from smoking for several weeks prior to surgery and during the first few weeks following surgery. Impaired circulation due to smoking can delay healing and cause sloughing of the skin and unsightly scarring. A surgeon might even recommend that no one smoke in the patient's presence following delicate free flap reconstruction or replantation surgery.

Aspirin interferes with platelet agglutination and can predispose the patient to intraoperative bleeding and postoperative hematoma. Patients should avoid taking aspirin or products containing aspirin for several days before surgery.

Nutritional status affects wound healing. Most plastic surgery patients are in good general health. It would be unlikely for a surgeon to accept an individual in poor general health and with deficient nutritional status for an elective procedure. When possible, reconstructive procedures are usually delayed until the general health and nutritional status of the patient are appropriate for good healing. However, it is always important to include the principles of good nutrition in patient education.

Oxygen is a requirement for wound healing. Under normal circumstances, tissue oxygenation is dependent on good circulation. Positioning and restrictive dressings or clothing can impair blood flow to a healing body part. Vigilance on the part of the health care professional and appropriate patient teaching can avoid this type of complication in wound healing.

Anatomy of the Skin

The appearance of the skin in different parts of the body varies widely in color, texture, thickness, and the presence of adjunctive structures such as hair follicles and sweat glands. Successful plastic surgical procedures rely on using tissue as much like the original as possible, for both optimal appearance and optimal function.

The skin is composed of two main layers. The thinner, outer layer, the *epidermis*, contains layers of epithelial cells. The thicker, inner layer, the *dermis*, is composed primarily of connective tissue with elastic and collagen fibers. The dermis also contains lymphatics, nerves, and small perforating vessels from the subcutaneous tissue. Hair follicles, sweat glands, and sebaceous glands are also located in the dermis (Fig. 16-1).

The aging of skin is a process of atrophy. As elastic fibers degenerate the skin loses resilience. Loss of collagen bundles results in both thinning of the skin and a decrease in tensile strength, making the skin more fragile. As the skin thins and adherence to underlying tissues loosens, folds or wrinkles develop. The fine, shallow wrinkles disappear when the skin is stretched, but the deep, coarser wrinkles remain.

Aging of the face begins by age 30. The most significant changes take place predominantly in the face. The progression is gradual, starting with redundancy of the upper eyelids, the fine laugh lines around the eyes, and a

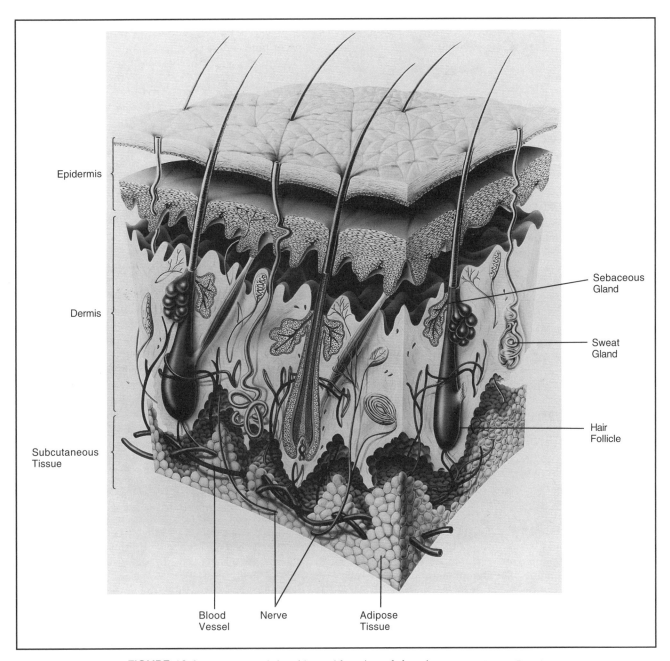

FIGURE 16-1 Anatomy of the skin: epidermis and dermis. (Artist: Vincent Perez)

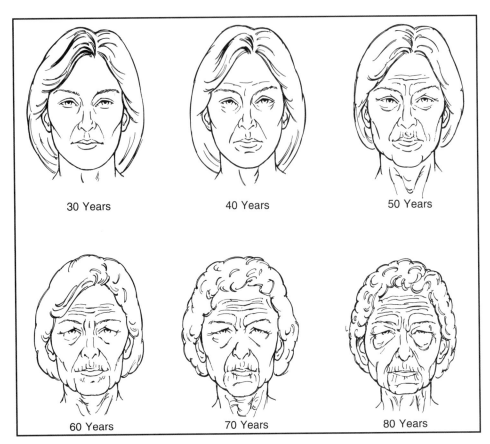

FIGURE 16-2 Facial changes resulting from the aging process.

deepening of the nasolabial grooves. Later, the forehead begins to wrinkle, followed by wrinkling of the neck (Barton, 1991) (Fig. 16-2).

Closure for Minimal Scarring

Plastic surgeons attempt to create the most aesthetic scar possible, regardless of the surgical procedure. When possible, incisions are positioned where they are hidden by normal body structures. For example, the incision for an augmentation mammaplasty is hidden in the inframammary fold; an abdominoplasty incision, while very long, is placed low enough to be hidden by panties or a bathing suit.

For the most aesthetic scarring, the size and direction of an incision should always follow the body's lines of minimal tension. These are lines formed by habitual expression and lines of skin relaxation that accompany movement of parts of the body. Straight line incisions tend to contract and pucker during wound healing. When possible, the contractile forces should be distributed in more than one direction. The fundamental technique in plastic surgery for the release of linear contractures is the Z-plasty, or the transposition of two triangular flaps (Fig. 16-3). When tissue is excised leaving a round defect, the wound is elongated to avoid puckering and to create a better scar (Fig. 16-4).

Synthetic Implants

Synthetic implants are made of material that has been designed for use in medical application. These materials should be noncarcinogenic, mechanically reliable, and capable of withstanding long-term stability. Most synthetic implants used for soft tissue augmentation are made of plastic and silicone, whereas those for bone are made of methyl methacrylate, Silastic, demineralized bone paste, and polyethylene. The major advantages of using synthetic devices include the greater flexibility to contour and mold, ample quantity, and ease of use. Disadvantages mainly include the increased chance of infection and rejection.

Some implants are under increased scrutiny due to legal issues related to complications. Some breast implants, for example, are available only for research protocols.

Nursing considerations for synthetic implants

1. The implant should be handled according to the manufacturer's instructions.
2. Some surgeon's soak or impregnate implants with an antibiotic solution.
3. Documentation regarding the implant information, such as size, description, and identifying numbers, must be recorded in the intraoperative record.
4. Some manufacturers provide an implant information card to be carried by the patient. The card should be

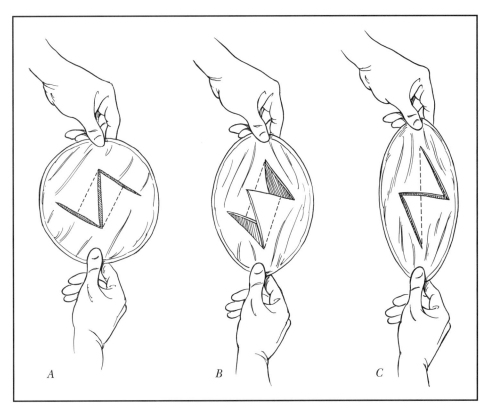

FIGURE 16-3 Illustration of the Z-plasty technique. Two triangular flaps are elevated and transposed to elongate and relax a scar by interrupting the lines of tension.

placed in the chart to be given to the patient prior to discharge.

Tissue Expansion

Tissue expansion is a safe, reliable, and cost-effective procedure to stretch the tissues adjacent to a defect in order to increase the amount of tissue available for reconstruction. The well-vascularized tissue produced through expansion will have the appropriate characteristics (e.g., texture, color, sensation, hair-bearing qualities) to reconstruct the defect. Expanding adjacent tissue also avoids a donor site defect.

The expander itself is a soft, pliable pouch with a self-sealing inflation reservoir that is either connected to the pouch by a tube or may be incorporated into the pouch itself. Tissue expanders are handled in the same manner as prosthetic implants. Expanders come in many sizes and shapes (Fig. 16-5). They can also be custom designed to address specific needs. The surgeon positions the expander and implants the valve subcutaneously a short distance away. The expander is injected at regular intervals with isotonic saline by inserting a needle into the valve. Serial injections are done in the doctor's office using strict aseptic technique. The patient experiences little discomfort beyond the needle stick and a feeling of initial tightness or fullness, which subsides as the tissue expands.

The major disadvantage is related to time. Tissue expansion takes place over a period of months, depending on the elasticity of the tissue being expanded and the amount of tissue needed for reconstruction. In many cases, more than one expander is placed around the defect to provide sufficient tissue. The patient will experience a period of disfigurement as the expander increases in size, particularly if it is in a location not easily hidden by clothing. Support and encouragement are needed at this time.

COSMETIC SURGERY PROCEDURES

Cosmetic surgical procedures are elective procedures, generally performed because the patient desires to change or improve a part of the body. Many of the procedures involve the face, and a patient may have several procedures, such as rhytidectomy, blepharoplasty, and brow lift, done over time or in one session. A unique relationship will exist between the patient and the perioperative nurse as the patient is supported in a nonjudgmental manner while undergoing surgery to alter appearances. Often, when procedures are done in a physician's office or outpatient clinic, the same nurse will be able to coordinate all perioperative care and teaching, including administration of intravenous conscious sedation.

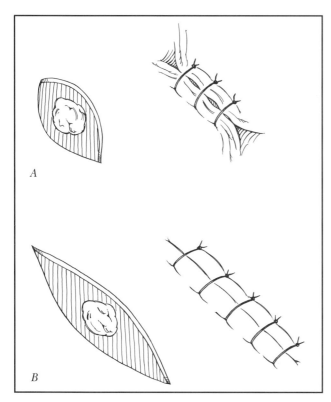

FIGURE 16-4 Closing a round defect results in a puckered scar (*A*). Elongating the excision results in a more aesthetic closure (*B*).

Face, Brow, and Lid Surgery

Perioperative nursing considerations

1. A rhytidectomy can last several hours, especially if it involves one or more additional procedures such as blepharoplasty, submental lipectomy, or coronal brow lift. The nurse must consider the patient's physical comfort and well-being. A warming blanket and pressure-relieving mattress may be indicated, especially if the procedure is done under general anesthesia, which results in vasodilation and loss of body heat.
2. If the procedure is done under local anesthesia with intravenous conscious sedation, the nurse must be prepared to monitor the patient appropriately and provide emotional support.
3. While the patient is under general anesthesia, the nurse shares in the responsibility for positioning the patient, protecting the patient from injury related to positioning, and maintaining an appropriate body temperature (not allowing the patient to get too warm or too cold).
4. The patient's hair may be clipped along the incision line and secured with rubber bands.
5. If the surgeon marks the patient's face preoperatively, the nurse must take care to preserve the markings during the preoperative skin preparation.
6. It is essential to protect the patient's eyes during the preoperative skin prep and during the surgical procedure

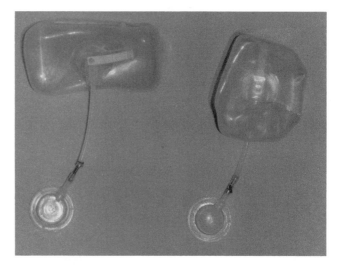

FIGURE 16-5 Tissue expanders come in a variety of shapes and sizes.

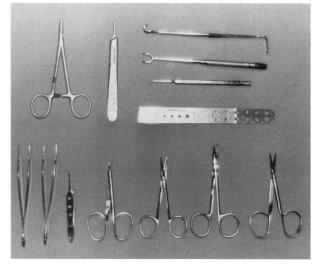

FIGURE 16-6 Instruments for eye lid surgery: *top row:* Webster needle holder, #3 knife handle, Senn retractor, double hook, ruler; *bottom row:* Adson forcep with teeth, smooth Adson forcep, Bishop Harmon forcep, strabismus scissors, straight iris scissors, Stevens tenotomy scissors, curved iris scissors.

7. The surgeon may inject the operative site with a local anesthetic containing epinephrine to promote vasoconstriction and control hemostasis. Because the face is very vascular, infection is a rare complication.
8. A light source will be necessary to support a fiber-optic headlight or lighted retractors.
9. Postoperatively, the patient's head should be elevated to reduce swelling. The patient should avoid activities that increase blood pressure, such as lifting, straining, coughing, sneezing, and vomiting, that could promote hematoma formation. Postanesthesia nausea must be controlled.
10. Instrumentation is fine and delicate, much like that used in ophthalmic and microvascular surgery (Fig. 16-6).

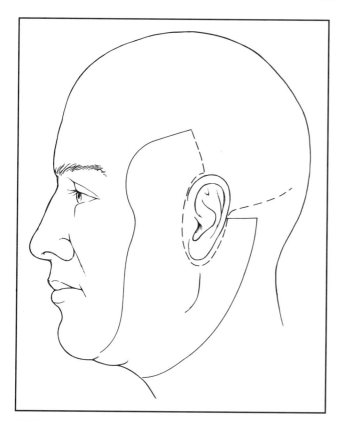

FIGURE 16-7 Proposed facelift incision and area of undermining.

11. Care must be taken to protect the eyes from the cleansing agent used for the preoperative skin preparation.

Rhytidectomy

A rhytidectomy, or facelift, first performed in the early 1900s, is one of the most commonly performed surgical procedures. Patients with sagging, wrinkled facial appearance resulting from sun exposure, weight loss, or the aging process frequently look older than their years and tired or worried. A facelift can produce a softening of the creases and tightening of the face and neck.

Key steps

1. Incisions are made in the temporal region hidden in the hairline, extending in front of the ear, around the lobe, and into the hair toward the back of the head (Fig. 16-7).
2. The skin and subcutaneous tissue are undermined and elevated, exposing the underlying tissues.
3. The parotid gland, facial nerve branches, and external jugular vein can be visualized and carefully avoided once the superficial musculoaponeurotic system (SMAS) is elevated (Fig. 16-8,*A* and *B*).
4. The SMAS and platysma are tightened, and excess fat is excised or suctioned.
5. Facial and neck skin is redraped over the tightened facial structures.

6. Redundant skin is excised, and the flaps are secured in place. Sutures are used where incision lines are visible; staples can be used in the hairline (Fig. 16-8,*C*). Suture used in the repair should be undyed, because dyed suture may be visible through translucent skin and appear as a blemish.
7. Drains may be used to prevent hematoma or seroma formation.
8. A bulky pressure dressing is applied to promote adherence of redraped skin to the underlying tissues and to prevent development of hematoma or seroma.

Coronal brow lift

The normal aging process can cause transverse forehead wrinkling, brow ptosis, and glabellar wrinkling. The frontalis muscle, innervated by the frontal branch of the facial nerve, contracts to elevate the brow, producing wrinkles transversely across the forehead. Creases in the forehead become permanently engraved in the skin and frown lines develop between the eyebrows. This causes the patient to appear perpetually tired or sad. When a coronal brow lift is needed, it is usually performed in conjunction with a rhytidectomy. Following the removal of excess skin and adjustment of muscles of the forehead, the brow and forehead have a smooth and more youthful appearance.

Key steps

1. The preferred approach is a bicoronal incision that will be hidden by the patient's hair. The incision line is injected with epinephrine to promote vasoconstriction and reduce bleeding. Alternative incision sites include the hairline, mid-forehead, and supraciliary (Fig. 16-9).
2. The skin over the frontal and forehead area is undermined down to the level of the orbital rims.
3. The soft tissue attachment at or near the level of the supraorbital rim must be mobilized for an effective brow elevation (Hodges & Tebbetts, 1991).
4. Blunt dissection can be continued down to the tip of the nose if necessary.
5. The procerus, corrugator, and frontalis muscle activity is interrupted to reduce the ability to produce forehead wrinkling.
6. The skin is redraped over the forehead. Excess skin is removed and the flap is sutured or stapled into place. The surgeon is careful to avoid excess tension on the flap to reduce the possibility of vascular compromise and hair loss.
7. The bulky facelift pressure dressing provides compression to stabilize the flap and minimize the formation of hematoma.

Mentoplasty/genioplasty (reshaping of the chin)

When the chin is receding or too prominent, it can be reshaped either in conjunction with a rhytidectomy or independently. The chin can be augmented either by inserting a prosthesis or by splitting and advancing the

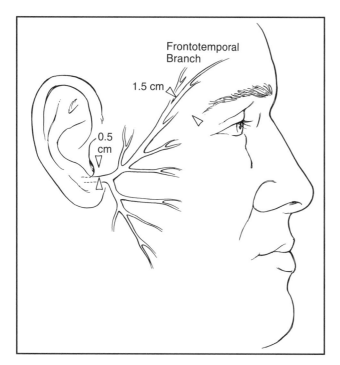

A

FIGURE 16-8 *A*, Branches of the facial nerve. *B*, Facial structures to identify and protect during a facelift. *C*, redraping of skin and completed closure following facelift.

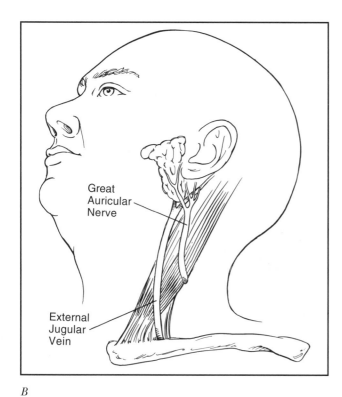

B

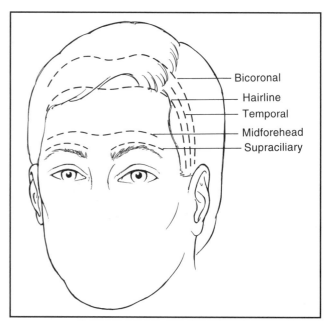

C

Blepharoplasty (eyelid lift)

Loss of elasticity of the eyelid skin and muscles during the aging process results in eyelid redundancy, or *blepharochalasia*, usually more extreme in the upper eyelids. Blepharochalasia is derived from the Greek words *blepharon*, meaning eyelid, and *chalasis*, meaning relax-

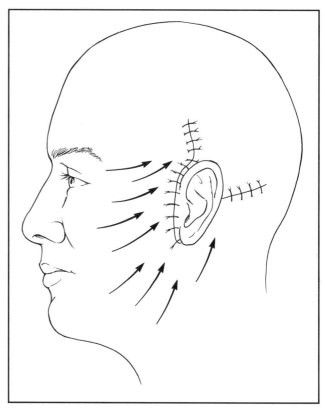

FIGURE 16-9 Incision alternatives for a brow lift.

mental process of the mandible. Reduction or contouring of a prominent chin can be accomplished by recontouring the mental process. Soft tissue is usually not recontoured.

ation. Blepharochalasia make the patient look perpetually tired or sad.

Severe blepharochalasia may obstruct the patient's vision. Before a blepharoplasty, the patient may be asked to see an ophthalmologist to determine if there is any ocular symptomatology.

Depending on the type of blepharochalasia, a patient may have an upper blepharoplasty, involving only upper eyelid redundancy; a lower blepharoplasty, involving only the lower eyelids; or a quadrilateral blepharoplasty, involving all four eyelids. Blepharoplasty is frequently performed at the same time as a rhytidectomy.

Key steps

1. Incisions are placed in the upper eyelid fold and below the ciliary margin of the lower lid (Fig. 16-10). This approach conceals scars in the natural crease of the eyelid (Hodges & Tebbetts, 1991).
2. Excess skin and muscle are resected.
3. Periorbital fat is trimmed, using meticulous hemostasis.
4. Incisions are closed, using a very fine nonabsorbable suture.
5. Ophthalmic antibiotic ointment is applied to incision lines.
6. Iced saline dressings applied immediately postoperatively serve to control edema.

Chemical peel

Fine, crosshatched wrinkles around the eyes and lips cannot be eliminated by rhytidectomy or blepharoplasty. A chemical peel procedure is, in effect, a controlled chemical burning of the epidermis, the top layer of the skin. The peel eliminates the superficial, fine wrinkles and leaves new, smoother skin.

Hypopigmentation can occur following a chemical peel, producing a line of demarcation between the peeled and unpeeled skin. Fair-complexioned people are better candidates for chemical peel, as they will exhibit less color contrast between normal and treated skin. Asians, Blacks, and people of Mediterranean descent may heal with permanent pigmentary changes. Following a peel, the new skin is extremely photosensitive and the patient must avoid sun exposure by using sun block and a head covering.

A degreasing agent is used to remove oils from the skin that would impede the penetration of the peel solution. The peel solution is extremely caustic. It is imperative that the patient's eyes be protected during the procedure. Alcohol must be available to neutralize the peel solution should it come in contact inadvertently with the patient or staff (study the Material Safety Data Sheet for phenol for explicit instructions). Postoperative patient instructions include keeping the head elevated on pillows to reduce swelling and avoiding sun exposure, which aggravates the tendency for pigment alteration.

Key steps

1. Phenol is the most commonly used agent for the chemical peel procedure. Phenol, also known as carbolic

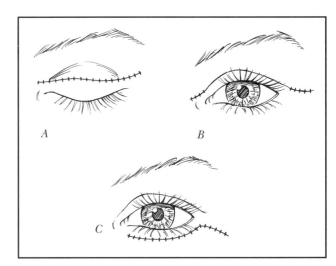

FIGURE 16-10 Location for blepharoplasty incisions.

acid, is a protein precipitant. It causes denaturation and coagulation of the surface keratin. Croton oil is added to the solution to act as a skin irritant, causing secondary collagen formation. The peel solution also contains liquid soap to act as a surfactant, which lowers surface tension and aids in skin and pore penetration (Barton, 1991).
2. Chemical peel solution is applied evenly and slowly with cotton applicators. It is important to work slowly as the concentration of phenol in the blood and the development of arrhythmias are interrelated.
3. The treated areas may be covered with waterproof tape to prevent evaporation and increase chemical penetration for a deeper peel.

Dermabrasion

Patients with irregularities of the skin surface such as acne pitting or scarring are candidates for dermabrasion. Dermabrasion is a sanding procedure for the epidermis that makes scarring less visible by evening out the skin surface. Sanding produces a fine spray of blood and skin. Ensure protection for the eyes of the patient and the surgical team.

Key steps

1. A local anesthetic agent with epinephrine may be injected to control bleeding.
2. Skin may be frozen with a refrigerant such as ethyl chloride to stiffen it, providing a firmer working surface for the dermabrader.
3. An abrasive wheel or burr is attached to a powered surgical instrument (Fig. 16-11). The surgeon abrades or sands the epidermis. The result appears similar to an abrasion or a superficial burn.
4. A sponge soaked with a local anesthetic agent containing epinephrine may be used to blot the skin after sanding, promoting hemostasis.
5. Antibiotic ointment and nonadherent dressings may be applied. These are removed on the first postoperative day.

6. Crusts form in 2 to 3 days and begin to separate within 2 weeks. The new skin will remain pink for 6 to 8 weeks.
7. Protection from the sun is imperative to prevent permanent discoloration.

Surgery to Shape the Nose

The nose is the most prominent facial feature. Reshaping of the nose (*rhinoplasty*) is a common plastic surgical procedure that may involve reshaping the tip, removing a dorsal hump, reducing or augmenting the overall size, or reshaping the overall contour of the nose. Difficulty in breathing due to obstructed nasal airway may also be an indicator for surgery. Septal reconstruction (*septoplasty*) involves restructuring of the septum that divides the two nasal passages. In conjunction with recontouring of the nose, the procedure is called *septorhinoplasty*. A *turbinectomy* may be required if the anterior turbinates are involved in airway obstruction.

The nose is composed of cartilage, bone, and soft tissue. The nasal bones—small, paired oblong bones—form the bridge of the nose. The middle portion of the nose is

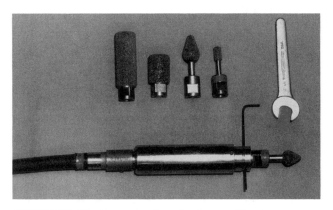

FIGURE 16-11 Dermabrader wheels are affixed to a powered surgical instrument.

called the dorsum. The nares, or nasal orifices, are formed by bilateral thin plates of alar cartilage (Fig. 16-12). The vestibule, immediately inside the nares, is lined with skin and has hairs called *vibrissae*. The nasal cavities are lined with mucous membrane. Separating the two nasal cavities are a thin column of cartilage, very thin ethmoid bone, and a thin, flat vomer bone. The anterior part of the cartilaginous septum is the columella. Turbinates are scroll-shaped bones that project medially from the lateral walls of the nasal cavity. They humidify and regulate nasal air flow. The function of the nose is independent of its size and shape (Moore, 1985).

Rhinoplasty can involve removal of bone and cartilage from a dorsal hump, reshaping the nasal tip, augmentation of a saddle deformity, reduction or augmentation of cartilage of the columella, excision of skin to diminish the size of the nares, and breaking and repositioning the nasal bones. A combination of techniques is required to address specific nasal deformities.

Most plastic surgeons strive for a natural looking nose that has a higher dorsal profile, less tip elevation, and less sculpturing of the alar cartilages (Byrd, 1991). When the restructuring of the nose fits the facial structure well, the changes may go unnoticed by observers because the "new nose" appears so natural. It is important to explain to the patient that the edema from surgical trauma subsides very gradually and the ultimate results of the procedure may not be evident for up to a year.

Perioperative nursing considerations

1. Rhinoplasty is usually done on an outpatient basis.
2. Rhinoplasty is performed with the patient in the supine position. The surgeon's preference card will indicate his preference for sitting or standing for the procedure.
3. Local anesthesia with intravenous sedation is preferred. There is increased potential for intraoperative bleeding with general anesthesia.

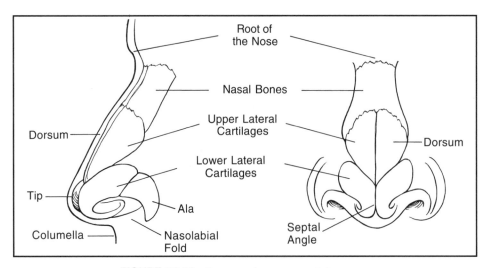

FIGURE 16-12 Structural anatomy of the nose.

4. A goal of preoperative patient preparation is to reduce the anxiety caused by the disconcerting sounds and the pressure that the patient can experience during the procedure.
5. Rhinoplasty instruments are unique adaptations of bone and cartilage instruments. They are used by ENT surgeons as well.
6. A light source will be needed if the surgeon uses a head light or fiberoptic instruments.
7. Splint material may be used, depending on the surgeon's preference.
8. The patient's head should be elevated postoperatively to reduce swelling.
9. Postoperative instructions should include directions to change the drip pad under the nose frequently and to observe the color and amount of drainage. Drainage should be blood-tinged and should not represent frank bleeding. Initially, the patient should sleep in the supine position to avoid putting pressure on the reconstructed nasal structures.

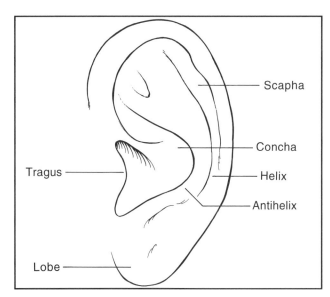

FIGURE 16-13   Anatomy of the external ear.

Rhinoplasty

Key steps

1. A local anesthetic agent with epinephrine is used for its vasoconstrictive effects, even with general anesthesia.
2. When possible, all incisions are made inside the nose to avoid external scars. Incisions just inside the rim of the ala expose bony cartilage structures. On occasion an open rhinoplasty—an external incision at the base of the columella—is necessary for adequate exposure.
3. The bony hump is reduced with nasal rasps, with a nasal saw, or with a chisel and mallet. The dorsum is trimmed of cartilage tissue. A rasp is used for final smoothing. A cartilage graft may be added to augment the dorsum.
4. To straighten or narrow the nose, osteotomies are performed at the bridge, using a chisel and mallet.
5. The nasal tip can be either reduced or altered. Alar cartilage is undermined and separated from the overlying skin. It is trimmed to the desired shape, and the mucosal flap is replaced.
6. Cartilage grafts, either from cartilage that has been removed from the nose or from the patient's ear, can be used in the reconstruction.
7. If a septal resection and septoplasty are indicated, the mucosa is elevated and the deviated cartilage and bone are resected and/or straightened, followed by replacement of the mucosal flap.
8. Both internal and external sutures, absorbable and nonabsorbable, are determined by physician preference.
9. Upon completion of the surgery, packing impregnated with an antibiotic ointment is usually placed in each nostril to maintain the reconstruction during the initial healing period.
10. An external splint may be fitted over the nose for protection. A small dressing is taped under the nose to absorb drainage.

External Ear Surgery

Only the outer ear is involved in an otoplasty procedure. The pinna or auricle, the shell-like part of the external ear, consists of a single elastic cartilage covered with a thin layer of skin. The structures of the outer ear are shown in Figure 16-13.

Ear prominence is usually a familial trait, the result of failure of the antihelix to develop or fold during fetal life. Individuals with protruding ears describe a history of peer ridicule, embarrassment, and self-consciousness. The majority of patients requiring otoplasty are male. Females tend to be less concerned with ear protrusion as they have the ability to cover their ears with a variety of hair styles. It is recommended that otoplasty not be considered before the ears attain about their adult size, usually by age 6. Although most otoplasty patients are children, results in adult patients are also excellent.

Perioperative nursing considerations

1. Explain everything to the child to allay fears and misconceptions.
2. Instruct the child and family not to remove or rearrange the dressing and to avoid pulling on the ears once the dressing has been removed.
3. Sensitivity to cold is a common side effect of otoplasty. Instruct the patient or the parents to protect the ears with earmuffs or scarf postoperatively.
4. Sensitivity to heat is also common. For 3 to 6 months postoperatively, ears may turn pink and swell in hot weather.

Otoplasty

Key steps

1. The ear is marked with methylene blue or a marking pen. At times, a hypodermic needle is used by dipping

the tip in methylene blue and passing it through the auricle to mark the cartilage.

2. A crescent-shaped incision is made behind the ear.
3. Cartilage is exposed by undermining the skin.
4. Cartilage is trimmed, thinned, and frequently scored to weaken it and "erase its memory."
5. Undyed, braided, nonabsorbent suture is used to suture the cartilage in place.
6. Absorbable suture is used to suture the skin into place.
7. The surgeon may elect to overcorrect the ear initially as the cartilage's "memory" might increase the postoperative projection slightly.
8. The surgeon may elect to use a drain to prevent fluid collection at the operative site. This is usually a small-diameter drain attached to a stopped vacuum tube (Fig. 16-14).
9. A bulky turban-like bandage with lots of cushioning around the ears is kept in place for 3 to 10 days.

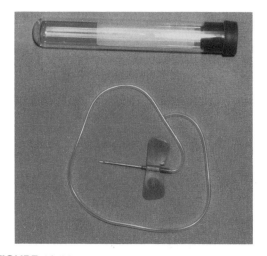

FIGURE 16-14 Small closed wound drainage system.

Surgery of the Breast

The breasts are envelopes of skin containing mammary glands and adipose tissue. They overlie the pectoralis muscle on the anterior surface of the chest from the second to the sixth ribs and from the edge of the sternum to the midaxillary line. Breast size is related to the amount of adipose tissue that surrounds the mammary glands. A network of ducts connect the mammary glands to the nipple (Fig. 16-15). The shape and size of breasts vary considerably among individuals, although the circular base of the breast is fairly constant (Moore, 1985).

Augmentation mammoplasty

For some women, small breasts have a negative impact on body image. Additionally, having breasts that are undersized in proportion to the rest of the body makes it difficult to obtain a proper fit in clothing. Aesthetically, augmentation mammoplasty can create fuller, more shapely breasts.

Augmentation mammoplasty is also indicated to compensate for the absence of breast and chest tissue in Poland's syndrome, and for hypomastia (failure of growth of the breast), which can be either unilateral or bilateral. Augmentation can also correct a mild ptosis by increasing the contents within the breast envelope. A sense of moderation and body proportion will guide the surgeon in deciding on the proper implant size.

Augmentation mammoplasty is the surgical placement of a breast prosthesis under the breast tissue (subglandular or prepectoral) or under the pectoralis muscle (subpectoral). The subpectoral approach produces an improved contour and softness of the breast, and the incidence of capsular contraction may be decreased.

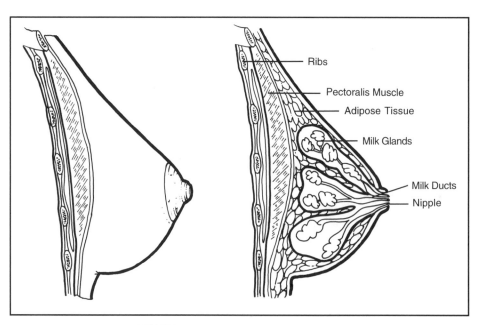

Ribs

Pectoralis Muscle

Adipose Tissue

Milk Glands

Milk Ducts

Nipple

FIGURE 16-15 Anatomy of the breast.

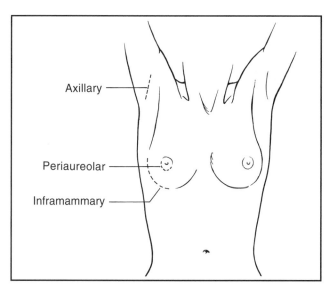

FIGURE 16-16 Incision alternatives for augmentation mammoplasty.

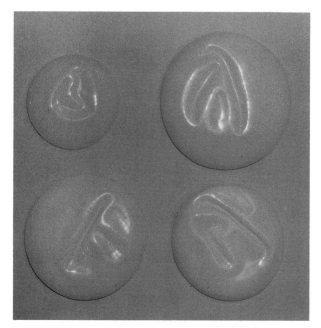

FIGURE 16-17 Trial mammary prostheses.

The procedure can be approached through a variety of incisions. The inframammary incision is technically the easiest approach for the surgeon and is hidden by the breast unless the arms are raised. It permits complete visualization of the submammary or subpectoral plane, for placement of the prosthesis. The circumareolar incision produces less visible scarring as it is easily camouflaged at the junction of the breast skin and areola. However, the incision may interfere with nipple sensation and the lactiferous ducts. The transaxillary incision is technically the most difficult approach as it is at a distance from the operative site. However, it produces a well-hidden scar (Fig. 16-16).

The following nursing considerations are specific to patients undergoing breast augmentation.

1. Selection of the mammary prostheses should be made in advance of surgery so that the appropriate type and sizes will be available at the time of surgery.
2. The procedure can be done with either general or local anesthesia and is most frequently done on an outpatient basis.
3. The procedure is performed in the supine position. The patient should be positioned so that the operating room bed can be elevated to a sitting position to allow the surgeon to evaluate the augmentation intraoperatively.
4. Though the incisions are small, the prepped area should include the entire chest (chin to umbilicus and bedside to bedside). For a transaxillary approach, in addition to the chest prep, the arms are prepped to the elbows in a circumferential manner.
5. A light source will be needed to support a headlight or fiberoptic retractors.

Key steps

1. The surgeon may use both sharp and blunt dissection to create the breast pocket.

2. Maintaining hemostasis throughout the procedure is essential to prevent postoperative hematoma.
3. The inferior edge of the pectoralis muscle is identified.
4. For subpectoral placement, the muscle is released from its costosternal attachments, and laterally to a point midway between the anterior and midaxillary lines, and the muscle is elevated.
5. Trial sizers (Fig. 16-17) may be placed in the newly created pockets to determine the appropriate size of prosthesis. The patient may be elevated to a sitting position and assessed from the foot of the bed and from both sides.
6. The patient is returned to the supine position for placement of the prostheses and for wound closure.
7. A mildly supportive dressing may be applied.

Reduction mammoplasty

Overly large breasts disproportionate to the rest of the body (macromastia) can cause significant physical discomfort. Patients complain of neck strain, headache, aching shoulders, low back pain, deep brassiere strap furrows, heavy anterior chest, poor posture, and paresthesia of the little fingers. Some patients experience chronic breast pain. When breasts are heavy and pendulous, skin in the inframammary region, rarely exposed to the air, is prone to maceration and dermatoses. A reduction mammoplasty is usually curative, with patients expressing satisfaction in their appearance and in the removal of previous physical symptoms.

Many women seek breast reduction for both physical and psychological reasons. A teenager with disproportionately large breasts may find that to be a troublesome source of embarrassment. It can be difficult for very large breasted women to find an appropriate selection of clothes that fit well.

The procedure should be performed after breast growth is completed. It is possible that the procedure can interfere with lactation. For this reason, this potential side effect should be discussed with patients of childbearing age.

Reduction mammoplasty can result in significant scarring. In time, the scars will mature and be less noticeable, but scarring should be discussed with patients preoperatively. Most patients feel that the scarring is less problematic than the relief of symptoms and having more normal body proportions that permit a much wider selection of clothing.

The following nursing considerations are specific to patients undergoing breast reduction.

1. The patient must be positioned so that she can be elevated to a sitting position intraoperatively.
2. The pattern of skin excision is marked on the breast preoperatively. There are several commercial patterning devices available. The surgeon's preference card should indicate what he uses. Patterns and marking equipment should be available for the surgeon to use before the patient is positioned and prepped.
3. It is essential that the markings be preserved during the preoperative skin preparation.
4. A scale must be available to weigh breast tissue so that tissue can be excised from each breast proportionally. The nurse may choose to write the amounts so that the surgeon can see them easily.

5. Tissue from the right and left breasts is sent to the laboratory separately. It is important to identify the location should pathology be discovered.
6. Blood loss may be significant. Weighing sponges and keeping close track of irrigation and the contents of the suction canister may be important.

Key steps

1. The breast skin is deepithelialized in an inverted "T" pattern (Fig. 16-18,*A*).
2. The nipple remains attached to a pedicle of tissue that contains its blood supply. On some occasions, when the pedicle is too long to provide adequate blood supply to the nipple, the nipple can be removed and reattached as a skin graft at the end of the procedure.
3. Tissue is excised in a pattern that is consistent from one breast to the other.
4. Breast tissue is weighed on a scale, and accurate accounts of tissue removed from each section of the breast are documented.
5. After the breast tissue has been excised bilaterally, the breasts are temporarily sutured and the patient is elevated to a semisitting position. The surgeon can assess the newly constructed breasts for size and symmetry. When the results are satisfactory, final closure follows (Fig. 16-18,*B*).
6. Drains are placed in the breast and attached to evacuators to prevent accumulation of fluid.

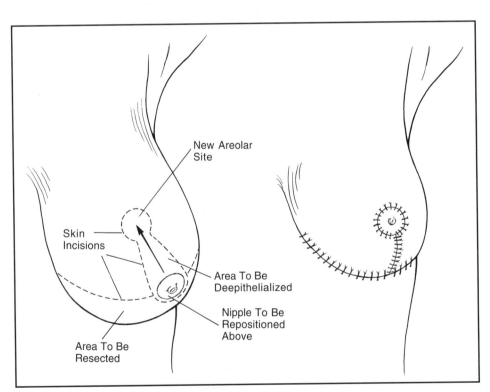

FIGURE 16-18 *Left,* Planned areas of deepithelialization and resection for reduction mammoplasty. Nipple will remain attached to a vascular pedicle. *Right,* Nipple will be elevated to a new position. Final reduction mammoplasty closure represents an inverted "T."

7. A supportive dressing is applied. Some surgeons put minimal dressings over the incisions and have the patient wear a brassiere purchased to use as a support dressing postoperatively.

Mastopexy (breast lift)

Mastopexy is the procedure of choice for sagging breasts where there is a redundancy of skin but not an excess of breast tissue. Mastopexy lifts the breast by excising redundant skin and reconstructing contour and symmetry.

One approach to mastopexy is to excise skin in a pattern identical to a breast reduction. The breast is de-epithelialized, the nipple is elevated into its new position, and the skin edges are brought together with no excision of breast tissue. The pattern of scarring will be the same as a reduction and should be discussed with the patient preoperatively. As the procedure involves the removal of skin only, there is little blood loss and no need to weigh tissue or sponges.

Miscellaneous Cosmetic Surgery Procedures

Liposuction (suction assisted lipectomy, suction lipectomy)

The predisposition to increased collection of fatty deposits in certain areas of the body is determined by sex, age, and race. Women have a thicker subcutaneous layer than do men and with a higher fat concentration. Women typically accumulate fat in the lower trunk: hips, upper thighs, and buttocks areas (Fig. 16-19). Men accumulate fat in abdominal girth, the upper abdomen, and the up-

per torso. The proportion of adipose tissue in the trunk area increases with age in both sexes.

There are two layers of subcutaneous or adipose tissue. The superficial layer consists of compact, well-organized fat cells and is continuous throughout the body. This layer is spared in liposuction. The deep layer of adipose tissue, the target of liposuction, consists of looser, haphazard, irregular fat cells. The function of these fat cells is padding and energy storage. The deeper layer carries intervening fibrous septa that contain small vessels and nerves that innervate and nourish the skin.

Liposuction is a body-contouring procedure that removes fatty deposits. It is performed frequently in conjunction with other procedures to achieve optimal contouring. The procedure involves the removal of fat under negative pressure, by means of a cannula inserted through small, hidden incisions. The cannula is blunt and comes in a variety of sizes and designs (Fig. 16-20,*A*). The cannula and tubing are attached to a generator that produces 1 atmosphere of negative pressure (Fig. 16-20,*B*).

The cannula is passed back and forth through the deep subcutaneous layer. The cannula is held with the perforations facing the muscle to avoid removing the su-

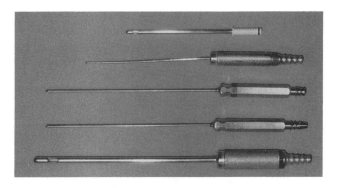

A

FIGURE 16-20 *A,* Cannulas for liposuction come in a wide variety of sizes and shapes. *B,* The suction lipectomy generator creates 1 atmosphere of negative pressure.

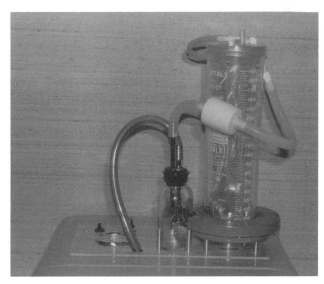

B

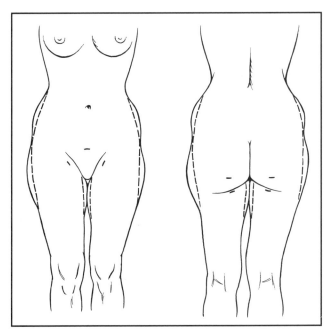

FIGURE 16-19 Patterns of female lipodystrophy; common areas for liposuction.

perficial layer of fat, which can contour irregularities. The blunt tip leaves the intervening fibrous septa intact. Criss-cross tunneling ensures more even removal of fat (Fig. 16-21). Postoperatively, the patient must wear a compression garment continuously for approximately 10 days. This compression of the skin collapses the tunnels and promotes recontouring of the tissues, and it stabilizes the surgical area to prevent shearing. The compression garment also helps to prevents fluid collection and reduce edema.

As a general rule, for every 150 ml of tissue removed, the patient's hematocrit can be expected to drop about 1%. The volume of tissue that can be removed safely must be determined before the procedure begins. Customarily, three times the equivalent of fat removed is replaced with intravenous fluid.

The following information is specific to patients undergoing liposuction.

1. The room temperature is raised to ensure patient comfort. Frequently, large areas of the body are exposed, especially during the preoperative skin preparation.
2. For extensive procedures, the operating room bed can be prepared with a warming blanket to maintain body temperature.
3. If the procedure is not extensive, the nurse may be responsible for monitoring the patient under intravenous conscious sedation.
4. Suction equipment includes a generator that creates 1 atmosphere of negative pressure, suction cannulae in sizes appropriate to the areas being suctioned, and suction tubing specifically designed for liposuction procedures.
5. The areas to be suctioned are marked while the patient is standing. For extensive procedures, the preoperative skin prep may be done with the patient standing next to the operating room bed.
   - Solution should be at body temperature to prevent chilling the patient.
   - Windows may be covered to respect the patient's privacy.
   - The patient is assisted onto the bed.
   - If the patient's position must be changed, the application of antimicrobial solution and draping must be repeated.
6. Intraoperatively, the amount of tissue removed is monitored carefully to avoid hypovolemia. The surgeon and anesthesia provider, if present, should be informed periodically of the amount of tissue in the suction canister.
7. Monitoring the amount of tissue removed from bilateral structures is important. To ensure symmetry, similar amounts of tissue are removed from each side.

Key steps

1. Areas to be suctioned are injected with a local anesthetic containing epinephrine to control bleeding.
2. Small incisions (1 to 2 cm) are made where the scars will be hidden.

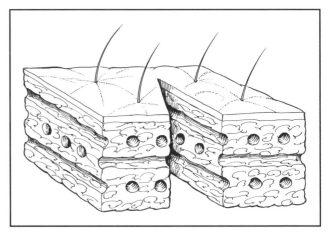

FIGURE 16-21 Criss-cross tunneling ensures more even removal of fat.

3. The suction machine is activated after the cannula has been inserted, and tunneling proceeds in a fan-like manner. Criss-cross technique requires a second incision distant from the first.
4. The amount of fat suctioned from each site is measured and recorded to compare with the same site bilaterally.
5. The total amount of adipose tissue removed should not exceed the amount determined prior to the procedure. Removing more may require a blood transfusion. Fluid intake must also be monitored carefully.
6. All incisions are closed and dressings applied to skin closure areas where necessary.
7. A compression garment is applied to be left in place for approximately 10 days to aid in preventing shearing and for contouring and controlling edema.

Abdominoplasty

Abdominoplasty is the repair of the abdominal wall, including skin, fat, muscle, and fascia. In addition, a diastasis (separation) of the rectus muscles can result from an incomplete closure of a previous abdominal surgery or pregnancy. Muscular support can be tightened if muscles have been stretched or weakened. Tightening of the muscles flattens the abdominal bulges and supports fascial weakness.

Massive weight loss can result in a pendulous apron of skin and fat (pannus) that hangs loosely from the lower abdomen. Patients with this condition complain of excessive perspiring and chafing with dermatitis and localized infection under the pannus tissue fold.

The surgeon assesses the extent of tissue redundancy with the patient standing. Muscle diastasis is evaluated with the patient supine while raising the head and shoulders slightly off the examining table.

The following nursing considerations are specific to patients undergoing abdominoplasty.

1. Preoperative markings are essential to proper closure. It is important to preserve the markings during the preoperative skin prep.

2. The patient's hospital bed should be brought to the operating room. It should be arranged in a lawn chair position and should be outfitted with a trapeze attachment to facilitate the patient's repositioning postoperatively.

3. An indwelling urinary catheter will be inserted for the surgical procedure to preclude distention of the bladder and lower abdominal wall.

4. The patient will be in a flexed position at the end of the surgical procedure. Moving the patient directly into the bed, which has been flexed as well, will protect the suture line and reduce the number of times the patient must be transferred postoperatively.

5. The patient will be out of bed as early as the evening of surgery, but will remain in a stooped position when standing to protect the suture line.

Key steps

1. The surgeon usually makes a low transverse incision, which can be hidden by underwear or a swim suit (Fig. 16-22,*A*).

2. The incision line is marked to outline the flap and to aid in resection and closure.

3. The abdominal wall flap is undermined to the level of the umbilicus.

4. The umbilicus is incised as an ellipse with a sufficient amount of subcutaneous tissue to ensure vascularization.

5. The abdominal flap is divided to the umbilicus and dissection continues to the upper portion of the abdomen. The flap is elevated to the xiphoid process and laterally above the costal margin.

6. Diastasis of the rectus muscle is corrected. A synthetic mesh can be used for additional support.

7. Redundant fat is removed by dissection and/or with suction lipectomy for contour and ease of closure.

8. The stalk of the umbilicus is sutured to the muscle fascia. A heavy suture facilitates location of the umbilical stalk for replantation in the abdominal flap (anteriosuperior location).

9. The operating room table is flexed, and the abdominal flap is redraped over the abdomen.

10. The old umbilical site is advanced to the midline symphysis marking and fixed with temporary suture.

11. Redundant abdominal skin and subcutaneous tissue are excised, drains are placed, and the flap is sutured into place.

12. The umbilicus is located under the flap. A new umbilical site is created in the flap, and the umbilicus is sutured into its new position (Fig. 16-22,*B*).

13. The incision line is dressed and a supportive dressing, garment, or abdominal binder is placed to support the reconstruction. The patient remains in a flexed

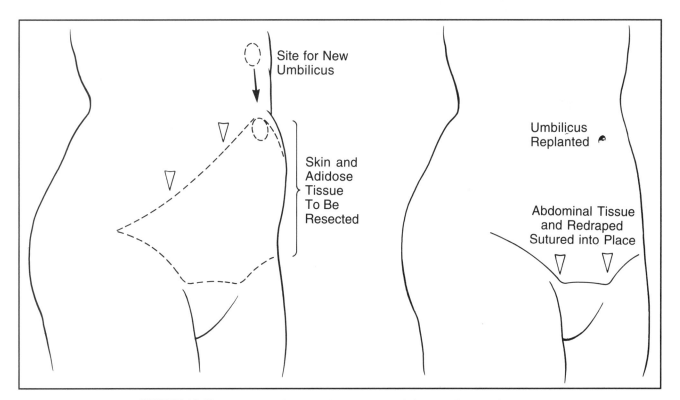

FIGURE 16-22   *Left,* Low abdominal incision for abdominoplasty and section of tissue to be resected. The original umbilical site will be excised with the flap. *Right,* Following resection of abdominal tissue, the umbilicus is replanted and the lower abdominal incision closed.

position for several days postoperatively to relieve tension on the suture line.

RECONSTRUCTIVE SURGERY

Reconstructive surgical procedures are performed to repair or replace a part of the body that has been injured by trauma or burns, or to correct a congenital deformity. Often, multiple procedures are required to obtain the desired outcome. Care of patients having reconstructive surgery requires extensive multidisciplinary coordination. Physical therapists, occupational therapists, speech therapists, social workers, nutritionists, surgeons, and nurses will be involved in determining the timing for each subsequent procedure. Patients having reconstructive surgery because of trauma from a motor vehicle accident may not be close to their home and may require additional support from the multidisciplinary team.

Many reconstructive surgical procedures use grafts or flaps to repair the injured body part. Many different types of grafts and flaps are used.

Grafts

A simple graft is a piece of tissue—skin, bone, muscle, or fat—that has been completely separated from its blood supply and transferred to fill a defect elsewhere in the body. The graft tissue survives by the rapid growth of vessels from the recipient site into the graft. Graft tissue can be used successfully only if the recipient site has a good blood supply and the surrounding tissues are healthy.

The technique of grafting skin was initially developed in 1869 when a French surgeon, Reverdin, discovered that tiny pieces of a patient's skin could be "planted" in a denuded area and would eventually "take," grow, and cover the area. Reverdin's grafts were *split-thickness skin grafts (STSG)*, which are comprised of epidermis and varying amounts of dermis and therefore can be of varying thicknesses (Fig. 16-23). Very thin grafts are indicated where there is poor vascularization at the recipient site. They are used extensively to resurface burns because they "take" well.

STSG shrink as they heal. If an STSG were used to resurface an area of flexion, contracture would occur as the graft healed and shrank. Thicker STSGs and *full-thickness skin grafts (FTSG)*, popularized in the 1890s, contain epidermis and a significant amount of dermis. They provide better coverage but require a healthier recipient wound bed in order to survive. FTSG are indicated to resurface areas of flexion and where tissue bulk is needed for well-padded coverage of superficial defects.

Tissue grafts taken from the same individual are called *autografts.* Autografts are intended for permanent reconstruction. *Homografts* are grafts taken from other individuals of the same species. When an individual has large areas to be resurfaced, such as extensive burned areas, and has few available donor sites for grafting, skin from other individuals can be used. Homograft skin lasts for 3

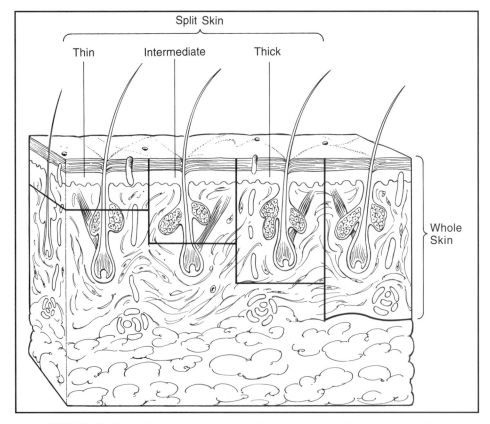

FIGURE 16-23 Split-thickness and full-thickness skin grafts.

to 10 weeks; it stimulates epithelialization and leaves a clean, granulating wound bed for further reconstruction. *Xenografts* or heterografts are taken from other species and are utilized only for temporary coverage. Porcine grafts are an example of xenografts commonly used when extensive temporary protection of a defect is needed.

Skin grafts are harvested with a dermatome (literally *skin knife*). Dermatomes come in varying sizes and degrees of sophistication. Some are powered (electric, air-powered, or battery) (Fig. 16-24,*A*); others are handheld (Humbe knife, Watson knife, Gouillian knife (Fig. 16-24,*B*). Most dermatomes can be preset for both the size and the thickness of graft desired.

Skin grafts can be expanded to cover a defect larger than the graft. A mesh graft dermatome scores a graft with a pattern of tiny slits (Fig. 16-25). The pattern of slits creates a Japanese lantern effect, permitting the graft to be stretched from 1.5 times to 9 times its original size. This is beneficial when large defects require resurfacing.

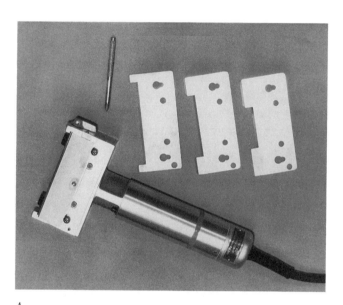

A
FIGURE 16-24 *A,* Powered dermatome with templates that determine the width of the skin graft taken. *B,* Hand-held dermatome.

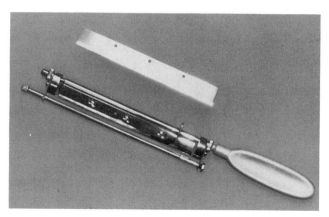

B

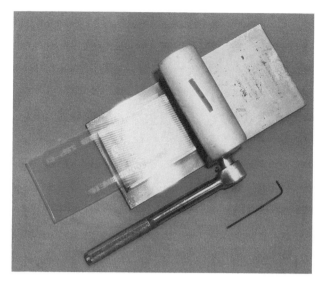

FIGURE 16-25 The skin graft is spread out on the dermacarrier, which determines the pattern of slits made as it passes through the meshgraft dermatome. The degree of expansion depends on the size of the dermacarrier.

The meshed graft can also be contoured easily over an irregular defect. One disadvantage of a meshed graft is that it heals with a waffled appearance. When possible, surgeons avoid using meshed grafts in areas like the face and hands where an aesthetic appearance is important.

Skin grafts can be removed repeatedly from the same donor site. Regenerating epithelium covering a split-thickness donor site achieves maximum thickness in 14 to 16 days. The same donor site can be used approximately every three weeks when the patient requires extensive grafting.

Reconstructive surgery utilizes other graft tissue as well. Bone grafts can be used following resection of a bony tumor or traumatic loss of bone as well as to reconstruct congenital defects involving absent or deficient bony structures. Cartilage grafts are used to provide support in nasal reconstruction and a framework for reconstruction of the ear. Nerve and tendon grafts replace damaged structures in traumatic injuries. Nerve grafts are also used in reconstructive procedures involving uninnervated muscle (e.g., facial paralysis).

Perioperative nursing considerations

1. Grafting involves two operative areas: the donor site and the recipient site. A donor site accessible to the recipient site will be selected if possible.
2. Positioning must allow access to both sites, if possible. Some procedures will require repositioning and redraping following the procurement of the skin graft.
3. The donor site is considered the cleaner of the two areas. The donor site is prepped first. The skin prep tray can be divided to prep both sites with a change of gloves, or two separate prep trays can be used.
4. Because the donor site is considered cleaner, the graft will usually be procured before the recipient site is addressed.

5. The graft tissue must be handled carefully and protected while the recipient site is being prepared for grafting. Skin grafts should be folded dermis to dermis to prevent drying, and folded in a moist gauze sponge.

6. Bleeding or hematoma beneath the graft is the most important cause of graft failure. Meticulous hemostasis at the recipient site is important before application of the graft. Postoperatively, any collection of fluid must be evacuated immediately.

7. The second most important cause of graft failure is mechanical injury. The graft site is usually immobilized with a bolster dressing or a splint if it is in an area of flexion (Fig. 16-26).

8. Patient teaching must include the importance of protecting the grafted site and careful observation for signs of fluid collection under the graft. The patient must be encouraged to call the surgeon's office if there is any indication that the graft is not healing appropriately.

Flaps

A *flap* is a section of vascularized tissue nourished by its own blood supply. When inset into a defect, it brings nourishment to support the reconstruction initially. Ingrowth of vessels from the recipient site promotes the healing process.

Local flaps are elevated, then rotated or advanced to reconstruct a defect in the same area. *Delayed flaps* are elevated, inset, and divided in a second procedure at a later time when vascularity at the recipient site has been established. The delayed flap technique is used only in selected procedures (e.g., Abbe flap for reconstruction of the lip). Advances in microsurgical technology have made the discomfort and inconvenience of delayed flap reconstruction unnecessary.

Microsurgical techniques permit the surgeon to select tissue of the appropriate size from any area of the body and transport it as a *free flap* to reconstruct a defect of any size. In a sophisticated one-stage procedure, the surgeon can reconstruct a defect in a distant area of the body. The donor tissue is completely detached from its blood supply and anastomosed to a new blood supply at the recipient site.

Flaps are identified by the type of tissues involved. *Cutaneous* flaps contain skin and subcutaneous tissue. They are used throughout the body to reconstruct defects created by the surgical removal of diseased tissue (e.g., skin cancers) and in scar revisions. *Muscle* flaps can be used to cover, protect, and nourish defects where vascularity is poor (e.g., deep pressure ulcers, exposed tendon and bone). In many cases, muscle flaps can actually promote healing in difficult wounds like chronic pressure ulcers and osteomyelitis. *Osseous* flaps are sections of vascularized bone, which can be fashioned to replace portions of bony structures (e.g., mandible). *Omental* flaps, vascularized sections of omentum, can provide protection and nourishment in areas adjacent to the abdomen (e.g., sternal defects).

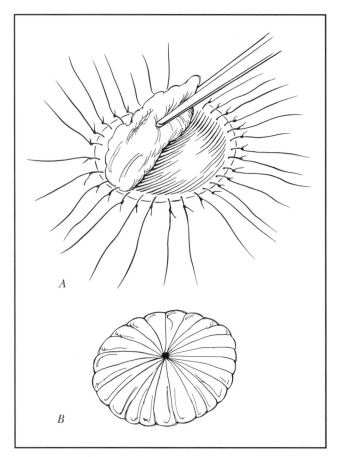

FIGURE 16-26 A bolster dressing may be applied over a skin graft to provide even compression of the graft on the recipient site and to discourage an accumulation of fluid under the graft.

Some flaps are composed of several types of tissue and provide even more versatility in the reconstruction of defects. The *myocutaneous* (or *musculocutaneous*) flap contains skin, subcutaneous tissue, and muscle. This flap is appropriate where bulk is needed to reconstruct a defect. Myocutaneous flaps are used frequently in breast reconstruction following mastectomy.

The *osseomyocutaneous* flap contains skin, subcutaneous tissue, muscle, and bone. Such a flap can be designed to replace an entire anatomical structure. For instance, in mandibular reconstruction for ameloblastoma, an osseomyocutaneous flap from the iliac area can replace an entire section of the lower jaw. A *fasciocutaneous* flap, such as the gluteal thigh flap, contains skin, subcutaneous tissue, and supporting fascia. It is the most commonly used flap in the reconstruction of ischial pressure ulcers.

Flaps are also described by the method of mobilization of the flap tissue to reconstruct a defect. An *advancement* flap is undermined on two or three sides and advanced (or stretched) to reconstruct an adjacent defect. This flap is most successful where there is some redundancy of skin, found more frequently in the very young and in the aged. A *rotation* flap is elevated and rotated to cover an adjacent defect. The donor defect can be closed primarily, if small, or resurfaced with a skin graft.

An *island* flap is tissue that is elevated and left connected to the body by only an artery and a vein. It is usually tunneled under a bridge of tissue and inset into a defect. If it is small enough, the donor site is closed primarily, or it can be resurfaced with a skin graft. A *pedicle* is based on a "stalk" or pedicle that contains the tissue's nourishing vessels and nerves. The flap is very mobile and can be rotated into defects somewhat distant from the donor site. It is essential to avoid twisting, kinking, stretching, or compressing the pedicle, which would interrupt the flap's blood supply and cause the death of the flap tissue. The latissimus dorsi flap is an excellent example of a pedicle flap. It is elevated from the back and can be rotated to reconstruct a missing breast or a chest wall defect. Sensibility is retained at the recipient site when an innervated muscle is used for reconstruction.

A *transposition* flap transposes tissue to alter the lines of tension and produce a more relaxed scar. The Z-plasty is one of the most widely used techniques in plastic surgery. Instead of a straight line incision, which can contract and produce an ugly scar, two triangular flaps of tissue are transposed and sutured in a Z-pattern (see Fig. 16-3).

When planning reconstruction with flaps or grafts, the surgeon evaluates several criteria. Morbidity at the donor site is a consideration, as is expendability of the donor tissue. For example, a latissimus flap would be a poor choice for a swimmer as this muscle acts as an abductor and medial rotator of the arm. The surgeon strives to create the most cosmetically acceptable scar. Table 16-1 describes muscles most commonly used in flaps.

Perioperative nursing considerations

1. The microscope and other equipment should be checked to ensure that they are in working order prior to the patient's arrival.
2. The room temperature should be maintained at 75 to 80° F because too cool a temperature can cause vasoconstriction and jeopardize flap viability.
3. Protect the patient from the physical stresses of a long procedure. Provide a pressure-relieving pad and a warming blanket for the bed. Protect skin and bony prominences carefully.
4. An indwelling urinary catheter will be inserted; monitor fluid output.
5. A Doppler may be used preoperatively to identify vessels at the recipient site.
6. Some surgeons, prior to prepping, may outline the graft and identify donor and recipient arteries and veins with marking pens for photographs (Goodman, 1988),
7. Patient positioning depends on the donor and recipient graft sites.
8. The surgeons may use two electrosurgical units. Follow the manufacturer's guidelines carefully (see Chapter 23 in Volume 1 on electrosurgery).
9. The procedure will require skin preps at two sites, which should be done separately, beginning with the donor site.

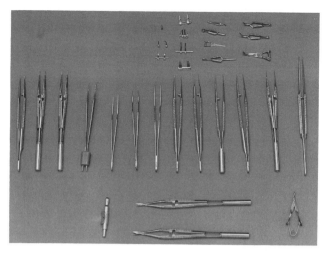

FIGURE 16-27 Microvascular instruments are small and delicate. They require meticulous cleaning, gentle handling, and protection during storage. Instruments: microvascular clamps, bulldog clamps, forceps, spring handle barrel forceps (2), bipolar forceps, jeweler's forceps, curved forceps, iris forceps, barrel forceps (4), spring handle forceps, barrel handle forceps, suction adaptor, spring handle scissors (2), microvascular clamp applier.

10. The draping technique will depend on positioning and can require some creative use of draping materials.
11. There may be two surgical teams operating simultaneously—one on the donor site and the other on the recipient site. In this event, separate sterile instrument set-ups will be required. Take care that cross-contamination between the two sets does not occur.
12. Ensuring the safety and sterility of the procured flap until time for implantation is of the utmost importance.
13. Postoperatively the donor site is kept elevated and warm to reduce vasospasm and increase circulation.
14. The major postoperative complication is vascular compromise to the flap site. A thorough postoperative vascular assessment is crucial. If inadequate or questionable blood supply is suspected, the surgeon must be notified immediately so action can be taken for flap survival.
15. Special attention needs to be given to the microscope and the microsurgical instruments (Fig. 16-27), which are costly and easily damaged. The microscope must be wiped clean and the lens cleaned with lens paper to avoid scratches. After cleaning, the microscope should be covered to protect it from dust, and stored in a safe place, out of the way of traffic. The microinstruments should be individually cleaned as soon as possible. Avoid bending the delicate tips. Check the instruments frequently for bent tips and burrs and to ensure that the jaws of needle holders close adequately. The instruments with extremely fine tips should be stored with their points protected in a cushioned container that provides instrument immobility.

Table 16-1 Muscles Most Commonly Used in Flaps*

The temporalis muscle aids in mastication. Its function is expendable because of other surrounding muscles. The maxillary artery, through two branches, supplies blood. It is used in cases of facial paralysis. The nerve supply, from branches of the temporal nerve, is maintained. The temporalis fascia has been used in fascial flaps for defects in the leg and the hand.

The sternocleidomastoid muscle, from the head of the clavicle to insertion of the mastoid process, has three sources of segmental blood supply. This muscle is used to cover intraoral defects and tracheostomy defects.

The platysma muscle covers the lower margin of the mandible. It is supplied from small branches of the facial artery and the superior thyroid arteries. It is used for intraoral defects.

The trapezius muscle is triangular in shape and elevates the scapula and shoulder. It is ideal for coverage of upper thoracic and cervical spine defects.

The pectoralis muscle covers an extensive area over the chest wall. It has multiple sources of blood supply, including the thoracoacromial artery and perforating arteries from the internal mammary artery. This muscle can be used to cover defects over the shoulder, or it can be transferred to the midline of the sternum for partial coverage of post-mediastinal wound infections. Its versatility leads to its use in head and neck reconstruction, including intraoral defects. The pectoralis muscle is the flap of choice for coverage of pharyngeal fistulas and reconstruction of the esophagus. Some disadvantages include aesthetic deformity and bulkiness in intraoral transposition, causing difficulty in swallowing. The advantages of using the pectoralis muscle exceed any risks of impairment.

The latissimus dorsi muscle is a rectangular muscle whose function is primarily as an abductor and medial rotator of the arm. It is supplied by the thoracodorsal artery. The distal portion of the muscle is supplied by the paravertebral posterior perforating vessels. The nerve to this muscle is the thoracodorsal nerve. This muscle has great versatility. It can be used for reconstruction of the breast, chest wall, head and neck region, shoulder, arm, axilla, back, scapula, and abdomen. Its long vascular pedicle allows it to swing as a pendulum and cover many defects within its reach. This flap has become the most favored donor muscle in free flaps. Its advantages include ease of elevation, safety, and reliability. If the thoracodorsal artery has been ligated, the muscle can survive with the blood supply from a branch of the serratus anterior vessels. The disadvantages of this muscle flap include winging of the scapula and some flattening of the back.

The serratus anterior muscle is supplied by the lateral thoracic artery and a branch of the thoracodorsal artery. It is

used for intrathoracic coverage of broncho-pleural fistulas. The major disadvantage of using this muscle is the need to retract the latissimus dorsi and portions of the pectoralis major muscle to obtain access to it.

The rectus abdominis muscle and musculocutaneous units are supplied by the superior and inferior epigastric arteries. The muscle alone is quite suited for coverage of post-mediastinal wound infections. In addition, it can cover smaller defects in the lower chest wall and pacemakers inserted in the abdominal wall. It is most popular in breast reconstruction, providing enough bulk to allow reconstruction without an implant. The loss of one rectus abdominis muscle is well tolerated, in contrast to using two muscles, which may show some loss of pelvic tilt. Some other disadvantages include asymmetric bulging and/or hernia.

The gluteus maximus muscle is quadrilateral in shape and supplied by the inferior and superior gluteal vessels. This muscle has been used for coverage of sacral or ischial defects in paraplegics. The simplest way to cover the sacrum is with a turnover or advancement flap. This muscle, along with a skin island flap, can also be used in ambulatory patients with similar defects.

The gracilis muscle is a totally expendable muscle. It is supplied by a branch of the saphenous artery. It is used to reconstruct perineal defects or ischial pressure ulcer defects. Some disadvantages include the limited extent of its pivot and unreliability of the distal third of the skin flap.

The tensor fascia lata muscle is a small muscle supplied by a branch of the profunda femoris. It originates from the greater trochanter of the femur and is innervated by the inferior branch of the gluteal nerve. This muscle is used for coverage of trochanteric pressure ulcers, reconstruction of the abdominal wall, and defects in the medial thigh. However, it has been found that the use of this muscle as a flap in the athlete causes instability to the knee.

The rectus femoris muscle insets into the patellar tendon and extends the knee. It is supplied by the lateral circumflex femoral vessels. It is used for reconstruction of lower abdominal defects, to resurface post-radiation ulcerations in the perineum, or after groin dissections.

The gastrocnemius muscle is supplied by the sural artery and the sural nerve. It is used as a muscle flap to avoid a defect in the posterior calf. This muscle is most likely used to cover exposed bone over the proximal one-third of the tibia.

*From Vasconez, L. O., McCraw, J. B., & Camargos, A. G. (1991). Muscle, musculocutaneous, and fasciocutaneous flaps. In *Grabb & Smith's plastic surgery* (4th ed.). Boston: Little, Brown & Co.

Microvascular free flap

Microvascular free flaps permit immediate and complete coverage of almost any defect in a one-stage operation. The surgeon can select tissue of appropriate color, thickness, texture, and sensation from anywhere in the body to reconstruct a defect or replace a missing body part. The procedure requires specialized instrumentation and equipment and is lengthy, but advances in microscope technology and microvascular techniques have enabled surgeons to reconstruct defects previously impossible to repair.

Key steps

1. Although either site (donor or recipient) may be prepared first, the recipient site is often started first. The defect is explored and the arteries and veins that will feed the flap are identified and marked with microclamps. The advantage of having the recipient site and vessels ready is that it allows for immediate anastomosis of vasculature after the flap is procured, thereby decreasing the period of time the flap is without continuous blood supply (Goodman, 1988).

2. The donor flap is then procured. The flap may need trimming or thinning to "fit" the recipient site. The last dissection to remove the flap from the donor site is dividing the vessels that feed the donor tissue.

3. If the donor site is prepared first, ischemic time must be kept to a minimum. The flap must be kept in an iced, normal saline slush until the recipient site is ready.

4. Once the flap is correctly positioned at the recipient site, it is loosely sutured into place to immobilize it and prevent any rotation of the flap while the anastomosis is being done.

5. The anastomosis takes place using the microscope and microsurgery instruments. Suture type and size depend on vessel size and surgeon preference. A heparinized, normal saline solution may be used to flush vessels. Peripheral vasodilators may also be used.

6. Following the anastomosis, flap vascularity is assessed by noting the color and temperature of the flap. Often a sterile laser Doppler will be used, as it is a more reliable tool to assess perfusion. A preoperative Doppler study of the recipient site may have been done to obtain a baseline measurement to be compared to intraoperative or postoperative studies.

7. Hemostasis is maintained throughout the procedure by applying pressure or using hemostatic agents. Postoperative bleeding and hematoma formation can threaten graft viability.

8. Drains may be placed to prevent fluid accumulation.

9. The choice of dressing material varies with surgeon preference. Some prefer a pressure dressing to encourage venous return. Others will use an exposure technique to allow visibility and detection of hematomas. Still others prefer to apply moist, sterile saline sponges to keep the skin moist until revascularization occurs. A cast may be applied in some cases to immobilize extremities that have required flap surgery.

Replantation Surgery

The goals of replantation surgery are to restore function to the amputated part, achieve primary healing, if possible, with minimal scar formation, and provide an optimal environment for subsequent surgery (McCarthy, May, & Littler, 1990).

Of particular importance, especially if the patient is not located near a transplantation center and will be travelling a distance for surgery, is to instruct the patient/family member regarding care of the amputated part. Instructions should include directions not to warm, freeze, or pack the part in dry ice but to place the dry, amputated part in a plastic bag, seal it, and place it in a container of crushed ice for transport.

Replantation surgery involves the replanting of a severed finger, hand, toe, foot, or an entire limb. With advanced microsurgical techniques, surgeons are able to replant severed parts that were once discarded and restore function to appendages that previously remained useless following less sophisticated surgical repair.

The decision to proceed with replantation surgery must involve the patient. The procedure is long and complex, and the patient will require a long period of rehabilitation to achieve maximum use of the replanted part.

Factors affecting the decision to replant

1. Patient's age, general health, and occupational needs; replantation is more successful in younger patients than in older.

2. Ischemic time since amputation; the shorter the time from amputation to replantation, the greater the chances of success. Generally, distal amputated parts (i.e., fingers, hands, and toes) can withstand a greater ischemic time before irreversible change takes place.

3. Mechanism of amputation and the associated tissue trauma; clean, sharp amputations can be repaired more successfully than crushing injuries.

4. Degree of amputation; incomplete amputations can be replanted more successfully than complete amputations because they have intact subcutaneous venous circulation in the remaining skin.

5. Need for the amputated part; the replanted part must have potential usefulness. The thumb is the most important digit and should generally be replanted first (Marsh, 1989). If debridement leaves the thumb too short, there are alternatives to repair. One alternative is to attach another amputated finger to the thumb position. Another option is to preserve the stump of the thumb and cover it with a soft tissue flap to facilitate a later toe transfer. Other guidelines to follow are to complete one digital reattachment before starting another and that the long or ring finger position is more useful than an index finger position, therefore leaving an index finger to be replanted last (Marsh, 1989).

6. Contraindications to replantation include:
   • Irreversible loss of blood supply
   • Unstable condition of the patient
   • Prolonged warm ischemia
   • Severe crushing injury
   • Multiple fractures of the digit/limb

Perioperative nursing considerations

1. The patient and family will need a significant amount of psychological support.

2. All of the responsibilities of a microsurgical procedure apply to replantation procedures.

3. Prior to applying the tourniquet, the extremity is padded with several layers of soft cast padding. The cuff is

then applied snugly around the extremity. Inflation of the tourniquet does not occur until the procedure is ready to start and the surgeon asks that the tourniquet be inflated. The perioperative nurse documents tourniquet location, time of inflation, pressure setting, deflation time, and subsequent reinflation and deflation times.

4. The patient should keep the affected appendage elevated postoperatively to prevent edema. A sling may be used if an arm is involved.

5. Postoperatively, dressings must be checked carefully and circulation assessed. In addition, the replantation site should be assessed for edema, infection, and joint stiffness. The original dressing may remain for 5 to 10 days postoperatively.

Replantation of an amputated part

Key steps

1. The amputated part usually accompanies the patient into the operating room suite. Cleansing of the amputated part is done on a separate sterile surface with lactated Ringer's or 0.9 normal saline instead of water, which causes lysis of the cells.

2. Anesthetic options include local, regional blocks, intravenous sedation, or general anesthesia.

3. Tourniquet time varies but does not usually exceed 2 hours.

4. Initially, an exploration of the wound is necessary, including the skin, bones, joints, nerves, tendons, and vessels.

5. Both the amputated part and the stump are debrided; the damaged and contaminated tissue is removed along with loose bone fragments.

6. Skeletal fixation is usually done first to provide a fixed, stable frame for subsequent repair of smaller structures. Fixation may be accomplished by K-wires, interosseous wires, pins, plates, and screws, depending on the part amputated. Shortening of the bone may be necessary prior to fixation to allow for a tension-free closure and repair of blood vessels and nerves. Bone grafting may also be necessary.

7. Tendon and ligament repair usually follow the bony repair. The surgeon takes care to decrease the occurrence of adhesions and scar tissue between the joints to avoid inhibition of movement.

8. Microsurgical repair includes the veins, arteries, and nerves and, except for large structures, is accomplished with the aid of a microscope. The order of repair of these structures is situation-dependent. It is preferable, initially, to repair one or more veins to provide sufficient venous return, therefore decreasing edema and promoting circulation. If the ischemia time has been lengthy, the surgeon may repair an artery first to promote perfusion of the part. However, repairing an artery first makes subsequent repair of veins and nerves more difficult due to excessive bleeding.

9. Next, the nerves are repaired, and finally, the artery. A heparinized normal saline flush may be used to flush the vessels. Peripheral vasodilators may be necessary as well.

10. Following vessel reanastomosis, hemostatic agents may be necessary to control bleeding. A sterile Doppler may be used to determine vascularity.

11. Soft tissue and skin coverage are the last to be addressed. When there has been significant tissue loss, free tissue flaps or skin grafting may be necessary to augment defects and to ensure closure. The surgeon should attempt to cover the vessel anastomosis with local tissue. If there is questionable muscle viability, primary closure should be avoided.

12. Dressings can include compressive dressings to minimize edema, splints and casts to immobilize the reconstruction, and soft dressings to protect the wound. With any dressing, avoid constriction of the tissues, which may impair blood flow and jeopardize the reconstruction.

Toe-to-thumb transfer

The hand is a critical part of the body in function and image. The thumb accounts for 40% to 50% of hand function. An individual's ability to power grip and twist grip is due to the strength and mobility of the thumb. The thumb is required for the manipulation of small objects.

The anatomy of the great toe is nearly identical to the anatomy of the thumb. The toe provides the new thumb with tendon, bone, and nerves. The function and characteristic of the thumb can be restored with profound success.

The loss of the great toe is not a functional problem. There is very little alteration of normal gait patterns. Patients tolerate the absence of the toe with no ill effects. Participating in hiking, skiing, tennis, basketball, and football is accomplished with ease.

CLEFT LIP AND PALATE SURGERY

Cleft Lip

Cleft lip is one of the more common congenital anomalies. It is the result of incomplete fusion of the facial processes during embryonic development. A unilateral cleft is usually located below the center of one nostril (Fig. 16-28,*A*). Bilateral clefts occur beneath both nostrils (Fig. 16-28,*B*). Midline clefts are rare. Cleft lip can occur alone or in conjunction with a cleft palate. Clefts range from a slight indentation in the lip to a full, open cleavage involving skin, muscle, and bone.

The normal lip is composed of skin, the orbicularis muscle, and mucous membranes. A cleft deformity produces a distortion of Cupid's bow, the normal bow-shape of the superior ridge of the upper lip, and can involve the absence of philtral ridges, the medial groove(s) on the exterior surface of the upper lip. More severe clefts distort the lower portion of the nose.

The goal of cleft lip repair is to restore a symmetrically functional and aesthetically natural lip. Long-term objec-

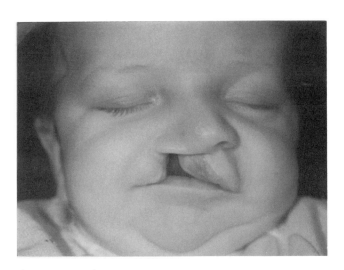

A

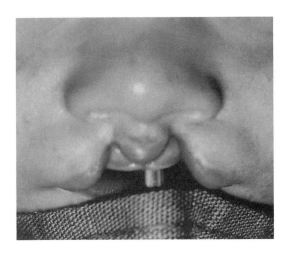

B

FIGURE 16-28 *A,* A unilateral cleft lip occurs under one nostril. *B,* A bilateral cleft lip occurs under both nostrils.

tives of cleft lip repair include reconstructing a functional speech mechanism, separating the nasal and oral cavities, encouraging adequate growth of the facial skeleton, and reconstructing the cosmetic features of the lip and nose to achieve an aesthetic appearance.

Surgical closure of the lip is usually performed when the patient is between 1 and 3 months of age. Some surgeons elect to repair cleft lips within the first few days of birth to facilitate feeding and to minimize the parents' psychological trauma. Others delay surgery until the infant is older. A common determinant of the appropriate time for repair is the "rule of 10's"—10 weeks of age, 10 grams of hemoglobin, and 10 pounds of body weight. Possible advantages of delaying the procedure include increased weight of the infant and a red blood cell count closer to normal. There is also more time for complete preoperative evaluation and detection of other anomalies. Anesthetic risks may be lower than in the neonatal period, and the larger facial structures of an older infant may permit a better definitive repair. There is also more time to teach the parents, for them to comprehend the situation, and to promote realistic expectations for the future.

Secondary surgery may be necessary to further correct any remaining deformity, to correct deficiencies secondary to bone growth, to revise scar tissue, or to improve the appearance if the muscles of the lip were not well positioned and approximated during the primary lip closure. Frequently, subsequent procedures are required to revise scarring.

Cleft lip repair approximates the cleft edges while preserving or reconstructing natural landmarks such as the Cupid's bow and philtral ridges. There are three techniques for cleft repair: straight line closure (lip adhesion), rotation-advancement closure, and flap closure. Straight line closure is the easiest repair. It is usually reserved for smaller clefts, or as an interim procedure to allow for improved feeding until more definite surgery can be performed. The straight line closure can result in a contracted scar, which requires revision.

The rotation advancement closure technique is the most common. Advantages include minimal tissue loss, allowance for replacement of missing anatomy such as various nasal structures, and the ability of the surgeon to make adjustments throughout the procedure. Disadvantages include the need to remove excess mucosa and manipulate the nostrils. This approach is not appropriate for wide clefts (Sauter, 1989).

Flap closure involves the use of triangular or rectangular flaps and requires exact measurements. Advantages include an optimal cosmetic appearance, minimal tissue waste, and preservation of Cupid's bow. This technique can be used successfully on wide clefts. Disadvantages include the complicated measurements required, the degree of surgical difficulty, and a resulting zigzag scar.

Perioperative nursing considerations

1. Offer psychological support for the parents and communicate with them as often as possible during the surgical procedure.
2. Prepare the room for pediatric surgery:
   • Raise room temperature prior to bringing the child in.
   • Ensure that all preparatory activities have been completed prior to the arrival of the child so that attention can be focused on the child and the process of anesthesia induction.
3. The patient is placed in a supine position, taking care to preserve body alignment and prevent injury.
4. The procedure is performed under general anesthesia. The oral endotracheal tube is placed directly over the center of the lower lip so that it does not distort the anatomy.
5. Prior to the skin prep, the surgeon may mark landmarks important to the surgical repair. Be sure to preserve these markings when prepping.
6. The surgeon may inject local anesthesia with epinephrine to promote hemostasis. He or she will inject carefully to avoid distorting the anatomy.
7. The surgeon's preference card should indicate if he or she operates standing or sitting.

8. Arm or elbow restraints may be applied while the patient is still anesthetized to prevent self-injury to the lip postoperatively.

9. Two potential complications are airway obstruction secondary to edema and bleeding.

10. The Logan bow is left in place for a few days and sutures are usually removed 3 to 9 days postoperatively.

Bilateral cleft lip repair

Surgical repair of the bilateral cleft lip is more complex than repair of the unilateral cleft lip, not only because of the presence of two clefts but also because of the probability that displacement of the primary palate has occurred. Depending on the severity of the deformity, the repair may be done in two or more stages.

If the cleft is very wide, with a great deal of alveolar displacement, lip adhesion surgery may be performed as an initial procedure. Definitive repair is performed once the tissues have softened, usually in about 3 months.

In staged reconstruction, when there is no palatal involvement, the first-stage procedure may reduce the bilateral cleft to the unilateral cleft lip. If both clefts are repaired at the same time, the second cleft may be closed under sufficient tension to cause wound dehiscence or spreading of the scar. For this reason, the widest side is usually closed first.

With a staged reconstruction, the initial repair allows for increased blood supply and promotes growth of the prolabium (the central portion of the upper lip). Also, during this first stage, precise measurements and plans for repair of the second cleft can be made. The second stage, closure of the remaining cleft, is usually done 3 to 4 months following the initial surgery when the tissues of the first closure have softened.

If the palate is involved, the surgeon may opt to repair the anterior palate, depending on the severity, during the time of the lip repair, in which case the palatal repair is done first. The alternative is to repair the defects in two separate operations.

Key steps

1. Normal landmarks are identified and marked. Markings are made with a marking pen or the patient is tattooed with a needle dipped in methylene blue.

2. The surgeon may inject the area with a local anesthetic agent containing epinephrine to aid in hemostasis. Injection will be done sparingly to avoid distortion of the lip tissues.

3. Incisions are made along the markings.

4. The dissection follows and includes primarily the muscle but may include the nasal structures, anterior palate, and premaxilla.

5. Closure is done in three layers: the muscle and mucosa are sutured with an absorbable suture, and the lip is sutured with a nonabsorbable suture. Upon near completion of the repair, the skin edges are trimmed as perfectly as possible and sutured, ensuring that the lip is united and balanced.

6. A Logan bow (a small curved metal frame) may be used and is applied to the lip to relieve tension on the incision. It is held in place by narrow adhesive strips. An adhesive bandage covering the incision may be all that is used.

Cleft Palate

A cleft palate defect results from incomplete fusion of palatal tissues during embryonic development, resulting in a fissure through the roof of the mouth. A cleft may involve only the soft palate or may extend through both hard and soft palates into the nose and include the alveolar ridge of the maxilla. Most often, a cleft palate occurs in conjunction with a cleft lip, but on occasion occurs as a distinct deformity. A cleft palate occurring alone has a different embryonic etiology than the cleft palate associated with a cleft lip.

The bony or hard palate forms barrier between the nasal and oral cavities. Posterior to the hard palate is the soft palate, which is necessary for the production of normal speech sounds. The alveolar ridge of the maxilla borders the hard palate. The cleft forms a passageway between the nasopharynx and the nose. Clefting of the palate occurs in the midline and may involve only the soft palate or may extend through both hard and soft palates into the nose and include the alveolar ridge of the maxilla.

The primary goal of cleft palate surgery is to provide adequate palate function for the development and maintenance for normal speech (Marsh, 1989). While the cleft lip is more common, the cleft palate is a more serious anomaly. It can be associated with malnutrition, dental malocclusion, deficiencies in dental growth, eustachian tube malfunction, deafness, and airway obstruction. Cleft palate patients can have difficulty speaking, feeding, and hearing, and may have altered perceptions of taste and smell (McCarthy, 1990a).

Surgical closure of the palate is ideally performed when the patient is between 12 and 18 months of age to provide the best opportunity for the development of normal speech. If surgery is performed after the child learns to talk, a guttural tone produced by the deformity may become habitual and can persist after repair of the cleft has made normal speech possible.

Perioperative nursing considerations

1. The patient is placed in the supine position. Protect the patient's anatomy and preserve body temperature. After intubation, a shoulder roll is positioned to tilt the head backward for better visibility.

2. The surgical prep includes the nose and mouth.

3. A heavy suture is placed in the tongue at the end of the procedure. Traction on this suture can help to maintain an adequate airway.

4. Instructing the parents in the care of the postoperative palate patient is very important.
   - *Nothing* should be allowed into the mouth except the tip of a spoon for feeding.
   - Very soft foods and liquids are best for several days.

- The bolster is usually removed on the first postoperative day.
5. An oronasal fistula may develop during the healing period, requiring a second procedure.

Cleft palate repair

Key steps

1. The procedure is done under general anesthesia.
2. An oral endotracheal tube is placed directly over the center of the lower lip.
3. The surgeon may inject the palatal tissues with local anesthesia with epinephrine either before or after positioning a self-retaining mouth gag (Fig. 16-29) over the endotracheal tube.
4. Incisions are made in the palate and muscle. Dissection includes the soft palate, muscles, and preparation of the flaps.
5. The palatal incisions are closed with one layer of sutures on the nasal mucosa and another on the oral mucosa. The flaps are sutured with an absorbable suture. A bolster dressing may be sutured against the palate to provide compression and stabilize the repair (see Fig. 16-26).
6. At the end of the procedure, a heavy, nonabsorbable suture is placed deep in the tongue and taped loosely to the cheek. Tension can be applied on this suture to help maintain an adequate airway postoperatively in the event of an upper airway obstruction. A nasal airway may also be inserted and taped securely in place for the same purpose.
7. Arm or elbow splints may be applied to prevent the child from injuring the operative site.

CRANIOFACIAL SURGERY

Craniofacial surgery involves procedures to address cranial as well as facial skeletal structures. Patients may have complex congenital anomalies or defects secondary to trauma and tumor resections.

Surgical Procedures

Maxillofacial procedures

Micrognathia (receding chin) and *prognathia* (protruding chin) are deformities that involve the mandible and/or maxilla. The deformity can be one of size or relative position of the facial bones. Causes include a genetic tendency, direct trauma, sucking of the thumb, and an increased or decreased growth pattern of the mandible itself or of the adjacent facial bones. These deformities can result in difficulty with chewing or speaking, periodontal disease, temporomandibular joint dysfunction, and abnormal dental occlusion.

Orthognathic surgery addresses the relative positions of the mandible and maxilla. Mandibular and/or maxillary

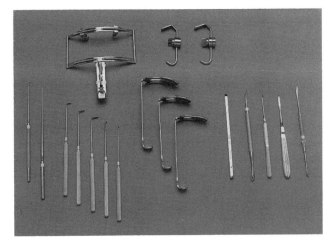

FIGURE 16-29   Palate instruments include a self-retaining mouth gag to provide adequate exposure of the operative site, nerve hooks, retractors, elevators, osteotome, periosteal elevator, septal knife, Joseph elevator, and a Freer elevator.

osteotomies with advancement or recession of the bones may be required. Small plates and screws are frequently used to secure the bone fragments into optimal position following osteotomy. The result is a stable reconstruction that usually does not require intermaxillary fixation (IMF). IMF requires the application of arch bars that hold a configuration of wires and elastics to maintain the new skeletal alignment by holding the jaw together until the surgical procedure has healed (Stever, Addante, & Strong, 1989).

Craniofacial reconstruction following trauma

Traumatic injuries may involve multiple facial fractures that can be unstable, especially if the bone has been shattered into many fragments. The segments are often displaced or dislocated. Some segments of bone may be so severely damaged that any form of fixation is almost impossible. Skin and soft tissue may be missing, in addition to the bone injury. Reconstruction may involve the use of small plates and screws (Fig. 16-30) to maintain the alignment of bony fragments. Table 16-2 describes methods of internal fixation. Augmentation with autogenous grafts or synthetic implants may be required to restore contour and replace missing structures. Performing the reconstructive surgery as a one-stage procedure addressing all of the defects can prevent the development of secondary deformities (Marsh, 1989).

A Le Fort fracture is a general term for a maxillary fracture. Differentiation between types of Le Fort fractures is based on points of structural weakness of the maxilla and serves to identify the pattern of midfacial fractures. This organization of maxillary fractures is known as the *Le Fort classification* (see Table 16-3).

General principles

1. Facial injuries are repaired as soon as possible, providing the patient's condition is medically stable. Facial edema and discomfort are reduced with early repair.

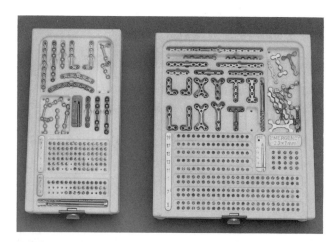

FIGURE 16-30 Various sizes, shapes, and thicknesses of plates and screws are used for stable fixation of facial bones.

TABLE 16-2 Methods of Internal Fixation

Interosseous wiring—usually used for relatively stable, localized, and undisplaced fractures of the cranium and some eye fractures. Wire is not as useful in severe, unstable fractures secondary to the ability for the bone to rotate around the wire, yielding a less than rigid fixation.

Lag screws—provide fixation by securing two bones on top of one another. Holes are made in the outer and inner bones to match the outer and inner diameters of the screw. The technique using lag screws is sometimes referred to as *interfragmentary compression* of the bone. As this method may also cause some rotation of bone, usually more than one lag screw is used to provide adequate bony fixation. Lag screws are usually used on fractures of the midface and mandible and can be used along with miniplates and reconstructive plates.

Miniplates and screws—used primarily for upper and midfacial injuries. This method provides three-dimensional stability (i.e., there is no bone rotation). The miniplate is fixed at each end to relatively stable bone segments with miniscrews; and the bone segments are then anchored to the middle of the plate, again with miniscrews.

Compression plates—because these plates are stronger than the miniplates they are often used for mandibular fractures. They produce compression at the fracture site.

Reconstruction plates—these are specially designed plates that are bendable and mimic the shape of the mandible. These plates are often used along with miniplates, lag screws, and compression plates.

TABLE 16-3 Le Fort Fractures

Le Fort I level fracture: a fracture above the teeth, including the alveolar processes of the maxilla (that portion of the maxilla containing the tooth sockets) and possibly the roof of the mouth. The fracture extends in a horizontal fashion across the base of the maxillary sinuses.

Le Fort level I stabilization is accomplished by intermaxillary fixation of the mandible, a procedure involving a configuration of wires and elastics that maintain the new skeletal alignment by holding the jaw together (Steuer, 1989) and/or open reduction technique that may allow early or immediate mobilization. If the palate is fractured, open reduction will be required along with the use of a palatal splint. The primary consideration in this fracture is to reestablish a functional dental occlusion as early as possible.

Le Fort II level fracture: a fracture of the upper maxilla, also known as the pyramidal fracture because of the general shape and configuration of the fracture. Other affected structures are the medial orbit, including the tear duct system, nose, and ethmoid. These fractures may be associated with dural lacerations, cerebrospinal fluid fistulas, and damage to the anterior portions of the brain.

Le Fort III level fracture: a fracture that extends across the bridge of the nose and floor of the orbits, yielding a complete separation of the midface from the cranium, also known as *craniofacial dysfunction*. These fractures, like those of the Le Fort II, may be associated with dural lacerations, cerebrospinal fluid fistulas, and damage to the anterior portions of the brain.

Le Fort II and III fracture stabilization is accomplished by interfragment wiring and intermaxillary fixation and open reduction of the frontal bone, zygoma, orbit, and nasoethmoid–orbital area. Bone grafting may be necessary if the injury is severe and there is a large amount of bone missing. The primary considerations in this fracture are reestablishment of midfacial height and facial projection.

Le Fort IV level fracture: a fracture involving the frontal bone.

The goal of the Le Fort IV fracture treatment is to reestablish midfacial height. This is accomplished by stabilization of the fractures.

ment, which could lead to severe secondary deformities. Fractures are reduced and fixed internally to adjacent fragments and to areas of intact craniofacial skeleton.

5. All severely damaged or missing bone is replaced and the defects are augmented, if feasible, by immediate grafting. Bone grafting may be delayed if there is an infected or contaminated wound or in the absence of adequate soft tissue cover.

Craniosynostosis

The cranial bones enclosing and protecting the brain and its associated structures include occipital, parietal, frontal, temporal, sphenoid, and ethmoid bones. These bones are united at lines of union, called "sutures," in an

2. Consultation with other disciplines (e.g., ophthalmology, ENT) may be warranted when the injuries are extensive.

3. To minimize facial scarring, the surgeon attempts to utilize the preexisting lacerations to provide direct visualization of the involved facial anatomy.

4. All fractures are directly exposed and examined to avoid missing an unreduced fracture or displaced frag-

immovable articulation. Normally the bones of a newborn infant's skull are separated, and the sutures are also separated by a layer of fibrous tissue where growth later takes place. Craniosynostosis (or craniostenosis) is the premature fusion of one or more cranial sutures before or shortly after birth. Growth of adjoining bones is stopped, with a subsequent reduction in the diameter of the skull in that direction. Compensatory growth or enlargement occurs where the sutures have remained open, resulting in a deformity of the skull. In addition, varying degrees of brain damage and mental retardation can occur secondary to the increased intracranial pressure. Hydrocephalus and visual abnormalities may occur as well.

Surgical treatment of craniosynostosis should be done as early as is feasible to avoid both the physical trauma or increased intracranial pressure and the psychological and social trauma associated with craniofacial deformities.

Crouzon's disease and Apert's syndrome

Facial clefts are congenital defects that appear to be associated with an increased incidence of congenital malformations, intellectual impairment, hearing impairments, speech difficulties, and psychological problems. Two of the more common are Crouzon's disease and Apert's syndrome.

Crouzon's disease is characterized by craniosynostosis involving the coronal, sagittal, and lambdoid sutures, resulting in brachycephaly and acrocephaly. While there is usually increased intracranial pressure, mental retardation occurs in only 20% of children with this syndrome. The forehead appears to bulge forward over the face due to the midface retrusion caused by maxillary hypoplasia. The nose arches and appears beak-like. Bulging of the eyes (exorbitism) is due to the inadequacy of shallow orbits to house the eye structures. Approximately 80% of Crouzon's patients suffer some degree of optic nerve damage.

Apert's syndrome involves anomalies of the head and extremities and bilateral symmetric syndactyly of the hands and/or feet. Syndactyly usually consists of a bony fusion of the second, third, and fourth fingers or toes, with a single common nail (Fig. 16-31,*A* and *B*). The craniofacial deformities are similar to Crouzon's disease (craniosynostosis, exorbitism, and midface retrusion). Other characteristics particular to Apert's syndrome are acne, eye paralysis, asymmetry of the exorbitism, ptosis, overhanging of the forehead with a transverse frontal skin furrow, and enlargement of the ear lobes (McCarthy, 1990b).

Hypertelorism, which grossly deforms the patient's appearance, is an abnormal increase in the bony distance between the eyes. Dystopia, a condition in which one eye is higher than the other, may also be present. Hypertelorism is usually accompanied by binocular visual defects not always corrected by craniofacial surgery. Hearing can be impaired due to anomalies of the eustachian tubes and otitis media, even without the presence of a cleft palate.

Surgery for craniofacial anomalies is complex. In addition to the physiological and mental aspects of the syn-

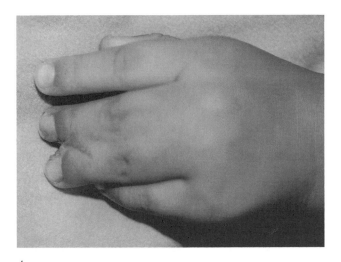

A

FIGURE 16-31 Syndactyly before (*A*) and after (*B*) surgical repair.

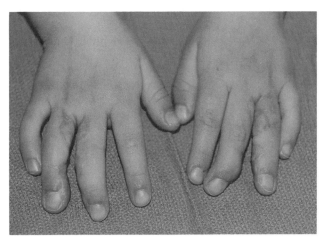

B

drome, the psychological impact on both patient and family must be addressed. A surgical endeavor of this magnitude must be addressed by a multidisciplinary team of specialists. The team includes representation from plastic surgery, neurology, neurosurgery, anesthesiology, ophthalmology, orthodontics, otolaryngology, psychology, psychiatry, radiology, speech pathology, social services, nutrition support, and nursing.

Craniofacial surgery has many goals. Relieving increased intracranial pressure permits normal brain development. Improving cosmetic appearance and restoring the anatomy to a satisfactory form help to improve the patient's physiological function. The overall goal is a significant improvement in the patient's quality of life.

Preoperative planning for patients undergoing craniofacial surgery is extensive. Diagnostic testing includes in-depth ophthalmologic evaluations, radiographic studies, computed tomography (CT) scans, and dental examinations. In the case of traumatic injury, time frequently allows for no more than X-rays and a possible CT or magnetic resonance imaging (MRI) scan. These studies help to establish the degree of deformity and determine the type of surgical correction needed.

Surgery for craniosynostosis is usually a one-stage procedure. The two major goals for early surgery are to decompress the intracranial space, alleviating the increased intracranial pressure, preventing visual problems, and permitting normal mental development; and to achieve a satisfactory craniofacial form. Craniofacial surgery for most of the other anomalies involves a series of procedures performed at various stages of the child's development.

Cranial microsomia

Cranial microsomia is a syndrome characterized by asymmetry in both position and size of facial structures. Deformities vary in extent and degree and may involve only one side of the face (hemifacial microsomia) or both sides (bilateral microsomia). The ear is usually microtic (not completely formed) and displaced. Mandibular structures may be abnormal or absent. Facial paralysis and dental abnormalities may also be involved. Deformities of the nervous system may be involved as well.

Surgical repair involves the reconstruction of several different types of tissue and is usually done in several stages. Surgical decisions depend on the age of the patient and the extent of the skeletal and soft tissue deficiency. In general, the more severe the pathological condition, the more extensive will be the surgical procedure and the younger the patient at the time of surgery (McCarthy, 1990b). Surgery is usually done on only one area at a time, and some stages, depending on the success of the original procedure, the timing, and skeletal growth, may need to be repeated. Goals of surgical intervention include soft tissue augmentation, corrective jaw surgery, and restructuring of craniofacial bone deformities. Nonsurgical devices such as splints and functional orthodontic appliances may be used preoperatively in conjunction with surgery.

Mandibulofacial dysostosis (Treacher Collins syndrome)

Mandibulofacial dysostosis involves malar and mandibular hypoplasia. The lower eyelids may be notched and there may be a partial to total absence of lower lashes. The patient is characterized as chinless, with laterally drooping eyelids, a slanted position of the eyes, and a sad facial expression.

Other problems associated with this syndrome include external ear deformities with or without middle ear anomalies that may cause hearing loss and subsequent impairment of speech and intellectual development. There is usually underdevelopment of the body, probably related to chronic respiratory deficiency (Marsh, 1989). Mental retardation usually does not occur.

Correction of the deformities involved in Treacher Collins syndrome require a series of surgical procedures. Surgical repair involves malar and maxillary reconstruction, mandibular reconstruction, correction of eyelid de-

formities, and reconstruction of the ear. Timing of surgery is important, involving determination of normal facial growth and psychological impact of the deformity on the patient and family. Generally the bony reconstruction precedes soft tissue corrections.

Down syndrome

Because of the increased life expectancy and the improved health care for persons with Down syndrome, there is increasing emphasis on their integration into society and provision of vocational training. These factors have increased the importance of improving the appearance, speech, and eating behaviors of the individual with Down syndrome.

Functional corrections include reducing the size of the large, protruding tongue with a wedge excision of the anterior section. An ophthalmic surgeon can correct strabismus. Pharyngopalatoplasty (corrective surgery of the pharynx and palate) can relieve possible obstructive sleep apnea, and adenoidectomy and tonsillectomy improve the airway.

Aesthetic corrections include repairs of the nose, eyes, cheekbones, lower lip, and chin. Rhinoplasty can correct the "saddle nose" appearance, which is the flattened bridge area between the eyes. The repair of the epicanthal folds and the upward slanting of the eyes can be done in conjunction with the rhinoplasty. The slanting is corrected by detaching one of the lateral tendons of the eye and reinserting it in a lower position. The flattened cheekbone and the smallness of the chin or lack of chin projection can be augmented with a prosthetic implant. The hanging lower lip sometimes disappears as the Down syndrome child grows older, especially with the help of physiotherapy or speech therapy. If the redundant lip persists, a wedge excision of the lip can improve the appearance.

SUMMARY

Plastic surgery involves a broad range of procedures and varied opportunities for the perioperative nurse. Whether the patient is having a cosmetic procedure in a physician's office or multistaged reconstructive surgery in a large operating suite of a tertiary care facility, the goal is to achieve the most normal appearance possible and restore the patient's function to the highest degree possible. The healing process; knowledge of skin, grafts, and flaps; and wound closures are critical to each procedure.

The perioperative nurse will have a special supporting relationship with many patients having plastic surgery. By understanding the surgical procedure and the supplies, equipment, and instruments required, the nurse will be able to meet the patient's and family's needs as well as manage the sophisticated technology associated with the surgical procedure.

REFERENCES

Barton, F. E. (1991). The aging face: Rhytidectomy and adjunctive procedures. *Selected Readings in Plastic Surgery, 6* (19).

Byrd, H. S. (1991). Rhinoplasty. *Selected Readings in Plastic Surgery, 6* (17).

Goodman, T. (1988). Grafts and flaps in plastic surgery. *AORN Journal, 48,* 650–663.

McCarthy, J. G. (Ed.) (1990a). *Plastic surgery: Cleft lip and palate and craniofacial anomalies* (vol. 4). Philadelphia: W. B. Saunders.

McCarthy, J. G. (Ed.) (1990b). *Plastic surgery: The face* (vol. 3). Philadelphia: W. B. Saunders.

McCarthy, J. G., May, J. W. Jr., & Littler, W. J. (Eds.) (1990). *Plastic surgery: The hand. (Part I, vol. 7).* Philadelphia: W. B. Saunders.

Marsh, J. L. (1989). *Current therapy in plastic and reconstructive surgery: Head and neck.* Toronto: B. C. Decker

Sauter, S. K. (1989). Cleft lips and palates. *AORN Journal, 50,* 813–824.

Steuer, K. Addante, R. R., & Strong, J. (1989). Orthognathic surgery. *AORN Journal, 50,* 536–551.

Burns, A. J., & Ornstein, H. H. (1990). Pressure sores. *Selected Readings in Plastic Surgery, 5* (39).

Chen, Z. W., & Chen, Z. R. (1991). Reconstruction of the thumb and digit by toe to hand transplantation. *World Journal of Surgery, 15* (4).

Goodman, T. (Ed.) (1989). *Core curriculum for plastic and reconstructive surgical nursing.* Pitman, NJ: Anthony J. Jannetti, Inc.

Goodman, T., & White, S. (1988). Microvascular revascularization. *AORN Journal, 48,* 666–676.

Hodges, P. L. (1990). Principles of flaps. *Selected Readings in Plastic Surgery, 6* (3).

Hodges, P. L., and Tebbetts, J. B. (1991), Blepharoplasty and Browlift, *Selected Readings in Plastic Surgery, 6* (18).

Kelton, P. L. (1990). Principles of skin grafts. *Selected Readings in Plastic Surgery, 6* (2).

Kunert, P. (1991). Structure and construction: The system of skin flaps. *Annals of Plastic Surgery,* 509–516.

Moore, K. L. (1985). *Clinically oriented anatomy (2nd ed.).* Baltimore: Williams & Wilkins.

Snively, S. L. (1991). Deformities of the external ear and their correction. *Selected Readings in Plastic Surgery, 6* (14).

Spicer, T. E. (1989). Reduction mammoplasty and mastopexy. *Selected Readings in Plastic Surgery, 5* (29).

Vasconez, L. O., McCraw, J. B., & Camargos, A. G. (1991). Muscle, musculocutaneous, and fasciocutaneous flaps. In *Grabb & Smith's plastic surgery (4th ed.).* Boston, Little, Brown & Co.

ADDITIONAL READINGS

Agris, J., & Varon, J. (1983). *Suction assisted lipectomy: Clinical atlas.* Houston: Terrico.

Aston, S. J., & Smith, J. W. (1991). *Grabb and Smith's plastic surgery (4th ed.).* Boston: Little, Brown & Co.

PART III

Special Information

Minimally Invasive Surgery

Key Concepts

- Minimally invasive techniques for surgery represent a dramatic revolution. The innovations of minimally invasive surgery pose challenges not only for surgeons but for nursing and ancillary staff as well.

- Minimally invasive surgery is possible because of a series of technological breakthroughs, including miniaturized rigid and flexible optical systems, insufflation, electrosurgery and lasers, and miniaturized instrumentation.

- Applications of minimally invasive surgery are spreading rapidly. Gynecologists were the first laparoscopists, and orthopaedic surgeons have long used endoscopic techniques. Recently, the techniques have been adopted by a wide variety of other specialties, including general surgery and cardiovascular surgery.

- Minimally invasive surgery is fueling the shift to outpatient surgery, which may change the very nature of hospitals.

- Much of the surgical training for laparoscopic surgery is taking place outside academic medical centers. This underlines the importance of a strong hospital credentialing process.

- Minimally invasive surgery means significant changes for operating room staff and will require added resources for service planning, education, staffing, and supply management.

- A strong focus on patient education and discharge planning is necessary because patients spend little time at the facility.

- Understanding each component in the endoscopic surgery armamentarium is essential for persons who assist with minimally invasive surgery.

- Endoscopes and endoscopic instrumentation pose a challenge for infection control because they are difficult to clean, disinfect, and maintain.

INTRODUCTION

In recent years, surgery has experienced a dramatic revolution unlike any since the introduction of general anesthesia and antibiotics. For many common procedures, patients no longer need a large incision. Instead, surgeons can operate through tiny incisions using an endoscope while watching their progress through a lens or on a video screen. Because the operations cause less trauma, patients have less pain and discomfort, a shorter hospital stay, and much more rapid recovery than with conventional surgery. As patients have learned of these benefits, they have eagerly sought out surgeons to perform them, and this surgical revolution has spread with unprecedented speed.

These innovations have produced challenges not only for surgeons but for nursing and ancillary staff as well. Staff must be trained to assist with the new procedures, which involve very technical equipment. New supplies and equipment must be evaluated and purchased. Operating room suites must be redesigned to accommodate the advanced equipment. The hospital must shift its patient care focus because many patients who once needed inpatient surgery now arrive the morning of their procedure and may go home the same day. This shift requires dramatic changes in program planning, including facilities, admitting procedures, patient teaching, and recovery. Meeting these challenges requires a multidisciplinary, interactive approach to patient care.

Nursing's role in the revolution of minimally invasive surgery is to manage the technology by obtaining knowledge and skills necessary to operate and care for the equipment and to teach others these skills. Nurses must also be prepared to teach patients and their families about their surgical procedure and how the technology minimizes hospital stay and contributes to a more rapid recovery than with more invasive methods.

Care of the equipment and instrumentation is a challenge due to the many channels, grooves, curves, and delicate nature of scopes and associated instruments. Nurses must create the systems and procedures to use in caring for the technology, and then must train ancillary staff to perform that care.

The nurse must also learn new ways to prepare and position the patient for some of the new procedures and must identify associated hazards in order to provide a safe environment.

Descriptions of two minimally invasive surgical procedures are provided as examples. Additional descriptions of minimally invasive surgical procedures can be found throughout this volume, especially in Chapters 7, 9, 11, and 12.

THE HISTORY OF ENDOSCOPY

The recent revolution in surgery would not have been possible without a series of technological breakthroughs. Surgeons have been able to experiment with and to per-

TABLE 17-1. Milestones in Endoscopy

1805 Bozzini examined the urethra with a tube and candlelight.
1843 Desormeaux invented the first effective endoscope.
1869 Pantaleoni designed the first hysteroscope, a "uteroscope." Light source was a kerosene lamp or a candle.
1901 Kelling performed celioscopy on a living dog.
1910 Jacobeus performed the first laparoscopy on a human.
1911 Bernheim was the first in the United States to view the peritoneal cavity using a proctoscope.
1918 Getze developed the automatic spring needle. Takagai performed knee arthroplasty on a cadaver, using a cystoscope.
1920 Ordnoff developed the pyramidal point on a trocar.
1921 Bircher introduced the Jacobeus laparoscope into the knee, terming it "arthroendoscopy."
1928 Bovie developed the electrosurgical cauterization unit.
1929 Kalk devised the foroblique lens; second puncture for controlled liver biopsy.
1932 Schindler introduced the first semiflexible gastroscope.
1934 Ruddock reported on 900 peritoneoscopy procedures.
1938 Verres developed the modified spring needle to induce pneumothorax.
1940 TeLinde described culdoscopy.
1947 Palmer introduced the endouterine cannula.
1952 Fourestier, Gladu, and Vulmiere developed the quartz rod external light source.
1953 Thomsen took color photographs of cul de sac.
1965 The Wolf Company developed the electronic flash.
1967 Hopkins lens system was introduced.
1968 Cohen and Fear rekindled laparoscopy in the United States.
1969 Lumina optic system was introduced.

(Data from Phillips, J. [Ed.]. [1977] *Laparoscopy* [pp. 15–16]. Baltimore: Williams & Wilkins, 1977, adapted from Gaskin et al.)

fect new techniques because of developments in light sources, optics and photography, insufflation, energy sources, and instrumentation.

The history of endoscopy dates back to the 1800s (Table 17-1). According to Hirschowitz (1988), a leader in endoscopy, understanding the development of the technology requires an examination of endoscopy before fiberoptics were available. The first documented attempt at endoscopy was by Bozzini, an obstetrician, in 1805 (Wheeless & Katayama, 1985; Russell, 1988; Gaskin et al., 1991). Interestingly, Bozzini was censured by the medical faculty of Vienna for being too inquisitive in attempting to observe the interior of the urethra of a living patient with a simple tube and candlelight. The instrument at that time was called a *Lichtleiter* (Fig. 17-1).

Desormeaux (called the father of endoscopy) invented the first effective endoscope in 1843 (Gaskin et al., 1991). In 1869 Pantaleoni designed a uteroscope (an early hysteroscope) similar to an instrument Desomeaux had developed in 1865 for examination of the urinary bladder. Pantaleoni's uteroscope consisted of a small, straight, narrow tube that could easily be inserted into the urethra or uterus. The light came from a kerosene lamp or a candle

(Russell, 1988). These innovations were followed by Brunton's development of the otoscope, Langlebert's development of the urethroscope, and Nitze's invention of the cystoscope (Gaskin et al., 1991). Nitze, in cooperation with the Leiter company, built the first optical lens into the instrument (Russell, 1988).

The first laparoscopies were performed in 1901 by von Ott in Petrograd, when he inspected a patient's peritoneal cavity with a head mirror and a speculum introduced through a small abdominal incision, and by Kelling in Dresden, when he introduced a cystoscope into the abdominal cavity of a dog (Filipe et al., 1991; Gaskin et al., 1991; Davis, 1992). Others credit Jacobeus of Stockholm for the first abdominal endoscopy in the human body. In 1910, he described the inspection of three body cavities, peritoneal (laparoscopy), pleural, and pericardial (Filipi et al., 1991; Gaskin et al., 1991). In the United States, Bernheim was the first physician to view the peritoneal cavity using a proctoscope in 1911 (Gaskin et al., 1991).

Takagi of Tokyo University in Japan first successfully applied the principles of endoscopy to the knee joint when, in 1918, he viewed the interior of a cadaver knee using a cystoscope. Bircher introduced the Jacobeus laparoscope into the knee in 1921, calling the technique arthroendoscopy. Watanabe and Ikeuchi performed the first arthroscopic meniscectomy in 1962. Early operative procedures done under arthroscopic control were somewhat limited by the equipment available at that time. Biopsies, removal of loose bodies, and trimming of menisci were all that was possible with the early equipment (Jackson, 1991).

The first gastric endoscopes, called electroscopes, were produced nearly 80 years ago by Bruening (Fig. 17-2). Because they were difficult to pass into the stomach, Schindler introduced the first semiflexible gastroscope in 1932. Half of the instrument could be flexed for introduction, but once in the stomach, the device had to be straight to accommodate the 50 or more lenses spaced along the shaft. Hirschowitz (1988) comments, "Gastroscopy with the Schindler instrument required good training, a good assistant, and a patient with a compliant anatomy approaching that of a sword swallower" (Fig. 17-3).

Optics, Lighting, and Photography

Over the past 90 years, manufacturers have invented, improved, and miniaturized rigid and flexible optical systems that have improved diagnostic and therapeutic capabilities of instrumentation while reducing trauma to patients. Urologists began examining the urinary tract in the nineteenth century with fairly crude instrumentation. In 1929 Kalk devised a new lens system that permitted oblique (132-degree) viewing (Gaskin et al., 1991). This advance transformed laparoscopy into an effective diagnostic and surgical procedure (Wheeless & Katayama, 1985). By 1967 British physicist Harold H. Hopkins had developed a superior lens system using large, rod-shaped,

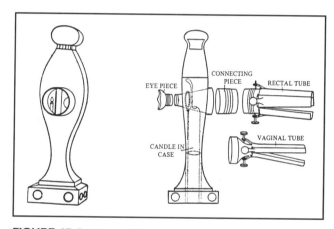

FIGURE 17-1   Bozzini lamp. Note lighted candle. (From Berry, L. H. [1974]. *Gastrointestinal pan-endoscopy.* Springfield, IL: Charles C Thomas. Reprinted with permission.)

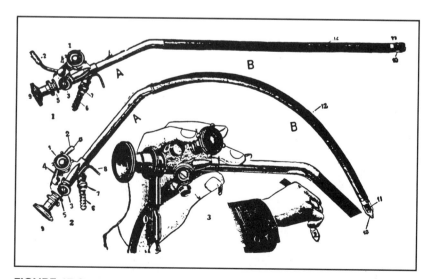

FIGURE 17-2   Bruening's electroscope was one of the first to use electric illumination, about 1907. (From Berry, L. H. [1974]. *Gastrointestinal pan-endoscopy.* Springfield, IL: Charles C Thomas. Reprinted with permission.)

quartz lenses that vastly improved image brightness and clarity (Gaskin et al., 1991). His principles are still utilized in laparoscopes today (Talamini & Gadacz, 1991). In the 1970s, a flexible fiberoptic endoscope was invented that conducted the images from inside the body through thousands of flexible glass fibers rather than rigid rod lenses.

The earliest source of endoscopic lighting was the incandescent bulb. The introduction of fiberoptic (cold) light sources in the early 1960s eliminated the risk of bowel burns caused by incandescent lighting (Talamini & Gadacz, 1991). The fiberoptic cable consists of an inner core of glass known as cladding. The hot light source enters one end of the fiberoptic cable and is repeatedly and totally reflected from the lateral surfaces until it emerges at the opposite end as cold light (Gaskin et al., 1991). In the 1970s, high-intensity halogen light sources enhanced endoscopic photography. Most recently, the xenon vapor light source has been utilized.

In 1934 Carl Schroeder produced the first pictures taken through a hysteroscope (Russell, 1988), but photography was not really feasible until fiberoptic technology was developed because of the low level of illumination from the small light bulb and loss of much light through the many lenses (Hirschowitz, 1988). Laparoscopic cinematography was developed in the late 1960s. A xenon vapor source, color film of appropriate speed, and finally, the development of the Lumina optic system in 1969 allowed enhancement of full-screen color movies. The Lumina system had narrow diameters with optics at the top, allowing a 160-degree angle for oblique vision, surrounded by glass fibers for the transmission of cold light (Gaskin et al., 1991).

The first commercially successful medical color video system was introduced in 1972. The system, which employed fiberoptics to transfer a microscopic image to an 18-pound, three-tube video camera, was used primarily for teaching. These cameras were large, complex, and too heavy to be attached directly to an endoscope. A smaller camera weighing about 4 pounds became available the next year. For the first time, the camera could be attached directly to the microscope or endoscope, eliminating the need for the fiberoptic image guide. A dramatic advance, this camera was simple to operate yet offered high performance.

The first truly miniature camera, brought to market in 1975, measured only 2 inches by 2 inches by 8 inches and weighed a little more than a pound. This practical innovation allowed the camera to be attached directly to the endoscope and afforded a good range of movement for the surgeon. By 1980 cameras small enough to hold in the palm of the hand provided a full range of natural color with excellent resolution. Solid-state technology now enables cameras to be less than 2 inches on a side and weigh about 3 ounces (Fig. 17-4). Cameras have also been made waterproof, so they can be soaked in liquid disinfectants.

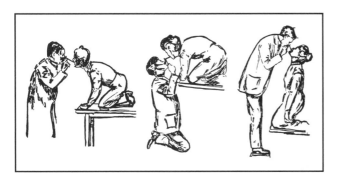

FIGURE 17-3 Three successive positions used to introduce a rigid gastroscope in the early 1920s. (From Berry, L. H. [1974] *Gastrointestinal pan-endoscopy.* Springfield, IL: Charles C Thomas. Reprinted with permission.)

Insufflation

The first attempts at laparoscopy in humans were initiated without pneumoperitoneum (insufflation) (Gaskin et al., 1991). In 1920 Ordnoff developed a trocar with a pyramidal point, making access to the abdominal cavity easier. He also developed an automatic trocar sheath valve that prevented the escape of gas (Fig. 17-5). In 1938 Verres adapted an automatic spring needle for safe puncture and gas insufflation of the abdomen that is still used today (Fig. 17-6).

Carbon dioxide gas is used for insufflation because of its quick absorption. In 1977, Kurt Semm introduced the carbon dioxide pneumautomatic insufflator (Gaskin et

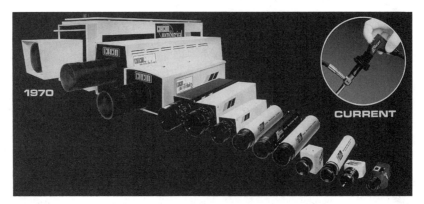

FIGURE 17-4 Advancements in video technology. (Courtesy of Circon ACMI Corp.)

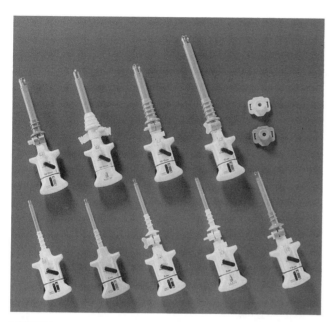

FIGURE 17-5 Endopath disposable surgical trocars with adjustable stability threads (grippers) and disposable trocar reducers. (Courtesy of Ethicon Endo-Surgery, Cincinnati, OH.)

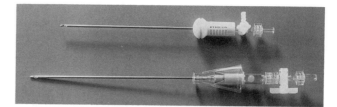

FIGURE 17-6 Disposable Endopath pneumoperitoneum needle and ultra Verres needle needed for insufflation. (Courtesy of Ethicon Endo-Surgery, Cincinnati, OH.)

al., 1991). Before that time, air was introduced into the peritoneal cavity with a syringe (Talamini & Gadacz, 1991).

Energy Sources

Advances in cautery and energy sources also contributed to the development of endoscopy. Electrocautery or laser energy is used to dissect tissue. Either energy modality also achieves adequate hemostasis of small blood vessels (Talamini & Gadacz, 1991). In 1928, an electrosurgical unit designed by Bovie was first used intraoperatively for the control of bleeding (Gaskin et al., 1991). Originally, only unipolar coagulation devices were available to control bleeding. Later, bipolar grasping forceps (Kleppinger forceps) were developed, providing for safer hemostasis.

Whereas electrocautery uses microwave wavelength energy to produce heat that can dissect and coagulate tissue, lasers use photons to dissect and coagulate tissue. A major advantage of lasers is that they produce less lateral tissue damage than electrocautery (Talamini & Gadacz, 1991).

Lasers, which had already been used in gynecology, were introduced to laparoscopic surgery by Bruhat et al. (in 1979) in France, by Tadir et al. (in 1991) in Israel, and by Daniell & Brown (in 1982) in the United States. This technique allowed more complicated laparoscopic operations, particularly extensive adhesiolysis and the destruction of endometriosis foci (Gordon & Magos, 1989).

Instrumentation

In 1925 a hysteroscope was developed by Harold F. Seymour in England that had three channels, one for the light and two for suction or irrigation, as needed (Russell,

1988). The culdoscope was used extensively to visualize the pelvic organs from 1949 to 1967. The culdoscope was introduced into the cul de sac after puncturing the posterior fornix. The patient was placed in the knee–chest position, allowing air to rush in by suction. Culdoscopy now has been almost completely replaced by laparoscopy (Mattingly & Thompson, 1985).

Palmer, a Frenchman, developed the endouterine cannula in 1947, along with a number of other instruments that modernized laparoscopy. Palmer, who used the term "gynecological celioscopy" rather than "laparoscopy," preferred this procedure to culdoscopy because it reduced the risk of pelvic infection (Mattingly & Thompson, 1985). Patrick Steptoe, an English gynecologist, described the necessary instrumentation and techniques, especially those for sterilization, and wrote the first textbook on laparoscopy (Davis, 1992).

The term "operative pelviscopy" was coined by Kurt Semm of Germany, who pioneered a series of technological advances that led to more complicated therapeutic laparoscopic procedures. He created an innovative heat transfer system, thermocoagulation, for sterilization procedures. To provide accurate and easy transection of tissues, he invented the hook scissors. In 1969, Semm designed a "uterus vacuum mobilizer" for improved manipulation and laparoscopic visualization of reproductive organs. He also perfected the Endoloop applicator, a device designed to prevent loss of intraperitoneal insufflated carbon dioxide when sutures are inserted into the peritoneal cavity. Semm also perfected intra- and extracorporeal knot-tying techniques and instruments that enabled surgeons to perform these maneuvers. He then developed an irrigation and aspiration apparatus to prevent tube clogging. He developed an automatic abdominal insufflator and pressure monitor. Many other instruments were then created, such as needleholders, cone-shaped trocars, microscissors, clip appliers, atraumatic forceps, and the Hasson cannula (Filipe et al., 1991; Davis, 1992). Consequently, laparoscopic operations grew to include techniques of tubal ligation, salpingostomy, salpingolysis, tumor biopsy and staging, incidental appendectomy, and more (Davis, 1992).

In 1986, with the invention of the computer chip video camera, assistants and others in the operating room could view the progress of the operation and help more effectively. This advance paved the way for development of laparoscopic cholecystectomy (Davis, 1992). In 1987, building on prior advances in gynecological and abdominal surgery, Phillippe Maurial of Lyon, France, per-

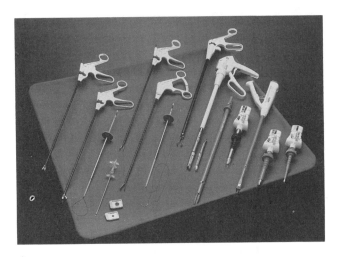

A

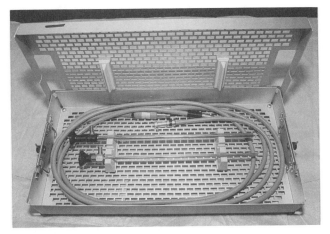

B

FIGURE 17-7   (*A*) Endoscopic instrumentation commonly used for laparoscopically assisted vaginal hysterectomies. (*B*) Five- and ten-millimeter zero-degree laparoscopes with light cords in instrument pan. Disposable Endopath (*C*) endoscopic instruments, (*D*) instrument tips, and (*E*) electrosurgery suction and irrigation devices. (*F*) Endopath rotating multiple clip applier used for endoscopic applications. (*G*) Endopath disposable retractor. (*H*) Instrument pan with reusable instruments. (*I*) SurgiTie used for pedicle ligation (commonly used for laparoscopic appendectomy) and SurgiWip used for endoscopic suturing. (*J*) Endo Catch used for capturing laparoscopically retrieved tissue (commonly appendix) or stones (commonly gallstones).   (*C* through *G* courtesy of Ethicon Endo-Surgery, Cincinnati, OH; *A*, *I*, and *J* courtesy of United States Surgical Corporation; *B* courtesy of Smith & Nephew Dyonics Inc.)

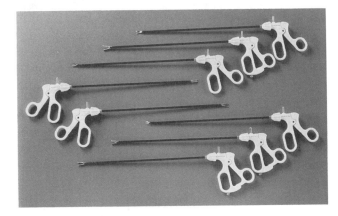

C

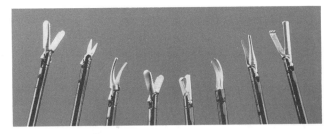

D

formed the first laparoscopic cholecystectomy. In June 1988, McKernan and Saye performed the first laparoscopic cholecystectomy in the United States, utilizing the argon laser. Other noteworthy surgeons pioneering this technique include Dubois of Paris and Reddick of Nashville, Tennessee (Gaskin et al., 1991; Davis, 1992).

Challenges for the future include continued development of more versatile operative endoscopic instruments and techniques and refinement of indications for procedures (Davis, 1992) (Fig. 17-7).

APPLICATIONS

Because major advances in endoscopic surgery occurred in several specialties, it is difficult to be certain which branch of surgery was the first to apply them. Laparoscopic cholecystectomy has attracted the most attention because gallbladder removal, one of the most common procedures in the United States, is performed more than 500,000 times each year. Whereas patients used to need 6 weeks to recover from major abdominal surgery, now they can be back to work in about a week.

By the year 2000, industry experts predict that 80% of abdominal surgeries will be endoscopic (American Hospi-

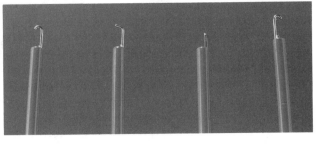

E

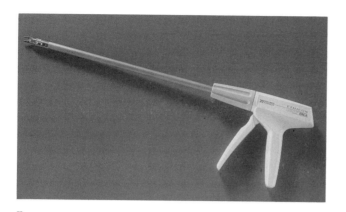

F

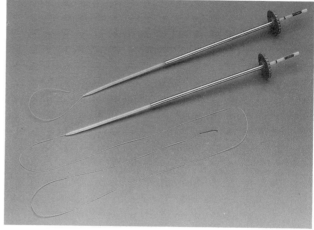

I

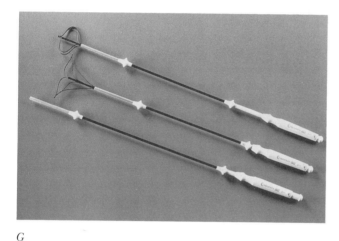

G

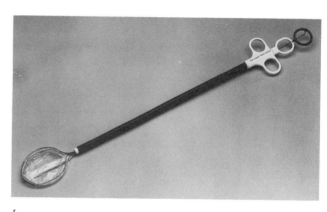

J

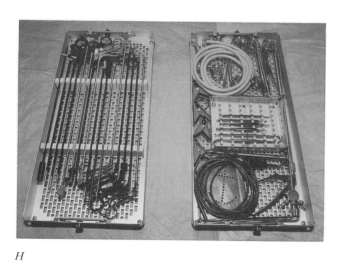

H

tal Association, 1992). Laparoscopic cholecystectomy has replaced open surgery as the gold standard for symptomatic gallbladder disease (Soper, 1992). An advisory panel of the National Institutes of Health (NIH) in 1992 endorsed the procedure as a safe and effective surgical treatment for gallbladder removal (NIH, 1992).

Endoscopic technique is spreading to other general surgery procedures as well, though more slowly than for cholecystectomy. In 1992 it is estimated that 15% of appendectomies and 5% of hernia repairs were being done laparoscopically. Though fewer than 1% of colectomies, vagotomies, and Nissen fundoplications were being done by this method, these figures are expected to increase dramatically (McKernan, 1992).

Surgeons from a variety of specialties are applying the techniques of minimally invasive surgery (Table 17-2). The frontiers appear to be limited only by the imagination of current and future innovators. The first laparoscopists were gynecologists, who have long used the instrument for endometriosis and tubal ligations. They are now performing laparoscopic-assisted hysterectomies. In urology, the time is rapidly approaching when open surgery will no longer be needed. Nonsurgical introduction of stents and drains, extracorporeal shock wave lithotripsy, advances in ureteroscopy, and use of pulsed-dye laser lithotripsy all offer alternatives to difficult open surgeries (Fig. 17-8). Investigators have performed and are refining endoscopic techniques for nephrectomy, herniorrhaphy, bowel resection, adhesiolysis, and vagotomy. Thoracoscopy, once a common procedure that fell into disuse, is being revived for diagnosis and treatment of malignant pleural effusions, treatment of bullous disease of the lung, biopsy of abnormal lung tissue, and staging of lung cancer (Davis, 1992).

TABLE 17-2 Examples of Minimally Invasive Surgery Applications

Endoscopic surgery

General surgery
Appendectomy
Bowel resection
Cholecystectomy
Choledocholithotomy
Hernia repair
Lymph node staging for Hodgkin's disease
Lysis of adhesions
Placement of catheters
Proximal gastric vagotomy

Gynecology
Bilateral tubal ligation
Drilling of polycystic ovaries
Ectopic pregnancy
Laparoscopic-assisted hysterectomy
Myomectomy
Neosalpingostomy
Oophorectomy
Ovarian cystectomy
Presacral neurectomy
Salpingectomy
Uterosacral nerve ablation
Vaporization of endometriosis

Orthopaedic Surgery
Abrasion arthroplasty
Anterior and posterior cruciate ligament reconstruction
Carpal tunnel release
Debridement/resection of osteophytes
Intraarticular fracture (femoral and tibial condyles)
Ligament repair
Meniscectomy

Patellar realignment
Shoulder decompression and rotator cuff repair
Synovectomy
Temporomandibular joint treatment

Thoracic surgery
Ablation of bleb
Hiatal hernia repair
Lobectomy
Pericardial window
Placement of internal cardiac defibrillator electrodes
Pleurodesis
Thoracic sympathectomy
Vagotomy
Wedge resection of the lung

Urology
Lymphadenectomy
Localization of undescended testes
Nephrectomy

Other minimally invasive surgery applications

Cardiovascular surgery
Atherectomy
Peripheral angioplasty
Vascular stent placement

Urology
Extracorporeal shock wave lithotripsy
Ureteroscopy with pulsed-dye laser

Neurosurgery
Laser percutaneous disc decompression

The arthroscope has dramatically changed orthopaedic surgery (Johnson, 1986). Arthroscopic surgery is possible for virtually every joint, including procedures such as arthroscopic meniscectomy, meniscus repair, abrasion arthroplasty, anterior and posterior cruciate ligament reconstruction, temporomandibular joint treatment, shoulder decompression repair, and carpal tunnel release (Fig. 17-9).

Cardiology and cardiovascular surgery are embracing a range of new catheter-based procedures, including laser angioplasty, atherectomy, and stents. From an even broader perspective, minimally invasive therapy eventually may include treatments at the molecular and genetic level that eliminate surgery altogether (American Hospital Association, 1991). A molecular therapeutic approach may eventually eliminate gross excision of some cancers. Computed tomography (CT) and magnetic resonance imaging (MRI) are eliminating the need for many invasive brain studies and helping to make neurosurgery more precise.

IMPACT

Such a dramatic revolution in surgery inevitably has a profound effect on an entire institution, especially its operating room department. Minimally invasive surgery is accelerating the trend toward outpatient surgery. In 1990, the number of outpatient surgeries for the first time surpassed that of inpatient surgeries in the nation's community hospitals (American Hospital Association, 1992). Many patients who once needed inpatient surgery now do not come to the hospital at all. They may have their surgery performed in an outpatient facility or even in a physician's office. Short-stay alternatives are evolving for patients who need hospital care for only a day or two.

Impact on the Hospital

With the major shift to outpatient procedures, the whole nature of the hospital may change. Some experts think the acute care hospital will evolve into a large intensive

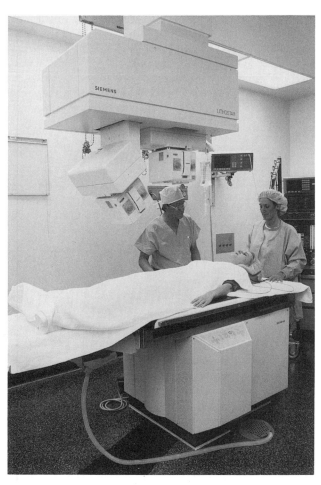

FIGURE 17-8 Preparing for an extracorporeal shock wave lithotripsy treatment using the Siemens Lithostar. (Printed with permission of Siemens Medical Systems, Inc.)

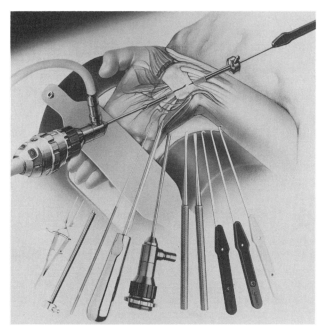

FIGURE 17-9 An arthroscopic carpal tunnel release using the Dyonics Ectra system. (Courtesy of Smith & Nephew Dyonics Inc.)

care unit for the most severely ill patients (Coile, 1991). Satellite facilities surrounding the hospital will provide a range of other health services, including outpatient care, ambulatory surgery, transitional care, and long-term care. "Except for major regional institutions, the acute-care hospital as we know it will probably not survive," contends health care strategist Jeff Goldsmith in the *Harvard Business Review.* "The successful hospital of the future will reach out into homes and residential communities as much as it depends on the sick to cross its threshold for help. This is the radical prescription in store for hospitals."

New types of institutions are already appearing. Some major medical centers are electing to "unbundle" (separate) all their outpatient services, including surgery, from the main hospital. They are building large new centers specifically geared to ambulatory services, emphasizing efficiency, convenience, and service in an aesthetically pleasing environment. Examples of these are the Johns Hopkins Outpatient Center in Baltimore, a nine-story, 450,000–square foot facility, and St Luke's Medical Tower, part of the St Luke's system in Houston, with 27 floors and 1 million square feet.

The hospital administration must be fully aware of the new technology and must support changes that will allow the hospital to maintain a competitive position. The technology is expensive, both as a capital expenditure and for operating expenses such as replacements, repairs, service contracts, and continuous staff training. Hospitals frequently hire outside consultants to assist with the necessary changes. A consultant may be able to act as a nonthreatening agent of change in making decisions about corporate direction or negotiating conflicts.

In this new climate, hospitals must plan strategically to refocus care for patients who are predominantly ambulatory. If hospitals hope to compete with outpatient settings, they must emphasize efficiency, convenience, quality, and service, not only for patients and families but for physicians, too.

Economic Impact

Procedures that minimize trauma and shorten recovery would seem to be less costly. For example, less traumatic gallbladder surgery may effect savings for society as a whole by minimizing days lost from work. One researcher estimated an employer would save about $3000 in wages alone when an employee who earns $25,000 a year has laparoscopic cholecystectomy instead of an open procedure (Stoker et al., 1992).

But the jury is still out on costs to the health care system. Though patient stays for laparoscopic cholecystectomy are shorter, costs of equipment and instruments are higher, and the new procedures frequently require additional operating room personnel. A recent study compared results and costs for 280 patients having laparoscopic surgery with those for 304 patients who had a traditional open procedure. Despite a shorter stay, laparoscopic surgery had much higher hospital costs (average $5541 per patient) than conventional surgery (average $4436 per patient). The higher costs were attributed to operating room costs, which were 63% of the total for laparoscopic procedures and 39% for conventional surgery. The initial laparoscopic surgery required a longer time in the operating room, as well as more expensive equipment, including disposable trocars and clip appliers.

Impact on the Operating Room Department

Although minimally invasive surgery is more convenient and comfortable for patients, it has not made life easier for operating room managers and their staffs. Procedures such as cholecystectomy, once routine, now can be logistical nightmares. Surgeons and nurses alike must learn a whole new way of performing surgery, with an array of advanced technology. In planning for this massive change, operating room departments must consider facilities, staffing, and technology.

Many hospitals are reorganizing surgery facilities to accommodate better the volume of outpatients and same-day admissions. Several models are emerging (American Hospital Association, 1992). No one model is right for every situation, experts point out, and facilities must evaluate a number of variables when developing a plan appropriate for their needs. Blends of these options are common. The models include

1. integrated inpatient and outpatient operating room suites;
2. hospital-based outpatient surgery centers (on campus); and
3. hospital-based free-standing outpatient surgery centers.

Also growing rapidly is the number of independent free-standing surgery centers. Free-standing centers, both hospital-owned and independent, grew from 964 in 1988 to 1690 in 1992 (Henderson, 1994). Hospitals' share of outpatient surgery declined from more than 90% in 1985 to 83% in 1990 (American Hospital Association, 1992).

Integrated inpatient and outpatient operating room suites

The economical and practical solution may be to combine inpatient and outpatient surgery in a single suite. Potential advantages of an integrated suite include construction savings (assuming the hospital has enough operating rooms to accommodate volume), surgeon convenience, flexibility, and shared resources (Patterson, 1992). Many hospitals find that physicians who perform both inpatient and outpatient procedures prefer to schedule all their procedures in the same suite so they do not have to shuttle between two locations.

Experts emphasize, however, that to work well for outpatients this arrangement must provide a well–thought out system for patients to enter the system. Ideally, the hospital will have a separate outpatient surgery admissions area with its own entrance and waiting area, where patients come both for testing and for preparation on the day of surgery. The traditional arrangement, which requires patients to travel all over the hospital for their presurgical testing, is inconsistent with today's emphasis on efficiency and service.

Separate outpatient surgery units

Another possible arrangement is to have a separate outpatient surgery unit within the hospital or to build a separate surgery center on or off the hospital campus. Again, the decision rests on the hospital's existing facilities and strategic objectives.

Advantages of a separate unit, say experts, are marketing, pricing, aesthetics, and greater efficiency (Patterson, 1992). A separate facility can position itself in the market as being specifically designed for outpatients. Package pricing is easier because supply use is more readily monitored and controlled. Outpatient surgical personnel are accustomed to a fast pace and rapid turnover of cases, and the schedule is less likely to be interrupted by emergencies than in an inpatient facility. Also, anesthesia providers are geared to faster-acting anesthetic agents and more rapid recovery of patients.

Separate operating room units may have disadvantages as well. Some centers have found that their outpatient operating rooms, built several years ago, are no longer large enough for today's technologically sophisticated cases. As a result, they lack scheduling flexibility. Physicians may find it cumbersome to move back and forth between two suites even if they are under the same roof. Off-campus surgery centers do best, planners advise, if they are tailored to a single specialty such as ophthalmology, sports medicine, or plastic surgery that has sufficient volume to keep them busy. (See Chapter 33, Volume 1 for more details on same-day surgery.)

Impact on Surgeons

In many specialties in the near future surgeons will have to be able to operate through an endoscope. The change is a major one. Surgeons who for years have performed conventional surgery suddenly must learn a new way of doing surgery. Rather than directly visualizing and touching the surgical field, they must learn to operate in two dimensions while watching a video monitor and manipulating instruments in opposition. One surgeon has compared the challenge of performing endosurgery to learning to drive a car backward, full speed, while watching in the rear view mirror.

Physician credentialing for laparoscopic surgery

Much of the learning for endoscopic techniques is taking place outside the academic medical centers where surgical education typically occurs. Many surgeons are learning in short laparoscopy courses, where, ideally, they practice on animals in the laboratory. Shortly thereafter, they may begin operating on humans.

Though in expert hands laparoscopic cholecystectomy is considered safe, the complication rate during a surgeon's early procedures is higher than that for conventional surgery. A large study of 1518 patients having laparoscopic gallbladder procedures found a 2.2% incidence of bile duct injury in the first 13 patients operated on by each surgical group. The rate dropped to 0.1% in subsequent patients, the same as for open surgery (Southern Surgeons Club, 1991). This finding was confirmed by another study, which found that 10 of 12 bile duct injuries occurred during a surgeon's first dozen or so cases (Davidoff et al., 1992).

Reports of complications from the procedure began to appear in late 1991 and 1992. The New York State health department, gathering data from hospitals in the state, estimated a surgical error rate of 2% for laparoscopic cholecystectomy. From August 1990 to June 1992, the department recorded 192 laparoscopic procedures resulting in injury. Seven patients died (*Health Facilities Series*, 1992). Injuries included cuts to the common and hepatic bile ducts, the aorta and other major vessels, and organs such as the liver and small bowel. A number of reports also appeared in the medical literature by surgeons who treated complications of patients who had been referred to them (Cheslyn-Curtis et al., 1992; Davidoff et al., 1992; Hawasli & Lloyd, 1991; Moossa et al., 1992; Rossi, 1992; Wolfe et al., 1991).

Laparoscopic cholecystectomy has become fertile ground for malpractice litigation. A commentary in the *Archives of Surgery* predicted a "firestorm of litigation" as plaintiff's attorneys take on bile duct injury cases (Rossi, 1992). Bile duct injury from routine gallbladder surgery traditionally has been a leading cause of malpractice claims (Kern, 1992).

Because so many surgeons are receiving their laparoscopic training in midcareer, hospitals, through their medical staff credentialing committees, bear a heavy responsibility for making certain surgeons are prepared for the new procedures. That role will become increasingly important as laparoscopic techniques spread to other applications. Though nurse managers are not directly involved in physician credentialing, they often have an administrative role in monitoring surgeons' credentials for procedures that are scheduled. Managers also should be aware that, under the legal doctrine of corporate liability, a health care facility can be held liable separately from physicians for harm to patients.

Credentialing committees need to establish standards to ensure that surgeons who undertake laparoscopic surgery are qualified to do so. If surgeons have not received such training in a residency program, they should have taken an approved, well-designed course; have hands-on animal experience; and if appropriate, have performed a certain number of procedures under an expert proctor. Setting credentialing standards can be difficult because of the lack of precedent for midcareer surgical training. There is little oversight for orthopaedic courses and no consensus on the type or extent of proctoring that should be expected. Opinions differ about whether surgeons should be credentialed separately for each new laparoscopic procedure they undertake (Meyer, 1992b).

Professional statements and guidelines provide hospitals some assistance in formulating credentialing policies. For laparoscopic courses, the American Medical Association and the AHA recommend use of a standard report form developed for recording course content and physician performance.

The American College of Surgeons said in a 1990 statement, "For optimal quality patient care, laparoscopic cholecystectomy should be performed by surgeons who are qualified to perform open cholecystectomy." The college believes only such surgeons have the skills to perform biliary tract procedures, to determine the best method for gallbladder removal, and to treat complications.

Concerned about complications in New York State, the health department in 1992 took the unprecedented step of issuing detailed guidelines to hospitals on laparoscopic cholecystectomy. The guidelines specified that surgeons who do the procedure must have attended a course including direct experience with animals. Before receiving full credentials for laparoscopic cholecystectomy, surgeons must assist at least five to ten procedures under a surgeon credentialed for the procedure and then must act as responsible surgeon under direct supervision until competency is attained (Health Facilities Series, 1992).

The Society of American Gastrointestinal Endoscopic Surgeons (SAGES) has three guidelines covering privileges for laparoscopic general surgery, clinical application of laparoscopic cholecystectomy, and courses seeking SAGES endorsement. The privileging guidelines say proctoring is desirable but do not say it must be done. Procedural details are left to the hospital credentialing body (SAGES, 1992a) (Fig. 17-10). Two expert laparoscopists suggested expert supervision for a surgeon's first 12 to 50 procedures (Way, 1992; Braasch, 1992). A national registry for laparoscopic surgery has been established at Temple University in Philadelphia.

Though credentialing for advanced laparoscopic procedures is controversial, particular concern has been raised by one of the new procedures, laparoscopic colon resection. The American Society of Colon and Rectal Surgeons has warned that the technique is unproven and that its complication rate may exceed that of traditional therapy. For that reason, the society said laparoscopic resection should be done only in controlled environments where safety and efficacy can be evaluated. It stopped short of suggesting the procedure be limited to clinical trials. The society has established a registry for laparoscopic colectomy (American Society of Colon and Rectal Surgeons, 1991).

Impact on nursing and operating room personnel

Minimally invasive surgery means significant changes for the operating room staff. The salary budget will increase because the staff needs additional time for education, program planning, and equipment management. Additional staffing is needed for surgical cases as well. For example, unless a robotical mechanical arm is utilized an additional scrub person is needed to operate the camera for endoscopic cases, and an additional nurse is required

FIGURE 17-10 Privileging Guidelines for Laparoscopic General Surgery

Guidelines for granting privileges for laparoscopic general surgery have been developed by the Society of American Gastrointestinal Endocopic Surgeons (SAGES).

For a surgeon who has not had residency or fellowship training or documented prior experience in laparoscopic surgery, the training process should be similar to a residency experience, including didactics, hands-on animal experience, participation as a first assistant, and performance of the operation under proctorship.

Minimum requirements for training should be:

- Completion of an approved residency in general surgery, with privileging in the comparable open procedure for which laparoscopic privileges are being sought.
- Privileging in diagnostic laparoscopy.
- Training in laparoscopic general surgery by an experienced laparoscopic surgeon or completion of a university-sponsored or academic society–recognized didactic course, which includes instruction in handling and use of laparoscopic instrumentation, principles of safe trocar insertion, establishment of safe peritoneal access, laparoscopic tissue handling, knot tying, equipment utilization (e.g., staplers), as well as animal experience in specific categories of procedure for which the applicant desires privileges. The individual must demonstrate to the satisfaction of an experienced physician course director or preceptor that he or she can perform a given procedure from beginning to end in an animal model. Such proficiency for each category of procedure in question must be documented in writing by the physician course director. The course content and procedures taught should clearly include material specific to the category of procedure for which privileges are sought. Attendance at short courses that do not provide supervised hands-on training or documentation of proficiency is not an acceptable substitute.
- Experience as first assistant to a previously privileged individual performing the category of the laparoscopic procedures for which privileges are being sought in patients; documentation to be provided by the privileged individual.
- Proctoring by a laparoscopic surgeon experienced in the same or similar procedure(s) until proficiency has been observed and documented in writing.

SAGES also has guidelines for courses seeking its endorsement as well as for diagnostic and gastrointestinal endoscopy.
(Excerpted with permission from Society of American Gastrointestinal Endoscopic Surgeons. [1992]. *Granting of Privileges for Laparoscopic (Peritoneoscopic) General Surgery.* Los Angeles, SAGES.)

if a laser is used. Because the circulating nurse typically is responsible for monitoring the safety of all personnel in the operating room suite, that person must be thoroughly familiar with the equipment and its proper use.

Seminars on new technology may require travel, an additional expense. New employees require extended orientation periods to learn new procedures. New orientation programs and in-service sessions must be developed to meet the changing needs of current and new staff. Staff must also be trained for the ongoing maintenance of equipment. All this educational preparation should be documented for quality assessment purposes.

Supply management also takes additional time. The staff must work with surgeons to standardize supplies and equipment. They need to evaluate whether disposable or reusable instruments are used, and they must plan for

managing the supply inventory. Many facilities have computerized their surgical inventories for effective monitoring. Computerization of inventory requires a large initial investment because personnel are needed to enter and maintain the data.

Time is needed for planning patient education, updating policies and procedures, and conducting quality-monitoring activities. It is critical that staff have time to interact with members of other hospital departments to provide coordinated, quality care to patients.

On the other hand, surgical innovations bring benefits to the staff as well. Financial, management, and clinical skills are refined in the process of developing minimally invasive services. And with the new technological demands, surgical nurses have become more educated, knowledgeable, skilled, and, thus, empowered.

PATIENT EDUCATION

Candidates for minimally invasive surgery must be thoroughly oriented to and educated in their procedure. Because patients spend little time at the facility before surgery and are dismissed shortly after the surgical procedure, a new approach to preoperative teaching is needed. Many outpatient surgery centers arrange for nurses to call patients before the day of surgery to obtain a nursing history. At that time, the nurse collects pertinent historical medical and surgical data and communicates any concerns to the anesthesia provider and surgeon. A letter should also be mailed to the patient before surgery that explains the procedure and provides preoperative instructions (Figs. 17-11, 17-12). A map showing where the facility is located and a floor plan with facility locations can be enclosed.

Some institutions have established preoperative clinics, where patients can come before the day of surgery for diagnostic testing and anesthesia evaluation. A few institutions have begun to send registered nurses to the patient's home for a preoperative evaluation. Whatever the procedure, a thorough preoperative evaluation is required.

Discharge planning is also essential for minimally invasive surgery. This process can be initiated during preoperative teaching. Written home instructions are mandatory to describe follow-up care (Figs. 17-13, 17-14). Many facilities include in their plan of care a postoperative phone call; some include a postoperative home visit by a registered nurse. In many cases, a discharge planner facilitates the planning.

MANAGING THE TECHNOLOGY

Managing the technology associated with minimally invasive surgery is a nursing responsibility, often done in collaboration with other disciplines such as surgeons, materials management personnel, biomedical engineers, and central processing department.

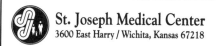

St. Joseph Medical Center
3600 East Harry / Wichita, Kansas 67218

Dear **JOHN DOE:**

Your physician has scheduled you for **LAPAROSCOPIC CHOLECYSTECTOMY WITH CHOLANGIOGRAM POSSIBLE OPEN CHOLECYSTECTOMY** at St Joseph Medical Center on **MONDAY MARCH 1, 1993** at approximately **7:30 AM**. So that your surgery may start on time, please check in at the Registration Desk in the front lobby at **5:30 AM**. Please park your car in the main lot in front of the hospital on Harry Street, and enter through the front door.

In order for us to obtain a **medical history**, you need to call us at **689-5356** between the hours of **9:00 A.M.** and **4:00 P. M.,** Monday through Friday. If you have a history of (**and/or** take medications for) blood pressure problems, diabetes, heart or lung disease, be certain to inform us because we have special instructions for you! If you have had a previous anesthetic and experienced any problems, inform us so that we may correctly plan for your care. If we do not hear from you , we will call you one or two day before your scheduled surgery.

The enclosed list of instructions must be followed to ensure proper care and safety. If we can be of any additional assistance, please do not hesitate to call us.

Patricia A. Kusnerus R.N.
Patricia A. Simmons R.N.
ST. JOSEPH SURGERY DEPARTMENT

Blending technology and family care . . . for life.
Member CSJ Health System of Wichita.

FIGURE 17-11 Sample preadmission letter to patient. (Courtesy of St. Joseph Medical Center, Wichita, KS.)

This section describes necessary equipment, design of the operating room, placement of equipment within the room, care of instruments and equipment, and the process for disinfection and sterilization.

Endoscopy Equipment and Instrumentation

With endoscopic procedures, operating rooms have entered a new age in therapeutic technology. An endo-scopic equipment cart has become standard equipment in most operating rooms. An understanding of each component on the endoscopy cart is absolutely essential for persons assisting with minimally invasive endoscopy procedures. Staff must thoroughly understand the purpose, use, and complications associated with this complex, delicate equipment and instrumentation. This section describes the major types of endoscopy equipment.

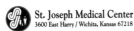

St. Joseph Medical Center
3600 East Harry / Wichita, Kansas 67218

Please bring a list of your medications to the hospital with you.

Do not eat or drink anything after Midnight, INCLUDING WATER, unless otherwise instructed.

Arrange in advance for a responsible adult to drive you home upon your dismissal.

Wear comfortable clothing that will allow for easy dressing and undressing.

Dentures or partial plates must be removed prior to coming to the operating room.

Nail polish and makeup should not be worn.

Please leave all valuables at home, jewelry and rings must be removed.

Bring your special insurance forms/cards.

Blending technology and family care . . . for life.
Member CSJ Health System of Wichita.

FIGURE 17-12   The patient instruction list enclosed with the patient preadmission letter.   (Courtesy of St. Joseph Medical Center, Wichita, KS.)

Endoscopy carts

Two carts should be used to house the essential equipment for endoscopic surgery (Table 17-3; Fig. 17-15). The first cart contains the primary equipment, and the second the slave video monitor. The primary cart typically has an enclosed area to protect the delicate video equipment, insufflation equipment, and other components. The cart should be durable (usually of steel construction), easily movable (usually on casters), have a turntable platform on top for the video monitor, contain four enclosed shelves, and be equipped with a hospital-grade outlet strip with a cord at least 15 feet long, terminating in a hospital-grade, operating room–compatible plug. Primary cart components typically include a video monitor, one or two dual-head video camera systems (each with single or dual camera head) with a picture-in-picture attachment, a color video printer, videocassette (VCR) and still video recorder, a universal light source, an automatic carbon dioxide insufflator with an attached carbon dioxide tank, a bipolar generator, and possibly an irrigation and aspiration device. Two camera systems used with a video mixer afford picture-in-picture capability.

The secondary cart should also be of durable construction and easily movable. Since it houses only the slave monitor, the cart can be open, and shelves are optional.

Video camera system

The video camera system should provide surgeons with advanced video technology for all endoscopic procedures. The video system is a chain of components that affords visualization inside the body. The basic chain consists of the high-intensity light source, fiberoptic or liquid light guide, flexible or rigid endoscope, miniature video camera, monitor, and videotape recorder.

Miniature color video cameras now are widely used for all types of endoscopic procedures. Attached to the endoscope, these cameras convert the optical image viewed by the endoscope into electrical signals displayed on a high-resolution color monitor. Endoscopic clip-on cameras weigh about 3 ounces and are about 1.5 inches cubed. A dual-head camera system is essential. Accessory control buttons on the camera head give the surgeon or camera holder control of printers, still image recorders, VCRs, and camera sensitivity. A dual–camera head input provides the ability to switch quickly and easily between different scopes.

Modern cameras utilize a one- or three-chip technology. The chips, technically termed charge-coupled devices (CCDs), are solid-state sensors composed of tiny light-sensitive pieces of silicon called pixels. The pixels emit electrical impulses that are transmitted through the system to the video monitor. In one-chip cameras, a single CCD is responsible for the image, which is broken into red, green, and blue color bands by a special filter. A three-chip camera dispenses with the filter, directing each of the red, green, and blue color bands to its respective receptor chip. Both one- and three-chip cameras are available in three formats: NTSC, S-VHS (Super VHS), or RGB (red, green, blue). By separating luminance (light) and chrominance (color) information, the S-VHS format reduces problems of "dot crawl" and video distortion. Further improvements in image sharpness and color rendition are offered by the professional RGB format, which provides separate signal paths for the three color components along the entire route to the monitor.

The next generation of cameras will employ computerized digital technology. Rather than providing a continuous (analog) image, these cameras will translate the image into thousands of tiny digitized bits. Digitized pictures can be manipulated to provide dual images, split screens, and freeze frames. Images can also be stored for later retrieval. Beyond digital technology are three-dimensional video and virtual reality with remote technology, which will enhance the surgical team's visualization potential even further.

New integrated systems have also become available in which the camera is permanently attached to the endoscope. These systems can deliver clear, bright images without the inconvenience of focusing and fogging at the scope-camera connection. Some scopes also have built-in lens-washing and irrigation systems (Fig. 17-16). This feature allows for washing of the distal lens to remove fog and debris and provides an irrigation channel to rinse the operative site.

PHYSICIANS ORDER		ST. JOSEPH MEDICAL CENTER ● WICHITA, KS. 67218			
DATE	TIME	ORDERS	NOTE: Specify route of Administration on Medication Orders	R$_X$**	**ANTIMICROBIAL**

R$_X$** Authorization is given for the dispensing of a generic (Therapeutic) equivalent medication as governed by the Pharmacy & Therapeutics Committee UNLESS THIS COLUMN IS CHECKED NEXT TO THE ORDERED MEDICATION.

Drug _____

Date _____

Duration _____

_____ Prophylactic

_____ Empiric

_____ Therapeutic

POST-OP LAPAROSCOPIC CHOLECYSTECTOMY ORDERS

1. ROUTINE V.S.

2. UP AD LIB

3. CLEAR LIQUID PROGRESSIVE DIET

4. IV TO HEPARIN LOCK

5. DC NG AND FOLEY

6. MS 4-8 MG IV Q 2 HRS PRN PAIN

7. PERCOCET 1-2 TABS Q 3-4 HRS PRN PAIN

8. REGLAN 10 MG. IV Q 4 HRS NAUSEA

9. MAY TAKE OWN MEDS.

10. STRAIGHT CATH IF UNABLE TO VOID

11. GIVE PATIENT THEIR GALLSTONES. MAY DISMISS WHEN
    ABLE TO EAT, VOID, AMBULATE AND WHEN PAIN IS
    CONTROLLED WITH PERCOCET. CALL ME FOR
    OUTPATIENT OBSERVATION ORDERS OR ADMISSION AS
    AN INPATIENT.

Drug _____

Date _____

Duration _____

_____ Prophylactic

_____ Empiric

_____ Therapeutic

Drug _____

Date _____

Duration _____

_____ Prophylactic

_____ Empiric

_____ Therapeutic

APPROPRIATE USAGE:

Prophylactic - Surgery or invasive procedure

Empiric - Diagnosis or pathogen not confirmed

Therapeutic - Documented infection or known pathogen

DRUG ALLERGIES	SO458 REV 11/91		UNIT	ROOM

PATIENT NAME - PLATE IMPRESSION

PATIENT NAME - HAND WRITTEN

Pink Copy - Original - Retain on Chart

Yellow Copy - Duplicate - PHARMACY COPY

PHYSICIAN'S ORDERS

FIGURE 17-13   Routine postoperative laparoscopic orders.   (Courtesy of St. Joseph Medical Center, Wichita, KS.)

1. ☐ Prescription sent home with patient. Use as directed.
    ☐ If you have discomfort take Tylenol or Aspirin as you would at home for minor irritations.
    ☐ No prescription necessary.

2. **ACTIVITIES FOLLOWING A GENERAL ANESTHETIC OR SEDATION**
    ☐ Do not make important personal or business decisions or sign any legal documents for today.
    ☐ Do not drive or operate hazardous machinery today.
    ☐ Limit your activities for 24 hours. Do not engage in sports, heavy work, or heavy lifting until your
      physician gives you permission.
    ☐ When taking pain medications, be careful as you walk, drive, or climb stairs. Dizziness is not unusual.
    ☐ May resume normal activities.
    Diet
      ☐ Begin with liquids and light food (Jello, soups). Progress to your normal diet if you are not nauseated.
      ☐ Resume Normal Diet.
      ☐ Do not consume alcoholic beverages for a 24-hour period.

3. **WOUND CARE**
    A small amount of bright red blood is to be expected. Do NOT be alarmed. If you feel that the
    amount is excessive, call your doctor.
    ☐ Change dressings as necessary.
    ☐ Do not change your dressings until you are seen by your doctor.
    ☐ Keep dressings dry.
    ☐ May bathe or shower over wound.

4. **SPECIAL INSTRUCTIONS**
    ☐ Elevate affected extremity.
    ☐ Apply ice to the affected area.
    ☐ Apply heat to the affected area.

5. **FOLLOW-UP CARE:**
    You should see Dr. _____ on _____. Call the office for an appointment.

6. **OTHER INSTRUCTIONS**
    Specific complications to watch for:
      Fever over 101°F by mouth.
      Pain not relieved by the medication ordered.
      Increased redness, warmth, swelling, or hardness around the operative area.
      Inability to urinate.
    If any of the above complications occur, call the physician.

    Date: _____ Physician Signature _____

    I have received and understand these instructions. I also have been informed that if I have any questions or
    problems, I am to call my physician.

    Date: _____ Signature _____

PATIENT IDENTIFICATION

ST. JOSEPH MEDICAL CENTER
WICHITA, KANSAS 67218

**ADULT OUTPATIENT
DISCHARGE INSTRUCTIONS**
P-714   12/90

ORIGINAL: CHART   CANARY: PATIENT | PINK: INSURANCE   GOLDENROD: PHYSICIAN

FIGURE 17-14 Routine adult outpatient discharge instructions form.
(Courtesy of St. Joseph Medical Center, Wichita, KS.)

Other important characteristics of the integrated system include extreme light sensitivity for viewing inside dark body cavities and waterproof construction to withstand immersion in disinfecting solutions. Importantly, cameras should have universally interchangeable heads, to provide flexibility, instant backup, and fast replacement.

The correct combination of monitor and camera system is necessary to provide the desired degree of resolution. A three-chip camera requires a high-resolution monitor with 700 horizontal lines per inch to provide the enhanced image.

Replacement cameras are essential, whether they are additional purchases or "loaners" available from sales representatives. Couplers and adapters also are needed for the proper use of endoscopes, arthroscopes, and operating microscopes. A picture-in-picture attachment can be added to allow the surgeon and assistants to view two areas simultaneously on the monitor, using a dual camera system.

TABLE 17-3   Primary Endoscopy Cart Contents

Video camera system
Color video monitor
Videocassette recorder, still image recorder (with remote
  control)
Video printer
Universal light source
Automatic high-flow insufflator
Bipolar electrosurgical generator (optional)
Irrigation/aspiration device (optional)

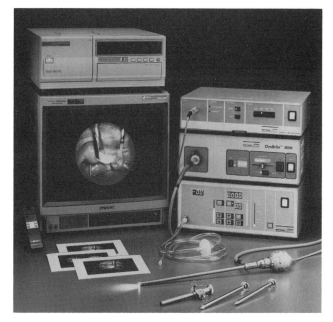

B

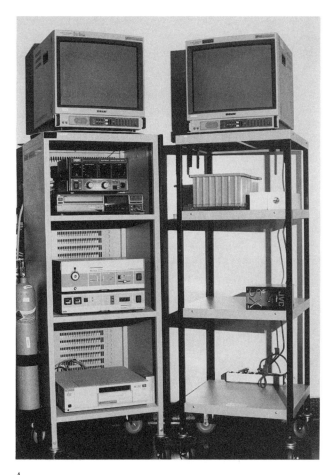

A

FIGURE 17-15   (*A*) Primary and secondary endoscopy
carts. The primary cart is shown with a single dual-head
camera system. (*B*) Video camera system shown with
printer, monitor, camera box, light source, insufflator,
videolaparoscope, reusable sheath, pyramidal trocar, and
conical trocar. (*C*) DyoCam 750 dual-head camera system.
(*B, C* courtesy of Smith & Nephew Dyonics Inc.)

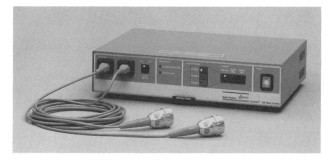

C

primary monitor. Features of a video monitor should include high resolution to ensure clear, detailed image display; bright, true-to-life color to permit superior
discrimination in the viewing field; compatibility with a
variety of inputs to provide versatility; and multiple out-
puts to permit use in a dual-monitor system. Monitors
should be of medical grade to provide the safety, quality,
and durability needed for daily use. A minimum 1-year
warranty should be considered when purchasing the
monitors.

Videocassette recorder, still image recorder, and video printer

A videocassette recorder is necessary to document
cases and to replay tapes for educational purposes. Some
surgeons record episodes of procedures and give the tape
to patients after surgery for education and information.
The recorder should offer options for frame-by-frame review, copying, or the addition of special effects.

A still-image recorder allows still images to be recorded
during surgery for disk storage and later playback. The

Color video monitors

A video monitor is needed for both primary and secondary endoscopy carts. The primary cart holds a 20-inch
color video monitor. The secondary cart has a stationary
video monitor, which should have the same features as the

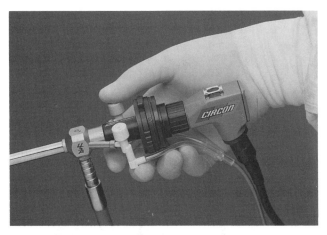

FIGURE 17-16 An advanced video hydrolaparoscope with integral operating site irrigation and antifog/antidebris scope tip cleaner. (Courtesy of Circon ACMI. Corp.)

recorder can print images in a multitude of combinations and quantities using a video printer. A video printer can save space by providing still image prints. An alternative to videotape documentation of procedures, the printer can record multiple images on a single page, depending on the size and amount of detail needed.

Universal light source

A universal light source is needed on the endoscopy cart to provide lighting for the endoscope. The standard light bulb produces 150 to 300 watts and requires a light cord at least 4 to 5 mm in diameter. As the cord diameter increases, so does the efficiency of light transmission, until the fiberglass bundle exceeds the diameter of that in the endoscope (Soderstrom, 1986). The light cable, scope, and light source must be compatible. New halogen metal halide or xenon light sources offer the brightness many surgeons demand.

Insufflation equipment

Visualizing the peritoneal cavity requires space in which to shine light and maneuver. In a standard laparotomy, this space is created by opening the abdomen and allowing room light and air into the cavity. In laparoscopic procedures this space is achieved by filling the peritoneal cavity with carbon dioxide that distends the abdominal wall and provides an area for light and manipulation. This condition is termed pneumoperitoneum. The pressure must not rise above 12 to 14 mm Hg, to prevent complications such as air embolus, damage to the diaphragm, and hemodynamic instability. A sophisticated high-flow insufflator has been developed that automatically delivers carbon dioxide from a high-pressure tank, through a regulator, and into the patient at predetermined flow rates. The new machines constantly monitor intraabdominal pressure, stop the flow once a certain pressure is reached, indicate the rate of flow of carbon dioxide into the abdomen, and record the total volume of gas delivered from the machine.

Rapid carbon dioxide insufflation into the abdomen is often necessary when smoke or a laser plume is being evacuated from the abdomen. Carbon dioxide is also lost through leaks around valves and gaskets and during exchange of instruments. Therefore, for laparoscopic general surgery, a high-flow insufflator capable of delivering at least 6 L of gas per minute is necessary, but a flow rate of 8 or 10 L per minute is preferable. Machines must be inspected frequently to ensure they are accurately calibrated because there is no backup system for regulating intraabdominal pressure (Talamini & Gadacz, 1991).

Bipolar electrosurgical generator

A bipolar electrosurgical generator, in addition to a unipolar generator, is utilized for gynecological procedures and for certain general procedures for coagulation. A bipolar forceps (when used exclusively during the case) eliminates the need for the dispersive electrode (ground pad) pad used in unipolar or monopolar electrosurgery.

Irrigation and aspiration device

An irrigation and aspiration device instills fluid at a high rate of flow that can dislodge loose material such as blood clots. A gauge regulates the irrigation pressure. Some instruments utilized with the machine are powered by pressurized carbon dioxide, which drives fluid from sterile reservoirs of irrigating solution.

Product Evaluation and Acquisition

Careful planning must take place before equipment is purchased so the components are compatible. It is desirable that equipment be standardized from room to room and from specialty to specialty. Purchase decisions must consider not only price but also service contracts and sales representative availability. If the hospital's biomedical engineering and maintenance staff are unable to repair equipment, service and repair arrangements need to be made with the manufacturer. Preventive maintenance procedures should be included in service contracts and monitored for implementation.

Design of the Operating Room

When building or renovating operating rooms, planners should allow for modifications that will accommodate future changes in endoscopic surgery. Ideally, every room should be equipped for endoscopic procedures with both primary and secondary endoscopy carts. In addition, one suite should be dedicated to arthroscopic and associated orthopaedic procedures because of the specific requirements of this specialty.

Some new operating room construction includes observation or viewing rooms. The viewing room and operating room are separated by glass panels, allowing observers to view the procedure (Fig. 17-17). Having a viewing room promotes in-service education for staff and

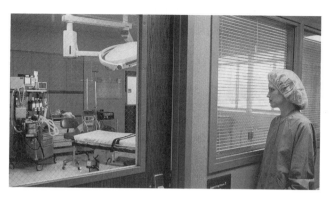

FIGURE 17-17 A minimally invasive surgical suite with a viewing window.

visitors. The viewing room can also be used for hospital public relations and promotional activities.

New operating rooms should not be less than 24 by 24 feet, to accommodate the ever-growing number of devices and equipment. If possible, there should be 15 to 16 feet between floors, allowing for a dropped ceiling with space above for electrical and television cables or other suspension systems. Electrical cords, rather than running across the floor, should drop from the ceiling and provide for a single connection to the power source at the table.

Ideally, the electrical system for each suite should be isolated from all other systems. Isolating the system prevents video interference from any microwave, electrocautery, or X-ray equipment in use adjacent to or on the same circuit. Loss of visualization can stop an operation. The arthroscopy room should also be lead-lined or be set off by distance and thick cement walls (Johnson, 1986). Multiple electrical outlets are needed because of the many pieces of power equipment that are used. Having a rheostat on the operating room lights allows them to be dimmed so they will not reflect on the video monitor. Proper air conditioning and humidity control are essential in operating rooms used for minimally invasive procedures.

If lasers are needed, the room should have a built-in smoke evacuation system connection to the suction system. The room may also need additional plumbing and special electrical wiring to accommodate lasers.

In states where floor drains are permissible, the drain should be directly under the operating room table, so that during arthroscopy or cystoscopy, water can be directed away from walking areas or cords on the floor. It is critical that large storage rooms be included in the design of a minimally invasive surgical setting. The entry to the storage area should be wide enough to allow delicate lasers, smoke evacuators, microscopes, and other equipment to be moved easily without bumping into doorways. Storage areas should have electrical outlets so that battery-operated equipment can be recharged when it is not in use.

Room Arrangement and Procedural Aspects for Endoscopic Surgery

The room arrangement for a routine laparoscopic cholecystectomy is shown in Figure 17-18. Placement of equip-

ment varies, depending on the area of focus inside the abdomen, the size of the room, and surgeon preference (Figs. 17-19 through 17-25). The procedure is described step by step in Box 17-1 (see page 470).

The arrangement for arthroscopic knee surgery is shown in Figures 17-26 through 17-29. Notice that the monitor and much of the equipment are stored on an over-bed table. A step-by-step description of an anterior cruciate ligament reconstruction is in Box 17-2 on page 473.

Care of Equipment

Endoscopic video equipment and instruments—delicate, expensive, and more fragile than standard items—must be cared for properly. Besides the obvious problem of breakage from dropping or excessive force, items can also be damaged during cleanup, takedown, scrubbing, sorting, and wrapping or packing. Continual education is essential to minimize breakage and maximize efficiency. The entire staff must be involved. Many operating rooms employ a video technician to maintain their endoscopy equipment. If no one is assigned to manage the endoscopy equipment and instrumentation, breakage is inevitable. The cost of repairing or replacing equipment and instrumentation will be exceedingly high and is unnecessary (Johnson, 1986).

Endoscope Sterilization and Disinfection

Endoscopes present a challenge for infection control. Their increased use has raised questions and controversies about the effectiveness of reprocessing. Many of these devices are made of materials that cannot withstand the heat and moisture of steam sterilization. Ethylene oxide sterilization often is impractical because of the long processing and aeration times.

The most common method for reprocessing endoscopes, high-level disinfection, is used by more than 90% of facilities in recent surveys (Gorse & Messner, 1991; Rutala et al., 1991a). Users who rely on high-level disinfection must be aware that the process is less lethal than sterilization. Sterilization is the complete elimination or destruction of all forms of microbial life. In contrast, high-level disinfection eliminates many or all pathogenic microorganisms, but not necessarily all microbial forms, such as bacterial spores, on inanimate objects. Typically, high-level disinfection for endoscopes involves soaking the devices in a liquid chemical sterilant and disinfectant, usually 2% activated glutaraldehyde, for 10 to 45 minutes, according to the manufacturer's instructions.

The confusion over sterilization and disinfection of endoscopes was underlined in three recent studies that found major gaps between professional recommendations for reprocessing and actual practice. In a three-state survey by the U.S. Food and Drug Administration (FDA), a number of fundamental disinfection and sterilization errors were observed (Kaczmarek et al., 1992). Among them were failure to monitor the time the device was exposed to the chemical germicide, failure to clean internal

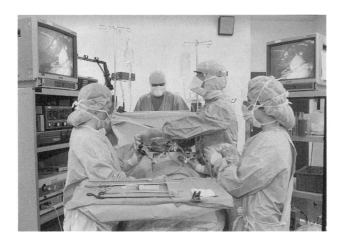

A

FIGURE 17-18   (*A*) A laparoscopic cholecystectomy in progress. (*B*) Operating room layout for laparoscopic cholecystectomy.   (*A*, Courtesy of St. Joseph Medical Center, Wichita, KS. *B*, Claire J. Sigler)

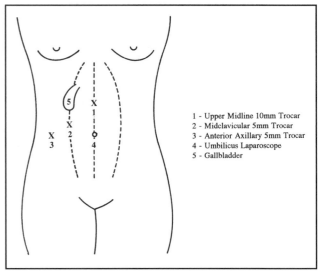

1 - Upper Midline 10mm Trocar
2 - Midclavicular 5mm Trocar
3 - Anterior Axillary 5mm Trocar
4 - Umbilicus Laparoscope
5 - Gallbladder

FIGURE 17-19   Trocar placement for laparoscopic cholecystectomy.   (Claire J. Sigler)

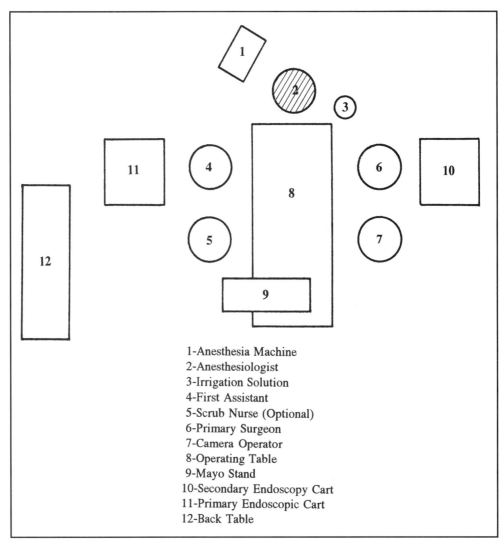

1-Anesthesia Machine
2-Anesthesiologist
3-Irrigation Solution
4-First Assistant
5-Scrub Nurse (Optional)
6-Primary Surgeon
7-Camera Operator
8-Operating Table
9-Mayo Stand
10-Secondary Endoscopy Cart
11-Primary Endoscopic Cart
12-Back Table

B

channels, not flushing all channels with disinfectant, not fully immersing the scope, and using the disinfectant beyond the date of expiration. More than three fourths (78%) of facilities did not sterilize biopsy forceps, though the Centers for Disease Control and Prevention (CDC) defines them as critical devices that require sterilization. The majority of facilities used sterilization rather than disinfection after an endoscope was used in patients with human immunodeficiency virus (HIV), hepatitis B virus (HBV), or tuberculosis infection, though that practice also is contrary to recommendations. Researchers who cultured scopes after they had been reprocessed found that almost one fourth of cultures from internal channels

of 71 gastrointestinal endoscopes grew 100,000 or more bacterial colonies. However, none of the cystoscopes or arthroscopes grew more than two colonies.

Two 1991 surveys found similar reprocessing flaws. A national survey of gasteroenterology nurses and associates with about 2000 respondents found that only two thirds were routinely using an enzymatic cleaner for decontamination. Fewer than half (48%) routinely used sterile water. Only 30% sterilized biopsy forceps. Most disinfected them. The respondents reported that the most negative influences on proper infection control practice were lack of administrative support and insufficient scopes (Gorse & Messner, 1991).

A survey of practices in North Carolina discovered that about half the hospitals were soaking endoscopes for less than 20 minutes—less than the time recommended to re-

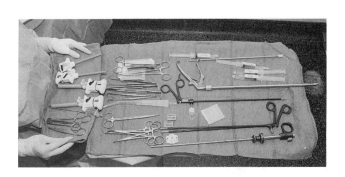

A

FIGURE 17-20 (*A*) Laparoscopic cholecystectomy Mayo tray. (*B*) Back table setup for laparoscopic cholecystectomy.

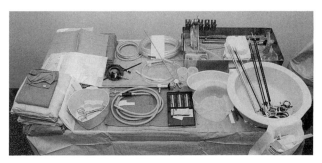

B

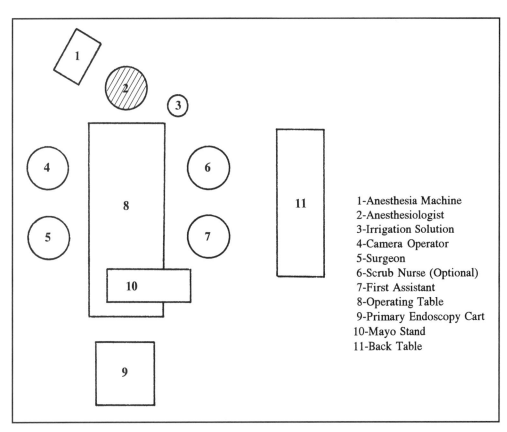

1-Anesthesia Machine
2-Anesthesiologist
3-Irrigation Solution
4-Camera Operator
5-Surgeon
6-Scrub Nurse (Optional)
7-First Assistant
8-Operating Table
9-Primary Endoscopy Cart
10-Mayo Stand
11-Back Table

FIGURE 17-21 Operating room layout for laparoscopic hernia repair.
(Claire J. Sigler)

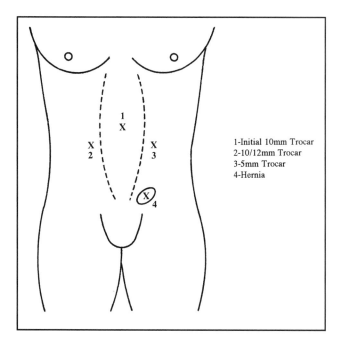

1-Initial 10mm Trocar
2-10/12mm Trocar
3-5mm Trocar
4-Hernia

FIGURE 17-22 Trocar placement for laparoscopic hernia repair. (Claire J. Sigler)

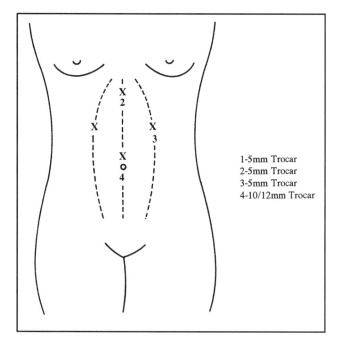

1-5mm Trocar
2-5mm Trocar
3-5mm Trocar
4-10/12mm Trocar

FIGURE 17-24 Trocar placement for laparoscopic bowel resection. (Claire J. Sigler)

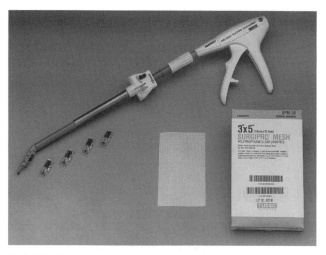

FIGURE 17-23 Multifire Endo Hernia (TM) with reloads and Surgipro mesh used for laparoscopic hernia repairs. (Courtesy of United States Surgical Corp.)

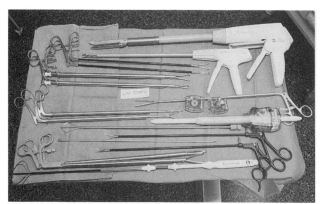

FIGURE 17-25 Laparoscopic bowel resection Mayo stand.

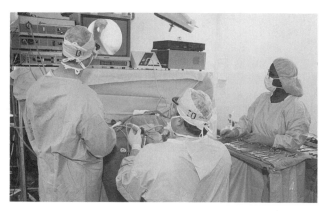

A

FIGURE 17-26 (*A*) Arthroscopic anterior cruciate ligament reconstruction in progress. (*B*) Operating room layout for an arthroscopic anterior cruciate ligament reconstruction. (*B*, Claire J. Sigler)

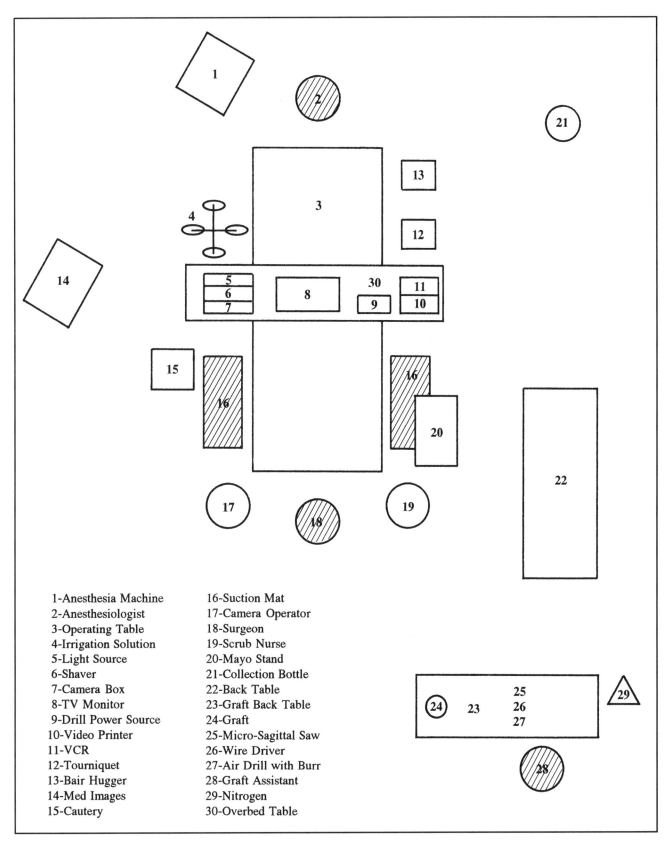

1-Anesthesia Machine
2-Anesthesiologist
3-Operating Table
4-Irrigation Solution
5-Light Source
6-Shaver
7-Camera Box
8-TV Monitor
9-Drill Power Source
10-Video Printer
11-VCR
12-Tourniquet
13-Bair Hugger
14-Med Images
15-Cautery

16-Suction Mat
17-Camera Operator
18-Surgeon
19-Scrub Nurse
20-Mayo Stand
21-Collection Bottle
22-Back Table
23-Graft Back Table
24-Graft
25-Micro-Sagittal Saw
26-Wire Driver
27-Air Drill with Burr
28-Graft Assistant
29-Nitrogen
30-Overbed Table

B

Box 17-1   Perioperative Nursing Considerations for Endoscopic Surgery (Laparoscopic Cholecystectomy)

Personnel
Circulating nurse
Scrub camera person (or robotical/mechanical arm)
Scrub first assistant
Laser nurse (if applicable)
Operating room
Supplies
   According to surgeon's preference
   Consider adequate backup, integrity and sterility of equipment
   Camera/light cord/instrument set (grasper/scissors/clipper)
   10-mm zero-degree telescope/5-mm zero-degree telescope
   Irrigation/suction setup
   Medications (antibiotic before incision/heparinized irrigation/ cholangiogram dye or contrast medium)
Equipment
   Video endoscopy cart
   20-inch TV monitor/VCR (audio and video)/high-flow insufflator/light source/camera unit/video printer
   Satellite TV monitor
   Electrosurgical unit and pedal
   High-level disinfection solution cart
   Backup CO_2 tank
   Laser (if applicable)
Location of equipment
   Video endoscopy cart on patient's right side toward head
   Satellite TV monitor on patient's left side toward head
   Electrosurgical unit and pedal on patient's left side toward head
Backtable
   Instrument set
   Basin set
   Drapes, gowns, gloves
   Electrosurgical cord, CO_2 hose, cystoirrigation tubing
   Light cable, camera or video drape for camera
   Sharps container
   Sponges
Mayo stand setup
   #11 blade
   Sharp towel clips
   CO_2 needle
   10-mm port × 2
   5-mm port × 2
   Reducer, 5.5-mm
   Endoscopic graspers
   Endoscopic scissor
   Endoscopic clipper
   Endoscopic cholangiocath setup
   Endoscopic electrosurgical hook, spatula
   Endoscopic suction-irrigation device
   Saline, dye syringes

Antifog solution
Instrumentation to remove gallbladder from umbilicus
   Hemostats, curved × 3
   Metz scissors
   Oral suction tip
   Senn retractors
   Army-Navy retractors
   Needle holder, 7-inch
   Tissue forcep with teeth
   Needle holder, 6-inch
   Adson forceps with teeth
Patient preparation
Assessment/identification
   Conduct interview, establish rapport, talk with family, identify surgeon.
Safety/comfort/position
   Transport patient, transfer to operating room bed.
   Provide comfort with warm blankets, touch, quiet.
Anesthesia induction/intraoperative period
   Stand by patient, assist anesthesia person with intubation.
   Monitor input and output and drugs (preincision antibiotic).
Nursing interventions
   Scout film
   Assess condition of skin; place Foley catheter, Salem sump drain; perform shave (if ordered); place electrosurgical grounding pad.
   Prepare skin above nipple line to pubis and from bedside to bedside, with emphasis on umbilicus.
   Monitor aseptic technique practices.
   Prioritize and anticipate activities, such as X-ray.
   Be knowledgeable about equipment purposes and functions; connect and turn off equipment.
   Contact family of delay or longer than anticipated case.
   Maintain accountability (medications, counts for sponges, instruments, and sharps).
   Communicate with team members and other nursing units who will be caring for the patient.
   Maintain laser safety (if applicable).
Step-by-step procedure for scrub person
1. Assist with draping patient.
2. Hand off to circulator:
      CO_2 tubing
      Light cord
      Suction tubing
      Electrosurgical cord
      Cysto flow tubing
3. Drape camera with circulating nurse assisting.
4. Hand surgeon No. 11 knife, hemostat, then towel clip. (Surgeon dissects then grasps fascia with towel clip.)
5. Hand surgeon Verres needle (Surgineedle). Insufflation begins.

Box 17-1 Continued

6. Hand surgeon 10-mm trocar, which is inserted, followed by 10-mm laparoscope for abdominal viewing.
7. Hand surgeon No. 11 knife to make three additional incisions (for one 10-mm trocar and two 5-mm trocars).
8. Pass endoscopic instruments as needed:
    Suction
    Electrosurgical instrument
    Graspers
    Scissors
    Clip applier
    Cholangiocatheter
    Stone basket
9. Assist as surgeon removes gallbladder through the 10-mm umbilical port using the 10-mm laparoscope in the upper midline port.

10. Hand surgeon a hemostat and Metz scissors when gallbladder is pulled up through 10-mm port. (Gallbladder remains grasped with grasper.)
11. Assist with suctioning gallbladder contents and retracting with a Senn retractor for easy removal of gallbladder.
12. Once gallbladder has been removed, pass closing suture.
13. Place dressings on patient ($\frac{1}{4}$-inch adhesive strips, one 2 by 2, and three small adhesive bandages).
14. Wash patient's abdomen and remove drapes.

Documentation
    Wound classification - II

By Darci Gressel, RN, section leader, operating rooms, and Debbie Keagy, RN, BSN perioperative nurse instructor, St. Joseph Medical Center, Wichita, Kansas.

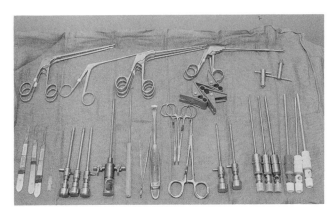

FIGURE 17-27 Mayo tray for arthroscopic anterior cruciate ligament reconstruction.

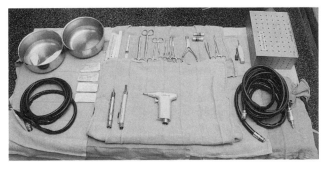

FIGURE 17-28 Graft table setup for arthroscopic anterior cruciate ligament reconstruction.

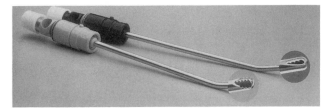

A

FIGURE 17-29 Instruments for arthroscopic anterior cruciate ligament reconstruction. (*A*) Curved incisor and Synovator. (*B*) Stonecutter used for notchplasty. (*C*) A Med Image machine used by surgeons for operative reports integrated with intraoperative pictures. (C, page 472) (*B*, courtesy Smith & Nephew Dyonics Inc.; *C*, courtesy of Med Images Inc.)

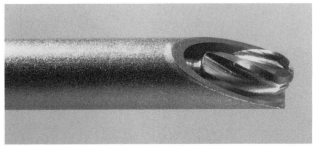

B

liably inactivate mycobacteria. Almost all hospitals disinfected at room temperature. More than half were rinsing scopes with tap water, though sterile water is recommended. And, as in the national survey, more than half of hospitals modified their disinfection process when the

previous endoscopy patient was known to have HIV, HBV, or tuberculosis (Rutala et al., 1991a).

Problems also have been found with endoscope washers. The CDC reported in 1991 on two hospitals that had traced endoscope contamination to automated reprocessing machines. The machines can become colonized with organisms such as *Pseudomonas aeruginosa* and *Mycobacterium chelonei*. Such colonizations can result in nosocomial infections or pseudoinfections (CDC, 1991). The FDA is

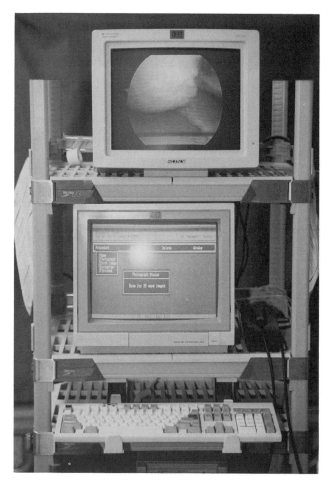

C

working with the American Society for Testing and Materials toward a standard for performance testing of endoscope-washing systems.

Developing a sound process

Developing a sound and safe procedure for endoscope reprocessing relies on a number of important factors. The user cannot always rely on detailed instructions from the manufacturer, as Favero and Bond point out in their recent chapter on chemical disinfection. Consistent and effective procedures, they say, "often depend highly on the knowledge and judgment of the responsible health-care practitioner" (Favero & Bond, 1991).

Voluntary guidelines may be helpful in this effort, including those of the CDC, Association of Operating Room Nurses (AORN), Association for Professionals in Infection Control and Epidemiology (APIC), Society of Gastroenterology Nurses and Associates (SGNA), and the British Society for Gastroenterology.

Sterilization or disinfection: selecting a process The Spaulding classification system for medical devices is an accepted and logical guide to selecting a method for reprocessing endoscopes. Spaulding divides medical devices into three broad categories—critical, semicritical,

and noncritical items—according to their potential for causing infection (Spaulding, 1972).

Critical items are those introduced directly into the bloodstream or other normally sterile areas of the body, such as surgical instruments, cardiac catheters, implants, and biopsy forceps. In the semicritical category are noninvasive flexible fiberoptic and rigid endoscopes, endotracheal tubes, anesthesia breathing circuits, and cystoscopes, because they come in contact with intact mucous membranes and ordinarily do not penetrate body surfaces. The third category, noncritical items, are those that do not usually touch the patient or touch only intact skin. Examples are crutches and blood pressure cuffs.

The Spaulding classification is the basis for the CDC's recommendations on cleaning, disinfecting, and sterilizing medical care equipment, contained in the *Guideline for Handwashing and Hospital Environmental Control, 1985* (CDC, 1985). Though not a regulatory agency, the CDC issues guidelines that are well accepted by the infection control community. The guideline states:

> Critical medical devices of patient-care equipment that enter normally sterile tissue or the vascular system or through which blood flows should be subjected to a sterilization procedure before each use.
>
> Laparoscopes, arthroscopes, and other scopes that enter normally sterile tissue should be subjected to a sterilization procedure before each use; if this is not feasible, they should receive at least high-level disinfection.
>
> Equipment that touches mucous membranes (e.g., endoscopes, endotracheal tubes, anesthesia breathing circuits, and respiratory therapy equipment) should receive high-level disinfection.

These are all Category I recommendations; that is, they are strongly supported by research and are considered effective.

In reality, for scopes, many facilities depend on high-level disinfection with a liquid sterilant/disinfectant because this process enables rapid turnaround of equipment that is often in high demand and short supply. A relatively new method involves sterilization with a peracetic acid formulation in an automated tabletop system. The system is designed to achieve sterilization in 20–30 minutes at temperatures that are moderate enough not to damage endoscopic equipment (Crow, 1992).

Infection control experts note that it is unnecessary to change the disinfection process after a scope is used on a patient known to have HIV infection. First, HIV is more easily inactivated than other more resistant organisms; thus, a sterilant/disinfectant that is EPA registered as active against a broad spectrum of organisms will be effective against HIV. Second, changing the process is inconsistent with universal precautions for prevention of transmission of bloodborne pathogens, precautions that assume that *every* patient is potentially infected. Finally, such a practice would not ensure special treatment of all scopes that treat an infected patient because not all such patients can be clinically identified. Using a different method for patients infected with certain diseases must indicate that the facility does not have confidence in its routine disinfection process. If that is the case, a more

Box 17-2 Diagnostic Arthroscopy and Arthroscopic Anterior Cruciate Ligament Reconstruction with Allograft

Equipment

Medical imaging machine

Endoscopic wall cart:

  Shaver

  Camera

  Video machine

  Printer

  Control panel

Tourniquet and tourniquet tester

Tourniquet cuff

Nitrogen hoses, three (need at least three sources of nitrogen)

Makar leg holder (for operative knee)

Allen stirrup, right or left (for nonoperative knee)

Blue aqua vac mats (two suction tubing 20-foot connected to wall suction)

Rolling sitting stools (one for graft table and one for surgeon)

Short backtable (for graft preparation)

Upper body hypothermia blanket

Patient positioning preparation and supplies

Supine position

Armboards:

  Foam pad under patient's arms

  Foam pad wrapped around patient's hands

Patient's heels hang off bed 1 inch (essential for Makar leg holder)

Nonoperative extremity in Allen stirrup with thermal cover

Allen stirrup attachments placed at patient's iliac crest (Allow for nonoperative knee in good alignment and out of surgeon's working space.)

Circulator duties

Position patient:

  Supine position

  Heels 1 inch off operating room bed

  Safety belt secure across chest

  Arms secured to armboards, foam pad under each arm and around hand (protection from endoscopic wall unit)

  Thermal cover over leg

  Nonoperative leg in Allen pad stirrup

Assist surgeon with application of tourniquet, Makar leg holder.

Drop foot of operating room bed.

Prepare skin of operative knee from Makar knee holder to ankle and circumference of the knee.

Hook up arthroscopic Y-tubing to 3000 ml 0.9% NaCl

Plug in:

  Light cord

  Camera

  Shaver

  Control panel

Assist surgeon in applying cooler wrap, knee brace.

Step-by-step procedure for scrub person

1. Assist with draping the patient.
2. Hand off tubing and cords to circulator.
3. Hand surgeon No. 11 knife for incision, then 5.5-mm cannula and trocar.
4. Hand surgeon shaver and basket forceps for debridement.
5. Hand surgeon shaver to begin notchplasty.
6. Pass following instruments as needed for debridement and preparation of femoral notch for Achilles tendon graft:

    5.5-mm full radius arthroscopic blade

    4.0-mm full burr acromionizer

    Acuflex small halfmoon rasp

    Basket forceps, 1.3-mm upbiter, 1.5-mm upbiter

    Straight 2.7-mm, straight 3.4-mm, and posterior upbiter forceps

7. Hand surgeon high-flow cannula.
8. Hand surgeon No. 10 blade for tibia incision, followed by small Weitlaner, periosteal elevator, and electrosurgical instrument.
9. Hand surgeon tibial aimer.
10. Surgeon removes tibial aimer, then drills guide pin into femur for stability.
11. Pass cannulated drills as surgeon drills to size of graft.
12. Hand surgeon pin puller to remove guide pin.
13. Hand surgeon shaver to debride and remove bone particles.
14. Hand surgeon bone plug, which is inserted into the bone tunnel.
15. Pass 5.8-mm obturator and cannula to insert 30-degree 4-mm arthroscope.
16. Hand surgeon femoral aimer loaded on 2.4-mm guide pin.
17. Pass endoscopic cannulated drills.
18. Hand surgeon pin extractor to remove guide pin.
19. Hand surgeon shaver to debride again.
20. Pass instruments to prepare tibia for graft:

    Straight gouge

    Mallet

    Large halfmoon rasp

21. Pass surgeon spade tip, passing pin loaded in small Jacob chuck as surgeon inserts pin through tibial tunnel through femoral graft site out of the knee.
22. Hand surgeon Achilles tendon graft.
23. Hand surgeon femoral driver to position graft in prepared notch.
24. Hand surgeon interference screw on screwdriver.
25. Hand first assistant soft tissue suture washer.

Box 17-2 Continued

26. Pass the following instruments as requested:
    3.5-mm drill bit
    Depth gauge
    6.5-mm tap
    6.5-mm low-profile cancellous screw on screw-driver
27. Hand surgeon mallet and staple driver loaded with 1.5-mm bone staple.
28. Pass the following instruments for applying bone graft as surgeon impacts bone chips around distal

end graft:
    Adson tissue forceps or Russian forceps
    Bone impactor
    Mallet
29. Once bone graft is impacted, pass closing suture.

By Edwina Blackman, RN, TNCC, section leader, operating rooms, St. Joseph Medical Center, Wichita, Kansas.

---

rigorous process should be used for all scopes (Rutala et al., 1991a; Favero, 1991).

Selecting a sterilant or disinfectant The product selected must be appropriate to the task. A number of chemicals, principally glutaraldehyde formulations, are commonly used for chemical sterilization and high-level disinfection. As Favero and Bond advise, "An essential property of a high-level disinfectant is a demonstrated level of activity against bacterial endospores." The ability to kill spores is an indicator of its power and activity against a range of organisms. If the contact time is long enough, the agent can act as a sterilant (Favero & Bond, 1991).

These chemicals are regulated by two government agencies, the U.S. Environmental Protection Agency (EPA) and the FDA. Under law, companies must register with the EPA any products that claim to be sanitizers, disinfectants, or disinfectants/sterilants. Manufacturers must submit data substantiating their label claims. The FDA, which has authority over medical devices, regulates chemical germicides used on devices as "accessories" to the device. The FDA is taking an active role in ensuring that the device design and reprocessing instructions are conducive to providing a device that is safe for use.

In late 1991, the EPA resumed independent validation testing of chemical sterilants and sporicides, which the agency had discontinued in 1982 because of a lack of funds. One impetus for the renewed testing was a highly critical 1990 report from the U.S. General Accounting Office, which found that the EPA lacked assurance that registered disinfectants were as effective as the companies claimed. Major reasons included scientific controversies over the test methods, which often yield inconsistent results, and lack of internal agency controls over quality and integrity of data submitted (U.S. General Accounting Office, 1990). The EPA has begun an effort to improve test methods.

Cleaning Meticulous cleaning of the endoscope is a critical step in reprocessing because unless the device is clean the disinfectant cannot reach all surfaces to do its work. Unfortunately, the intricate channels and interconnections in many scopes make them difficult, if not impossible, to clean. Experts have documented this fact by using a small rigid scope to examine and photograph the inside of a flexible fiberoptic scope that had been cleaned

and disinfected according to the manufacturer's directions. They found the channels still contained body substances, including feces and blood (Favero, 1991). Cross-infection has been documented when an inadequately cleaned device was sterilized with ethylene oxide (Babb, 1984).

The Society of Gastroenterology Nurses and Associates (SGNA) states in its guidelines that cleaning is probably the most important step in the disinfection process. The guidelines advise vigorous mechanical cleaning with an enzymatic detergent. Also, the user should have a good understanding of the scope's internal constructions, particularly access areas and channel interconnections. The best way to ensure consistency is to have staff who are well-trained in the procedures dedicated to the task of reprocessing endoscopes.

The SGNA guidelines state, "Scrupulous mechanical cleaning of all immersible parts of the endoscope, including all channels and removable parts, is imperative" (SGNA, 1990). Following cleaning, the scope and all channels are rinsed thoroughly with water. Excess water is removed to prevent dilution of the disinfectant. After removal of gross debris, all nonimmersible parts are cleaned with 70% alcohol–moistened pads.

AORN recommends that endoscopes be "disassembled, thoroughly cleaned with an endoscopic process or cleaned manually, and dried before sterilization or high-level disinfection" (AORN, 1994).

Certain videoscopes can be damaged by soaking in glutaraldehyde solution with surfactants. Users should check with the device manufacturer for specific instructions on reprocessing, to ensure an effective process and to prevent damage.

Contact time, concentration, and temperature Understanding and control of these three variables is essential to ensuring effective high-level disinfection. A scope that is immersed in an appropriate product may not be safe if the liquid is diluted, the temperature is too low, or the device is not left in long enough. Users must read carefully and understand the manufacturer's label to be sure the product is being used as directed. For example, a glutaraldehyde product may specify that liquid is to be at 25° C (77° F). The product may not be effective if it is cooler when used. Similarly, a product used to disinfect devices that were not thoroughly cleaned and dried may become laden with organic debris and diluted to the point where its effectiveness is compromised. And a product whose recommended shelf life has expired may likewise lose some of its microbicidal activity. The APIC (1990) guidelines advise that the minimum exposure time for 2% glutaraldehyde to kill *Mycobacterium tuberculosis* reliably is 20 minutes at room temperature (20° C or 68°F); however, users should check the manufacturer's label for the appropriate soaking time, which may vary from 10 to 45 minutes, depending on the desired level of disinfection or the temperature of the disinfectant.

Rinsing and storage   Glutaraldehyde-processed endoscopes must be rinsed after disinfection, to flush out toxic residues. Ideally rinsing should be done with sterile water rather than tap water, because tap water contains a variety of microorganisms. If tap water is used, SGNA (1990) advises, the scope should then be rinsed with 70% alcohol and dried with compressed air.

Alcohol rinse and drying are essential before storage, SGNA notes. Moist endoscopes stored overnight are a breeding ground for microorganisms. An outbreak of seven infections after endoscopic retrograde cholangiopancreatography (ERCP) was associated with overnight storage of endoscopes that had not been completely dried. One patient died (Classen et al., 1988). Felmingham found that even scopes that seemed adequately disinfected were heavily contaminated the next morning (Felmingham, 1985). Alcohol rinse and drying may also be considered necessary between cases in certain situations, as when a patient is immunosuppressed, when ERCP is done, or when a particular type of scope is used, such as a side-viewing scope with hard-to-dry areas (SGNA, 1990).

AORN (1994) also recommends that disinfected flexible or rigid endoscopes be thoroughly rinsed with sterile water and dried before storage.

Toxicity of glutaraldehyde   Glutaraldehyde is strongly irritating to the nose, eyes, and skin. It can cause allergic contact dermatitis from occasional or incidental exposure. The Occupational Safety and Health Administration (1990) has established a maximum allowable exposure limit for glutaraldehyde of 0.2 ppm. This limit is not to be exceeded at any time during the work day, even for a brief period. Employers must monitor workers' exposure, to ensure compliance. If the limit is exceeded, hospitals must supply workers with proper protective garb. The area where glutaraldehyde is used must be properly ventilated to evacuate fumes (Notarianni, 1992).

ANESTHESIA

The technique of laparoscopic surgery has the capability to decrease operative and anesthetic time, to shorten the duration of postsurgical convalescence, and to offer a favorable cosmetic final result. In addition there is the likelihood of diminished morbidity. The implications are that the anesthesia care team must use a technique that not only allows for optimal surgical conditions but also provides intraoperative patient comfort and safety and a rapid postoperative anesthetic recovery.

Anesthesia Techniques

General anesthesia

General anesthesia offers several advantages: muscle relaxants and nasogastric or orogastric tube placement with proper positioning can provide optimal surgical conditions; endotracheal intubation allows control of the airway and protection against aspiration of gastric contents; continuous end-tidal carbon dioxide monitoring facilitates early detection of carbon dioxide embolus, indicated by a transient but rapid rise in the end-tidal carbon dioxide, and monitors carbon dioxide absorption; use of an esophageal stethoscope may help in the detection of new heart murmurs that may signify a gas embolus (Hanley, 1992).

Although the effect is inconsistent, agents such as morphine, meperidine, and fentanyl have the potential to cause spasm of the sphincter of Oddi (Radnay et al., 1980); therefore, perioperative use of narcotics to provide analgesia for cholecystectomy is controversial. Difficult visualization of the distal common bile duct may thus occur during intraoperative cholangiography.

Regional anesthesia

Thoracic epidural anesthesia with a segmental nerve block of T2–L1 is an acceptable technique for laparoscopic cholecystectomy (Hanley, 1992). Advantages of this technique are that the patient is awake, protective airway reflexes are intact, and postoperative anesthesia recovery may be shorter. Intraoperative intravenous supplementation may become necessary, as carbon dioxide insufflation can cause irritation of the diaphragm, significant nausea and vomiting, and referred pain in the distribution of the phrenic nerve. Respiratory compromise secondary to intercostal paralysis, patient position, and increased intraabdominal pressure from carbon dioxide favors controlled ventilation and general anesthesia.

Spinal anesthesia, with advantages similar to those of thoracic epidural anesthesia, may also be used for laparoscopic surgery. A continuous spinal anesthetic may be indicated for lengthy procedures.

Local anesthesia

Local anesthesia, with or without sedation, has been used for laparoscopic liver biopsy, staging laparoscopy for malignant disease, and diagnostic gynecologic laparoscopy (Beilin et at., 1986; Shane, 1983).

Combination anesthesia

Total intravenous anesthesia (TIVA) implies that all the components of general anesthesia are injected intravenously; unconsciousness and amnesia are produced by sedative-hypnotic drugs; sympathetic reflex response to surgery is decreased or abolished by analgesic drugs; and muscle relaxation is provided, when needed, by nondepolarizing muscle relaxants. The lungs are ventilated with oxygen-enriched air (Fragen, 1991).

Several combinations of drugs and techniques are available for TIVA. Hay (1993) suggests for routine ASA I patients undergoing short to medium length cases propofol and alfentanil hydrochloride, plus mivacurium chloride as the neuromuscular blocker and midazolam as a preoperative medication for amnesia augmentation. This combination provides patients with a rapid, pleasant induction as well as residual analgesia when they are awake postoperatively.

General anesthesia with block (regional, local infiltration, interarticular, etc.) offers postoperative pain relief, decreased anesthesia requirements, relaxation at the surgical site, quicker recovery, and faster dismissal.

Complications

Carbon dioxide embolus

If large amounts of carbon dioxide gain access to the central venous circulation through open venous channels, or if splanchnic blood flow is reduced by excessive intraabdominal pressures or peripheral vasoconstriction, severe hemodynamic and respiratory compromise can result (Hanley, 1992). Symptoms of a gaseous embolus are a sudden and profound decrease in blood pressure, cardiac dysrhythmia, a mill wheel or other new-onset heart murmur, cyanosis, pulmonary edema, and an increase in end-tidal carbon dioxide as the gas embolizes. The incidence of gas emboli where high intraabdominal insufflation pressure is used is significantly higher than with lower insufflation pressure.

The response to embolization is immediately to deflate the peritoneum, place the patient in left lateral decubitus position with the head below the level of the right atrium (Durant's position), and obtain intravenous access to the central circulation to aspirate gas from the heart.

Subcutaneous emphysema

The prevalence of subcutaneous emphysema during laparoscopy is between 0.43% and 2.0% (Kalhan & Reaney, 1990). It may occur by two mechanisms: (1) as a result of improper positioning of the Veress needle, or (2) in the neck, face, or chest wall, in conjunction with pneumothorax, pneumomediastinum, or both. Carbon dioxide may diffuse through weak points in the diaphragm and enter the mediastinum. Pneumothorax and pneumomediastinum need to be detected and treated in the early stages by inserting a chest tube to prevent life-threatening changes. As soon as subcutaneous emphysema is suspected a chest radiograph is obtained to rule out pneumomediastinum or pneumothorax. Increased end-tidal carbon dioxide, which continues to rise and cannot be lowered by increased tidal volume or rate of ventilation, is diagnostic, as is decreased lung-thorax compliance. Visualization of the head and neck with palpation of crepitus is also indicative of this phenomenon. Facial and conjunctival subcutaneous emphysema may be noted. Decompression of the pneumoperitoneum and termination of the procedure are indicated. Muscle relaxants are reversed and the patient is ventilated with oxygen. Within 15 to 20 minutes there should be visible signs of a decrease in facial and conjunctival swelling. The patient is allowed to awaken. If oxygen saturation and vital signs are well-maintained, extubate and transport the patient to the recovery room.

Gastric reflux

Patients who have a history of diabetes complicated by gastroparesis, hiatal hernia, obesity, or any type of gastric outlet obstruction are at higher risk for aspiration of gastric contents. The increased intraabdominal pressure associated with pneumoperitoneum may be enough to increase the risk of passive reflux of gastric contents (Duffy, 1979). A nasogastric or orogastric tube may be passed to decompress the stomach of its contents, thus lowering the risk of visceral puncture during pneumoperitoneum, improving laparoscopic visualization, minimizing the risk of aspiration, and reducing the risk of postoperative vomiting. Intravenous metoclopramide, 10 mg, given preoperatively may promote gastric emptying. Metoclopramide given near the end of the operative procedure may provide for reduced postoperative nausea and vomiting.

Miscellaneous

Other complications that must be considered and treated if present include cardiovascular collapse (hemorrhage, pulmonary embolism, myocardial infarction), perforation of the viscera (bowel or bladder), peritonitis, abdominal wall hematoma, cellulitis, and transient ileus.

In the current outpatient setting in which anesthesia providers find themselves practicing, the emphasis is on providing anesthesia with hemodynamic and respiratory stability, appropriate muscle relaxation, intraoperative and postoperative patient analgesia, and a rapid postanesthesia recovery time. Patients want to be awake and pain-free. They want to go home the same day and want to feel like doing so. Hospitals and surgeons expect patients to be happy with their anesthesia as well as with the overall health care experience. Overall, a good outcome requires an alert anesthesia team that is willing to accord high priority to cooperation and communication among the members of the health care team, to ensure a successful patient outcome. (See Chapter 32, Volume 1 for more details on anesthesia.)

SUMMARY

Minimally invasive surgery has not only changed the way surgery is done, it has changed the way that hospitals prepare, admit, and care for patients. The perioperative nurse is challenged to manage the technology associated with minimally invasive surgery; educate others in the care and handling of the technology, equipment, and instrumentation; and manage the patient's care in a compressed time frame.

This chapter has described the history of endoscopy, implications of minimally invasive surgery, and the impact on hospitals, operating rooms, surgeons, and operating room personnel. Education for patients is identified.

Technology management is detailed to provide information related to purchase, care, and storage of the multiple pieces of equipment. The disinfection and sterilization process is specifically detailed. Finally, anesthesia considerations and complications are described.

Applications and uses for minimally invasive surgery will continue to expand, as will advances in the associated technology. The perioperative nurse can use the information in this chapter to develop systems for managing the technology and patient care today and in the future.

REFERENCES

Allen, J., et al. (1987). *Pseudomonas* infection of the biliary system resulting from use of a contaminated endoscope. *Gastroenterology, 92,* 759–763.

American Hospital Association. (1991). *Meditrends: 1991–1992.* Chicago, Author.

American Hospital Association. (1992). *Ambulatory care trendlines: Ambulatory surgery.* Chicago: Author.

American Society of Colon and Rectal Surgeons. (1991). *Colon and rectal surgeons adopt position on laparoscopic colectomy.* Palatine, IL: Author.

Association of Operating Room Nurses. (1994). Recommended practices: Care of instruments, scopes, and powered surgical instruments. *Standards and recommended practices.* Denver, CO.

Association of Operating Room Nurses. (1994). Recommended practices: Disinfection. *Standards and recommended practices.* Denver, CO: Author.

Association for Practitioners in Infection Control. (1990). APIC guideline for selection and use of disinfectants. *American Journal of Infection Control, 18,* 99–117.

Babb, J., Bradley, C., & Ayliffe, G. (1984). Comparison of automated systems for the cleaning and disinfection of flexible fiberoptic endoscopes. *Journal of Hospital Infection, 5,* 213–226.

Beilin, B., Vatashsky, E., & Aaronson, H. B. (1986). Conscious sedation for laparoscopy. *Israel Journal of Medical Science, 22,* 346–349.

Braasch, J. W. (1992). Laparoscopic cholecystectomy and other procedures. *Archives of Surgery, 127,* 887.

British Society of Gastroenterology. (1988). Cleaning and disinfection of equipment for gastrointestinal flexible endoscopy: Interim recommendations of a working party. *Gut, 29,* 1134–1151.

Burke, M. (1992). New surgical technologies reshape hospital strategies. *Hospitals, 66,* 30–42.

Centers for Disease Control. (1985). *Guideline for handwashing and hospital environment control, 1985.* Atlanta, Author.

Centers for Disease Control. (1991). Nosocomial infection and pseudoinfection from contaminated endoscopes and bronchoscopes: Wisconsin and Missouri. *Morbidity and Mortality Weekly Report, 40,* 675–678.

Cheslyn-Curtis, S., Emberton, M., Ahmed H., et al. (1992). Bile duct injury following laparoscopic cholecystectomy. *British Journal of Surgery, 79,* 231–232.

Classen, D. C., Jacobson, J. A., Burke, J. P., et al. (1988). Serious *Pseudomonas* infections associated with endoscopic retrograde cholangiopancreatography. *American Journal of Medicine, 84,* 590–596.

Coile, C. R. (October 1991). Hospitals of the future: Architecture and design for the year 2000. *Hospital Strategy Report, 3,* 9.

Cole, E. C., Rutala, W. A., Nessen, L., et al. (1990). Effect of methodology, dilution, and exposure time on the tuberculocidal activity of glutaraldehyde-based disinfectants. *Applied and Environmental Microbiology, 56,* 1813–1817.

Crow, S. (1992). Peracetic acid sterilization: A timely development for a busy healthcare industry. *Infection Control and Hospital Epidemiology, 13,* 111–113.

Davidoff, A. M., Pappas, T. N., Murray, E. A., et al. (1992). Mechanisms of major biliary injury during laparoscopic cholecystectomy. *Annals of Surgery, 215,* 196–202.

Davis, C. J. (1992). A history of endoscopic surgery. *Surgical Laparoscopy and Endoscopy, 2,* 16–23.

Duffy, B. L. (1979). Regurgitation during pelvic laparoscopy. *British Journal of Anaesthesia, 51,* 1089–1090.

Favero, M. S. (1991). Strategies for disinfection and sterilization of endoscopes: The gap between basic principles and actual practice. *Infection Control and Hospital Epidemiology, 12,* 279–281.

Favero, M. S., & Bond W. W. (1991). Chemical disinfection of medical and surgical materials. In S. S. Block (Ed.). *Disinfection, sterilization, and preservation* (4th ed.). Philadelphia: Lea & Febiger.

Felmingham, D. (1985). Disinfection of gastrointestinal fibrescopes: An evaluation of the Pauldrach Endocleaner, and various chemical agents. *Journal of Hospital Infection, 6,* 379–388.

Filipi, C. J., Fitzgibbons, R. G., & Salerno, G. M. (1991). Historical review: Diagnostic laparoscopy to laparoscopic cholecystectomy and beyond. In K. A. Zucker (Ed.). *Surgical laparoscopy.* St Louis: Quality Medical.

Fragen, R. K. (1991). Total intravenous anesthesia. *Drug infusions in anesthesiology* (pp. 129–145). New York: Raven Press.

Gaskin, T. A., Isobe, J. H., et al. (1991). Laparoscopy and the general surgeon. *Surgical Clinics of North America, 71,* 1085–1097.

Goldsmith, J. (May/June 1989). A radical prescription for hospitals. *Harvard Business Review, 67,* 104–111.

Gordon, A. G., & Magos, A. L. (1989). Development of laparoscopic surgery. *Balliere's Clinical Obstetrics and Gynaecology, 3,* 429–449.

Gorse, G. J., & Messner, R. L. (1991). Infection control practices in gastrointestinal endoscopy in the United States: A national survey. *Infection Control and Hospital Epidemiology, 12,* 289–296.

Hanley, E. S. (1992). Anesthesia for laparoscopic surgery. *Surgical Clinics of North America, 72,* 1013–1019.

Hawasli, A. and Lloyd, L. R. (1991). Laparoscopic cholecystectomy: Learning curve: Report of 50 patients. *American Surgeon, 57,* 542–545.

Hay, J. R. (1993). *A plus anesthesia.* Unpublished work, University of Kansas School of Medicine, Wichita, 1993.

Health facilities series: H-18. Laparoscopic surgery. (1992). Albany: State of New York Department of Health.

Henderson, J. (January 1994). Health reform gains speed in a scrambling market. *SMG Market Letter,* 1–3.

Hirschowitz, B. I. (1988). Development and application of fiberoptic endoscopy. *Cancer, 61,* 1935–1941.

Jackson, R. W. (1991). History of arthroscopy. In J. B. McGinty (Ed.). *Operative arthroscopy.* New York: Raven Press.

Johnson, L. L. (1986). *Arthroscopic surgery principles and practice* (3rd ed). St. Louis: C. V. Mosby.

Kaczmarek, R. G., Moore, R. M., McCrohan, J., et al. (1992). Multistate investigation of the actual disinfection/sterilization of endoscopes in health care facilities. *American Journal of Medicine, 92,* 257–261.

Kalhan, S. B., & Reaney, J. A. (1990). Pneumomediastinum and subcutaneous emphysema during laparoscopy. *Cleveland Clinic Journal of Medicine, 57,* 639–642.

Kern, K. A. (1992). Risk management goals involving injury to the common bile duct during laparoscopic cholecystectomy. *American Journal of Surgery, 163,* 551–552.

Martin, M. A., & Reichelderfer, M. (1994). APIC guidelines for infection prevention and control in flexible endoscopy. *American Journal of Infection Control,* 22:19–38.

Mattingly, R. G., & Thompson, J. D. (1985). *TeLinde's operative gynecology* (6th ed). Philadelphia: J.B. Lippincott.

McKernan, B. (1992). Personal communication.

Meyer, H. (July 2, 1992). Shooting the learning curve. *American Medical News, 35,* 3.

Meyer, H. (May 4, 1992). Surgical self-regulation under fire. *American Medical News, 35,* 1.

Moossa, A. R., Easter, D. W., VanSonnenberg, E., et al. (1992). Laparoscopic injuries to the bile duct. *Annals of Surgery, 215,* 203–208.

National Institutes of Health. Office of Medical Applications of Research. (1992). *Consensus development conference statement: Gallstones and laparoscopic cholecystectomy.* Bethesda, MD: NIH, OMAR.

Notarianni, G. L. (July 1992). Glutaraldehyde overexposure: Myth or reality? One hospital-wide study. *Journal of Healthcare Materiel Management, 10,* 20–34.

Occupational Safety and Health Administration. (1990). *OSHA safety and health standards.* 29 CFR 1910.1000. Washington, DC: Author.

Patterson, P. (April 1992). Shift to OP surgery key issue in redesign. *OR Manager, 8,* 8–10.

Radnay, P. A., Brodman, E., & Mankikar, D. (1980). The effect of equinalgesic doses of fentanyl, morphine, meperidine and pentazocine on common bile duct pressure. *Anaesthetist, 29,* 26–29.

Reichert, M. M. (1991). Automatic waters/disinfectors for flexible endoscopes. *Infection Control and Hospital Epidemiology, 12,* 497–499.

Rossi, R. L., Schirmer, W. J., Braasch, J. W., et al. (1992). Laparoscopic bile duct injuries: Risk factors, recognition, and repair. *Archives of Surgery, 127,* 596–602.

Russell, A. D. (1990). Bacterial spores and chemical sporicidal agents. *Clinical Microbiology Reviews, 3,* 99–119.

Russell, J. B. (1988). History and development of hysteroscopy. *Obstetrics and Gynecology Clinics of North America, 15,* 1–11.

Rutala, W. A., Clontz, E. P., Weber, D. J., et al. (1991a). Disinfection practices of endoscopes and other semicritical items. *Infection Control and Hospital Epidemiology, 12,* 282–288.

Rutala, W. A., Cole, E. C., Wannamaker, N. S., et al. (1991b). Inactivation of *Mycobacterium tuberculosis* and *Mycobacterium bovis* by 14 hospital disinfectants. *American Journal of Medicine, 92 (suppl 3B),* 267S–271S.

Schaffner, M. (1990). Infection control issues in the gastrointestinal endoscopy unit. *Gastroenterology Nursing, 11,* 279–284.

Shane, S. M. (1983). *Conscious sedation for ambulatory surgery.* Baltimore: University Press.

Society of Gastroenterology Nurses and Associates. (1990). *Recommended guidelines for infection control in gastrointestinal endoscopy settings.* Rochester, NY: Author.

Society of American Gastrointestinal Endoscopic Surgeons. (1992). *Granting of privileges for laparoscopic (peritoneoscopic) general surgery.* Los Angeles: Author.

Society of American Gastrointestinal Endoscopic Surgeons. (1991). *Guidelines for submission of continuing medical education programs seeking SAGES endorsement for laparoscopic surgery courses.* Los Angeles: SAGES.

Society of American Gastrointestinal Endoscopic Surgeons. (1990). *Role of laparoscopic cholecystectomy: Guidelines for clinical application.* Los Angeles: Author.

Soderstrom, R. M. (1986). Laparoscopic sterilization: Equipment and procedures. In G. I. Zatuchni, J. J. Daly, & J. J. Sciarra (Eds.). *Gynecology and obstetrics* (rev ed., Vol. 6). Philadelphia: Harper & Row.

Soper, N. J., Stockmann, P. T., Dunnegan, D. L., et al. (1992). Laparoscopic cholecystectomy: The new "gold standard"? *Archives of Surgery, 127,* 917–923.

Southern Surgeons Club. (1991). A prospective analysis of 1518 laparoscopic cholecystectomies. *New England Journal of Medicine, 324,* 1073–1078.

Spaulding, E. H. (1972). Chemical disinfection and antisepsis in the hospital. *Journal of Hospital Research, 9,* 5–31.

Stoker, M. E., Vose, J., O'Mara, P., et al. (1992). Laparoscopic cholecystectomy: A clinical and financial analysis of 280 operations. *Archives of Surgery, 127,* 589–595.

Talamini, M. A., & Gadacz, T. R. (1991). Laparoscopic equipment and instrumentation. In K. A. Zucker (Ed.). *Surgical laparoscopy.* St. Louis: Quality Medical Publishing.

Targeting treatment. (June 1990). *Architectural Record, 178,* 87–89.

U.S. General Accounting Office. (1990). *Disinfectants: EPA lacks assurance they work.* Washington, DC: Author.

Way, L. W. (1992). Bile duct injury during laparoscopic cholecystectomy. *Annals of Surgery, 215,* 195.

Wheeless, C. B., & Katayama, K. P. (1985). Laparoscopy and tubal sterilization. In R. F. Mattingly and F. D. Thompson (Eds.). *TeLinde's operative gynecology* (6th ed). Philadelphia: J.B. Lippincott.

Wolfe, B. M., Gardiner, B. N., Leary, B. F., et al. (1991). Endoscopic cholecystectomy: An analysis of complications. *Archives of Surgery, 126,* 1192–1198.

Chapter 18

Pediatric Surgery

Key Concepts

- Many factors contribute to advances in the care of pediatric surgical patients, including advances in diagnostic technology and surgical techniques, creation of surgical instrumentation and equipment specific to children, the growth of pediatric anesthesia as a subspecialty, advances in pediatric intensive care, and family-centered approaches to care.

- Pediatric caregivers should have a general knowledge of growth and development when caring for a child.

- Pediatric patients differ, anatomically and physiologically, from adult patients. Neonates and infants grow and change rapidly and differ the most significantly.

- Pediatric patients have a greater potential than adults for alterations in fluid balance, thermoregulation, and skin integrity.

- Effective preoperative preparation for hospitalization and surgery reduces anxiety and fear for both child and parents. Preparation modalities and the types of information given are determined by the age of the child.

- Parents play an important role in caring for the child during hospitalization. Efforts should be made to minimize separation whenever possible.

- Age, size, and weight are important factors to consider when planning intraoperative care.

INTRODUCTION

The perioperative nurse who cares for pediatric patients has a special challenge to provide care for individuals who, often, cannot communicate their needs, concerns, or fears. The pediatric nurse will develop a special trusting relationship with the child and family in order to best meet the child's needs.

It has often been said that children are not small adults. This chapter identifies the differences between children and adults and how the unique needs of the pediatric patient are met in the operating room. Developmental stages from infancy to adolescence are described, as are anatomical and physiological differences. Interventions based on these differences are identified.

Nurses who care for the pediatric patient have significant involvement with the family. Family-centered care, a parent or parents present at anesthesia induction, and a surgical liaison program are described as programs to facilitate family involvement.

Perioperative nursing care planning is identified for selected pediatric surgical procedures. Other surgical procedures that may be performed on children and adults, such as tonsillectomy or open reduction of a fracture, are described in chapters devoted to the surgical specialty. Cardiac procedures, neurosurgical procedures, and some plastic-reconstructive procedures are described in those procedural chapters.

Not all perioperative nurses will have an opportunity to care for pediatric patients. Others may provide limited care. In smaller community hospitals, pediatric surgery may be for only selected procedures. The principles identified in this chapter can be implemented in any setting where children have surgery.

HISTORICAL PERSPECTIVES

The recognition of the specific nature of children's diseases dates back to the middle of the eighteenth century. In 1802, the first children's hospital (Hôpital des Enfants Malades, Paris) was founded by Napoleon Bonaparte (Anagnostapoulas, 1986). During the mid-nineteenth century, a number of children's hospitals were founded (Children's Hospital, Boston; Great Ormond Street and the Hospital for Sick Children, London; St. Annespital, Vienna), where the foundations for pediatric surgical subspecialties would later be laid (Elrempreis, 1986).

Modern pediatric surgery has been practiced for three generations. A small number of pioneers began their work shortly after World War I. The number has grown to thousands in the past generation.

One modern pioneer was Denis-Browne (1892–1967), the father of British pediatric surgery. An Australian surgeon of Irish descent who moved to England at the end of World War I, he became a member of the Royal College of Surgeons and joined the staff of Great Ormond Street. He was the first surgeon in England to confine his practice to pediatric surgery. Denis-Browne's research into the etiology of congenital defects spanned his lifetime. He further evolved the theory of mechanical deformations due to external pressure on the fetus, particularly with those of orthopaedic origin. (The modern term "orthopaedics" stems from Greek words for *straight* and *child*.) He identified methods of treatment comprised of selectively applied pressures and controlled movements. His use of splints revolutionized the treatment of congenital hip displacement and scoliosis. Denis-Browne's studies of anatomy and physiology formed the basis for operations for cleft palate, tonsillectomy, inguinal hernia, hypospadias, imperforate anus, and pyloric stenosis. He improved neonatal intestinal surgery by introducing end-to-back anastomosis. Denis-Browne had a great impact on the development of general surgery in infants and children. He was the first routinely to employ transverse abdominal incisions. Denis-Browne's interests were not limited to surgery. He studied anesthesia, pre- and postoperative management, and surgical instrumentation. He devised instruments for use in pediatric surgery that still bear his name today (Rickham, 1986).

Surgery for infants and children in the United States began with Dr. William Ladd, of Boston Children's Hospital. Born to a merchant family in Boston in 1880, he was educated at Harvard and joined the staff of Children's Hospital in 1910 (Bill, 1986). Along with his general surgery and gynecology practice, he occasionally operated on children.

Dr. Ladd volunteered his services after the great disaster following the explosion of a munitions ship in Halifax, Nova Scotia, in 1917 that injured more than 9000 persons, among them many children. After this experience with injured children, Ladd resolved to dedicate his career to the care of pediatric surgical patients.

Ladd's early papers described surgical interventions and outcomes for children with intussusception and pyloric stenosis. His recommendations and innovations much reduced mortality rates in pediatric surgery. Ladd emphasized the importance of diagnosis, early operation, careful provision of anesthesia, and gentle supportive care for children before, during, and after surgery. Ladd was a pioneer in the treatment of cleft lip and palate, biliary atresia, rectal anomalies, and bladder extrophy. He influenced improvement in the care of almost all common types of pediatric disease that were treatable by surgery (Goldbloom, 1986; Randolph, 1985).

Dr. Ladd demonstrated the need for the specialty of children's surgery and trained several men to carry on his work. Three notable examples were Dr. Robert E. Gross, Dr. C. Everett Koop, and Dr. Herbert E. Coe. Dr. Ladd occupied the first chair of pediatric surgery in the United States (Bill, 1986).

Dr. Ladd's leadership was passed on to Dr. Robert Gross, who had great mechanical insight and who, as a resident, worked out the first closure for patent ductus arteriosus. Dr. Gross introduced the era of modern reconstructive vascular surgery using aortic homografts. His contributions to the literature include the landmark textbook *Abdominal Surgery of Infants and Children* in 1941 (written with Dr. Ladd), *The Surgery of Infancy and Childhood* (1952), and *An Atlas of Children's Surgery*. Other major contributions included leadership in showing the surgical world that newborn infants with life-threatening anomalies could be operated on successfully. Dr. Gross trained pediatric residents who would later practice and teach pediatric surgery across the country and around the world (Randolph, 1985).

The continuing rapid advances in pediatric surgery can be attributed to many factors (Clotworthy, 1986). The growing numbers of pediatric specialists, and the subsequently reduced ratio of patients to physicians, has made possible enormous developments in research, techniques, materials, and technology related to pediatrics and pediatric surgery (Clotworthy, 1986). Pediatric anesthesia has grown as a subspecialty, accompanied by improvements in anesthesia techniques and agents. There have been ongoing improvements in surgical technology and pediatric instrumentation. There is better understanding of pediatric physiology and pathology, especially of congenital malformations. More accurate and timely diagnoses are made possible by prenatal ultrasonography, computed axial tomography, and magnetic resonance imaging. Advances in understanding and technology in pediatric intensive care and nutritional support have allowed younger patients with more complex problems to be considered as candidates for surgery (Randolph, 1985).

The history of pediatric surgery is still being written, as more research, publications, and advances in techniques are developed. Organ transplantation is accomplished more frequently and in younger children. The scarcity of livers suitable for transplantation into pediatric patients has led to techniques for transplantation of segmental liver resections from related living donors. Techniques have also been devised to detect malformations in fetuses, which have led to the development of procedures that can be accomplished in utero and increasing numbers of procedures that are performed immediately after delivery. Advances in pediatric surgical technique, along with the forces of technology, legislation, and reimbursement, will provide challenges for the future.

GROWTH AND DEVELOPMENT

A general knowledge of growth and development is necessary in caring for infants, children, and adolescents. Each child's patterns of growth and development are somewhat peculiar, but it is possible to generalize about age groups.

Growth implies changes in size of the body as a whole or of its separate parts. *Development* describes the differentiation in changes in bodily function, including structural, emotional, and social interactions.

The perioperative nurse takes into account the child's developmental stage to prepare the child for surgery and to interact best with the child and family during the perioperative period.

Age group classification in the pediatric patient is generalized and varies a bit from textbook to textbook, as there are no clear boundaries. Children in any age group develop at different rates. The developmental needs and tasks of each group can be studied in detail by reading the

theories of Piaget, Erikson, Maslow, and Freud (Kaplan & Saddocka, 1988).

The *premature* infant is usually categorized as one born prior to 37 weeks' gestation. The premature infant is discussed in the section on anatomical and physiological differences.

Neonate is the term used to describe the infant in the first month after birth. Infancy is usually described as the period from the time of birth until age 1 year. During that time the child is first oriented to interactions that meet physiological needs such as hunger and comfort. Once those needs are met, the infant focuses on social interactions between parents and siblings, which become the foundation for lifetime relationships. By the end of infancy, the child is beginning to develop language.

Early childhood constitutes the toddler and preschool-age child. The toddler period spans late infancy until after age 2 years. The preschool age ends near 5 years, before entry into kindergarten. This developmental phase includes language development and locomotion.

Middle childhood encompasses the time from kindergarten through the mid–school-age years (third or fourth grade). The child is less egocentric and develops relationships with adults outside of the family through school activities. The child learns to adapt to new environments and experiences.

Late childhood is the later half of the school-age period (about age 8 to 12 years), when children increasingly encounter new situations and refine motor and social skills. They are becoming increasingly independent.

Adolescence begins at puberty, a time when the child is maturing physically, socially, and sexually. Onset of adolescence is usually defined as the appearance of secondary sex characteristics, and adolescence ends with the cessation of growth.

Key concepts in growth and development are described by Mott, James, and Sperhac (1990). The ones that should be given special consideration for children undergoing surgery are listed according to developmental stage.

Developmental Stages

Infancy

- Infancy is the developmental phase from birth until the beginning of language.
- Parents' behaviors relate to their perception of the infant's state of health and to their ability to provide for the infant's needs.
- Play is an important part of infancy. The infant develops gross and fine motor skills through play and practices new skills that reflect cognitive growth.
- The objects of play include the infant's own body and toys. Play can be exploratory, repetitive, or symbolic in content.
- The cognitive-perceptual pattern includes the infant's use of sensory organs (eyes, ears, nose, mouth, skin) to mediate perception and learning through the attachment of meaning to stimulus.

- Initially infants communicate by crying, but they rapidly add cooing, babbling, and then words.
- Erikson pointed out the foundation of trust established between parent and infant and its relation to the gratification of basic needs.
- Temperament is a factor in the infant's responses to caregivers and to changes in the environment.
- The role-relationship pattern defines the infant's emotional bond with the parent. Stranger anxiety and separation anxiety are manifested as part of this pattern.
- A variety of interacting variables influence how infants cope with developmental and situational stress. These variables include age, temperament, previous experiences, and supportive adults.
- The parent's values/belief pattern guides decisions concerning parenting and conveys expectations of behavior to the infant.

Early childhood

- Early childhood encompasses the developmental phase between early language and locomotion and formal school in kindergarten.
- The child's concept of health correlates with cognitive ability, experiences with illness, and parental attitudes.
- The health perception or health management pattern includes learning about basic self-care activities.
- The activity-exercise pattern emphasizes experiences with objects in the environment that promote mastery of many gross and fine motor skills.
- Play enhances all types of learning and all aspects of development through the use and practice of motor, cognitive, and social skills.
- The child engages in various types of play; solitary, onlooker, parallel, and—by the end of early childhood—associative and cooperative play.
- According to learning theorists, cognitive development during early childhood involves imitation and increased attention span for information processing.
- Early childhood is characterized by incessant questioning, as the child learns about the organization and functioning of the environment.
- The child fuses fantasy and reality in seeking to understand the world, but increasingly learns to distinguish between them.
- Erikson describes this as a time of developing autonomy and initiative, leading to either a positive or a negative sense of self.
- Adults who support a child's questions, needs for increased reassurance, and expression of initiative help to foster the child's self-concept.
- The parents' role in protecting and educating the child changes as the child gains independence and spends time away from home.
- Parents can minimize common behavior problems in early childhood, such as anger and aggression, by placing consistent, clearly defined limits.
- In the coping–stress tolerance pattern, coping strategies are ways the child responds to either environmental stress or self-disequilibrium.

Middle childhood

- Middle childhood is characterized by the child's movement away from the home and family as a primary resource and toward school, peers, and community.
- Physiological changes include increased muscle mass and slower pumping action of the heart, increased lung tissue and transition to vesicular breath sounds, and increased antibody protection in defense against foreign antigens.
- The child's concept of health is related to physical experience and capacity for activity. The child has a good understanding of the external body but vague ideas about the structure and function of internal body parts.
- The health perception–health management pattern includes learning about and participating in self-care activities related to hygiene, dress, nutrition, and exercise.
- As part of the activity-exercise pattern, the child perfects gross motor skills and uses them in combinations.
- The child refines the fine motor skills and uses them in writing, model building, crafts, and projects.
- Play becomes more organized, and games involve groups and competition. The child knows where fantasy leaves off and reality begins.
- Play provides the opportunity for children to cope with disappointment and to control emotions.
- According to the information-processing theorist, the advance in cognitive skills during middle childhood is related to increased attention span and improved memory.
- During middle childhood there is a dramatic increase in the child's vocabulary, articulation skills, and correct use of grammar.
- Self-concept continues to develop as a result of social interaction with a wider variety of people.
- Fears at the beginning of middle childhood are concerned with personal safety and unexpected experiences, and at the end of middle childhood with performance.
- Aggression and anger are best handled with parental consistency, clear limits, and avoidance of power struggles with the child.
- In the coping–stress tolerance pattern, children continue to use coping strategies that they previously found to be helpful for reducing stress. Some adopt new strategies as they struggle to cope with multiple, sometimes conflicting, requests and expectations.

Late childhood

- Late childhood is a time of coordinating, perfecting, and using the skills gained through earlier experiences and a time of increased independence as the child spends more time away from home—at school, clubs, lessons, and play.
- The child's concept of health becomes more sophisticated with development. The child gains an understanding of the human body and the physiological functions of the internal organs.

- The health perception–health management pattern includes defining health and illness in specific terms, as existing within the body and as manifested in activity.
- Play during late childhood enables children to learn more about themselves, their interests, and their abilities.
- Major changes occur in the child's cognitive-perceptual pattern. Piaget refers to this stage as the concrete operational phase.
- Late childhood is characterized by a general centering of cognitive thought processes. The child can take the perspective of another and can reverse or reconstruct an event or problem to reach a solution.
- The child's longer attention span facilitates organization of information for later retrieval. Improvements in long-term memory allow children to use and apply previously learned material more efficiently.
- Children use language to express thought, explain logic, and communicate new knowledge.
- Personality development continues. The concept of industry includes self-control, cooperation, and compromise.
- Self-esteem increases when the child positively evaluates accomplishments. Success is judged by self-satisfaction and the recognition received from others.
- Children with high self-esteem are less likely to conform than children with low self-esteem.
- The family remains a significant influence in the child's life but is more in the background as peers and other adults assume importance.
- Continued development occurs as children become more sophisticated in their use of coping strategies.
- The child is able to confront stress and use skills of logic and communication to remove stress. Sometimes maladaptive strategies of aggression, depression, or withdrawal and denial are used in reaction to stress.

Adolescence

- Adolescence involves changes in the self-concept that affect the person's interactions with family, community, school, and peers.
- The onset of puberty is a major transition. Some of the physical and psychological as well as physiological reasons are given as causes for illness.
- The adolescent formalizes attitudes and beliefs about health.
- According to Piaget, the adolescent has the ability to think abstractly, to propose hypotheses, and to manipulate ideas and concepts.
- Learning is best achieved when the adolescent is an active participant in an environment conducive to learning. Memory ability is at its peak, and motivation to learn is high when the adolescent is interested in the subject matter.
- Language development is linked to maturation of cognitive skills, the ability to express thoughts, and an expanded vocabulary.
- Self-concept involves sexuality, leader-follower roles, responses to authority, values, emotional control, self-esteem, belonging, asceticism, self-assertion, and daydreaming.
- The adolescent acquires independence, a sense of self in relation to others, and the skill to assume adult roles. Peers become increasingly important.
- Stresses increase during adolescence, and coping strategies must be equal to the challenge. Adolescents perfect previously used strategies and add intellectualization to their repertoire.

ANATOMICAL AND PHYSIOLOGICAL DIFFERENCES

Premature infants, neonates, infants, children, and adolescents all differ anatomically and physiologically (including their responses to pharmaceuticals) from each other and from adults. It is neonates and infants who possess the most distinctive and rapidly changing characteristics and who differ most significantly from adults. Cardiopulmonary system changes are most marked, but maturational changes are evident in all systems. Anatomical and physiological differences that demand the most consideration when caring for pediatric patients in surgery are described next.

Size

Size, the most obvious difference between adults and children, varies not only at different ages but within age groups. The difference in proportion of body structure is marked in pediatric patients, especially in infancy.

Weight, height, and surface area are all variables. Harris (1957) described a normal 7-pound infant as "1/3.3 the size of an adult in length, having 1/9 an adult's body surface area, and 1/21 an adult's weight" (Fig. 18-1). The difference in body surface is most significant because of its relationship to basal metabolic activity, which affects fluid and nutrition requirements (Smith, 1980).

Respiration

Upper airway The pediatric airway differs from the adult airway, particularly in younger children. The size and position of the airway allow it to become more easily obstructed. The relatively large tongue occupies the majority of the mouth and oropharynx. The infant's neck is short; the chin often touches the chest. The infant's epiglottis is shorter and narrower than the broad, flat epiglottis of the adult. The vocal cords are short and concave, and canted back rather than perpendicular to the axis of the trachea. The younger child's cricoid cartilage is the narrowest part of the airway; in older children and adults the vocal cords are.

The airway is probably the structure most likely to cause danger to pediatric patients. During anesthesia induction, glottic spasm may cause mild or moderate glottic closure. This is often aborted by manual pressure on the breathing bag and may require a muscle relaxant. After

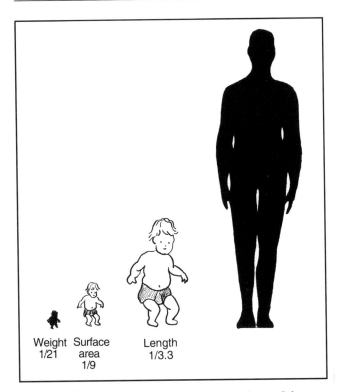

Weight 1/21 Surface area 1/9 Length 1/3.3

FIGURE 18-1 A comparison of the proportions of the newborn and adult with respect to weight, surface area, and length. (Adapted from Harris, J. S. [1957]. *Annals New York Academy of Science, 6,* 966.)

tracheal extubation, spasm can reoccur suddenly requiring reintubation to prevent hypoxia. The risk of airway problems is greater in the postanesthesia care unit, where sudden airway obstruction or ventilatory depression may go unnoticed. Infants who have undergone repair of cleft lip or palate or other oral surgery are particularly prone to upper airway obstruction.

For intubation, a long, straight-bladed laryngoscope is preferred for children younger than school age, owing to their higher and more anterior larynx. When holding the mask to the face, it is important for the anesthesiologist to avoid unnecessary pressure to the submandibular soft tissues that could result in obstruction.

Lower airway The thoracic cage differs among infants, children, and adults. The thorax of infants is small and the sternum soft. The ribs of younger children are more horizontal, rising less during inspiration. Because the child has less anteroposterior movement of the ribs during inspiration, the mechanical movement of the diaphragm is more important.

Thermoregulation

Changes in body temperature occur more rapidly in pediatric patients and carry more risk than for adults. Infants and children cannot sustain body temperature as well as adults in cold environments. Heat loss occurs through radiation, convection, and conduction, and there is more heat loss as a result of the high ratio of surface area to body weight and lack of subcutaneous fat. The

epidermis and dermis of children are thinner. Children perspire less than adults and thus have a less effective cooling mechanism. For infants and young children undergoing surgery, the danger is primarily from hypothermia; older children have a tendency toward hyperthermia. Common causes of hyperthermia are dehydration, fever related to primary disease, heated environment and drapes, release of toxic material into the bloodstream, and blood transfusion reactions.

Body temperature is monitored by probes, which may be placed in the rectum, esophagus, ear, or axilla. For infants who weigh less than 3 kg the rectum is avoided to prevent perforation.

Cardiovascular system

Immediately after birth, the cardiovascular system undergoes a series of complex changes that do not end for several years. The younger the child, the more pronounced are the cardiovascular differences.

A newborn's heart rate is 120 to 180 beats per minute. Gradually it decreases until about age 4 years, when it falls below 100 beats per minute. A child's blood pressure is slightly less than that of an adult, and the hemoglobin concentration diminishes from age 3 months to 3 years. The immature sympathetic nervous system in the developing myocardium may manifest an altered response to vasoactive drugs. Vasoconstrictive response during hemorrhage is less pronounced in infants.

Tachycardia is seldom useful as a sign of blood loss in children, since they normally have a rapid pulse. Blood pressure is a valuable indication of changing blood volume. Accurate blood loss measurement is difficult but more important for young patients, as relatively small losses are risky. During surgery a precordial or esophageal stethoscope is an accurate and easy to use monitor for the assessment of heart rate, ventilation, and cardiac rhythm.

Fluid and electrolytes

There are critical differences between children and adults in fluid metabolism. The percentage of total body water content and fluids in extracellular space is higher in children. Fluid and electrolyte status is more precarious in children and there is greater danger of both dehydration and fluid excess. There is greater daily exchange of water and more limited ability to handle sodium and other electrolytes. The younger the child, the more water is needed to excrete metabolic waste. Close attention to intraoperative fluid management is essential, particularly for children younger than 2 years.

Methods used for thermoregulation (e.g., radiant warmers and increased room temperature) as well as fever can increase insensible fluid loss to dangerous levels in children who are improperly monitored.

Nervous system

Infants, children, and adults differ in their central nervous system responses. The brain of a neonate is relatively large. The permanent level and position of the spinal cord within the dural sheath are not fixed until the end of the first year, an important factor when considering spinal anesthesia.

Urinary tract

Anatomically, kidneys do not attain their final fixed internal structural relationships until the body is fully grown. Though they are anatomically mature after 2 weeks, the structures do not assume their final size and proportion until growth is completed. Adult functional level is attained by the end of age one month.

Response to drugs

Responses to pharmaceuticals may differ in pediatric patients and in adults. Neonates may require smaller doses of barbiturates and opiates for anesthesia induction, owing to the immaturity of the blood-brain barrier and to decreased ability to metabolize drugs. Children older than 5 years may require larger doses of thiopental per kilogram of body weight than adults. Hepatic and renal clearance of many drugs during the neonatal period is decreased, but it may be increased in older children. Uptake of inhaled anesthetics is more rapid in infants than in older children and adults.

Malignant hyperthermia

Although malignant hyperthermia is not limited to pediatric patients (reported age range 2 months to 70 years) its incidence is significantly higher in children and young adults. Malignant hyperthermia results in susceptible patients after injection of succinylcholine or inhalation of a volatile anesthetic such as halothane, which are triggering agents. One half of susceptible patients exhibit symptoms during their first anesthesia.

The speed at which malignant hyperthermia develops and the high incidence of death justify precautions and early intervention. Early clinical signs of malignant hyperthermia include hypermetabolic signs such as tachycardia, other cardiac dysrhythmias, hypercarbia, tachypnea, skeletal muscle rigidity, hypercalcemia, and metabolic and respiratory acidosis. Elevated body temperature is a late secondary symptom (Gregory, 1989).

Successful treatment depends on early diagnosis. Potential for malignant hyperthermia can be identified in the medical and family history. There is increased risk for patients with some neuromuscular disorders. Previous anesthesia experiences can indicate susceptibility.

If potential susceptibility is identified, anesthetic triggering agents and drugs that might mask symptoms are avoided. Regional anesthesia may be considered. Administration of nitrous oxide and oxygen should be accomplished with an anesthesia machine that has never been used to administer volatile anesthetics, to avoid triggering by residual agent. Dantrolene should be readily available to be given intravenously.

If malignant hyperthermia is suspected, the elective surgical procedure and administration of anesthesia should be terminated. The patient is then hyperventilated with 100% oxygen. Metabolic acidosis is corrected with sodium bicarbonate, hydration, and maintenance of urine output. Cooling is facilitated by the utilization of cooled intravenous therapy and gastric lavage (Gregory, 1989). (See Chapter 32 in Volume 1 for more information.)

The premature infant

The most marked anatomical and physiological differences from adults are seen in infants, particularly neonates. These differences are even more pronounced in premature infants, requiring diligent assessment and interventions to respond to needs dictated by their immaturity and fragility.

The physical characteristics, behaviors, and needs of premature infants vary with the degree of prematurity. Most infants born before 27 or 28 weeks' gestation are physiologically too immature to survive. Infants past 37 weeks' gestation usually are not defined as premature.

The younger the gestational age, the larger the skin surface–body weight ratio and the larger the head is in proportion to the body. Skin is thin, with visible blood vessels and little subcutaneous fat. The thin skin is easily damaged or broken. Glucose must be provided to make up for the inability to store glycogen in the liver.

The immaturity of the respiratory tract and insufficient surfactant can result in collapse of alveoli on expiration and respiratory distress syndrome (hyaline membrane disease). There may be decreased motility in the gastrointestinal system, and sucking and swallowing reflexes may be inadequate. Feeding by gavage or intravenous or central lines may be necessary.

Fetal circulation may persist if oxygen levels are low at the time of delivery. Persistent patent ductus arteriosus or intermittent patent ductus arteriosus may be present. Reduced glomerular filtration rate, renal tubular absorption, and excretion may result in fluid retention, poor excretion of drugs, low urine output, or metabolic acidosis. Limited drug clearance can cause drugs to accumulate in the body.

Thermoregulation is particularly important when caring for premature infants. Temperature is maintained by placing the infant in a heating unit with a heat-sensitive probe taped to the abdomen. Great care is taken to avoid burns. Careful handwashing is necessary before touching infants because their immune system is immature. Positioning and padding are crucial to preventing skin breakdown. Small amounts of paper tape may be used to anchor lines, drains, and dressings.

Premature infants often require oxygen therapy administered with a combination of humidity and warmth. Mechanical ventilation may be necessary if the infant is unable to breathe for himself. The infant may have difficulty clearing airway secretions if reflexes are immature. Care must be taken to use low-pressure suction to protect the delicate mucous membranes.

Pediatric regional anesthesia

Spinal, caudal, and epidural regional anesthetic blocks are accepted as alternatives to general anesthesia in premature infants. Premature infants are predisposed to potentially life-threatening respiratory problems, owing to their poorly developed respiratory control (Schwartz,

Eisenkraft, & Dolgin, 1988). Regional anesthesia is also a method of choice for older infants and children with compromised respiratory function. It may be used in abdominal, perineal, inguinal, and lower extremity surgery.

The advantages of anesthesia for infants are similar to those for adults. There is relief of postoperative pain, decreased narcotic requirement, more rapid return to an alert state, and minimal interference with laryngeal function, coughing ability, and respiratory performance.

Education and teaching are key factors to parents' acceptance of regional anesthesia for their premature infant. The teaching should include the information that regional anesthesia is often preferred for specific medical conditions where general anesthesia may be associated with an increased rate of complications, such as postoperative apnea, in premature infants (Moss & Hatch, 1991). The disadvantages of spinal anesthesia in infants are failures due to technical difficulties and the limited duration of the anesthesia. In premature infants there may also be a lengthier recovery period in the postanesthesia care unit (PACU), for observing apnea, airway obstruction, or pulmonary complications.

During the insertion of the epidural catheter and spinal tap for regional anesthesia the perioperative nurse provides proper positioning, safety and comfort measures to the premature infant. To facilitate catheter insertion, the infant is placed in a sitting position, with the nurse supporting the infant while arching the infant's spinal column and maintaining a patent upper airway. This position helps expose the vertebrae and facilitates accurate placement of the spinal catheter. Once the spinal anesthetic has been administered, the infant is placed supine with the legs safely secured to minimize untoward movement.

NURSING CONSIDERATIONS

Preoperative Preparation

Much in the literature supports the argument that hospitalization and surgery cause much stress for children and their parents. Child anxiety, fear, and maternal anxiety have all been found to influence the child's response to medical care (Bates & Broome, 1986). Melamed and Siegal (1975) noted that the stress is so great that 10% to 35% of children exhibit immediate or longer-term emotional and behavioral problems—night terrors, increased dependency, regression, loss of toilet training, eating disturbances, and increased fearfulness.

A young child's hospital-related fears focus on being in a new environment, disruption of routines, painful procedures, body mutilation, and abandonment and separation. Preschool children may perceive hospitalization as punishment. Intervention through preparation and support for children who are scheduled for surgery can acknowledge fears and prevent short- and long-term problems related to the surgical experience.

Parents also need education, support, and reinforcement. When both parent and child are psychologically prepared and offered emotional support, the child adapts better to the surgical experience and recovery. Children are very adept at picking up parental cues, and parents' anxiety and fear cause anxiety in the child.

Many hospitals and surgicenters provide preadmission programs that offer preoperative preparation for hospitalization and surgery. Often, they are presented by surgical suite staff. A variety of modalities of preparation are used. Preparatory booklets, films, puppet shows, slide shows, and tours are some modalities that are effective for different age groups. The preparation is focused on factual information about the purpose and timing of events. The child is encouraged to communicate and express fears and to establish trust in and familiarity with the surgical staff.

Play is the work of children. Effective learning takes place through play. Play deals with emotional release by giving the young child an outlet for expression and needs. When the child has limited verbal skills, it can be the most effective means of communication. Play sessions prior to surgery, involving hospital equipment such as blood pressure cuffs, stethoscopes, masks, and surgical gloves, can help children master the situation. Threat can be alleviated with stories or demonstrations with toys or stuffed animals. Play is one of the few ways a child can manipulate or control a situation, and it can help in coping with stress. Preoperative rehearsal play has been shown to reduce anxiety in children (Burstein & Meichenbaum, 1979).

The age of the child should influence the type of information given and when it should be provided. Infants and younger toddlers generally are not cognitively able to comprehend detailed procedural information or anticipate events. Older toddlers can be given a simple description of what will happen immediately before the event. Older children seems to benefit from preparation several days before the event so they have time to think about how they will respond and what actions or behaviors can be used to cope with the experience (Melamed et al., 1976).

In order to establish trust it is important that the child be given factual information. Children who are not given factual information fantasize fearfully about an upcoming event. Using easily understood words that have meaning but do not instill fear and anxiety is important. Telling a child that he will be "put to sleep" could suggest either fear of waking, as from normal sleep, or an association with the family dog's being "put to sleep" and never returning.

When preparing a parent, it is important to remember that if the parent perceives surgery as a threat to the child, the parent's anxiety may interfere with the ability to retain information.

Adequate preparation of both child and parent allows the child to better adapt to the surgical experience and recovery and enhances development of coping strategies that will benefit both.

Family-Centered Care

During the past two decades, systems of care for children and families have evolved into a family-centered care model. This philosophy of care emerged as a response to the changing health care needs of infants and children and in recognition of the integral role of the family in providing comprehensive care (Rushton, 1990). It is important that parents retain the caregiver role for the child. The emphasis on a family-centered approach and the need for informed parental participation will continue to increase as children receiving surgical care have shorter hospitalizations owing to changing reimbursement patterns. The numbers of children who are admitted on the day of surgery and who have shorter postoperative admission periods or same-day surgery continue to grow.

A young child's hospital-related fears focus on separation from parents. Traditionally, parents and children were separated during the immediate preoperative, intraoperative, and postoperative phases of care. There are opportunities in each of these phases when a parent can, and should be allowed to, stay with their child to support the child and participate in care. All efforts should be made to minimize the amount of time that children and parents are separated.

Preoperative Phase

Parents should accompany the child to the surgical suite and be allowed to stay as long as possible, and during any preparations, examinations, or interviews. Many hospitals provide a preoperative holding room or area where patients wait before anesthesia. This is often where the family and child are interviewed by anesthesia and operating room nursing staff (Fig. 18-2). Last-minute chart review is accomplished, and final preparations are made before transfer to the operating room. There is mutual interchange of information, and child and parent are able to communicate fears and questions. This is a time when trust in caregivers is established.

Intraoperative Phase

"Parent-present" anesthesia induction

Separation at the time of surgery is very stressful for both parent and child. With age-appropriate children the parents' presence during induction of anesthesia is allowed in a growing number of surgical suites. When a parent is present during the induction of anesthesia, the parent retains some control over the child and can support and reassure the child through the experience. Initial induction of anesthesia can be accomplished in the preoperative holding room, the induction room, or the actual operating room. Typically, sedation using rectal Brevital, intramuscular ketamine, or oral or intranasal Versed is administered in the preoperative holding room. A major advantage, especially for younger children, is that the parent can rock or cuddle the child as the child goes to sleep. The child is not aware of the separation when the anesthesia provider and perioperative nurse accompany the child to the operating room.

Induction of anesthesia using a mask is accomplished either in an induction room or in an operating room. A

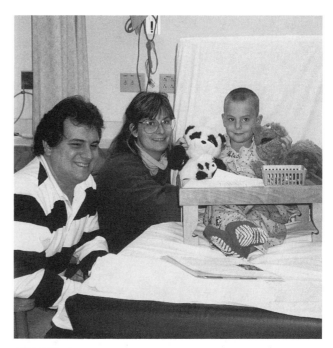

FIGURE 18-2 Parents wait with their son in the preoperative holding area in the surgical suite.

parent can accompany the child to either area. If the operating room is to be the site of induction, the parent changes into appropriate operating room attire. Parent and child are prepared for the sequence of events and the equipment, personnel, and environment. The parent may hold the child during the mask induction and offer verbal support. The parent knows what works for the child and how the child copes best (Fig. 18-3).

The parent or child can help the anesthesiologist hold the mask, gradually bringing it closer to the child's face as the child becomes more sedated. When the child is "asleep," the parent is escorted from the operating room. The parent usually maintains composure during the induction but may show distress or cry after leaving the child. These reactions are common on separation, even when the child does not have the benefit of the parent's presence. An escort helps the parent find the changing area and find other family members.

Many anesthesia and perioperative staff are initially skeptical about parent-present induction but they quickly accept the concept after realizing the great benefits to the child, parents, and caregivers. Parents are pleased to have participated and supported the child through a time of high anxiety. Induction is most likely to go more smoothly with the parent present. The emergence from anesthesia is also smoother, as children tend to "wake up" in the same state in which they go "to sleep." It is recognized that there are times when parent-present induction is not useful. Infants do not appear to require parental support during induction of anesthesia. Adolescents can tolerate having an intravenous line placed and can be given intravenous sedation before they are transferred to the operating room. Parental fear, distress, or inadequacy may be a contraindication. Most emergency situations, except a

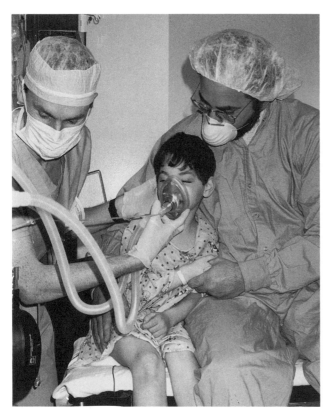

FIGURE 18-3 A father supports his child as they and the anesthesia provider watch the bag inflate and deflate during mask induction of anesthesia.

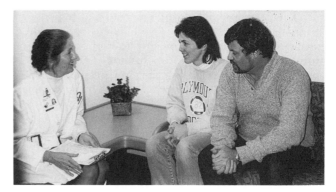

FIGURE 18-4 The surgical liaison nurse gives families frequent progress reports as the child is undergoing surgery.

child with epiglottitis, are not appropriate for parent-present induction.

Surgical liaison programs

Parents are very stressed and anxious waiting for surgery to be completed and before receiving communication from the surgeon about the events of surgery and the outcome. Some centers provide personnel who support the parents during surgery. An excellent example of provision of such a parent liaison program is described by Mitiguy (1986). The surgical liaison nurse meets the family in the preoperative holding room. This nurse reports to the family periodically throughout the surgery, communicating with the surgeon and perioperative nurse during the procedure. The surgical liaison nurse describes surgical milestones such as, "Your son went to sleep easily and surgery is under way" or "Your child is now off cardiopulmonary bypass and is doing well." The surgical liaison nurse helps families cope during this time (Fig. 18-4).

The surgical liaison nurse communicates the expected time of arrival into the PACU. She views the patient before escorting parents to the PACU to better prepare the parents for their child's appearance.

It is ideal to have a family waiting room adjacent to the surgical suite to facilitate communication during and after surgery. Most families prefer to stay in the waiting room throughout surgery and are best served by an area that is divided into a television area and a quiet area. Vending machines are important for nourishment. Some families who have a long wait leave the area if they are given a beeper by the surgical liaison nurse. It is preferable to have a nurse in the surgical liaison role, as the nurse has a thorough understanding of anatomy, physiology, anesthesia, surgical interventions, and medical terminology. She can interpret information in a way that is understandable to parents. The nurse also has skills for coping, crisis intervention, and teaching. Some centers use volunteers in an adaptation of this role, who can also provide support and general information to the family and can serve as escorts.

Postoperative Phase

Many parents wish to be with their child as soon as surgery is completed. A child relates and responds better to the familiar and usual parental support than to unfamiliar nursing and medical personnel. Waking up in the high-tech PACU, where other patients are at different stages of emergence from anesthesia, and hearing strange sounds can be very frightening for the child without a parent present.

When vital signs are stable, airway obstruction is not a threat, and when the child is wakening, the parents may join the child. Parents are prepared so that they will leave promptly, if asked, to meet the needs of the child, other patients, or unit activity. In most situations, the parent may stay until the child is recovered from anesthesia and discharged to the nursing unit, or, quite often, to home. The parent can hold, cuddle, and, in some situations, feed the child. Parental presence is also an important adjunct to postoperative pain management (Fig. 18-5).

Although hospitalization and surgery can be very anxiety provoking and traumatic for parents and children, opportunities for parental presence and encouraging parental involvement have been most often shown to provide a more positive experience with less anxiety for both.

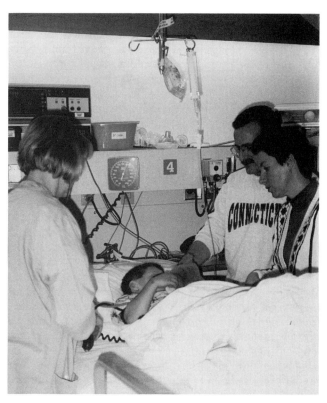

FIGURE 18-5 The parents' presence in the PACU comforts both parents and child.

General Information

The perioperative nurse caring for the pediatric patient views the patient in the context of the physiological and psychological variables unique to pediatric patients. The nurse should have an understanding of the growth and development norms for each age group.

Increased admissions on the day of surgery due to changing reimbursement practices have provided additional challenges for perioperative nurses in the assessment and planning of surgical patient care (see Chapter 27 in Volume 1). Often, initial anesthesia and nursing assessments and preoperative preparation are accomplished on an outpatient basis, days before surgery, and by a team who are not the caregivers on the day of surgery. In this situation, planning may begin when the perioperative nurse reviews the operative schedule. The nurse identifies the surgical procedure, planned anesthetic, and the age of the child.

Age is important to consider when planning for the setup of the surgical case. Age and size are determinants for selection of instrument kits, positioning device, and any size-variable equipment such as electrosurgical grounding pads, blood pressure cuff, pneumatic tourniquets, or sutures. Amounts and sizes of operative supplies vary with the age of the patient. Because of this there may be dual inventories. Even draping material depends on the size of the patient. Adult laparotomy sheets with large fenestrations for teenagers need to be stocked along with sheets with smaller fenestrations for infants. Various sizes

of stockinettes, Esmarch's bandages, and dressings are also required. Venosets with burettes are a necessary supply, along with adult drip venosets.

Appropriate positional supports are determined by the patient's size. Instead of blankets to make positioning rolls, towels may be used. The perioperative nurse is aware that the anatomical structures and tissue of the pediatric patient must be handled gently. The tissue is often fragile and cannot tolerate pressure from retractors or rough handling. To protect the tissue, instruments selected to be used in pediatric surgery are often similar to those used for adults, only smaller, lighter, and finer. The age of the patient is not the only determining factor in instrument size. The weight of the patient is also considered by the perioperative nurse when selecting instruments, sutures, and supplies. Microvascular fistula instruments are used when caring for infants, especially for handling the bowel of a premature infant with necrotizing enterocolitis. Smaller retractor blades are routinely used, along with shorter hand-held or self-retaining retractors. Vessel loops or strabismus hooks may be used for retraction of vascular structures.

Diverse sizes of pediatric patients dictate that various sizes, types, and lengths of instruments need to be available in a pediatric operating room. Pediatric patients require the same type of sutures as adults, only in smaller sizes and with smaller needles. Appropriate-sized absorbable and nonabsorbable sutures are used on delicate and fragile tissue in infants and children. Mineral oil may be used to lubricate sutures for easier passage and to decrease tissue tethering, especially on bowel. Skin is closed subcuticularly to avoid the removal of skin staples, a stressful and painful procedure for young children.

Age usually indicates the developmental stage. Knowledge of the developmental stage helps the nurse plan strategies to prepare the child for events and to help the child cope with stress. If patients receive their preoperative medical, anesthesia, or nursing workup in a preadmission center, it is suggested that "special needs" or individual considerations or requests be communicated to the operating room nursing staff the day before the scheduled surgery, to further assist in planning.

Key concepts related to developmental differences in different age groups to be considered for the surgical patient have already been outlined. General fears and emotional needs of the age groups to be considered by the perioperative nurse are kept in mind as the nurse guides and supports the child through the preoperative, intraoperative, and postoperative phases of care.

Up to 6 months of age, children appear to be relatively unaffected by parental separation and psychological fear of hospitalization, though the parents will most likely feel an effect of separation. If this anxiety is communicated to the child it may cause child distress. After 6 months of age the child is apt to have anxiety related to separation from parents. Such anxiety often increases with age.

Toddlers (after infancy until age 2 years) and pre–school-aged children fear separation and abandonment, the dark, mutilation, monsters and ghosts, intrusive procedures, and the unknown. Separation from a parent may be interpreted as abandonment. Without a parent, the child is often terrified by unfamiliar surgical staff dressed in unusual clothing and masks.

A toddler is believed to be developing mastery and the formation of a general image of and trust in self. Toddlers enjoy using their muscles and voices. Hospitalization and surgery restrict the basic tendencies and needs if body movements are controlled and the child is exposed to uncomfortable and intrusive procedure. This age group should be allowed to protest, cry, and resist. Toddlers and pre–school-aged children have not developed coping mechanisms that would help them through strange and frightening experiences.

School-aged children and adolescents fear disability, loss of a body part, disfigurement, and loss of status with friends. Adolescents are emotionally labile and can have great fears about surgical procedures, anesthesia, intraoperative awakening, and death. They may display fearful, aggressive, or explosive behavior. Self-esteem and body image are of particular concern for this age group. Rebellion and challenging adults and authority figures are not unusual behavior. Adolescents fluctuate between identifying themselves as children or as adults. What appears to be rejection of reassurance and comfort given by a caregiver or parent may be a result of not wanting to look like a child who needs help from adults, even if that is the case.

Preoperatively, the perioperative nurse alters the environment to meet the physiological needs of the pediatric patient. The nurse caring for an infant ensures that warming devices such as heating blankets, heat and extremity wraps, and radiant heaters are available. Room temperature is increased to a level that staff can tolerate. Blood warmers and warmed solutions are made available.

The perioperative nurse begins her nursing assessment during the preoperative phase. It is ideal for the nurse to begin assessment on the unit, where patient and family are less anxious and can be well prepared for events of each phase of the perioperative experience. If the patient is admitted before the day of surgery, ample time is available to gather information and educate patients and family and allow planning in advance of the surgery. The perioperative nurse has the ability to, and benefit of, communication with the primary nurse and can review nursing diagnoses, the care plan, and the medical and surgical status.

As most patients are now admitted on the day of surgery, the nurse usually meets the patient and family for the first time just before surgery, usually in a preoperative holding room.

The perioperative nurse introduces herself to the patient and family and verifies the identity of the patient and NPO status and checks for allergies. The nurse relies on preadmission staff and surgeons to have communicated special considerations before this opportunity for nursing assessment. The medical history and pertinent clinical data are reviewed, and the presence and accuracy of surgical and anesthesia informed consents are verified. Most of the data and information needed have been documented in the medical record by the surgeon, the primary nurse, or the staff in the preadmission center. The parents can provide additional information. Many centers with a significant population of same-day surgical patients have instituted preoperative telephone calls as an initial step in preparation for surgery and planning for care. Preoperative telephone calls have also been found to reduce the cancellation rate (Kleinfeldt, 1990).

Psychological aspects of care must be emphasized for pediatric patients. The nurse relates to the child in a way that is appropriate for the developmental level and engages the family and child in conversation in a way that establishes trust and confidence. The patient and family are reassured and prepared for procedures, sequence of events, and settings. If a parent is to be present for induction of anesthesia, the parent is prepared for the experience.

Nursing Diagnoses

The nurse identifies nursing diagnoses pertinent to pediatric patients undergoing surgery and anesthesia. Pediatric patients are at *increased risk for knowledge deficit, anxiety related to psychological effects of surgery, high risk for ineffective thermoregulation, high risk for impaired skin integrity, high risk for fluid and electrolyte deficit, high risk for injury due to positioning,* and *high risk for fluid deficit related to blood loss.* Premature infants have a higher risk of heat loss and impaired skin integrity.

Pediatric patients share diagnoses common to all surgical patients, including potential for infection due to surgical procedure, potential for electrosurgical burns, potential for retention of a foreign body in the surgical wound, and potential for embarrassment and loss of dignity.

Goals are set and interventions planned according to nursing diagnoses. All pertinent information is recorded on the preoperative assessment section of the operative record. Standardized intraoperative care plans or age-related or specialty care plans may be used to plan and implement nursing care.

Interventions

The perioperative nurse recognizes the developmental differences in children, understands their specific fears, and thus relates to the child in a meaningful and reassuring way that minimizes psychological trauma. The child is encouraged to keep a favorite stuffed animal, toy, or blanket with him. Efforts are made to allay parents' anxiety, minimize parental-child separation, and include parental presence and participation in care whenever possible.

The operating room is kept quiet and comfortable with minimum traffic and stimulation to the child. The nursing goal is to decrease the potential for anxiety related to psychological effects of surgery.

Upon transfer to the operating room, the nurse continues to comfort and reassure the child. Pediatric patients may be more active before and during induction. The circulating nurse ensures that appropriate safety straps are applied and remains by the patient's side, assisting the anesthesiologist, from the time of transfer to the operating table, until the child is anesthetized.

Modesty is an issue, particularly with older children, and it should be preserved. Blankets and drapes cover the patient in the operating room. Children are allowed to wear underwear until they are anesthetized. When removed, underwear, like the child's other personal belongings, is labeled and kept in a clean, safe place. The nursing goal is to decrease embarrassment due to exposure.

Skin prep and other solutions are warmed to body temperature before use. Warming devices to warm patient, blood, and solutions are utilized. Patient and room temperature are monitored to meet the patient's and surgical needs. The patient's skin is not needlessly exposed. Warm blankets are applied before transfer to the PACU. The nursing goal is to decrease potential for loss of body heat.

Padding is placed beneath sensitive skin areas and on bony prominences. Body supports are used that conform to the size of the child. Shoulder supports are utilized, especially for the younger child, whose head is disproportionately large. The patient is protected from pooling of prep and other solutions after application.

The electrosurgery dispersion pad applied is the largest possible for the child, and bony or curved areas are avoided when selecting the site. There are pediatric- and premature infant–sized dispersive pads to be placed on infants when using electrosurgery units. There are different sizes to be used according to weight. A pad is available for premature infants up to 2.4 kg. Before applying a dispersive pad, the pediatric perioperative nurse must be familiar with the weight and size limits of each pad, as described on its package. Like an adult pad, the infant one should not be cut to fit the premature infant or overlapped on itself (see Chapter 23 in Volume 1).

Nonallergenic or nonreactive tape is used when indicated. Care is taken to avoid heavy draping or accidental pressure on the patient's body from instruments or members of the surgical team. Intravenous lines are stabilized with adequate anchoring and application of appropriate-sized boards to limbs. Wrinkles are smoothed out of bed sheets, padding, and other positioning devices. The nursing goal is to decrease the potential for alteration of skin integrity.

Proper body alignment is maintained using positioning supports appropriate to the patient's size. Rolls made from small towels are used for axilla rolls, and foam may be used instead of pillows. Gel pads may be placed under the whole infant to relieve potential pressure points during long procedures (see Chapter 28 in Volume 1).

The perioperative nurse preparing the medications should use small syringes to avoid overmedication. For premature infants even a 10-ml syringe may be too large for accurate dosing.

The circulating nurse is aware of the patient's laboratory values before the procedure (e.g., hematocrit, electrolytes). A Foley catheter is inserted after the administration of anesthesia if so requested by the anesthesiologist or surgeon. The nurse helps monitor intake, output, and blood loss by measuring drainage and laparotomy sponges. It is difficult, but important, to measure blood loss accurately, as a small amount of blood loss is significant in a young child. Blood loss on drapes should be estimated. Suction bottles used should have measurements in minute increments, and tubing should be narrow and as short as possible. All irrigation fluids and fluids used on sponges are measured. The nurse records fluid intake and output often and on a board visible to other members of the team. She assists with intravenous fluids and blood replacement as requested by the anesthesiologist. Intravenous fluids are usually administered through a burette, and blood products are warmed for administration. The nursing goal is for the patient to maintain adequate fluid during the surgical procedure.

Sponges, needles, and instruments are counted on all appropriate procedures, to avoid retention of a foreign body in the surgical wound. Nursing care includes creating and maintaining the sterile field, administering medication, and collecting, labeling, and recording specimens.

There is continual assessment and reassessment of patient care conditions and needs throughout the surgical procedure. The circulating nurse communicates with the family through the surgical liaison or primary nurse by telephone at intervals during the surgery. Delays or surgical milestones are reported, as is the expected time of arrival into the PACU.

The perioperative nurse documents care on the intraoperative record. Positioning, special padding precautions, heating units, surgical personnel, specific procedure times, surgical counts, and implanted items are recorded. The nurse records patient outcomes.

Evaluation

The perioperative nurse evaluates care continually throughout the surgical procedure. Care is also evaluated in the PACU and by receiving feedback from patient and family and other caregivers, including the primary nurse and the surgeon.

Cardiopulmonary status is monitored and assessed during and after emergence from anesthesia. Fluid status is determined and output recorded. The nurse observes for airway compromise and assists the anesthesia provider at this time, being ready to respond to urgent situations. The nurse remains by the child's side until transfer to a safe vehicle. The skin is checked for temperature, redness, especially at pressure points, reaction to skin prep or other solutions, and at the site of the electrosurgery pad. Elbows may be splinted to prevent infants from disturbing the incision, dressing, or drains. Airway and drainage tubes are secured and protected throughout the transfer.

The child is comforted and may need to be gently restrained to prevent rolling and potential injury en route to the PACU.

Report is given to the PACU nurse. The perioperative nurse reviews the patient's diagnosis, condition, and surgical course. She includes fluid replacement, output, blood loss, and replacement with blood products in the report. Medications and response to anesthesia are reported. Dressings, drainage tubes, and drainage amounts are described. The nurse transfers responsibility for the care of the patient's personal belongings to the PACU nurse. Any special needs, child or parental issues, or requests are discussed. The PACU nurse is informed of the relationship of family members who have accompanied the child. The perioperative nursing practice goals are reviewed and outcomes are reported.

Outcomes

Outcome goals and statements include patient and family manifested appropriate psychological responses to the surgical experience; vital signs are stable and urine output adequate owing to adequate fluid volume; patient is free of retained sponges, needles, and instruments; the patient's body temperature is not less than 36° C nor more than 37° C on arrival in the PACU; and the patient will not have a break in skin integrity or skin burns from the electrosurgical pad. Further evaluation can be made by the perioperative nurse caring for same-day surgery patients who often phones to get this information.

PEDIATRIC PROCEDURES

Pediatric surgery is not performed at all facilities, nor are all procedures performed in each facility that does pediatric surgery. The procedures described are those associated with a comprehensive pediatric service and include procedures for neonates. Complex, coordinated, multidisciplinary care is required for many of the patients who have congenital anomalies. This care is best provided at a facility that specializes in pediatrics. Procedures such as insertion of a central catheter, herniorrhaphy, and pyloromyotomy may be performed in a general hospital with trained pediatric surgeons and anesthesia personnel.

Many other procedures are performed on children and adults. Those procedures, such as tonsillectomy or open reduction of a fracture, are described in the chapter devoted to that surgical specialty.

Pediatric Surgery Classification

According to Atkinson and Kohn (1986), pediatric surgery can be classified into three categories—congenital anomalies, acquired disease, and trauma or accidents.

Congenital anomalies

Congenital anomalies may be diagnosed in utero by ultrasonography or soon after birth. These anomalies may alter the appearance of the newborn child, or they may interfere with the function and growth of an organ or structure. The type of anomaly and its location determine the need for immediate surgical intervention or the ability to delay the surgery until the neonate is stabilized. Congenital anomalies requiring emergency surgery involve the alimentary tract, circulatory system, or respiratory tract. Factors that may affect the decision to proceed with surgical intervention are prematurity, birth weight, and the complexity of the anomalies. These factors also affect the risk of infant mortality.

Acquired diseases

Acquired diseases include diseases that occur in life, such as neoplasms, bilateral inguinal hernias, benign lesions, and appendicitis. The cause of the condition determines the urgency of surgery.

Trauma

Trauma is the third category. Accidents are the leading cause of death in children. Blunt trauma is the most common group of injuries in children. It is estimated that approximately 90% of the life-threatening injuries in this age group are due to blunt trauma (Haller & Beaver, 1990). Often there is little evidence of external injury with blunt trauma, but the injury may be life threatening because it often involves multiple organs. Experienced health care professionals in pediatric emergency rooms are necessary to quickly evaluate, diagnose, and resuscitate the child if necessary, because the margin of error in treating traumatic injuries in the pediatric population is small. The ability to diagnose trauma in solid organs has been enhanced and expedited by computed axial tomography and a multidisciplinary, systematic evaluative approach. Often emergency surgery is not necessary. If the child is stable a more conservative approach is taken, but, as in adults, blunt head injuries require a more aggressive approach.

Penetrating trauma in the pediatric population accounts for approximately 10% of the abdominal injuries seen in the emergency room (Haller & Beaver, 1990). These injuries require an exploratory operation to control bleeding, examine the abdominal contents, and repair any perforations or injuries. Exploratory laparotomy is also performed when pediatric patients are physiologically unstable despite appropriate fluid resuscitation and medical management. (Further information about trauma surgery can be found in Chapter 19 in this volume)

Numerous surgical textbooks have been devoted to pediatric patients and surgery specific to them. In other chapters some pediatric surgeries performed by surgical subspecialties have been described (e.g., cleft lip repair, myelomeningocele repair, and spinal fusion). In recognition of the many advances in surgical intervention and techniques performed on neonates, this chapter includes surgical procedures for neonatal congenital anomalies and neoplastic diseases.

Surgery for Acquired Diseases

Central venous catheter placement

Long-term venous access is an indication for an indwelling central venous catheter or an implantable infusion port. The catheter may be used for general venous access, the administration of total parenteral nutrition (TPN), long-term intravenous medical treatment, or chemotherapeutic or antibiotic drug administration. The use of central venous catheters along with advances in the techniques of TPN have had much impact on the survival of pediatric surgical and medical patients (Guzzetta et al., 1989).

There are two types of central venous catheters, tunneled catheters and implanted ports. There are in turn two types of tunneled catheters, those that have to be heparinized regularly (Hickman and Broviac) and those with a valve (Groshong). The tunneled catheters are made of silicone, a flexible biocompatible material. They have a cuff that becomes embedded with fibroblasts within a few weeks after surgery. This embedding decreases the chance of accidental removal by anchoring the line internally. It also decreases the risk of ascending bacterial infection (Mott, James, & Sperhac, 1990). These catheters may also have a vitacollagen cuff with an antimicrobial agent. This agent acts as a physical barrier to bacteria by swelling to twice its original size once implanted, facilitating tissue growth into the collagen and releasing the antimicrobial agent until the cuff is embedded in the tissue (Camp-Sarrell, 1990).

The Groshong catheter has a slit valve on the side. When the valve is in the neutral or closed position blood does not flow back into it. This eliminates the need for daily heparinization and decreases the danger of air embolism (Hadaway, 1989).

Implantable infusion ports do not have any external parts. They are surgically implanted in a subcutaneous pocket of the chest wall. The infusion device includes a stainless steel or titanium port chamber that is attached to a Silastic central venous catheter. An external Huber needle is used to gain access to the port. Implantable ports are used mostly for chemotherapy or total parenteral nutrition.

Perioperative nursing considerations All catheters must be handled according to manufacturers' instructions. The catheter should not come in contact with glove powder, lint, or other foreign materials. Before the catheter is inserted the lumina are flushed and filled with an infusion solution. This solution may be heparinized saline, usually one unit of heparin per millimeter of saline, or 10% dextrose in saline. By flushing the catheter lumen, air bubbles are prevented from entering the circulatory system. It also prevents blood clots from forming in the catheter lumen (Stellar, 1991). The insertion of the catheter is normally scheduled for the operating room. If the premature infant or pediatric patient is too unstable to be transferred to the operating room the procedure may be performed percutaneously in the intensive care unit (Roberts & Gollow, 1990).

The patient is positioned supine with a roll under the shoulders to hyperextend the neck. The head is turned to the opposite side, to expose the incision area. The required instruments are a minor instrument tray plus fistula forceps, a probe to make the subcutaneous tunnel in the chest wall, and a mini-Beaver handle with No. 67 blade.

Key steps

1. A transverse incision is made over the lower portion of the sternocleidomastoid muscle.

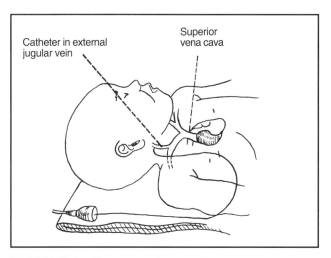

FIGURE 18-6 Placement of a central venous catheter into the external jugular vein. (From Coran, A. G. [1986]. Nutrition of the surgical patient. In K. Welch, J. Randolph, M. Ravitch, J. O'Neill, M. Rowe [Eds.]. *Pediatric surgery* [4th ed.]. Chicago: Mosby-Year Book.)

2. The external jugular vein is exposed. (The internal jugular vein or subclavian vein may also be used.)
3. A second incision is made in the chest wall, medial to the nipple. A subcutaneous tunnel is made between the two incisional sites.
4. The catheter is passed from the chest wall incision through the subcutaneous tunnel so that the tip of the catheter is at the neck incision.
5. An incision is made in the vein with the No. 67 knife blade. The heparinized, saline-flushed catheter is inserted into the vein and threaded to the junction of the superior vena cava and the right atrium.
6. Fluid is aspirated through the catheter to confirm placement and to observe if it flows easily. Fluoroscopy is also used to confirm catheter position.
7. The catheter is anchored to the chest wall with a nonabsorbable suture. The incisions are closed subcutaneously.
8. Each incision is covered with Steristrips, povidone ointment, and an occlusive transparent dressing. The catheter is securely taped to the patient.
9. The central venous catheter may be immediately connected to an infusion system with an air filter, or the heparinized line may be capped for transport to the PACU. Figure 18-6 illustrates placement of the line into the external jugular vein.

Patient outcome Postoperatively, the central venous catheter is used immediately. Complications may develop after insertion of such a catheter: sepsis, superior vena cava obstruction, chylothorax, right atrial thrombosis, hydrothorax, pericardial effusion, hemothorax, cardiac arrhythmias, and cardiac tamponade (Carey, 1989). Early recognition of these complications leads to early treatment and correction. The tunneling technique decreases the chances of the catheter's being dislodged owing to direct tension or stress on the catheter insertion site into the vein. Also, the risk of infection is less with a long-term central venous catheter than with a short-term catheter because of this same tunneling technique (Viall, 1990). When the line is not in use it is maintained by flushing with heparinized saline according to nursing policy procedures. The Groshong catheter does not need to be heparinized because of its valve.

Neoplastic disease resection

Cancer is the second leading cause of death in children (Guzzetta et al., 1989). The more common types of solid tumors are Wilms' tumor, neuroblastoma, teratoma, hepatoma, and rhabdomyosarcoma. The long-term survival rate has increased, owing to many medical advances: better diagnostic imaging, more effective chemotherapeutic agents, and team approaches to treatment that enlist the participation of oncologists, surgeons, radiologists, and pathologists. Multiinstitutional studies have advanced the crusade as well.

Wilms' tumor is the most common solid, intraabdominal tumor of children. An embryonal neoplasm of the kidney, it usually presents as an asymptomatic mass in the flank or upper abdomen. The tumor is often discovered while a parent is dressing or bathing a child or while a pediatrician is conducting a "well-baby" examination. It frequently occurs between age 1 and 3 years; the incidence of Wilms' is 1 in 250,000, and usually it is unilateral, though it can occur in both kidneys (Guzzetta et al., 1989).

Neuroblastoma, the second most common solid tumor of children, develops from neural crest cells originating in the adrenal glands, posterior mediastinum, or pelvis. It can develop along any of the sympathetic ganglia. Ninety percent occur before age 9 years, and 40% before age 2 years. Sixty-five percent of neuroblastomas are retroperitoneal tumors, and 65% of children with this tumor have metastatic disease at diagnosis (Guzzetta et al., 1989). Neuroblastoma appears as an asymptomatic abdominal mass; the child appears ill with weight loss, fatigue, and irritability.

The size of the tumor at presentation often dictates the course of treatment. Each type is managed differently, but the goal is to remove the tumor and provide appropriate chemotherapy or radiation therapy—or both—postoperatively. If the tumor is large, definitive surgery may be delayed until after chemotherapy or radiation. Chemotherapy shrinks the tumor and allows for more accurate and safer resection (Dykes et al., 1990).

Wilms' tumor resection: perioperative nursing considerations   Because many children with Wilms' tumor may have received a cardiotoxic chemotherapeutic drug, they must be examined by their oncologist and cleared for surgery. It may be necessary for them to have a thorough cardiac examination to determine the status of cardiac function.

All intravenous catheters and monitoring lines are placed in the upper extremities or neck because the inferior vena cava may be involved by tumor. Such involvement could require clamping of, or pressure on, the inferior vena cava, which would interfere with venous return. Preoperatively, a Wilms' tumor should not be palpated to avoid rupture and tumor cell spillage.

The patient is positioned supine, with a roll under the affected side. The entire abdomen and chest are prepped.

A major laparotomy instrument tray is used that contains larger retractors, vascular instruments, vessel loops, and titanium hemostatic ligature clips.

Key steps

1. A transabdominal incision maximizes exposure for removing the tumor, evaluating the contralateral kidney, and affording a general abdominal examination. A thoracoabdominal incision is made if the tumor extends to the chest cavity. To decrease the risk of tumor cell spillage, the incision for removal of Wilms' tumor is large enough to avoid manipulation as much as possible. Intraoperatively, the tumor is handled carefully to avoid tumor rupture.

2. The renal vein is identified. The vein is ligated before tumor dissection, to prevent tumor embolization from manipulation (Guzzetta et al., 1989).

3. Lymph nodes are removed and placed in separate specimen containers. They are labeled and identified by anatomical site in the abdomen.

4. The contralateral kidney is examined before the tumor is dissected and removed. Gerota's fascia is opened. The contralateral kidney is inspected and carefully palpated; any suspicious nodes are biopsied.

5. The colon and its mesentery are dissected off the tumor.

6. The ureter is identified and transected below the tumor.

7. The kidney and the tumor are removed. The adrenal gland may also be removed because of its proximity to the kidney. Tumor in the inferior vena cava must be removed. Vascular clamps that provide partial occlusion are necessary when the tumor is dissected from the inferior vena cava. Vascular sutures are used to repair any vascular dissection.

8. If there are no suspicious nodes, lymph node biopsy specimens are taken from the suprarenal, infrarenal, and pelvic areas. Tumor in any of these nodes determines tumor staging and what therapy is required.

9. The tumor site and any residual tumor are marked with titanium hemostatic ligature clips to identify tumor during postoperative radiation therapy.

10. The wound is irrigated with warm antibiotic solution and is closed with appropriate-sized absorbable sutures. The subcutaneous layer and subcuticular skin closures are completed with absorbable sutures. The incision is covered with Steristrips, a dry sterile dressing, and paper tape.

Patient outcome   Postoperatively, Wilms' tumor patients receive chemotherapy and radiation therapy appropriate to the stage of the lesion.

The histologic appearance of the lesion is an important indicator of prognosis because it defines the degree of anaplasia. Children with a favorable histological picture have an excellent prognosis; those who have "unfavorable histology," a poor one. The treatment is made as specific as possible to each child and disease present because fewer therapies result in a better quality of life with fewer residual side effects (D'Angio et al., 1989).

Bilateral Wilms' tumor is problematic, especially if there is local recurrence. The goal is to preserve renal tissue and to perform a bilateral nephrectomy only as the last resort (Halberg et al., 1991). Intraoperative radiation therapy may be beneficial at this stage. That combined with surgery offers obliteration of microscopic disease while maintaining renal function. Minimal radiation is delivered to normal tissue. This method of delivering radiation protects the child's future tissue growth, which can be compromised by radiation damage.

Treatment for neuroblastoma is surgical biopsy and removal, if possible. Often, though, the tumor is too large, and radiation therapy is necessary before surgical removal can be attempted. For Stage IV tumors, chemotherapy is administered in conjunction with radiotherapy.

For children with cancer, long-term survival is affected by their quality of life postoperatively and by strategies that enable them and their families to cope effectively.

Bilateral inguinal herniorrhaphy

Inguinal herniorrhaphy is the operation to repair an inguinal hernia. An inguinal hernia can develop in an infant owing to the failure of the processus vaginalis to close. A segment of the infant's intestine may descend into the patent processus vaginalis and produce an inguinal hernia. In utero, the male testes develop high in the posterior wall of the abdomen. They gradually descend into the scrotum before they enter the inguinal canal. The processus vaginalis projects downward but retains communication with the peritoneal cavity. If the upper part of the processus does not retain communication with the peritoneal cavity the remaining sac constitutes an indirect inguinal hernia (Stellar, 1991). In girls, the ligament extends from the uterus through the inguinal canal to its attachment in the labia majora. Weakness of the tissue around the ligament and increased abdominal pressure produce an inguinal hernia. A sliding hernia in an infant girl occurs when the ovary and fallopian tube make up one wall of the sac (Guzzetta et al., 1989).

The inguinal hernia is the most common surgical condition of infants and children. Half of all pediatric hernias in children occur before age 1 year (Moss & Hatch, 1991). An inguinal hernia appears as a bulge in the groin that may extend to the scrotum during crying and straining. On examination it is a smooth, firm mass that emerges through the external inguinal ring and enlarges with increased abdominal pressure. The hernia reduces spontaneously when the infant relaxes. Because the inguinal ring is narrow, infants are at risk for incarceration once the bowel has entered the sac. A hernia is repaired because there is a high risk of incarceration during the first months of life and early repair or repair before a premature infant goes home is recommended (Rowe & Lloyd, 1986). Incarcerated hernias are often manually reduced and repaired 24 to 48 hours later. If a hernia is nonreducible or there is obvious obstruction, an emergency operation is necessary to maintain the bowel's viability.

Most hernia repairs are scheduled as outpatient surgeries. The exceptions are high-risk newborn infants, premature infants, and older children with cardiac, respiratory, or other disorders that increase the risk of anesthesia. Figure 18-7,*A* illustrates different forms of inguinal hernias.

Perioperative nursing considerations The infant is positioned supine with a small towel roll under the lumbosacral region to extend the hips for better operative access. A minor instrument tray is used with small retractors, such as Children's Hospital double-ended and S-shaped retractors.

Key steps

1. A skin incision is made over the inguinal area (Fig. 18-7,*B*).
2. The subcutaneous fat is separated to expose Scarpa's fascia, which is picked up with a fine hemostat and incised. Small retractors are used for exposure.
3. The external ring is identified. The fatty layer is cleaned off the eternal oblique fascia (Fig. 18-7,*C*).
4. The external oblique fascia is opened with a No. 15 blade. Two forceps are used to grasp and separate the tissue (Fig. 18-7,*D*).
5. The hernia sac is grasped with a hemostat. After it is ascertained that the sac is empty, the hemostat is twisted and the sac is ligated with a nonabsorbable suture at the level of the internal ring (Fig. 18-7,*E–G*).
6. The excess sac is excised.
7. The inguinal canal is closed with nonabsorbable sutures.
8. In infant girls a hernia sac is sutured just above the sliding component. The entire stump is reduced into the abdominal cavity through the inguinal ring. Because there is no vas deferens or testicular vessels, the internal ring is sutured closed (Grosfeld et al., 1991).
9. Bupivacaine 0.25% is injected as an ilioinguinal/iliohypogastric nerve block or instillation method (Casey et al., 1990) prior to wound and subcuticular skin closure. The incision is covered with an occlusive dressing.

Routinely, the pediatric surgeon explores the contralateral side for inguinal hernia. This allows for discovery of and closure of a patent processus vaginalis. If bilateral inguinal herniorrhaphy is performed, the hernia sacs are placed in separate specimen containers and identified.

Patient outcome Reduction and surgical repair of an inguinal hernia eliminate the risk of bowel or ovarian ischemia and potential infarction of the herniated organ.

Surgery for Congenital Anomalies

Pyloromyotomy

Ramstedt's pyloromyotomy is the surgical procedure to correct hypertrophic pyloric stenosis, an overgrowth of the circular muscle of the pylorus, due to either hypertrophy or hyperplasia resulting in obstruction of the pyloric sphincter. The obstructed sphincter develops spasms,

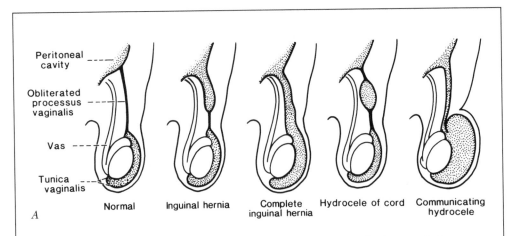

FIGURE 18-7 *A,* Different forms of inguinal hernia and hydrocele that result from failure of the processus vaginalis to obliterate completely. (Adapted from Rowe, M. I., & Lloyd, D. A. [1986]. *Inguinal hernia.* In K. Welch, et al., *Pediatric surgery.* Chicago: Mosby–Year Book.)

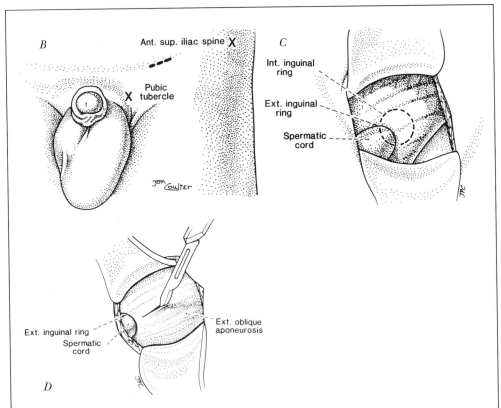

B, The incision is made in the skin crease above and lateral to the pubic tubercle, over the inguinal ring. *C,* Identification of the external ring. *D,* The external oblique fascia is opened. Tissue is grasped with two forceps.

which also affect the circular muscle. This stenosis results in severe narrowing of the pyloric canal between the stomach and duodenum. Peristaltic motions are not effective enough to move stomach contents through the obstructed pylorus, and the resulting inflammation and edema further reduce the size of the opening. Hypertro-

phic pyloric stenosis usually occurs between age 3 and 6 weeks and is more frequent in males than in females (Stringer & Brereton, 1990).

Infants with pyloric stenosis have a history of several days' nonbilious vomiting. The vomiting increases in frequency and may become projectile and blood streaked if

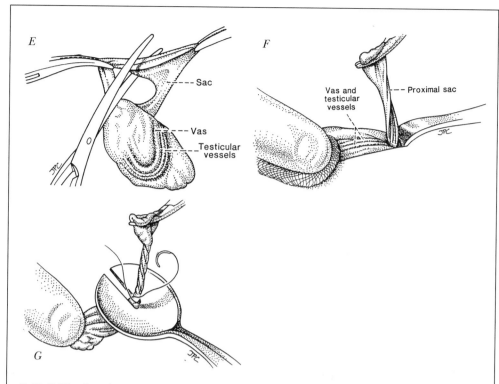

E, F, G, The hernia sac is grasped with forceps, twisted, and ligated. *G,* A grooved spoon is used to protect cord structures during suture ligation.

capillaries in the gastric mucosa are ruptured by frequent vomiting (Benson, 1986). When the infant is feeding, gastric peristalsis is visible across the upper abdomen from left to right. After each vomiting episode the infant appears hungry and immediately takes another feeding if one is offered. Dehydration and weight loss occur. Metabolic alkalosis develops owing to the loss of chloride and potassium during vomiting. On physical examination a small movable mass, the size of an olive, is felt in the infant's right upper abdominal quadrant.

Before surgery is undertaken sodium, chloride, potassium, and water losses must be restored. Surgery is not emergent, and the electrolyte imbalances and fluid balance are restored before surgery.

Perioperative nursing considerations Before anesthesia is administered suction is applied to the nasogastric tube the infant has had in place during hospitalization. This protects the infant against reflux of gastric contents around the tube during intubation. A minor instrument tray is used with a pyloric spreader and Wangensteen's forceps.

Key steps

1. An abdominal subcostal transverse skin incision is made with a No. 15 knife blade.
2. The rectus muscle is separated vertically, and the peritoneum is opened.
3. With two Wangensteen's forceps the surgeon delivers the hypertrophic pylorus.

4. With a warm, moist sponge the prepyloric area is grasped and rotated to expose the anterosuperior border of the hypertrophic pylorus.
5. Using a No. 15 blade, a partial incision is made along the length of the hypertrophic muscle in the pyloric mass through the circular serosa muscle (Fig. 18-8,*A*).
6. The back of a knife handle with the blade removed is used to spread the circular muscle incision. The pyloric spreader is used to complete the division of the submucosal fibers (Fig. 18-8,*B*).
7. The pyloric end of the stomach is returned to the abdomen.
8. The peritoneum and posterior and anterior rectus muscles are closed with absorbable suture. The subcutaneous layer and subcuticular skin closures are completed with absorbable sutures (Fig. 18-8,*C*).
9. Steristrips and a small sterile dressing with paper tape are placed over the incision.

Patient outcome Postoperatively, an intravenous catheter and nasogastric tube stay in place 12 hours. The nasogastric tube facilitates resolution of prepyloric edema and restitution of gastric tone. Small, frequent feedings of a diluted formula are offered to the infant. The volume of the feedings is gradually increased.

Repair of omphalocele or gastroschisis

An omphalocele is an abdominal wall defect in which a mass of bowel and viscera in the center of the abdomen is covered by a translucent membrane. A small omphalocele

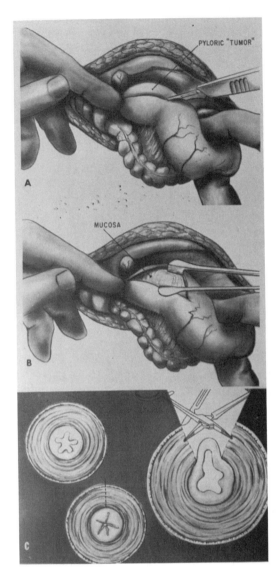

FIGURE 18-8 Pyloromyotomy. *A,* A partial incision is made through the hypertrophic muscle in the pyloric mass through the serosa circular muscle. *B,* The seromuscular layer is separated down to the submucosal base. *C,* A cross section illustrates the hypertrophic pylorus, the depth of incision, and the spreading of muscle to permit mucosa to herniate through the incision. (From Schwartz, S., et al. [1989]. *Principles of surgery* [5th ed.]. New York: McGraw-Hill.)

may involve only a loop of bowel; larger ones may include liver, spleen, and bowel. The abdominal contents are herniated into the umbilical cord. A gastroschisis is a large amount of viscera on the surface of an intact abdominal wall. With gastroschisis, the abdominal wall defect occurs at the right edge of the umbilicus and there is no visible sac (Guzzetta et al., 1989). Also, there may be intestinal malrotation and chemical serositis owing to the bowel's exposure to alkaline amniotic fluid (Shaw, 1990).

During fetal growth the midgut moves into the umbilical cord around the 6th to 10th week of embryonic development. The intestines continue to grow outside the abdominal wall and enter the abdomen around the 11th week. Omphalocele or gastroschisis develops when the intestines fail to enter the abdominal wall.

A neonate born with an omphalocele or gastroschisis requires immediate surgery to repair the anomaly. After birth, the abdominal defect is covered with warm, moist sterile bandages and Kerlex. The sterile protective covering is wrapped loosely to avoid rupture of the omphalocele sac and to avoid abdominal pressure that may interfere with abdominal venous return or respiratory function. Plastic wrap may be placed around the Kerlex, to keep the covering moist and to help maintain the infant's body temperature. Because of the extent of the exposed bowel, neonates may encounter complications that involve heat and fluid losses, increased need for calories, intestinal obstruction, or infection (Mott et al., 1990). The newborn infant with an abdominal wall defect also has increased fluid requirements because of the increased insensible loss that occurs due to bowel exposure (Yaster et al., 1989).

Perioperative nursing considerations The neonate is transferred to the operating room on a radiant warmer or in an Isolette and is placed supine on the operating room bed. The ambient temperature in the room is increased to help maintain the neonate's body temperature, which will tend to drop when viscera are exposed, especially once the protective bandages are removed. To avoid bowel distention that impedes returning the viscera into the abdominal cavity, nitrous oxide should not be administered for anesthesia.

The instruments required are a basic laparotomy tray and prosthetic material such as Silastic sheeting and Teflon mesh for constructing a protective "silo" covering if primary closure is not possible and staging procedures are required.

Key steps *Primary closure* is the ideal repair if it can be accomplished without compromising the patient's respiratory function, venous return in the inferior vena cava, or intestinal blood supply (Schuster, 1986). This is accomplished by dissecting the skin edges, removing the sac on an omphalocele, and returning the viscera into the abdomen. The abdomen is closed with appropriate-sized nonabsorbable sutures, absorbable subcutaneous closure, and a nylon skin closure. Primary closure often is not possible because the increased abdominal pressure may result in respiratory distress owing to increased pressure on the diaphragm and circulating interference due to compression on the inferior vena cava resulting in decreased return of blood to the heart.

Staged closure is similar for both omphalocele and gastroschisis. Prosthetic materials are necessary. Their purpose is to gradually allow the abdominal cavity's capacity to increase. The prosthetic sac is attached to the abdominal wall in the shape of a silo to protect exposed viscera.

Staged Closure

1. The moist protective sterile dressings are removed, and the complete defect is surgically prepped with warm povidone. The neonate is surgically draped using a laparotomy sheet with a small fenestration.
2. With a No. 15 knife blade, a skin flap is elevated around the omphalocele.

3. Teflon mesh is sutured with a nonabsorbable suture to each side of the medial edges of the rectus muscles.

4. Both edges of the mesh are brought up over the abdominal wall defect and sutured together to form a silo (Fig. 18-9).

5. Silastic sheeting is placed over the Teflon mesh. The sheeting protects the defect from fluid loss and keeps it moist.

6. If the defect is large and will require numerous procedures, a central venous catheter may be inserted.

7. Betadine ointment is applied to the suture lines. The whole abdominal defect is covered with dry sterile dressings and Kerlex. The infant is extubated and returned to the intensive care unit (ICU).

8. The staging of the procedure occurs 24 to 72 hours later, without anesthesia. The neonate is monitored by an anesthesia provider or intensivist if the procedure is done in the ICU. A malleable retractor is inserted through an opening in the mesh's suture line and placed on the omphalocele.

9. Gentle pressure is applied to the malleable retractor to press the defect farther into the abdomen. Another row of sutures is placed in the mesh. The anesthesiologist or intensivist monitors for circulatory and respiratory effects. The staging procedure is repeated every 24 to 72 hours until final closure is achieved.

10. Final closure of the defect occurs in the operating room and involves anesthetizing and intubating the infant for removal of the mesh and closing the abdominal cavity and fascia with nonabsorbable suture. The skin is closed with nylon. An umbilicus is created during the closure, if necessary.

11. The final incision is covered with povidone ointment, a dry sterile dressing, and paper tape.

Patient outcome After each staged procedure, respiratory and circulatory compromise may occur. The perioperative nurse must observe closely for signs and symptoms of compromise such as edema in the lower extremities, breathing difficulty, and cyanosis. Edema may occur in the infant because of the increase in extravascular volume caused by venous stasis secondary to increased abdominal pressure on the inferior vena cava.

Once the defect is completely repaired the infant may start to take small feedings.

Esophageal or tracheoesophageal atresia

Esophageal atresia (EA) and tracheoesophageal atresia (TEF) are congenital anomalies that result in a blind esophageal pouch or a fistula between trachea and esophagus. During gestational days 22 and 23 the esophagus and trachea are part of the ventral diverticulum of the foregut. The diverticulum continues to elongate with the growth of endodermal cells appearing on the lateral walls. This growth divides the foregut into tracheal and esophageal channels, and division is complete at day 34 to 36. At this time the submucosal and muscular layers of both anatomical structures are apparent (Guzzetta et al., 1989). EA develops when the cells of the embryonic foregut fail to

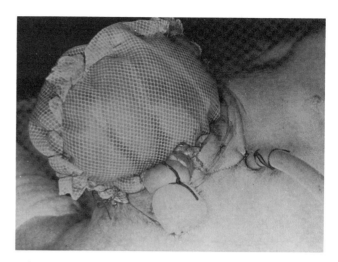

FIGURE 18-9 Silastic prosthesis provides temporary covering for gastroschisis. The remnant of the umbilicus is seen in the center of the photograph. (From Schwartz, S., et al. [1989]. *Principles of surgery* [5th ed.]. New York: McGraw-Hill.)

develop, leaving a blind pouch. TEF develops when the foregut fails to differentiate the separation between the esophagus and trachea, resulting in a fistula between the two (Mott et al., 1990).

Eighty-five percent of the defects are a blind-ended upper esophageal segment whose lower portion is connected to the trachea. This is a type C fistula (Guzzetta et al., 1989) (Fig. 18-10). The esophageal fistula usually joins the trachea at or just above the tracheal fistula. This fistula admits inspired air into the stomach, and gastric juices may flow back into the lungs.

In approximately 8% of infants with EA it is an isolated defect (Guzzetta et al., 1989). Surgical repair involves the creation of an esophagostomy of the upper esophageal pouch. The pouch is brought to the skin of the left side of the neck. This allows the saliva to drain and prevents aspiration. A gastrostomy is performed for feedings. During this postoperative period of growth and feeding, the infant should be offered a pacifier to facilitate the normal developmental stages that occur with sucking and the development of facial activity. At 1 year of age repair of the EA is accomplished. An esophageal-colon interposition or gastric tube may be performed. If successful dilatation of both esophageal ends occurred throughout the year, an end-to-end anastomosis may be accomplished, avoiding esophageal replacement.

The isolated H-type TEF accounts for only 4% of TEF (Guzzetta et al., 1989). This is an isolated congenital fistula that connects the normal trachea and the normal esophagus. A neonate with an H-type fistula does not have excessive secretions. The condition may first become evident after the first feeding, when choking, regurgitation, and perhaps cyanosis first appear. If the fistula is small the symptom may not be obvious, but recurrent pneumonia in the first few months of life is indicative of an H-type fistula. Definitive treatment is division of the fistula through an incision above the clavicle.

Other anomalies are often associated with EA or TEF that may threaten the neonate's survival. The most preva-

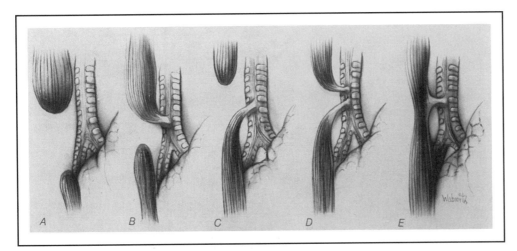

FIGURE 18-10 Five types of EA and TEF. *A,* EA and TEF. *B,* EA with TEF between proximal segment of esophagus and trachea. *C,* EA with TEF between distal esophagus and trachea. *D,* EA with fistula between both proximal and distal ends of esophagus and trachea. *E,* TEF without EA. (From Schwartz, S., et al. [1989]. *Principles of surgery* [5th ed.]. New York: McGraw-Hill.)

lent anomalies are cardiac defects and imperforate anus. These neonates may have vater syndrome—*v*ertebral defects, *a*nal atresia, *t*racheoesophageal fistula, *e*sophageal atresia, and *r*enal or *r*adial dysplasia.

In 1962, Waterson developed risk categories for infants with EA and TEF. Three classes were identified. Class A includes neonates whose birth weight was greater than 5½ pounds and who were well. Class B includes those whose birth weight was between 4 and 5½ pounds and who were well and those whose birth weight was greater but who had moderate aspiration pneumonia and other congenital anomalies. Class C includes infants whose birth weight was less than 4 pounds or whose birth weight was greater than 4 pounds but who had severe pneumonia and severe congenital anomalies.

For each class of patients there is a separate treatment plan. Class A neonates have surgery soon after birth with primary closure depending on the type of defect. For Class B infants surgery is deferred, except for insertion of a gastrostomy tube to decompress the stomach. The infant is stabilized, the aspiration pneumonia is treated, and surgical repair occurs as soon as the patient is stable. Infants in Class C require stabilization and must gain weight before surgical intervention is attempted. Affected neonates have excessive secretions and may become cyanotic and stop breathing because of the overflow of fluid from the esophageal pouch into the trachea and bronchus.

Owing to the many advances and improvements in pediatric surgery, Waterson's classes are no longer the only determinant of risk for anesthesia administration. Physiologic staging is also a major determining factor for deciding surgical intervention in all neonates with EA or tracheoesophageal fistula (Randolph, Newman, & Anderson, 1989). Immediate repair is advocated for all neonates whose cardiorespiratory status is stable, regardless of birth weight. If the cardiorespiratory status is unstable, surgery is delayed. Because the majority of these repairs are not delayed and staged, gastrostomy is avoided. Without the gastrostomy there is less chance of gastroesophageal reflux later (Randolph et al., 1989). A gastrostomy is required though if prolonged mechanical ventilation is necessary or there is cardiac instability.

An X-ray of a curled, radiopaque feeding tube placed in the esophagus verifies the atresia and identifies its level. Preoperative treatment of the infant includes a radi-

ant warmer, elevation of the head, antibiotic and intravenous therapy, and a Replogle tube placed in the upper pouch for drainage. Once the neonate's condition is stabilized, surgical intervention proceeds.

Perioperative nursing considerations The infant is placed in a lateral thoracotomy position with the left side down, using appropriate-sized protective padding and rolls.

A pediatric thoracotomy instrument tray is used to which are added a pediatric chest tube, Pleurevac, and Malecot catheter for gastrostomy tube in staged repair.

Key steps for c-type lesions

1. A retropleural thoracotomy is performed by making a right posterolateral incision through the fourth intercostal space. The intercostal muscle bundles are divided, and the pleura is dissected from the undersurface of the fourth and fifth ribs (Fig. 18-11,*A*)
2. The azygous vein is divided to expose the TEF. The posterior wall of the trachea protecting the vagus nerve is exposed by dissection (Fig. 18-11,*B*).
3. Traction is placed on a vessel loop that has been passed around the lower esophageal segment. This assists in identifying the fistula connecting the trachea.
4. The fistula is transected, leaving behind a 3-mm cuff that allows the fistula to be closed without compromising the tracheal lumen.
5. The fibrous portion of the fistula is excised from the lower segment of the esophagus. The open end is prepared for anastomosis (Fig. 18-11,*C*).
6. The blind upper pouch of the esophagus is located in the upper chest, and its lumen is exposed and incised. To assist in identifying the pouch, the anesthesia provider may gently push a catheter into the pouch.
7. Nonabsorbable fine suture corner stitches are placed, bringing the mucosal layer of the upper pouch to the entire thickness of the lower pouch. Interrupted sutures are placed around the pouch to complete the inside layer (Fig. 18-11,*D*).
8. The muscle of the upper pouch is brought down over the anastomosis and secured with fine interrupted nonabsorbable sutures in the wall of the lower seg-

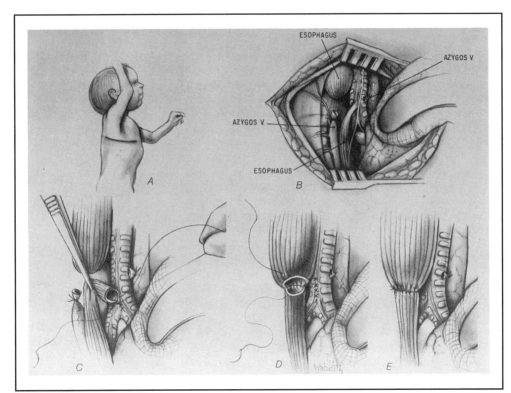

FIGURE 18-11 Repair of esophageal or transesophageal atresia. *A*, Right thoracotomy incision. *B*, The azygos vein is divided to expose the fistula. *C*, The fistula is transected and the defect in the trachea is closed. *D*, End-to-end anastomosis is accomplished between the proximal and distal esophagus. *E*, The anastomosis is completed. (From Schwartz, S., et al. [1989]. *Principles of surgery* [5th ed.]. New York: McGraw-Hill.)

ment of the esophagus (Fig. 18-11,*E*). The repair can also be accomplished in a single-layer suturing technique, with the interrupted sutures going through the full thickness of both upper and lower segments. The single-layer repair is the more popular closure of a C-type fistula (Poenaru, Laberge, Neilson, Nguyen, & Guttman, 1991). If the upper pouch needs to be lengthened, a circular myotomy may be made through all the layers except the mucosa of the esophagus.

9. A small extrapleural chest tube is inserted, secured to the skin with a nonabsorbable suture, and attached to a pediatric thoracic drainage system.

10. The muscle layers are closed with an appropriate-sized nonabsorbable suture. A subcutaneous layer and subcuticular skin closures are completed with an absorbable suture. Steristrips and a dry sterile dressing with paper tape are placed over the incision and the chest tube exit site.

11. A gastrostomy may be performed with a primary repair only if the infant has neurological impairment, is premature, or is not able to take oral feedings (Shaul, Schwartz, Marr, & Tyson, 1989). If a gastrostomy has not been done for a staged repair, it is avoided, lest it increase the risk of postoperative gastroesophageal reflux (Grosfeld, 1991).

Patient outcome Postoperatively, the sutured anastomosis line must heal properly to allow for maturation and growth. Hyperextension of the neck should be avoided, to prevent tension on the sutures. Placing the infant with the head elevated prevents gastric regurgitation, which also protects the suture line. Once it is healed, the infant is able to take oral feedings.

Congenital diaphragmatic hernia repair

A congenital diaphragmatic hernia (CDH) is an opening in the lateral segment of the diaphragm that lets abdominal contents slip into the thorax. The incidence is one in 4000 live births, and 85% to 90% of them occur in the left side of the thorax (Anderson, 1986). A diaphragmatic hernia on the left side may be filled with small intestine, spleen, stomach, the left lobe of the liver, or colon. With a hernia on the right side, the liver and small intestine may fill the chest cavity.

During intrauterine development, the pleuroperitoneal canal maintains the continuity of the pleural and abdominal cavities. If the diaphragm does not develop and close, a posterolateral defect occurs that is known as Bochdalek's hernia. Because the bowel lies in the chest cavity, the affected lung cannot mature, and the result is a hypoplastic lung. The ipsilateral lung may be underdeveloped because of mediastinal shift caused by the intrathoracic bowel. The abdominal cavity may be underdeveloped owing to the absence of abdominal contents during fetal life.

Congenital diaphragmatic hernias are often diagnosed prenatally with ultrasonography. Diagnosis before birth is beneficial. The mother can meet with a pediatric surgeon before delivery, and several specialist physicians—surgeon, obstetrician, high-risk neonatologist—can plan appropriate measures to facilitate safe delivery of the infant and transfer to a pediatric hospital. These measures may involve changing the delivery site, delivery method, or even the delivery date.

Surgical repair of CDH is one of the most urgent surgical procedures in newborns. After delivery, the bowel fills with air and the mediastinum shifts to the opposite side, compromising respiration in the better-developed lung. The negative thoracic pressure caused by the infant's crying may pull more intestines into the chest and further distend the chest cavity.

The clinical presentation of CDH in a newborn infant is immediate respiratory distress, which is caused by poor lung expansion secondary to lung hypoplastia and decreased number of alveoli. Respiratory distress is further increased by the intrathoracic presence of intestinal contents, the absence of negative intrathoracic pressure, and increased pulmonary artery pressure (Theorell, 1990). The chest wall may be barrel shaped or asymmetrical. Heart sounds are usually best heard on the right side. Shifting of the mediastinum interferes with venous return to the heart, and cardiac output may be impaired.

The neonate is intubated in the delivery room, to prevent gastric and bowel distention and assist in ventilation. A nasogastric tube is inserted to decompress the gastrointestinal tract and to prevent further bowel distention. An arterial line is inserted to measure arterial blood gases. The arterial line that is placed in the umbilical artery measures postductal blood gases. The arterial line placed in the radial artery measures preductal blood gases and helps determine the amount of right-to-left ductus arteriosus shunting that occurs (Anderson, 1986).

Perioperative nursing considerations The infant usually arrives in the operating room already intubated and with intravenous line and arterial lines in place. The infant is positioned supine.

A major pediatric thoracotomy instrument tray is requried, as is a chest drainage system and chest tube. Gore-Tex patches should be available for use if the diaphragm cannot be closed primarily.

Key steps

1. A subcostal incision is made on the side of the CDH.
2. The rib cage is retracted to expose the diaphragm and locate the abdominal contents that have herniated through the defect.
3. By gently retracting the bowel, the surgeon reduces the hernia.
4. A chest tube is inserted and anchored in place with a suture to the skin.
5. The posterior rim of the diaphragm is identified by dissecting the continuous layer of pleura and peritoneum off the rim. The muscle under the covering is unrolled; this will be the posterior rim of the diaphragm.
6. The diaphragm is closed by using absorbable sutures to close the anterior and the new posterior portions of the diaphragmatic muscle. If the defect is too large, a Gore-Tex patch is sutured in place to close it.
7. The abdominal cavity is closed with absorbable sutures. The abdomen may not be large enough to accommodate the replaced abdominal contents, in which case only the skin is closed, creating a ventral hernia that is repaired 10 to 14 days later. Suturing just the skin closed also allows intraabdominal pressure to be placed on the diaphragm and not just on the inferior vena cava.
9. A thoracic catheter is often placed in the contralateral side because of the high incidence of pneumothorax that may occur (Anderson, 1986).
10. The subcutaneous layer and subcuticular skin closures are completed with absorbable suture.
11. Povidone ointment is applied at the thoracic catheter exit sites. Steristrips and dry sterile dressings and paper tape cover the incision and catheters. The intubated neonate is transported directly to the pediatric ICU.

Patient outcome Postoperatively infants with minor defects progress well and are extubated after 1 day. Those with severe defects may appear to do well for a short time. This is called the "honeymoon period." Respiratory function is stable, with a low rate and pressure ventilator settings. Preductal and postductal blood gases are good. This period may last a few hours or a day; then the neonate's condition begins to deteriorate. Ventilation and oxygen needs are increased because of the development of persistent pulmonary hypertension (PPHN). PPHN is also referred to as persistent fetal circulation. The high pulmonary pressure is due to the hypoplastic lung and can be fatal.

In a normal newborn, the first breath expands the lungs. This action lowers pulmonary vascular resistance. As more blood flows to the heart's chambers, the pressures shift and the foramen ovale and ductus arteriosus close. With CDH the pressure in the right atrium is too high to allow blood to flow into the right ventricle, whence it goes to the lungs for oxygenation. The blood crosses the patent foramen ovale and enters the left atrium. The unoxygenated blood flows into the left ventricle and thence into the general circulation. PPHN causes any blood entering the right ventricle to be shunted from the pulmonary artery to the aorta via the patent ductus arteriosus. This results in a cyanotic neonate. The postoperative infant with PPHN is a candidate for extracorporeal membrane oxygenation (ECMO) (Gerraughty & Younie, 1987).

Extracorporeal membrane oxygenation

ECMO is a procedure that diverts the cardiac output away from the lungs. It is a form of partial cardiopulmonary bypass used for long-term support of respiratory or cardiac function. Currently, its most frequent use is for neonates with potentially reversible pulmonary disease who are at high risk of not surviving conventional treatment (White, Richardson & Raibstein, 1990; Roberts & Jones, 1990).

The purpose of ECMO is to allow the lungs to rest while the lungs heal. It allows the lungs to heal without subjecting them to high concentrations of oxygen from ventilatory support (Short & Lotze, 1988).

There are two methods of ECMO, venoarterial (VA) and venovenous (VV). Venoarterial ECMO supports cardiac function. It is most often used because cardiac function is compromised by the severity of the disease in most ECMO candidates (Roberts & Jones, 1990). Venovenous access avoids ligating the common carotid artery, but higher volume of blood flow is required to achieve gas exchange (Bartlett & Anderson, 1990).

The most successful candidates for ECMO have been infants at risk of developing PPHN. PPHN is characterized by cycles of hypoxia, acidosis, sustained pulmonary vascular resistance, and intrapulmonary and extrapulmonary right-to-left shunting (Rushton, 1990). ECMO is generally reserved for a population of neonates who have reversible lung disease, sepsis, or heart disease.

The primary indications for ECMO are meconium aspiration, respiratory distress syndrome, persistent fetal circulation, persistent pulmonary hypertension due to hypoplastic lung with congenital diaphragmatic hernia, and sepsis.

While infants are receiving ECMO their lungs do not participate in gas exchange. Blood flows by gravity drainage from the right internal jugular vein into the ECMO circuit, through the oxygenator and heat exchanger, and back into the patient via the right common carotid (Tuggle, 1991). Currently, ECMO is not used on premature infants because it requires systemic heparinization, and premature infants already are at increased risk of intracranial bleeds.

Each pediatric institution participating in ECMO develops a set of criteria to identify appropriate ECMO candidates. According to O'Rourke (1991) and Tuggle (1991), these criteria incude gestational age of 34 to 35 weeks, predicted mortality of 80% or greater, birth weight of at least 2000 g, no significant preexisting intraventricular hemorrhage, and no uncorrectable congenital heart disease or other anomaly that precludes a reasonable chance for survival.

Perioperative nurses participating in ECMO must demonstrate the ability to anticipate the needs of the patient, nurses, and physicians. These procedures are performed in the ICU because of the physical and mechanical difficulty of moving the infant once ECMO is instituted. In anticipation of patient requirements, all sterile supplies, sutures, instruments, electrosurgical unit, and headlight must be transported to the ICU. Electrical adapters are also necessary if equipment from the operating room has different electrical prongs than the receptacles in the ICU. Because the procedure is done in the intensive care unit, traffic control in and out of the bed space area is limited to necessary personnel only. Surgical hats and masks are worn by health care personnel near the bed space and sterile area. Before a neonate is placed on ECMO ultrasonography of the head is routinely performed to ensure that there is no intracranial hemorrhage. A major intraventricular bleed is a contraindication to proceeding with ECMO (Trento et al., 1988).

Perioperative nursing considerations The neonate is repositioned so that the head is at the foot of the radiant warmer bed, and an electrical dispersive pad is placed on the patient. The bed may also be elevated to help gravity drainage of the neonate's blood to the pump at floor level. The head is turned to the left, to expose the surgical site. A small towel roll may be placed under the shoulders to hyperextend the neck for better surgical access. Preparation of the sterile team and table takes place in the ICU.

Surgical draping is similar to that for any pediatric surgery involving the neck. A transparent plastic drape may be cut to fit the neonate's smaller neck space.

Equipment, supplies, and instrumentation A minor dissecting instrument tray with additional fistula forceps, fine scissors for dissection, a self-retaining hernia retractor, angled and straight Cooley neonatal vascular clamps, tubing clamps, a knife handle, and a No. 65 blade is used.

Key steps

1. An incision is made along the sternocleidomastoid muscle. The right carotid artery and the right internal jugular vein are isolated and identified with Vessel loops.
2. The neonate is systematically heparinized by the ICU nurse, with 30 to 50 units per kilogram of body weight, as determined by institutional protocol.
3. The carotid artery is ligated and secured with stay sutures and a Cooley neonatal vascular clamp. The sutures help prevent tearing and dissection of the arterial wall (Workman & Lentz, 1987).
4. A No. 8 or 10 Fr catheter with a single end hole is used for the arterial cannula. It is filled with heparinized saline and lubricated with a sterile lubricant. The carotid artery is incised with the knife blade. The cannula is placed in the carotid artery and advanced into the ascending aorta.
5. A No. 12 or 14 Fr multiholed drainage catheter is used for the venous cannula. It is filled with heparinized saline and lubricated also. After the internal jugular vein is incised the cannula is placed into the right internal jugular and advanced into the right atrium.
6. The cannulae are attached to the oxygenator pump tubing by having one surgeon unclamp one cannula at a time, allowing retrograde blood flow. The second surgeon connects the cannula to the tubing from the oxygenator while the scrub person fills the circuit connector with heparinized saline to eliminate any air bubbles (Fig. 18-12).
7. Both catheters are secured in the vessels with a ligature and secured again with a heavier ligature behind the ear, to prevent accidental decannulation.
8. The skin is closed with nylon.
9. The incision and cannula sites are covered with povidone ointment, sterile dressing, and foam tape. The sterile setup is maintained until an X-ray has confirmed the correct position of the cannulae.

In venovenous ECMO, blood is drained from and returned to the right side of the circulatory system. Venovenous ECMO offers respiratory support without cardiac support. There are two types of cannulae for venovenous ECMO; two catheters or one. Cannulation requiring two catheters involves placing one in the right atrium via the internal jugular and the second return catheter is placed in the femoral vein. Single-catheter cannulation uses a double-lumen catheter that allows continual outflow through the proximal port and inflow through the distal port. A single-lumen catheter may also be used for single-

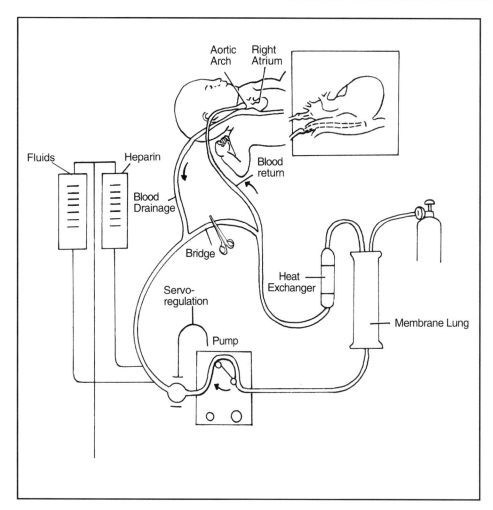

FIGURE 18-12 Extracorporeal life support circuit diagram in a typical neonatal application. (From Bartlett, R., & Anderson, H. L. [1990]. Extracorporeal life. In A. Coran and B. Harris [Eds.]. *Pediatric trauma: Proceedings of the 3rd conference.* Philadelphia: J. B. Lippincott.)

catheter venovenous ECMO. (This catheter is similar to the dialysis catheter that separates infusion flow patterns.)

How long an infant requires ECMO depends on the initial disease. According to the Extracorporeal Life Support Organization (ELSO) the average length of ECMO support for a neonate with meconium aspiration is 3 to 6 days and for congenital diaphragmatic hernia with PPHN 7 to 12 days (O'Rourke, 1991). ECMO normally is not sustained longer than 2 weeks because the complications override the benefits.

Once the decision is made to remove the infant from ECMO, the ECMO cycle is slowly decreased while the infant's ability to support gas exchange is evaluated. ECMO is removed when the infant can demonstrate acceptable levels of gas exchange with conventional ventilatory support. ECMO in neonates is effective because it breaks the persistent pulmonary hypertension cycle by supporting cardiopulmonary function and correcting acidosis. It allows the lungs to heal and to rest from high levels of oxygen and high positive-pressure ventilation (McDermott & Curley, 1990).

ECMO has complications and risks. The most common risk is the long-term effects of ligation and cannulation of the right common carotid artery. Neurologic assessment of these patients is still in the beginning testing levels because post-ECMO patients are young. Some institutions participating in ECMO now do carotid reconstruction at

the same time ECMO is removed (Moulton, 1991). Long-term follow-up is necessary to see if carotid reconstruction is beneficial. ECMO exposes the infant to blood products, and there is also the potential of mechanical problems to develop from the ECMO. If a neonate is not expected to survive being taken off ECMO, the perioperative nurse and ICU nurse should make every effort to keep the infant alive long enough for the parents to hold and comfort their child.

ECMO was first successful with neonates, and now it is beginning to be used to treat older children and adults with acute respiratory failure or cardiac failure. The conditions that may require support in these populations are the result of drowning, smoke inhalation, chemical aspiration, direct pulmonary contusion, pulmonary capillary injuries such as acute respiratory distress syndrome, and extrathoracic trauma (Bartlett & Anderson, 1990).

Heparin-bonded circuits are still in the developmental stages. This development will allow ECMO without systemic coagulation. If this occurs ECMO may be available for low–birth weight or premature infants who are not now candidates because of their already increased risk for intracranial hemorrhage (Hopkins & Cowell, 1991).

For a neonate with lung hypoplasia so severe that it cannot sustain respiratory function there is potential for ECMO to become a bridge to lung transplantation. A proposal put forth by Crombleholme et al (1990) states that

ECMO may provide temporary neonatal cardiopulmonary support, perhaps until a proper-sized lung is available. Further research is necessary to determine if this proposal is reasonable.

Biliary atresia and Kasai's procedure

Biliary atresia is obstruction or absence of a portion of the bile ducts. There are two types of bile duct obstruction, intrahepatic and extrahepatic. Intrahepatic biliary atresia, absence of bile ducts within the liver, can be treated only with liver transplantation. Extrahepatic biliary atresia is obstruction or absence of the main bile passages outside the liver. The most common type of blockage is complete atresia of extrahepatic structures. The incidence of biliary atresia in newborns is 1 in 20,000 (Guzzetta et al., 1989). Its cause is unknown, but evidence now indicates that it may be a viral infection that causes intrahepatic and extrahepatic bile duct obstruction from fibrosis (Grosfeld et al., 1989).

The newborn with biliary atresia shows signs of liver failure soon after birth, though this may go undetected because jaundice is not uncommon in newborns. Physiological newborn jaundice goes away without treatment soon after birth. Pathological jaundice with biliary atresia lasts more than 2 weeks and is associated with continued increases in the bilirubin value. The infant's urine is dark, and stools are lighter in color. Other signs are hepatomegaly, abdominal distention, malnutrition, and general failure to thrive. With more advanced disease, splenomegaly and portal hypertension develop, evidenced by prominent anteroabdominal wall veins.

Biliary atresia is not a static congenital anomaly. It is a progressive disease that results in total obliteration of the ducts because of the fibrous tissue (Lilly et al., 1989). The longer this anomaly goes uncorrected, the more permanent is the damage to the liver.

Extrahepatic biliary atresia has been divided into correctable and uncorrectable types (Lilly, 1986). The correctable category of biliary atresia includes proximal extrahepatic bile ducts associated with occluded distal ducts. The anomaly is corrected with an intestinal anastomosis of the Roux-en-Y limb of the jejunum to the proximal bile duct. The anastomosis occurs above the hepatic duct.

The uncorrectable category involves occluded proximal extrahepatic ducts resulting in no bile flow from the liver. The operation to correct this is hepatoportoenterostomy, also called Kasai's procedure, for the physician who discovered that there are microscopic patent biliary ductules at the porta hepatis, where the proximal ducts are occluded. These microscopic ductules allow passage of bile produced in the intrahepatic ductal system. With removal of the fibrous tissue at the porta hepatis, these microscopic channels are opened and bile flows into an anastomosed intestinal conduit, usually the Roux-en-Y limb.

Perioperative nursing considerations A major laparotomy instrument tray is used, with intestinal clamps, microvascular forceps and needle holders, and an abdominal self-retaining retractor. Biliary drainage catheters or Silas-

tic tubing and self-contained suction drains are needed. The infant is positioned supine. Two peripheral intravenous catheters and an arterial line are placed. An appropriate-sized urethral catheter is inserted.

Key steps

1. A left subcostal incision is made. The liver and ductal anatomy are exposed with meticulous dissection and hemostasis.
2. An intraoperative cholangiogram is performed. If the hepatic duct cannot be identified, the diagnosis of biliary atresia is confirmed.
3. After the extrahepatic duct remnant is identified, the biliary structures are dissected from the porta hepatis. Frozen section examination is performed to confirm the correct level for the hilar duct transection that will allow bile to drain through the microscopic ductules.
4. Fine, nonabsorbable sutures are placed on the lateral and posterior margins of the hilar duct and liver interface.
5. Biliary reconstruction is accomplished by the anastomosis of 20 cm of the Roux-en-Y limb of the jejunum to the transected ducts at the liver hilus, using the previously placed sutures (Fig. 18-13).
6. A small Silastic tube or T tube is placed in the Roux-en-Y limb and liver hilus anastomosis.
7. The end of the new biliary conduit is anastomosed to the intestinal tract. This step sometimes involves temporary exteriorization of the conduit to decrease the intraluminal pressure that the bile has to flow against when it is secreted into the Roux-en-Y limb. This may also decrease biliary stasis that could result in postoperative cholangitis. An intestinal conduit is not necessary if the gallbladder, cystic duct, and distal common duct are all present. This anastomosis also eliminates the risk of postoperative cholangitis.
8. The Silastic drain is brought out through the skin. A self-contained suction drain is placed for abdominal drainage and sutured to the skin to avoid accidental removal.
9. The abdomen is closed with appropriate-sized nonabsorbable sutures. The subcutaneous layer and subcuticular skin closures are completed with absorbable sutures.
10. Steristrips are applied and are covered with a dry sterile dressing. The drains are also taped securely to the skin.

Patient outcomes The necessary patient outcome for survival is for bile to flow from the liver into the intestinal tract. This allows proper liver function, nutrition, and growth. Autoanastomosis between the intestinal and ductal epithelial elements occurs within 4 to 6 weeks (Lilly, 1986). Factors associated with success of Kasai's procedure are the patient's age, presence of bile flow following the procedure, liver histology, the experince of the surgeon, and a technically adequate hepatoportoenterostomy procedure (Wood et al., 1990). The younger the infant, the more beneficial and successful the operation

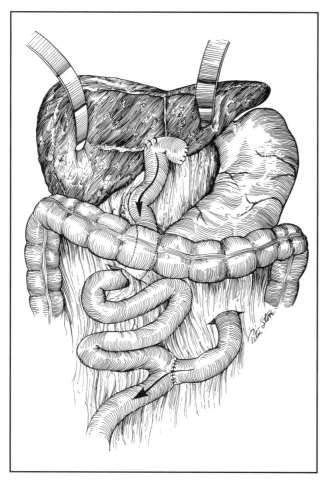

FIGURE 18-13 Operative diagram of Kasai's portoenterostomy for biliary atresia. An isolated limb of jejunum has been brought to the porta hepatis and anastomosed to the transected ducts. The Roux-en-Y principle has been used to restore intestinal continuity. The biliary conduit is usually vented externally. (From Schwartz, S., et al. [1989]. *Principles of surgery* [5th ed.]. New York: McGraw-Hill.)

will be. Operation within the first 2 months of life has a better prognosis, if the surgery is technically correct, because the liver will not have sustained permanent damage from entrapped bile. Because of these factors, infants with biliary atresia who need hepatoportoenterostomy should be cared for only at pediatric institutions experienced in the total care of these patients.

Kasai's procedure offers corrective palliative surgery for some infants, but others may have persistent and progressive liver diseases. If hepatoportoenterostomy is unsuccessful the infant continues to develop liver failure. The only treatment then is liver transplantation.

Indications for liver transplantation after Kasai's procedure are deteriorating liver function, growth failure, bleeding, sepsis related to hepatic compromise (Vacanti, Shamberger, Eraklis, & Lillehei, 1990), and uncorrected cholangitis resulting in cirrhosis of the liver. As the primary treatment for biliary atresia, liver transplantation may be indicated only for infants older than 4 months because their liver is already hard, enlarged, and permanently damaged (Kasai, Mochizuki, Ohkohchi, Chiba, &

Ohi, 1989; Grosfeld et al., 1989). It is the final treatment for biliary atresia when other interventions have failed.

Liver transplantation in pediatric patients is limited by the available number of donors. Organ size is the determining factor. Many patients die waiting for an organ of correct size. Orthotopic partial segmental organ transplantation has been instrumental in increasing the organ pool. Some pediatric medical centers are participating in living related segmental liver donation from a parent in response to the scarcity of cadaver organs. Other pediatric centers are combining Kasai's procedure with liver transplantation later, as needed (Vacanti et al., 1990). The surgical intervention of Kasai's procedure provides benefits to patients while they wait for a donor liver. Infants can grow because of improved nutritional status, and as they get older the pool of available donor organs becomes larger.

Endorectal pullthrough procedure

The definitive treatment for Hirschsprung's disease is one of the three endorectal pullthrough procedures. Hirschsprung's disease, the absence of autonomic parasympathetic cells (ganglion cells) in the distal alimentary tract, usually occurs in the rectum and rectosigmoid. The aganglionic colon does not permit normal peristalsis. Eighty percent of infants with Hirschsprung's disease are males, and the incidence is one in 5000 (Sieber, 1986).

Because of the absence of normal peristalsis, a functional defect occurs. Often neonates with Hirschsprung's disease do not pass meconium in the first 24 hours of life. Intestinal contents accumulate, and bowel distention develops proximal to the defect. Older infants have a history of constipation alternating with diarrhea, abdominal distention, and failure to thrive or poor nutrition. If the condition goes unrepaired the infant develops enterocolitis with explosive diarrhea, fever, and severe dehydration. Enterocolitis is the major cause of death in infants with Hirschsprung's disease. Early diagnosis and intervention decrease the incidence of enterocolitis.

The three modes of management for infants with Hirschsprung's disease depend on age and clinical manifestations. They are: (1) immediate pullthrough surgical intervention, (2) diverting enterostomy followed later by a pullthrough operation, and (3) (for infants older than 10 months and who have no enterocolitis) impaction removal, routine enemas, and a pullthrough operation (Foster, Cowan, & Wrenn, 1990).

Definitive diagnosis of Hirschsprung's disease is made by rectal suction biopsy. A barium enema identifies the transitional zone between the dilated proximal colon and the aganglionic distal segment. Initial treatment is colostomy to relieve the intestinal obstruction. The colostomy also allows time for the distended hypertrophic colon to return to its normal size before the definitive surgical repair is undertaken. The pullthrough operation of bringing normal bowel as low into the rectum as possible is usually deferred until the infant is 9 to 12 months old. During this time the colon returns to its normal size, to ease its passage through the infant's narrow pelvis, and it regains its tonicity. The infant returns also to a healthy nutritional state and gains weight.

There are three types of endorectal pullthrough surgical interventions for definitive treatment of Hirschsprung's disease. They are Soave's, Duhamel's, and Swenson's procedures (Fig. 18-14). Soave's procedure involves dissection of the rectal mucosa from the muscular sleeve. The ganglionic colon is brought through the sleeve and amputated at the anal level. The internal sphincter muscle is kept intact to preserve continence.

Hirschsprung's disease involving long segments of the colon is treated with Duhamel's procedure, which involves dissection in the retrorectal area, outside the rectum. The ganglionic colon is anastomosed posteriorly above the anus. The remaining anterior wall of the ganglionic colon and the posterior wall of the aganglionic rectum may be removed using an automatic stapling or suturing device. This is usually done to avoid accumulation of stool in the remaining aganglionic rectum (Guzzetta et al., 1989). If Duhamel's procedure is performed on an infant younger than 3 months, the anterior wall of the ganglionic colon and posterior wall of the aganglionic rectum are not dissected until later because the anus is too small for the stapling device (Hung, 1991; Carcassone, Guys, Morrison-Lacombe, & Kreitman, 1989).

In Swenson's procedure the aganglionic rectum is dissected in the lower pelvis and brought down to the anus. A perineal approach is done to anastomose the ganglionic colon to the anus. The initial colostomy is closed 4 to 6 weeks later, once the pelvic anastomosis is healed. Some studies have shown that if Swenson's procedure is done before age 3 months, the initial colostomy may not be necessary for abdominal decompression (Carcassone et al., 1989) (Fig. 18-14).

Perioperative nursing considerations A major laparotomy instrument tray is necessary, with bowel anastomosis clamps, Hegar dilators, small pole rectal retractors, and a urethral catheter. Once the patient is draped, a urethral catheter is inserted and kept on the sterile field. A collection system is maintained on the field, or the catheter is plugged and unplugged regularly for drainage and measurement. A separate instrument table may be used for the perineal dissection and anastomosis.

Preoperatively, the infant has a nasogastric tube. Nitrous oxide should not be administered so the bowel does not become distended.

The rectum may be irrigated with warm antibiotic solution. The infant is prepped extensively, from the nipples to the buttocks, including the genital and perineal areas and upper thighs. This preparation permits various changes in positioning for all stages of the surgery. The lower legs are wrapped with a sterile towel or sterile stockinette to allow them to stay in the sterile surgical field.

Key steps

1. A left paramedian incision involving the stoma is made. The stoma is freed from the abdominal wall, and the left colon is mobilized. The colon above the stoma is the proximal end of the resection if it has previously been identified as normal from a biopsy specimen. If aganglionic intestine has not been iden-

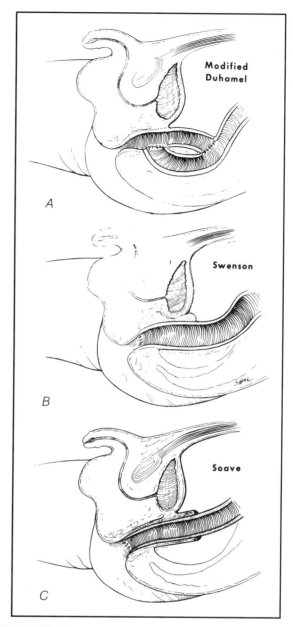

FIGURE 18-14 The three basic operations for surgical correction of Hirschsprung's disease. (From Schwartz, S., et al. [1989]. *Principles of surgery* [5th ed.]. New York: McGraw-Hill.)

tified this is done at this time by biopsy and frozen section examination. The involved colon is excised.
2. The blood supply to the rectum is preserved by dividing the mesocolon and vessels of the intestine close to the intestine.
3. The mucosal tube is dissected from the outer muscular layer and transected. Traction sutures are placed on the distal end of the tube, to facilitate the pullthrough motion.
4. The mucosa is stripped to the anus. Blunt finger dissection by the surgeon may help develop the presacral space.
5. The legs are lifted for the perineal dissection.
6. The anus is dilated with Hegar dilators; it may be retracted with pole retractors or Allis forceps.
7. Using electrosurgical cautery a circumferential inci-

sion is made in the anal mucosa. Scissors are used to complete the mucosal stripping.

8. A full-length hemostat is inserted into the rectum to grasp the traction sutures on the proximal colon. It is pulled through the rectal muscular sleeve, posterior to the rectum.
9. The seromuscular layers of the colon are sutured to the rectal muscular cuff with absorbable sutures. A Penrose drain may be placed to drain serous fluid.
10. The proximal edge of the rectal muscular cuff is sutured to the seromuscular layer of the colon.
11. The abdomen is irrigated with warm antibiotic solution and is closed with appropriate-sized absorbable sutures. The subcutaneous layer and subcuticular skin closures are completed with absorbable sutures. Steristrips and a dry sterile dressing are placed on the incision and covered with paper tape.

Patient outcome Postoperatively the infant may still have a proximal colostomy that was not closed intraoperatively. It is closed 4 to 6 weeks after the pelvic anastomosis has healed. Once the infant recovers successfully, normal bowel function is the desired patient outcome.

Intussusception reduction

Intussusception is an invagination of a portion of the intestine into itself. The invagination begins at or near the ileocecal valves (Ravitch, 1986). The ileum invaginates into the cecum and then the colon. An intestinal obstruction develops because two walls of the intestine are pressed against each other, causing inflammation, edema, and decreased blood flow.

Other types of intussusception are ileoileal (the ileum telescopes into another section of the ileum) and colocolic (the colon telescopes into another area of the colon, usually at the hepatic and splenic flexure or along the transverse colon) (Whaley & Wong, 1991). Intussusception occurs more frequently (3:2) in well-nourished males between age 8 and 12 months (Ravitch, 1986). It also is more prevalent in infants with cystic fibrosis or celiac disease.

Identifiable causes of intussusception are found in only 5% of cases. They include Meckel's diverticulum, intestinal polyps, and tumors (Mott et al., 1990). The most frequent cause may be hypertrophy of Peyer's patches in the terminal ileum secondary to viral infection (Guzzetta, 1989). The hypertrophic lymphatic patch becomes drawn into the lumen of the terminal ileum and progressively moves into the ascending and transverse colon.

Signs of intussusception appear suddenly. Infants cry from pain, drawing up the legs, and they vomit. They continue to have these bouts of abdominal pain, becoming apathetic, and may pass bloody "currant jelly" mucus rectally. The abdomen appears tender and distended. The presence of a sausage-shaped abdominal mass is a significant diagnostic finding (Bruce et al., 1987). Intussusception is fatal in 2 to 5 days if not reduced or surgically repaired because it can lead to hemorrhage, perforation, and peritonitis. An infant with intussusception must receive immediate medical treatment to limit damage to the bowel. There are two types of treatment, nonoperative and operative.

The nonoperative approach is attempted first unless the infant already shows signs of peritonitis. This treatment includes a barium enema for hydrostatic reduction of the intussusception and is the treatment of choice for most cases of intussusception. Many factors are related to the success of hydrostatic reduction—duration of signs, vomiting, age, absence of abdominal pain, rectal bleeding, small bowel obstruction, ileoileocolic intussusception, and the presence of a leading point. Rectal bleeding and presence of symptoms longer than 48 hours contribute significantly to the prediction of failure of hydrostatic reduction (Reijnen, Festen, & Van Roosmalen, 1990).

Hydrostatic reduction is contraindicated in infants who have a long history of symptoms, intestinal obstruction, peritonitis, obviously impaired intestinal viabilty, neonatal intussusception or in older children with recurrent intussusception and failed reduction (Bruce et al., 1987).

If the intussusception is not reducible, surgical intervention is necessary. Surgery is usually scheduled before the hydrostatic reduction is initiated, because of the urgency to protect the involved bowel if it is not reducible.

Perioperative nursing considerations Infants who need surgical intervention require intravenous fluids, aspiration of gastric contents, and antibiotics. According to Mark Ravitch (1986), the antibiotics are necessary because the vascular supply of the bowel may be jeopardized. Once the patient is anesthetized, the surgeon should palpate the abdomen because of the possibility of spontaneous reduction during transit to the operating room or during induction of anesthesia (Storey-Wilson, MacKinley, Prescott, & Hendrey, 1988).

The patient is positioned supine. An abdominal exploratory instrument tray is used; intestinal clamps are available if bowel resection is necessary.

Key steps

1. A right-side, lower quadrant incision is made.
2. The intussuscepted mass is delivered out of the wound.
3. Moist sponges are used to handle any bowel.
4. Reduction of the intussusception is accomplished by progressive gentle pressure on the bowel distal to the intussusception (Fig. 18-15).
5. Appendectomy is performed because the blood supply to the appendix may have been compromised.
6. If it is difficult to reduce the intussusception without pulling, bowel resection may be necessary to resect the bowel. Force may rupture the bowel, which could contaminate the wound and the peritoneal cavity.
7. The abdomen is irrigated with warm antibiotic solution.
8. The peritoneal cavity and muscle layers are closed with absorbable sutures. The subcutaneous layer and subcuticular skin closures are completed with absorbable sutures.
9. The incision is covered with Steristrips, a dry sterile dressing, and paper tape.

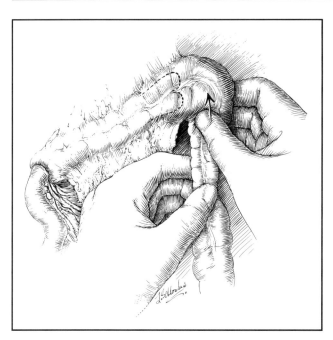

FIGURE 18-15   Manual reduction of intussusception.
(From Schwartz, S., et al. [1989]. *Principles of surgery* [5th ed.]. New York: McGraw-Hill.)

Patient outcome   Postoperatively, the nasogastric tube is kept in place until normal bowel activity is restored. The infant is given small feedings to facilitate normal bowel activity once it has begun.

Fetal Surgery

Advances in prenatal diagnoses—owing to improved ultrasonography and understanding of fetal pathophysiology from research in the animal laboratories—has led to greater interest in fetal surgery. Prenatal diagnosis and sonographic studies of fetuses have made it possible to understand the development of these defects and their clinical outcomes. It has also made it possible to begin to develop medical and surgical care that is specific to some of these defects.

Prenatal diagnosis of a congenital defect benefits the infant and the parents. Prenatal diagnosis can change prenatal treatment, the delivery date, and the delivery method. Parents can prepare themselves psychologically and begin to seek appropriate future care for their unborn child. When possible, many mothers of fetuses who have a life-threatening anomaly choose to deliver near a pediatric hospital where immediate care is available.

Fetal surgery has the potential, in years to come, of becoming a preventive medium in obstetrical practice (Levine, 1991). Early intervention through fetal surgery may alter the outcome of the anomaly for the newborn.

Perioperative nursing considerations

Very few centers are experienced in fetal surgery. It requires specially designed equipment and monitors for the fetus. It also involves anesthesia for the mother. The only medical centers that should be involved in fetal surgery are those whose professionals have studied the pathophysiology of the fetus in animal laboratories and have implemented that knowledge to develop a fetal surgery program.

Many factors must be examined if fetal surgery might be an option. The natural outcome of the anomaly must be evaluated, to determine if additional or irreversible damage will occur if the repair is delayed until after the fetus is born. The risk to the mother must also be identified, along with her reproductive future. In fetal surgery, the mother's safety is also a major consideration. Postoperatively, premature labor is a major concern.

Fetal surgery should be considered only (1) if the natural history of the condition inevitably leads to a severe handicap or to death, (2) the result can be altered by surgical intervention, and (3) the risk to the mother is small. Three fetal conditions are identified that meet these criteria: hydronephrosis, hydrocephalus, and congenital diaphragmatic hernia (Evans, Drugan, Manning, & Harrison, 1989; Harrison & Adzick, 1991). Only future research will determine the success of the interventions.

Patient outcome

A successful fetal surgery program requires cooperative and collaborative practice. A committed multidisciplinary team approach is required. This team includes, but is not limited to, an obstetrician, a skilled fetal sonographer, a skilled pediatric surgeon, a neonatologist, a perinatologist for high-risk obstetrics, skilled perioperative nurses, a review board, and ethicists.

SUMMARY

The perioperative nurse who cares for the pediatric patient has a special challenge as care is planned and provided. The nurse must not only understand the surgical procedure to be performed, and the associated equipment, supplies, and instrumentation used for each procedure, but must also understand growth and development and anatomical and physiological differences seen in infants and children. Temperature regulation, fluid and electrolyte balance, skin integrity, infection prevention, and prevention of injury due to positioning are areas for nursing intervention for all patients, but are more critical in pediatric patients because of their size. Appropriate interventions have been described.

This chapter has identified developmental stages of infants and children, anatomical and physiological differences, and family involvement with the care. Although many of the surgical procedures described are not performed in all facilities, the principles related to the care are appropriate to all pediatric patients in any setting.

REFERENCES

Aimo, P. A. (1987). Perioperative nursing documentation: Integrating nursing on the patient record. *AORN Journal, 46*, 73, 76–81, 84–86.

Anagnostapoulas, D., & Pellerin, D. (1986). The cradle of pediatric surgery. *Progress in Pediatric Surgery, 20*, 35–38.

Anard, K. J., & Hickey, P. R. (1987). Pain and its effect in the human neonate and fetus. *New England Journal of Medicine, 317*, 1321–1329.

Anderson, K. D. (1986). Diaphragmatic hernia. In K. J. Welch, J. G. Randolph, M. M. Ravitch, J. A. O'Neil, & M. I. Rowe (Eds.). *Pediatric surgery* (4th ed.). Chicago: Mosby–Year Book.

Atkinson, L., & Kohn, M. (1986). *Berry and Kohn's introduction to operating room technique* (6th ed.). New York: McGraw-Hill.

Bartlett, R., & Anderson, H. L. (1990). Extracorporeal life support in pediatric trauma. In A. G. Coran & B. H. Harris (Eds.). *Pediatric trauma: Proceedings of the third conference.* Philadelphia: J. B. Lippincott.

Bates, T. A., & Broome, M. (1986). Preparation of children for hospitalization and surgery: A review of the literature. *Journal of Pediatric Nursing, 1*(4), 230–239.

Behrman, R. E., & Vaughan, V. C. (1987). *Nelson textbook of pediatrics* (13th ed.). Philadelphia: W. B. Saunders.

Benson, C. D. (1986). Pyloric stenosis. In K. Welch, J. Randolph, M. Ravitch, J. O'Neil, & M. Rowe (Eds.). *Pediatric surgery* (4th ed.). Chicago: Mosby–Year Book.

Bill, H. (1986). William Ladd: Great pioneer of North American pediatric surgery. *Progress in Pediatric Surgery, 20*, 52.

Bruce, J., Huh, Y., Cooney, D. R., Karp, M. R., Allen, J. E., & Jewett, T. C. Jr. (1987). Intussusception: Evolution of current management. *Journal of Pediatric Gastroenterology and Nutrition, 6*, 663–674.

Burstein, S., & Meichenbaum, D. (1979). The work of worrying in children undergoing surgery. *Journal of Abnormal Child Psychology, 7*(2), 121–132.

Camp-Sarrell, D. (1990). Advanced central venous access. Selection catheters, devices, and nursing management. *Journal of Intravenous Nursing, 13*, 361–370.

Caracassone, B. M., Guys, J. M., Morrison-Lacombe, G., & Kreitman, B. (1989). Management of Hirschsprung's disease: Curative surgery before three months of age. *Journal of Pediatric Surgery, 24*, 1032–1034.

Carey, B. E. (1989). Major complications of central lines in neonates. *Neonates Network, 7*, 17–28.

Casey, W., Rice, L., Hannallah, R., Broadman, L., Norden, J., & Guzzetta, P. (1990). A comparison between bupivacaine: Instillation versus ilioinguinal/iliohypogastric nerve block for postoperative analgesics following inguinal herniorrhaphy in children. *Anesthesiology, 72*, 637–639.

Clotworthy, H. (1986). Robert E. Gross. *Progress in Pediatric Surgery, 20*, 76–84.

Cluroe, S. (1989). Congenital oesophageal abnormalities. *Nursing (London), 3*, 20–23.

Crombleholme, T. M., Adzick, N. S., Hardy, K., Longaker, M. T., Bradley, S. M., Duncan, B. W., Verrier, E. D., & Harrison, M. R. (1990). Pulmonary lobar transplantation in neonatal swine: A model for treatment of congenital diaphragmatic hernia. *Journal of Pediatric Surgery, 25*, 11–18.

D'Angio, G. I., Breslow, N., Beckwith, J. B., Evans, A., Baum, E., deLorimer, A., Fernbach, D., Hraborsky, E., Jones, B., Kelalis, P., Othersen, H. B., Tefft, M., & Thomas, R. M. (1989). Treatment of Wilms' tumor. Results of the third national Wilms' tumor study. *Cancer, 64*, 349–360.

D'Antonio, I. J. (1984). Therapeutic use of play in hospitals. *Nursing Clinics of North America, 19*, 351–358.

Dykes, E. H., Marwaha, R. K., Dicks-Mireaux, C., Sans, V., Risdon, R. A., Duffy, P. G., Ransley, P. G., & Pritchard, J. (1990). Risks and benefits of percutaneous biopsy and primary chemotherapy in advanced Wilms' disease. *Journal of Pediatric Surgery, 26*, 610–612.

Elrempreis, T. (1986). 100 years of pediatric surgery in Stockholm. *Progress in Pediatric Surgery, 20*, 17–33.

Evans, A. E., D'Angio, G. J., & Randolph, J. G. (1971). A proposed staging for children's with neuroblastoma. *Cancer, 27*, 374.

Evans, M. I., Drugan, A., Manning, F., & Harrison, M. (1989). Fetal surgery in the 1990s. *American Journal of Diseases of Children, 143*, 1431–1436.

Faust, J., & Melamed, B. (1984). Influence of arousal, previous experience, and age on surgery preparation of same day of surgery and in-hospital pediatric patients. *Journal of Clinical and Clinical Psychology, 52*, 359–365.

Firkins, V. L., & Jay, S. (1989). The neonate in surgery, perioperative nursing care. *AORN Journal, 50*, 1193–1210.

Foster, P., Cowan, G., & Wrenn, E. L. (1990). Twenty-five years, experience with Hirschsprung's disease. *Journal of Pediatric Surgery, 25*, 531–534.

Gerraughty, A. B., & Younie, L. J. (May 1987). ECMO, the artificial lung for gravely ill newborns. *American Journal of Nursing, 87*(5), 655–656, 658–659.

Gillis, A. (1990). Hospital preparation: The Children's Hospital Story. *Children's Health Care, 19*, 19–27.

Goldbloom, R. B. (1986). Halifax and the precipitate birth of pediatric surgery. *Pediatrics, 77*, 764.

Gregory, G. A. (1989). *Pediatric anesthesia*, New York: Churchill Livingstone.

Grosfeld, J. L. (1991). Inguinal hernia repair in the premature neonate. In J. Grosfeld (Ed.). *Common problems in pediatric surgery*. St. Louis: Mosby–Year Book.

Grosfeld, J. L., Fitzgerald, J. F., Predaina, R., West, K. W., Vane, D. W., & Rescorla, F. J. (1989). The efficiency of hepatoportoenterostomy in biliary atersia. *Surgery, 24*, 581–584.

Grosfeld, J. L., Minnick, K., Shedd, F., West, K. W., Rescorla, F. J., & Vane, D. W. (1991). Inguinal hernia in children: Factors affecting recurrence in 62 cases. *Journal of Pediatric Surgery, 26*, 283–287.

Guzzetta, P. C., Andersen, K. D., Altman, R. P., Newman, K. D., Eichelberger, M. R., & Randolph, J. (1989). Pediatriac Surgery. In S. Schwartz, G. T. Shires, & F. C. Spencer (Eds.). *Principles of surgery* (5th ed.). New York: McGraw-Hill.

Hadaway, L. C. (1989). Evaluation and use of advanced I.V. therapy. Part 1: Central venous access devices. *Journal of Intravenous Nursing, 12*, 73–82.

Halberg, F. E., Harrison, M. R., Salvatierra, O., Longaker, M. T., Wara, W. M., & Phillips, T. L. (1991). Intraoperative radiation therapy for Wilms' tumor in site or ex vivo. *Cancer, 67*, 2839–2843.

Haller, J. A. (1987). Preceptors and stewardship. Our heritage of excellence in pediatric surgery. *Journal of Pediatric Surgery, 22*, 1067–1075.

Haller, J. A., & Beaver, B. L. (1990). Overviews of pediatric trauma. In R. Touloukian (Ed.). *Pediatric trauma*. St. Louis: Mosby–Year Book.

Hansen, B. D., & Evans, M. L. (1981). Preparing a child. *Maternal-Child Health Nursing, 6*, 392–397.

Harris, J. S. (1957). Annals of the New York Academy of Science, *66*, 966.

Harrison, M., & Adzick, S. (1991). The fetus as a patient. Surgical considerations. *Annals of Surgery, 213*, 279–291.

Haskins, R. (1990). Perioperative teaching of parents: A unit-based study. *AORN Journal, 47*, 568, 588, 590.

Heiser, M. S., & Downes, J. J. (1980). Temperature regulation in the pediatric patient. *Seminars in Anesthesiology, 2*, 37.

Hershberger, A. K. (1981). Growth and development of the family with an infant: Maintaining wellness. In J. J. Tackett & M. Hunsberger (Eds.). *Family-centered care of children and adolescents.* Philadelphia: W. B. Saunders.

Holder, T. M., & Aschcroft, K. W. (1980). *Pediatric surgery.* Philadelphia: W. B. Saunders.

Holtzman, R. S. (1991). Pediatric anesthesia: Practical differences from adults. Unpublished manuscript.

Hopkins, S., & Cowell, R. (1991). Making sense of neonatal ECMO. *Nursing Times, 87,* 36–37.

Hung, W. (1991). Treatment of Hirschsprung's disease. *Journal of Pediatric Surgery, 26,* 849–852.

Joseph, V. T., & Sim, C. K. (1988). Problems and pitfalls in the management of Hirschsprung's disease. *Journal of Pediatric Surgery, 23,* 398–402.

Kaplan, H. I., & Sadock, B. J. (1988). *Synopsis of psychiatry: Behavioral sciences, clinical psychiatry* (5th ed.). Baltimore: Williams & Wilkins.

Kasai, M., Mochizuki, J., Ahkohcki, N., & Chiba, R. O. (1989). Surgical limitation for biliary atresia: Indications for liver transplantation. *Journal of Pediatric Surgery, 24,* 851–854.

Kleinfeldt, A. S. (1990). Preoperative phone calls: Reducing cancellations in pediatric day surgery. *AORN Journal, 51,* 1559–1561, 1563–1564.

Korsh, B. M. (1975). The child and the operating room. *Anesthesiology, 43,* 25.

Kosloske, A., & Stone, H. H. (1986). Surgical infections. In K. J. Welch, J. G. Randolph, M. M. Ravitch, J. A. O'Neil, & M. I. Rowe (Eds.). *Pediatric surgery.* Chicago: Mosby–Year Book.

Levine, A. (1991). Fetal surgery. *AORN Journal, 54,* 16–19, 22–27, 30–32.

Lilly, J. R. (1986). Biliary atresia. In K. J. Welch, J. G. Randolph, M. M. Ravitch, J. A. O'Neil, & M. I. Rowe (Eds.). *Pediatric surgery* (4th ed.). Chicago: Mosby–Year Book.

Lilly, J. R., Karrer, F. M., Hall, R. J., Stellin, G. P., Vasquez-Estevez, J. J., Greenholz, S. K., Waken, E. A., & Schroter, G. P. J. (1989). The surgery for biliary atresia. *Annals of Surgery, 210,* 289–294.

Lord, D. (1989, Summer). *National Association for the Welfare of Children in Hospitals,* Update No. 27, Guernsey Evening Press. Bethesda, MD: Association for the care of Children's Health.

McDermott, B. K., & Curley, M. A. (1990). Extracorporeal membrane oxygenation: Current use and future directions. *AACN Clinical Issues in Critical Care Nursing, 1,* 348–364.

Meeker, M. H., & Rothrock, J. C. (1991). *Alexander's care of the patient in surgery* (9th ed.). St. Louis: C. V. Mosby.

Melamed, B., Dearborn, M., & Hermecz, D. (1983). Necessary changes for surgery preparation: Age and previous experience. *Psychomatic Medicine, 45,* 517–525.

Melamed, B. G., Meyer, R., Gee, G., & Soule, L. (1976). The influence of time and type of preparation on children's adjustment to hospitalization. *Journal of Pediatric Psychology, 1,* 31–37.

Melamed, B., & Siegal, L. (1975). Reduction of anxiety in children facing hospitalization and surgery by use of filmed modeling. *Journal of Consulting and Clinical Psychology, 43,* 511–521.

Meng, A., & Zastouney, T. (1982). Preparation for hospitalization. A stress inoculation training program for parents and children. *Maternal-Child Health Nursing, 11,* 87–94.

Mitiguy, J. S. (1986). A surgical liaison program: Making the wait more bearable. *Maternal-Child Health Nursing, 11,* 388–392.

Moss, R. L., & Hatch, E. I. (1991). Inguinal hernia repair in early infancy. *The American Journal of Surgery, 161,* 596–599.

Mott, S. R., James, S. R., & Sperhac, A. M. (1990). *Nursing care of children and families* (2nd ed.). Redwood City, CA: Addison-Wesley Nursing.

Moulton, S. L., Lynch, F. P., Cornish, J. D., Bejar, R. F., Simko, A. J., & Krous, H. F. (1991). Carotid artery reconstruction following neonate extracorporeal membrane oxygenation. *Pediatric Surgery 26*(7).

Ogilvie, L. (1990). Hospitalization of children for surgery: The parents' view. *Children's Health Care, 19,* 49–56.

Ohi, B. R., Tseng, S., Kamiyama, T., & Chiba, T. (1990). Two point rectal mucosal biopsy for selection of Hirschsprung's disease. *Journal of Pediatric Surgery, 25,* 527–530.

O'Rourke, P. P. (1991). ECMO: Where have we been? Where are we going? *Respiratory Care, 36,* 683–694.

Piaget, J. (1952). *The origins of intelligence in children.* New York: International Universities.

Poenaru, D., Laberge, J., Neilson, I. R., Nguyen, L. T., & Guttman, F. M. (1991). A more than 25-year experience with end-to-end versus end-to-side repair for esophageal atresia. *Journal of Pediatric Surgery, 26,* 472–477.

Randolph, J. (1985). The first of the best. *Journal of Pediatric Surgery, 20,* 580–591.

Randolph, J. G. (1986). Esophageal atresia. In K. Welch, J. Randolph, M. Ravitch, J. O'Neil, & M. Rowe (Eds.). *Pediatric surgery* (4th ed.). Chicago: Mosby–Year Book.

Randolph, J. G., Newman, K. D., & Anderson, K. D. (1989). Current results in repair of esophageal atresia with tracheoesophageal fistula using physiologic status as a guide to therapy. *Annals of Surgery, 209,* 526–531.

Ravitch, M. (1986). Intussusception. In K. Welch, J. Randolph, M. Ravitch, J. O'Neil, & M. Rowe (Eds.). *Pediatric surgery* (4th ed.). Chicago: Mosby–Year Book.

Reijnen, J. A., Festen, C., & van Roosmalen, R. P. (1990). Intussusception: Factors related to treatment. *Archives of Disease in Childhood, 65,* 871–873.

Rickham, P. (1986). Preface. *Progress in Pediatric Surgery, 20,* v–vi.

Roberts, J. P., & Gollow, J. J. (1990). Central venous catheters in surgical neonates. *Journal of Pediatric Surgery, 25,* 632–634.

Roberts, P. H., & Jones, M. B. (1990). Extracorporeal membrane oxygenation and indications for cardiopulmonary bypass in the neonate. *Journal of Obstetric, Gynecologic, and Neonatal Nursing, 19,* 391–400.

Rowe, M. I., & Lloyd, D. A. (1986). Bilateral inguinal hernia. In K. Welch, J. Randolph, M. Ravitch, J. O'Neil, & M. Rowe (Eds.). *Pediatric surgery* (4th ed.). Chicago: Mosby–Year Book.

Rushton, C. H. (1990). Balancing the benefits and burdens of ECMO. The nurse's role. *Critical Care Nursing Clinics of North America, 2,* 481–491.

Schuster, S. R. (1986). Omphalocele and gastroschisis. In K. Welch, J. Randolph, M. Ravitch, J. O'Neil, and M. I. Rowe (Eds.). *Pediatric surgery* (4th ed.). Chicago: Mosby–Year Book.

Schwartz, N., Eisenkraft, B., & Dolgin, S. (1988). Spinal anesthesia for the high-risk infant. *The Mount Sinai Journal of Medicine, 55,* 399–403.

Shaul, D. B., Schwartz, M. Z., Marr, C. C., & Tyson, K. (1989). Primary repair without routine gastrostomy is the treatment of choice of neonates with esophageal atresia and tracheoesophageal fistula. *Archives of Surgery, 124,* 1188–1190.

Shaw, N. (1990). Common surgical problems in the newborn. *Journal of Perinatal and Neonatal Nursing, 3,* 50–65.

Short, B., & Lotze, A. (1988). Extracorporal membrane oxygenation therapy. *Pediatric Annals, 17,* 516–518, 520, 522–523.

Sieber, W. K. (1986). Hirschsprung's disease. In K. Welch, J. Randolph, M. Ravitch, J. O'Neil, & M. I. Rowe. (Eds.). *Pediatric surgery* (4th Ed.). Chicago: Mosby–Year Book.

Smith, R. M. (1980). *Anesthesia for infants and children.* St. Louis: C. V. Mosby.

Smith, R. M., & Harris, J. S. (1957). Special pediatric problems in fluid and electrolyte therapy in surgery. *Annals of the New York Academy of Science, 66,* 966.

Stanfield, V. (1987). Perioperative documentation: Integrating nursing diagnosis on the patient record. *AORN Journal, 46,* 699–701, 703–704.

Stellar, J. J. (1991). Pediatric surgery. In M. Meeker & J. Rothrock (Eds.). *Alexander's care of the patient in surgery* (9th ed.). Chicago: Mosby–Year Book.

Stoelting, R. K., Dierdorf, S. F., & McCammon, R. L. (Eds.). (1988). *Anesthesia and co-existing disease* (2nd ed.). New York: Churchill Livingstone.

Stoney-Wilson, D., Mackinley, G. A., Prescott, S., & Hendry, G. M. (1988). Intussusception: A surgical condition. *Journal of the Royal College of Surgeons of Edinburgh, 33*, 270–273.

Stringer, M. D., & Brereton, P. J. (1990). Current management of infantile hypertrophic pyloric stenosis. *British Journal of Hospital Medicine, 43*, 266–272.

Theorell, C. J. (1990). Congenital diaphragmatic hernia: A physiologic approach to management. *Journal of Perinatal and Neonatal Nursing, 3*, 66–79.

Trento, A., Thompson, A., Siewers, R., Orr, R. A., Kochanek, P., Fuhrman, B., Frattalone, J., Beerman, L. B., Fischer, D. R., Griffith, B. P., & Hardesty, R. L. (1988). Extracorporeal membrane oxygenation in children. *Journal of Thoracic Surgery, 96*, 542–547.

Tuggle, D. W. (1991). Advances in Pediatric Surgical Critical Care. *Surgical Clinics of North America, 71*, 877–886.

Vacanti, J. P., Shamberger, R. C., Eraklis, A., & Lillehei, C. W. (1990). The therapy of biliary atresia combining the Kasai portoenterostomy with liver transplantation: A single experience. *Journal of Pediatric Surgery, 25*, 149–152.

Viall, C. (1990). Your complete guide to central venous catheters. *Nursing '90, 20*, 34–42.

Visintainer, M. A., & Wolfes, J. A. (1975). Psychological preparation for pediatric patients. The effect on children's and parents' stress response and adjustment. *Pediatrics, 56*, 187–199.

Waterson, D. J., Bonham-Carter, R. E., & Aberdeen, E. (1962). Oesophageal atresia, tracheoesphageal fistula—a study of survival in 218 infants. *Lancet, 1*, 819.

Whaley, L., & Wong, D. (1991). *Nursing care of infants and children* (4th ed.). St. Louis: Mosby Book Company.

Wood, R. P., Langnas, A. K., Stratta, R. J., Pillen, T. J., Williams, L., Lindsay, S., Meigerd, D., & Shaw, B. W. Jr. (1980). Optimal therapy for patients with biliary atresia portenterostomy ("Kasai" procedures) versus primary transplantation. *Journal of Pediatric Surgery, 25*, 153–160.

Workman, E., & Lentz, D. (1987). Extracorporeal membrane oxygenation. Its use in neonatal respiratory failure. *AORN Journal, 45*, 725–738.

Yaster, M., Scherer, T., Stone, M., Maxwell, L., Schleien, C., Wetzel, R., Buck, J., Nichols, D., Colombian, P., Dudgeon, D., & Haller, J. (1989). Prediction of successful primary closure of congenital abdominal wall defects using intraoperative measurements. *Journal of Pediatric Surgery, 24*, 1217–1220.

ADDITIONAL READINGS

Alfieris, G., Wing, C. W., & Hoy, G. P. (1987). Securing Broviac catheters in children. *Journal of Pediatric Surgery, 22*, 825–826.

Bartlett, B. H., & Anderson, H. L. (1990). Extracorporeal life support in pediatric trauma. In A. Coran & B. Harris (Eds.). *Pediatric trauma, proceedings of the third conference.* Philadelphia: J. B. Lippincott.

Brooks, B. F. (1984). *Controversies in pediatric surgery.* Austin: University of Texas.

Chang, J., Janik, J. S., Burrington, J. D., Clark, D. R., Campbell, D. N., & Pappas, G. (1988). Extensive tumor resection under deep hypothermia and circulatory arrest. *Journal of Pediatric Surgery, 23*, 254–258.

Cloud, D. (1987). Major ambulatory surgery of the pediatric patient. *Surgical Clinics of North America, 67*, 805–807.

deLorimier, A. A., Adzick, N. S., & Harrison, M. R. (1991). Amnion inversin in the treatment of giant omphalocele. *Journal of Pediatric Surgery, 26*, 804–807.

Dienno, M. E. (1987). Esophageal atresia. Corrective procedures and nursing care. *AORN Journal, 45*, 1356–1361, 1364–1367.

Donnellan, W., & Cobb, L. M. (1991). Intraabdominal pyloromyotomy. *Journal of Pediatric Surgery, 26*, 174–175.

Eichelberger, M., & Randolph, J. G. (1986). Abdominal trauma. In K. J. Welch, J. G. Randolph, M. M. Ravitch, J. A. O'Neil, & M. I. Rowe (Eds.). *Pediatric surgery* (4th ed.). Chicago: Mosby-Year Book.

Frenter, S. (1987). Abdominal wall defects: Omphalocele and gastroschisis. *Neonatal Network, 6*, 29–41.

Goh, D. W., & Brereton, R. J. (1991). Success and failure with neonatal tracheo-esophageal anomalies. *British Journal of Surgery, 78*, 834–837.

Golladay, E. S., Broadwater, J. R., & Mollitt, D. L. (1987). Pyloric stenosis—a timed perspective. *Archives of Surgery, 122*, 825–826.

Gregory, G. A. (1989). *Pediatric anesthesia.* New York: Churchill Livingstone.

Hatch, E., & Baxter, R. (1987). Surgical options in the management of large omphalocele. *The American Journal of Surgery, 153*, 449–452.

Hoffman, M. A., Pearl, R. H., Superina, R. A., Wesson, D. E., Ein, S. H., Shandling, B., & Filler, R. M. (1988). Central venous catheters—no x-rays needed: A prospective study in 50 consecutive infants and children. *Journal of Pediatric Surgery, 23*, 1201–1203.

Kenner, C., Harjo, J., & Brueggemeyer, A. (1988). *Neonatal surgery: A nursing perspective.* Orlando: Grune & Stratton.

Koo, A. S., Koyle, M. A., Hurwitz, R. S., Weese, D., Applebaum, H., Fonkalsrud, E. W., & Ehrlich, R. M. (19xx). The necessity of contralateral surgical exploration in Wilms tumor with modern noninvasive imaging technique: A reassessment. *The Journal of Urology, 144*, 416–417.

Lally, K. P., Hardin, W. D., Boettcher, M., Shah, S. I., & Mahous, G. H. (1987). Broviac catheter insertion: Operating room or neonatal intensive care unit. *Journal of Pediatric Surgery, 22*, 823–824.

Ohri, S. K., Sacker, J. M., & Singh, P. (1991). Modified Ramstedt's pyloromyotomy for the treatment of infantile hypertrophic pyloric stenosis. *Journal of the Royal College of Surgeons of Edinburgh, 36*, 94–96.

Reed, R., St. Cyr, J., Tornebenes, S., & Whitmore, G. (1990). Improved cannulation method for extracorporeal membrane oxygenation. *Annals of Thoracic Surgery, 50*, 670–671.

Shah, A. (1991). Colotomy with minimum resection for advanced irreducible intussusception. *Journal of Pediatric Surgery, 26*, 42–43.

Soave, F. (1985). Endorectal pull-through: 20 years experience. *Journal of Pediatric Nursing, 15*, 93–100.

Tackett, J., & Hunsberger, M. (1981). *Family centered care of children and adolescents. Nursing concepts in children and adolescents.* Philadelphia: W. B. Saunders.

White, C., Richardson, C., & Raibstein, L. (1990). High-frequency ventilation and extracorporeal membrane oxygenation. *AACN Clinical Issues in Critical Care Nursing, 1*, 427–424.

Chapter 19

Trauma Surgery

Key Concepts

- The perioperative nurse provides an important link in the cycle of trauma care by caring for patients and their families during the operative phase.

- Trauma can be defined as injury to the body resulting from either an acute exposure to energy or a lack of essential agents, such as oxygen or heat.

- Trauma is a surgical disease. A key component in any system that provides definitive care to trauma patients is a surgical suite within a designated trauma center that is adequately staffed, appropriately equipped, and in a state of readiness.

- The impact of trauma on society is tremendous. It accounts for the majority of deaths in the first 40 years of life and results in direct and indirect costs totaling $158 billion to $180 billion per year.

- An understanding of the mechanics of injury provides an important clue in anticipating possible surgical interventions, particularly when preoperative information is limited.

- As in all other areas of professional nursing practice, the perioperative nurse utilizes the nursing process of assessment, planning, implementation, and evaluation as a deliberate, problem-solving approach to the care of the trauma patient.

- Caring for the family of the trauma patient can be accomplished by providing them with information at any point in the perioperative phase, by initiating contact with other resources (psychiatric nurse clinicians, social services, clergy members), and by providing solace after the death of the patient in the operating room.

- The trauma center is a regional resource facility and has an obligation to provide public education and awareness programs. As an integral part of the system, the perioperative nurse can be involved by participating in these programs through lectures, demonstrations, and facility tours.

INTRODUCTION

Patients who have severe or extensive injuries place unique demands on perioperative nurses. Nurses who care for trauma patients in the operating room must be highly competent in a wide range of surgical specialties, anticipate surgical procedures based on the mechanism of injury, work quickly under stressful conditions, and be flexible in rapidly changing situations. Trauma patients often arrive unexpectedly and rarely at a convenient time for a system used to handling scheduled, elective surgery. Adequate knowledge, experience, and preparation on the part of the nurse can make a crucial difference when time is of the essence.

This chapter discusses the types and mechanisms of trauma and care of the trauma patient in the operating room, using the nursing process approach.

DEFINITION OF TRAUMA

Trauma can be defined as injury to the body resulting from acute exposure to some form of energy or to a lack of essential agents such as oxygen and heat (Sheehy, 1989). Though the elasticity of tissue helps it absorb energy, injury results when this capability is overwhelmed. The insult may be limited to a single organ or system, as in a hip fracture, or it may involve multiple systems, as in a motor vehicle accident where head, chest, abdominal, and skeletal injuries all can result.

Unlike progressive disease, trauma is an acute event. Within seconds, a trauma patient's condition can shift from relative equilibrium to severe physiological stress. The degree of stress depends on such factors as the severity of the injury itself, the effectiveness of resuscitative attempts, age, and preexisting pathophysiology (Richardson & Rodriguez, 1987). Young children, older adults, and patients with a preexisting disease may succumb to stress sooner and are at higher risk for developing complications. On the other hand, the bodies of healthy older children and young adults can compensate longer, making detection of subtle injuries more difficult.

In addition to physiological stress, trauma patients and their families are placed under enormous psychological stress. The unexpectedness of traumatic injury leaves no time for the planning or preparation routinely afforded by elective surgery. Patients have little opportunity to comprehend fully the information about their condition, and the loss of control and confusion can be terrifying.

SOCIAL IMPACT OF TRAUMA

As a disease entity, trauma has a tremendous impact on society. Although it is largely preventable, trauma accounts for the majority of deaths in the first 40 years of life in the United States. Trauma-related deaths exceed 140,000 annually (Rice & McKenzie, 1989). Approximately 57 million people—one in four U.S. residents—sustain injuries each year. Of those, 54 million seek medical care for trauma-related injuries and 2.3 million require hospitalization. The economic effects of trauma morbidity and mortality are no less staggering, resulting in direct and indirect costs of $158 billion to $180 billion per year.

TRAUMA CARE DELIVERY SYSTEMS AND THE OPERATING SUITE

Deaths resulting from trauma exhibit trimodal distribution (Trunkey, 1982). In one group death happens within seconds of injury, usually as a result of major cerebral or vascular injury. Though some patients in this category may be saved if a rapid emergency transport system is available, only education and legislation on such issues as seatbelts, driving drunk, and firearms will have a major impact. The second group die within minutes to hours after injury—from intracranial hematomas or major hemorrhage from thoracic, abdominal, or skeletal trauma. Health care professionals refer to the "golden hour," the relatively brief window of opportunity from initial injury to definitive treatment in a trauma center. Rapid intervention and resuscitation, with an emphasis on control of blood loss, will reduce fatalities in this category. For the third group, deaths occurs several days to weeks after the initial injury and often result from sepsis or multisystem failure.

The aim of a trauma care delivery system is to increase the survivability and reduce the morbidity of all trauma victims. Such systems can be set up at the local, county, or state level. Well-planned and coordinated trauma care–delivery systems include prehospital stabilization and transport, communication networks, public educational programs, and designated hospital trauma centers. The American College of Surgeons Committee on Trauma (1990) and the Trauma Nursing Coalition (1992) have identified recommended guidelines for trauma care–delivery systems. These guidelines cover facilities, equipment, and personnel resources.

A key component of any system that provides definitive care to trauma patients is a dedicated surgical suite in a designated trauma center that is adequately staffed, appropriately equipped, and in a state of constant readiness. It is not always possible, however, to make such a unit available, owing to financial or staffing constraints. Traditionally, patients are resuscitated in the emergency department and then go to the operating room for surgical intervention. Patients who meet certain criteria, such as those whose hemorrhage or shock is attributable to a surgically correctable injury, may benefit from bypassing the emergency department to be admitted directly to the operating room (Rhodes & Brader, 1989). Some centers that see a significant number of such patients have a dedicated "resuscitation operating room" or a specialized trauma resuscitation area. Physicians and emergency department and operating room nurses staff the area and provide service in a multidisciplinary team approach (O'Connell, 1992).

Care of the trauma patient can be conceptualized as a cyclical process that begins with the traumatic event and continues through the resuscitation, operation, critical care, intermediate care, and rehabilitative phases (Veise-Berry, 1988). Throughout the trauma cycle the task of nurses is to identify and manage the human response to injury. In addition to their preexisting physiological state, each patient's response to injury is influenced by a variety of developmental, social, economic, and environmental factors. By focusing on the uniqueness of every person, a "generic" and haphazard approach to care is avoided. As responsibility for care of the patient flows from the emergency department, to the operating room, critical care units, and other areas, nurses ensure continuity of care, serving as patient advocates, ensuring that the needs of each patient, as an individual, are met (Trauma Nursing Coalition, 1992).

EXPERIENCE AND EDUCATION

The unique challenges of caring for the trauma patient population require a level of commitment above and beyond that routinely faced in the operating room. The emergent nature of such cases demands rapid and competent responses from all members of the surgical team. Experience and education (both initial and continuing) help ensure that expert care is provided.

Nurses who care for critically ill patients in the operating room should have considerable experience in general perioperative nursing. Rotation onto shifts that see a large number of trauma patients and taking of emergency calls should, ideally, be delayed until nurses with relatively little experience develop the necessary level of competence. In larger operating suites nurses often practice "by surgical specialty," but those who practice in trauma-intensive institutions must be competent in emergent procedures of all specialties. The alternative is to have, either in house or on call, a team of perioperative nurses *whose specialty is trauma*, in all surgical specialties. Such nurses are also expert at managing the emergent resuscitative needs of injured patients in the operating room. Once the patient's condition is stabilized, other staff members assume care, and the trauma team are free to be available for the next emergency (Schramm, 1990).

Continuing education provides nurses opportunities to maintain proficiency by periodically reviewing important concepts and practicing critical skills. When establishing an educational program, it is important to know what types of patients are encountered most frequently. A database can be developed to track case statistics. For example, a suburban medical center located near a major highway may handle more survivors of motor vehicle accidents. An inner city trauma center may see more violent crime–related injuries such as knife and gunshot wounds. In the first case appropriate education programs would emphasize blunt trauma; in the second, penetrating trauma.

Skill labs afford the chance to refine necessary psychomotor dexterities in an environment where life is not in the balance (Schramm, 1990). Practicing assembly and use of supplies, instruments, and equipment on a regular basis renders critical skills more routine, so responses flow more smoothly when an actual trauma patient is at hand. Educational sessions should also provide participants information about the location and availability of supplies, instrumentation, and equipment.

MECHANISM OF INJURY

In trauma, the causative agent or the precipitating event and its effects on tissue are called the mechanism of injury. Traumatic injury results when body tissue is stressed beyond its capacity to absorb energy. The response of tissue to stress is determined by a number of factors, including the energy of the insult and the resiliency of the tissue (Weigelt & McCormack, 1988).

Understanding the mechanics of injury provides important clues to anticipating possible surgical interventions, particularly when preoperative information is limited. A classic example of this is Waddell's triad of injuries that results when a child pedestrian is struck by a motor vehicle (Halpern, 1982). The child sustains (1) femur or lower leg fractures from the car bumper, (2) blunt chest or abdominal injuries from the hood of the car, and (3) a closed head injury as he or she lands after being thrown by the force of the impact (Fig. 19-1). Upon being notified of the impending arrival of such a patient in the operating room, the nurse could anticipate exploration of the chest and abdomen for bleeding, intracranial bolt placement for intraoperative monitoring, and eventual reduction of fractures.

Although a full discussion of the mechanics of injury is beyond the scope of this chapter, it is helpful to think of traumatic injuries in two broad categories, penetrating and blunt. A brief description of each group follows with selected examples of the more common injuries and potential surgical interventions.

Penetrating Trauma

Penetrating trauma occurs when there is a break in the skin and outer soft tissue layers. Sharp objects such as bullets and knives are the usual causes. Injury occurs to tissue that lies directly in the path of the object. In stab wounds, for example, damage is limited to the underlying tissues. Penetrating trauma resulting from high-velocity missiles, such as gunshot injuries, may cause more widespread damage. Small entrance wounds may be deceptive, as massive tissue destruction can occur to any organ in the missile's tract. Cavitation along the tract occurs as the kinetic energy transferred from the missile literally pushes the tissue out of its way. In addition, the tract itself may be erratic, owing to "tumbling effects" of the bullet (Mendelson, 1991).

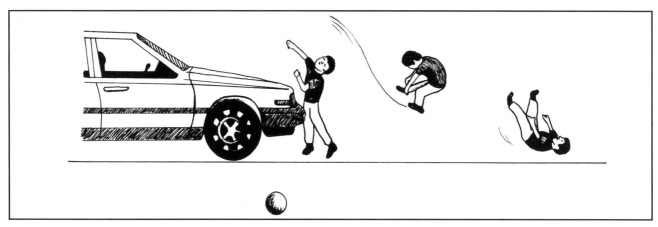

FIGURE 19-1 A triad of injuries often occurs when a child is struck by a motor vehicle: Leg fracture from bumper impact; blunt trauma to chest and/or abdomen from hood of vehicle; closed head injury from resulting fall.

Stab wounds to the abdomen may or may not require exploration. Careful wound inspection or laparoscopy may be performed to determine whether the peritoneum has been penetrated (Carnevale, Baron, & Delany, 1977). Patients who have obvious signs of shock or evisceration of omentum or bowel from the wound require exploratory laparotomy.

There should be a high index of suspicion of cardiac tamponade in patients with penetrating chest injuries. Patients who have cardiac arrest or quickly become hypotensive may require emergent thoracotomy. Otherwise, pericardiocentesis by the subxyphoid approach is often done (American College of Surgeons Committee on Trauma, 1989). Penetrating wounds to the chest can also result in hemopneumothorax on the affected side. An open thoracotomy may be necessary for patients with massive hemorrhage. Owing to movement of the diaphragm in respiration, wounds to the lower chest or upper abdomen can result in injuries to organs in either cavity.

Blunt Trauma

Blunt trauma occurs when energy applied over a large area is transferred to underlying structures without penetrating them. The mortality rate can be higher in blunt trauma, owing to the difficulty of diagnosing hidden injuries (Weigelt & McCormack, 1988). Deceleration injuries, direct blow, and shearing forces are common mechanisms of injury.

Closed head injuries are usually the result of falls, assault, or motor vehicle accident. Acute subdural hematoma has a high incidence of mortality and requires rapid evacuation. In the case of more diffuse brain injury in the presence of other injuries, an intracranial pressure-monitoring bolt may be placed for intraoperative and ongoing clinical management.

Blunt trauma to the chest is associated with such mechanisms as motor vehicle accidents and falls. Traumatic aortic rupture is the most common cause of death in

these patients (American College of Surgeons Committee on Trauma, 1989). Shearing of the aortic wall results from stretching of the ligamentum arteriosum following rapid deceleration. Generally, the diagnosis is made by arteriography. Patients who survive into the operating room undergo median sternotomy for direct repair or grafting of the aorta.

Blunt trauma to the abdomen most often involves the liver, spleen, or kidney. These solid viscera are prone to bursting and breakage from forced abdominal compression or organ motion. Deceleration injuries can cause stretching of vascular structures, with resulting tears. The surgeon may wish to evaluate intraabdominal injury through diagnostic peritoneal lavage (DPL). A peritoneal dialysis catheter is inserted into the peritoneal cavity through a small incision. Warmed saline or lactated Ringer's is instilled and then withdrawn and checked for blood. A positive result usually is an indication for abdominal exploration.

With experience, perioperative nurses can learn to utilize their knowledge of mechanisms of injury to predict possible surgical interventions. By anticipating these interventions, necessary equipment, supplies, and instrumentation can be prepared and the intraoperative course can proceed smoothly and uninterrupted.

CARE OF THE TRAUMA PATIENT IN THE OPERATING ROOM

The role of the perioperative trauma nurse is to provide optimal patient care by facilitating a seamless course throughout the preoperative, intraoperative, and postoperative phases. As in all other areas of professional nursing practice, the perioperative nurse utilizes the nursing process of assessment, planning, implementation, and evaluation as a deliberate, problem-solving approach to the care of the trauma patient (Bare, 1988).

Assessment

Care of the trauma patient in the operating room begins with obtaining as much information about the patient as possible. Report is taken from the nurse or paramedical person involved in the patient's immediate postinjury care. If the resuscitation takes place in the emergency department, and other staff are available to begin preparation in the operating room, a preoperative visit may be done simultaneously by the nurse and the anesthesia provider who will care for the patient in the operating room. This avoids unnecessary repetition. Particular attention is paid to mechanism of injury, hemodynamic stability, interventions already performed, and the patient's response to those interventions.

When time allows, rapid assessment is helpful in determining level of acuity and anticipating possible operative procedures. With practice, the nurse develops a systematic approach to assessment, so that it can be completed quickly. The goal is not to repeat the primary or secondary surveys that may already have been performed by the resuscitative team, but rather to glean information that may help the perioperative nurse manage the intraoperative course smoothly.

Before returning to the operating room, the nurse evaluating the patient should ascertain what blood products have been set up and where the family can be contacted postoperatively. When it is not practical for the nurse to leave the operating room, or when time is critical, as much of the information as possible can be obtained over the telephone from the emergency department nurse who is caring for the patient. Minimum information should include how the patient was injured, what surgical procedures are anticipated, the patient's hemodynamic stability, interventions performed in the emergency department, and whether the patient's family has been notified.

Planning

The planning stage begins once the nurse has obtained all available information. In concert with the surgeon and the anesthesia provider, priorities of care are determined with consideration for the most urgent injuries. When there are multiple injuries, the attending trauma surgeon determines the order in which the surgical interventions proceed, and the nurse organizes the operating room setup and preparation accordingly.

Implementation

Implementation of care starts by preparing the surgical environment. In the ideal setting, the trauma operating room should be set up to provide rapid resuscitation and surgical intervention. Airway management, fluid resuscitation, and hemodynamic monitoring equipment must be available for immediate use. Surgical supplies and instruments can be left wrapped and sterile but packaged so as to require minimal preparation once opened.

If no one operating room is dedicated for trauma patients, supplies and equipment can be kept on a trauma cart that can be present in, or brought to, any operating room. If the patient is to be resuscitated in the operating room, the cart should contain trays for intravenous access, chest tube insertion, diagnostic peritoneal lavage, and bladder catheterization. Specific instrumentation varies, depending on the patient's injuries, but patients with multiple injuries may require instruments for chest and abdominal exploration, as well as for vascular control. In addition, a tracheostomy tray should be available for patients who have airway problems.

Equipment should also be available to assist in the prevention and treatment of hypothermia and hypovolemia. Patients who have experienced prolonged exposure are at risk for hypothermia, which predisposes them to cardiac arrhythmias and prolonged bleeding time (Luna, 1987). The room temperature must be 75°F or higher. Other therapeutic measures include fluid warmers, warming blankets, convection heaters, use of warmed and humidified inspired gases, and warmed irrigation solutions (O'Connell, 1992).

Management of hypovolemia from blood loss is a major challenge in the treatment of trauma patients. Close communication with the blood bank is essential for patients who may have massive blood replacement requirements. In patients who have sustained blunt abdominal trauma, bleeding in the abdominal cavity may be temporarily controlled by tamponade. As the cavity is entered, bleeding resumes and the patient may exsanguinate quickly. Therefore blood products need to be in the room before the trauma surgeon enters the peritoneum. Rapid infusion devices that deliver at least 500 ml of blood per minute are commercially available. Devices that recover blood from the field for reinfusion (autotransfusion) should also be prepared and utilized when indicated.

Generic emergency carts should be available for electrocardiography, defibrillation, and drug administration. All supplies and equipment in the trauma operating room and in the trauma cart must be replaced at the end of each case and checked by a team member once every shift. This not only ensures that the equipment is in a constant state of readiness, it allows team members to be familiar with equipment contents and location.

Facilities that allow direct admission of the patient to the operating room should be designed to allow resuscitation to take place while the surgical equipment and instrumentation are being prepared. The instrument table is set up on one side of the room, away from the resuscitation area, to prevent contamination of the sterile field (Fig. 19-2). While the admitting team resuscitates the patient, the scrubbed person sets up equipment, maintains an accurate sponge count, and protects the integrity of the surgical field. The scrubbed person must be constantly aware of the patient's condition as resuscitative attempts continue, recognizing that if the patient suffers cardiac arrest, surgical intervention may proceed immediately (Butler & Campbell, 1988).

Initial life-support measures consist of airway management and ventilation and cervical spine immobilization. Large-bore intravenous access is established and blood samples sent for cross-matching and analysis. Obvious

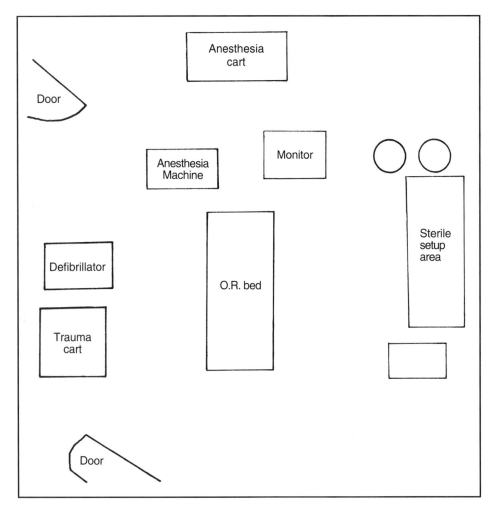

FIGURE 19-2   Trauma room setup.

sites of bleeding are controlled by manual compression or other methods. An overall assessment of the patient is conducted to identify injuries. Initial X-ray films are taken of the cervical spine, chest, and abdomen. Chest tubes may be placed in patients with thoracic injury. Once urologic trauma has been ruled out, the bladder is catheterized to monitor urine output. Patients with blunt trauma to the abdomen or penetrating trauma to the lower chest or abdomen are usually explored through a laparotomy approach. It is important for the perioperative nurse to realize that injuries may occur in both the abdominal and the thoracic cavities. In addition to supplies for the laparotomy, vascular and chest instrumentation (including a sternal saw and aortic clamps) must be readily available.

The surgical preparation of the patient with injuries to the chest and abdomen usually includes the area from at least the level of the suprasternal notch to midthigh (Mure & Brathwaite, 1991). This allows adequate exposure for left thoracotomy, median sternotomy, and vascular access in the groin for control of bleeding. A long midline incision from the xiphoid to below the umbilicus is used for a trauma laparotomy. If necessary the incision can be extended in multiple directions, providing exposure of the right and left diaphragm, the entire colon, and the genitourinary tract (Fig. 19-3).

As mentioned previously, large amounts of blood may be lost quickly when the peritoneum is entered. If the patient becomes hemodynamically unstable, aortic occlusion through a left thoracotomy may be necessary to control additional hemorrhage as well as provide adequate perfusion to the myocardium and cerebrum. With continued intraabdominal bleeding, the cavity is often packed with laparotomy pads to provide temporary hemostasis. Once bleeding is controlled and the patient is stable, surgical repair proceeds.

At the conclusion of the surgery the patient is transported to the receiving unit (postanesthesia or critical care) accompanied by the anesthesia provider, surgeon, and/or nurse. Report is given to the nurse who will be caring for the patient postoperatively. Included in the report is information obtained preoperatively, the surgical and nursing interventions performed intraoperatively, and the patient's course during surgery. Fluid volumes given, blood component transfusions, medications, estimated blood loss, and urine output are documented on the intraoperative record.

Evaluation

Evaluating the patient's responses to intervention should be a continuous process that is carried out by all members of the surgical team. As in elective surgery, a change in the patient's status noticed by one team member at any

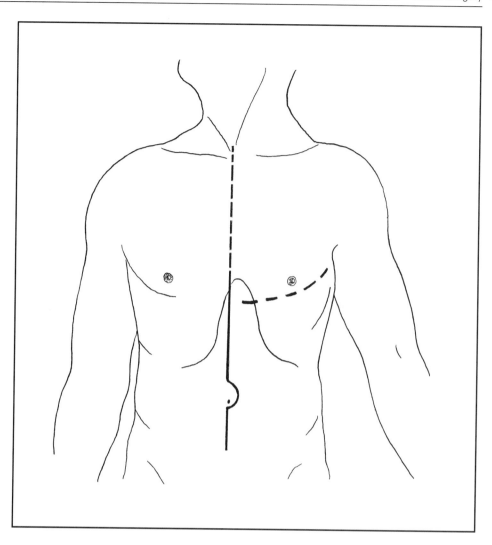

FIGURE 19-3 Trauma laparotomy incision with extensions to median sternotomy and lateral thoracotomy.

point during the process very often requires a response on the part of the other team members. In critically ill patients, changes are frequently more dramatic and require a faster response. Therefore, continuous communication between all members of the surgical team is essential.

In addition to providing immediate feedback on care during specific interventions, the evaluation process is utilized as an ongoing method of quality monitoring. Quality-monitoring programs are required for some reimbursement mechanisms and for Joint Commission on Accreditation of Healthcare Organizations accreditation. Most trauma centers are also required to maintain a trauma registry. The registry is a database that integrates medical, nursing, and trauma systems information. The data obtained through the trauma registry drive the periodic review, or surveillance system, so that an acceptable standard of care is attained (American College of Surgeons Committee on Trauma, 1990). Examples of data pertaining to the operating room to record in the trauma registry might include:

• Time elapsed between patient's arrival at the trauma center and arrival in the operating room

• Time elapsed from notification of anesthesia and nursing personnel to their arrival (if not inhouse)
• Adequate intraoperative documentation: Patient identification, level of consciousness on arrival, injuries sustained, preoperative medication and/or blood administered, traction in place, location of invasive lines, positioning

CARING FOR THE FAMILY OF THE TRAUMA PATIENT

Though the role of the perioperative trauma nurse most often involves the clinical care of the trauma patient, opportunities occasionally arise when the nurse interacts with the patient's family or significant others. Examples of such opportunities include:

• Witnessing consent from the parents of a child
• Providing information and support to the patient's family at any point in the perioperative phase
• Providing solace after the death of the patient in the operating room

Owing to the sudden and unexpected nature of traumatic injury, the course of events often contributes to a loss of control for the family. From the time the traumatic event first occurs until the patient is well stabilized in the critical care unit, family members are often relegated to the waiting room. Lack of information about the status of the patient increases feelings of helplessness.

The perioperative nurse frequently is the first contact for family members, especially if they arrive after the surgery begins. The receiving of information, even if it is limited to knowing the patient is in the operating room and receiving the best possible care, affords the waiting family some sense of control and may alleviate some of their anxiety (Clochesy, Breu, Cardin, Rudy, & Whittaker, 1993). It is often helpful to ask the family to designate one member as the contact person for communications. This is especially true with large or extended families, or when contact will be by telephone. Since family members do not always process information easily or correctly in a crisis situation, it is important for the perioperative nurse to present information in a slow and nontechnical manner. The nurse should recognize that family members placed in crisis often exhibit behaviors that are uncharacteristic of them (Solursh, 1990). Issues of guilt or anger may be operative, depending on the relationship of the patient to the family member before the injury.

Whether or not loss of life occurs, family members experience a sense of loss and separation. Early identification of the grief process and intervention by the nurse may help prevent the development of psychological pathology (Haber, Hoskins, Leach, & Sideleau, 1987). Specific interventions include empathetic listening and allowing expression of feelings. Other resources available to the family are social services, psychiatric nurse clinicians, and clergy. The nurse should take the responsibility of summoning and initiating contact with these support services when the family remains in crisis.

PUBLIC RELATIONS

Regional trauma centers have an obligation to develop public education and outreach programs. Emphasis should be placed on injury prevention and enhancing public awareness of the regional trauma system. The perioperative nurse can be an integral part of the system by participating in these programs through lectures, demonstrations, and facility tours.

Trauma centers also play a key role in local disasters that involve mass casualties. Although most medical centers have internal and external disaster plans, they may not always be coordinated with those of outside agencies and authorities. Ideally, the trauma center should be integrated with the dispatch office of the local emergency medical systems agency. Local or city mock disaster drills involving all aspects of the emergency medical system can help test the ability of the system to coordinate and deliver care under extreme circumstances. Performed on an annual basis, practice drills also provide an opportunity to enhance public safety awareness.

The operating room suite in the trauma center must develop disaster contingency plans that are in concert with the hospital's disaster plan. Included within the plan are command and control designations, strategies to free resources on short notice, and a mechanism for expanding personnel as needed.

Occasionally the trauma patient is a public figure, or the events surrounding the incident are sensationalistic enough to attract the news media. In the course of caring for the patient, the perioperative nurse may be contacted by reporters seeking information for a story. Most hospitals have guidelines that cover what information may be released and under what conditions, and who is authorized to do so. Protection of patient confidentiality is the overriding concern.

SUMMARY

The perioperative trauma nurse plays an important role in a system dedicated to the comprehensive care of critically injured patients. Trauma is sudden and unpredictable, and often it claims as its victims the most productive members of society. Utilizing the nursing process, the nurse draws on a specific body of knowledge that includes an understanding of trauma and its mechanisms of injury. When the patient's condition dictates direct admission to the operating room, the perioperative trauma nurse assists in the resuscitative efforts as part of a multidisciplinary team. The nurse also facilitates the organization of definitive surgical interventions by managing and coordinating the perioperative environment.

The focus of all nurses who care for trauma patients is managing the human response to injury while aiming for the final goal of restoration of health, or when necessary, the support of a dignified death. The perioperative trauma nurse provides an important link in the trauma cycle by supporting these patients and their families during the intraoperative phase of care.

REFERENCES

American College of Surgeons Committee on Trauma. (1989). *Advanced trauma life support student manual.* Chicago: Author.

American College of Surgeons Committee on Trauma. (1990). *Resources for optimal care of the injured patient.* Chicago: Author.

Bare, B. G. (1988). The nursing process. In L. S. Brunner & D. S. Suddarth (Eds.). *Textbook of medical-surgical nursing.* Philadelphia: J. B. Lippincott.

Beechley, M. (1988). Developing trauma care systems: The trauma nurse coordinator. *Journal of Nursing Administration, 18,* 7, 8, 34–42.

Butler, V., & Campbell, S. E. (1988). Resuscitation in the operating room. *Trauma Quarterly, 5,* 57–61.

Carnevale, M. D., Baron, N., & Delany, H. M. (1977). Peritoneoscopy as an aid in the diagnosis of abdominal trauma: A preliminary report. *Journal of Trauma, 17,* 634–638.

Clochesy, J. M., Breu, C., Cardin, S., Rudy, E. B., & Whittaker, A. A. (1993). *Critical Care Nursing.* Philadelphia, W. B. Saunders.

DeKeyser, F. G., Paratore, A., & Camp, L. (1993). Trauma nurse coordinator: Three unique roles. *Nursing Management, 24,* 56A–56H.

Haber, J., Hoskins, P. P., Leach, A. M., & Sideleau, B. F. (1987). *Comprehensive psychiatric nursing* (3rd ed.). New York: McGraw-Hill.

Halpern, J. S. (1982). Patterns of trauma. *Journal of Emergency Nursing, 8,* 170–175.

Luna, G. (1987). Incidence and effect of hypothermia in seriously injured patients. *Journal of Trauma, 27,* 1014–1018.

Mendelson, J. A. (1991). The relationship between mechanisms of wounding and principles of treatment of missile wounds. *Journal of Trauma, 31,* 1181–1202.

Mure, A. J., & Brathwaite, C. E. M. (1991). Errors and complications in abdominal trauma. *Trauma Quarterly, 8,* 49–75.

Norris, M. K. G. (1991). The clinical nurse specialist: Developing the case manager role. *Dimensions in Critical Care Nursing, 10,* 346–353.

O'Connell, W. D. (1992). The resuscitation OR: Priorities for the perioperative trauma nurse. *Today's O.R. Nurse, 14,* 9–12.

Rice, D. P., & McKenzie, E. J. (1989). *Cost of injury in the United States: A report to Congress.* San Francisco: Institute for Health and Aging, University of California and Injury Prevention Center, The John Hopkins University.

Richardson, J. D., & Rodriguez, J. L. (1987). The metabolic consequences of injury. In J. D. Richardson, H. C. Polk, and L. M. Flint (Eds.). *Trauma: Clinical care and pathophysiology.* Chicago: Year Book.

Rhodes, M., & Brader, A. (1989). Direct transport to the operating room for resuscitation of trauma patients. *Journal of Trauma, 29,* 907–915.

Schramm, C. A. (1990). Enhancing trauma skills. *AORN Journal, 52,* 847–850.

Sheehy, S. B. (1989). *Manual of clinical trauma care: The first hour.* St. Louis: C. V. Mosby

Solursh, D. C. (1990). The family of the trauma victim. *Nursing Clinics of North America, 25,* 155–162.

Trauma Nursing Coalition. (1992). *Resource document: Nursing care of the trauma patient.* Denver: Association of Operating Room Nurses.

Trunkey, D. D. (1982). The value of trauma centers. *Bulletin of the American College of Surgeons,* Chicago: American College of Surgeons, *67,* 20–23.

Veise-Berry, S. (1988). Evolution of the trauma cycle. In V. D. Cardona, P. D. Hurn, P. J. Bastnagel-Mason, A. M. Scanlon-Schilpp, and S. W. Veise-Berry (Eds.). *Trauma nursing: From resuscitation through rehabilitation.* Philadelphia: W. B. Saunders.

Weigelt, J. A., & McCormack, A. (1988). Mechanism of injury. In V. D. Cardona, P. D. Hurn, P. J. Bastnagel-Mason, A. M. Scanlon-Schilpp, and S. W. Veise-Berry (Eds.). *Trauma nursing: From resuscitation through rehabilitation.* Philadelphia: W. B. Saunders.

Chapter 20

Oncologic Surgery

Key Concepts

- Adjuvant therapy combines surgery for cancer with radiation, chemotherapy, and/or biotherapy to destroy cancer cells that have metastasized from the primary tumor site.
- Cancer surgery is performed for both diagnosis and treatment of the disease.
- Reconstruction and rehabilitation are new aspects of cancer surgery that can improve the quality of life for oncology patients.
- Caring for a cancer patient perioperatively requires careful planning, use of the nursing process, and the ability to adjust to rapidly changing situations.
- Tissue specimens obtained during cancer surgery must be meticulously labeled and handled according to the test required.

INTRODUCTION

Surgery is the oldest known treatment for cancer. Records from the Egyptian middle kingdom in 1600 B.C. describe surgical removal of tumors. The modern era of surgical treatment began in 1809, when Dr. Ephraim McDowell removed a 22-pound ovarian tumor from Jane Todd Crawford, who lived another 30 years. Subsequently, the introduction of general anesthesia and the principles of antisepsis enhanced the tolerance of the patient for treatment and the survival rate of patients undergoing surgical removal of tumors.

Surgical treatment of cancer is necessarily limited to tumor cells that can be visualized and resected. Unfortunately, by the time most cancers are diagnosed and are visible as tumors, micrometastasis has already occurred. For the patient to be cured, it is most common now to use surgery in combination with other treatment modalities. Such adjuvant therapies include radiation, chemotherapy, and biotherapy.

This chapter covers adjuvant therapy, purposes of cancer surgery, and the perioperative nursing that is an inherent part of the treatment modalities. The reader should refer to other chapters in Volumes 1 and 2 for general principles of perioperative nursing and surgical procedures that may be a part of oncologic surgery.

ADJUVANT THERAPY

Adjuvant therapy is treatment of cancer that combines radiation, chemotherapy, and/or biotherapy with surgery. The overall goal is to destroy metastatic cells along with the primary tumor.

Radiation

Radiation, ionizing and non-ionizing, is used for localized treatment of cancer lesions. Non-ionizing radiation produced by lasers is used to directly and immediately obliterate tumors. Laser radiation can be directed through an endoscope to destroy tumors within hollow organs such as the bronchus, the bladder, or the colon, without the necessity for surgical incision. Surface lesions on the skin, cervix, and vocal cords may be treated with laser radiation with little pain, bleeding, or scarring, often on an outpatient basis. Lasers are also used to remove tumors in the brain and to resect lung tumors. Rapid advances in laser technology and innovative surgeons have very quickly increased the applications for the treatment of cancer.

Laser light, used in combination with a light-sensitizing drug and oxygen, has a cytotoxic effect. This property is being used in a form of treatment called photodynamic therapy to treat superficial tumors growing on the surfaces of many different organs (Dachowski & DeLaney, 1992).

Ionizing radiation causes changes in the chromosome structure of cells that kill them immediately or render them unable to divide and reproduce. The effects of ionizing radiation are more pronounced on rapidly dividing cells and on poorly differentiated ones. This is why radiation can be used effectively on cancer cells. It does have an adverse effect on normal cells, but such cells have the ability to repair themselves more effectively than cancer cells can. The effect on normal cells accounts for the adverse side effects that result from radiation therapy. The susceptibility of rapidly dividing cells to the effects of radiation also explains why shielding the reproductive organs of the patient and the health care team is important when ionizing radiation is in use.

Ionizing radiation is delivered by several different methods: nonsealed systemic sources, external beam radiation (teletherapy), and placement of sealed and nonsealed internal sources (brachytherapy). Nonsealed systemic sources are radioactive isotopes that have affinity for certain types of cells. They may be injected intravenously or ingested orally. This treatment is often used for cancer of the thyroid gland. These sources render the patient and the patient's body secretions radioactive for a period of time. The short half-life of these isotopes allows them to be dissipated in a few weeks.

Teletherapy is delivered to a specific area of the body from a machine such as a cobalt-60 device or a linear accelerator. The treatment dose is delivered daily over a period of several weeks. This system of divided dosing is designed to deliver a maximum dose to the tumor while minimizing damage to overlying and adjacent normal tissues. Recently, more effective external beam radiation for abdominal tumors has been delivered by intraoperative radiation therapy, for which treatment the abdominal cavity is opened and the tumor exposed. The area around the tumor is shielded with pieces of lead foil. The patient is then moved to an area containing the radiation delivery machine, which may be located either in the operating room suite or in the radiation therapy department. A sterile cone is placed over the tumor and aligned with the radiation delivery device (Fig. 20-1). A maximum dose of radiation can then be delivered directly to the tumor with much less damage to surrounding tissues.

Brachytherapy involves the implantation of a radioactive source near the tumor area to deliver radiation over a period of time. A common example of brachytherapy is the use of afterloading tandem and ovoids to provide radiation for the treatment of cervical cancer (Fig. 20-2). These carriers are placed into the vagina and cervix while the patient is under general anesthesia. Proper placement is verified by radiography, and the devices are held in place with vaginal packing (Fig. 20-3). The actual radioactive source is placed into the carriers after the patient has been returned to her room.

Chemotherapy

Chemotherapy is a form of cancer treatment that is undergoing rapid advancement and new applications. Chemotherapeutic agents are cytotoxic drugs that work in a variety of ways on specific cell types during various phases of the cell life cycle. Some drugs are used to destroy only specific types of cancer cells. Study of tumor biology determines drug treatment plans that are based on specific drugs or drug combinations given over a rigidly pre-scribed time frame to achieve maximum effect. Chemotherapy almost never occurs concurrently with surgical treatment. If a patient undergoing chemotherapy does have surgery, it is very important for the members of the surgical team to strictly observe universal precautions, to avoid the cytotoxic effects from contact with these drugs that will be contained in the blood and body fluids of the patient.

Biotherapy

Biotherapy, the newest modality for the treatment of cancer, includes agents that have been derived from biological sources or that affect biological responses (Rieger, 1991). These agents are of three major types: those that enhance the host's defense against the tumor, those that are tumoricidal, and those that modify the biological behavior of the tumor (Mayer, 1989). Examples of biotherapeutic agents in use are interferon, interleukins, colony-stimulating factors, and monoclonal antibodies.

FIGURE 20-1 Placement of sterile cone in preparation for intraoperative radiation therapy. Linear accelerator is over the patient. (Courtesy of the University of Texas M.D. Anderson Cancer Center, Houston, TX.)

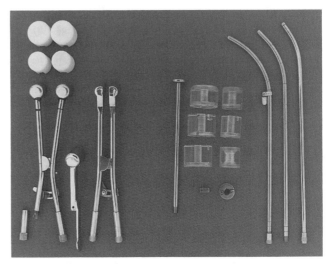

FIGURE 20-2 Afterloading devices for delivery of radiation to the uterus, cervix, and vagina. (Courtesy of the University of Texas M.D. Anderson Cancer Center, Houston, TX.)

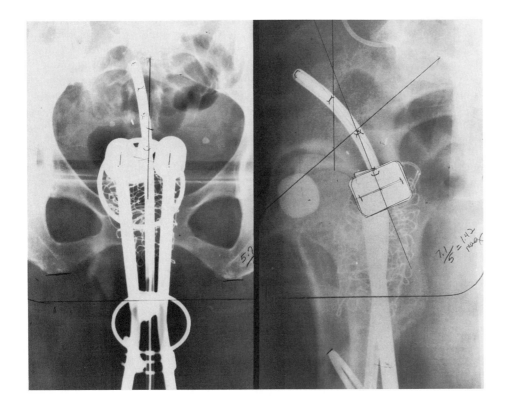

FIGURE 20-3 Radiographs verifying proper placement of tandem and ovoid devices. (Courtesy of the University of Texas M.D. Anderson Cancer Center, Houston, TX.)

DECISION FOR SURGICAL INTERVENTION

Surgical intervention for the treatment of cancer is a decision made after careful examination of all of the features of the case of the individual patient in question. The type and location of the tumor are some of the first considerations. If the tumor is inaccessible or is so invasive of surrounding tissues as to be nonresectable, surgery may not be an option. Surgical cure depends on the ability to remove all cancer cells. Since most malignant tumors are not encapsulated, this may prove to be difficult or impossible. If no adjuvant therapy is available to treat the remaining cancer cells, surgery may not be the treatment selected for that patient; however, patients with very large tumors usually respond most favorably to surgery because such tumors may have a necrotic center. Since the effects of radiation and chemotherapy depend on an adequate blood supply, they are not effective for necrotic tissue. If a tumor has already metastasized extensively, and the prognosis is poor, surgery may not be the best treatment. Some cancers, such as leukemias and lymphomas, are disseminated by nature and so cannot be treated by surgery.

When selecting surgery as a cancer treatment option, the health care team, the patient, and the patient's family must also consider the quality of life that would be achieved by the surgical intervention. Some people prefer to live out the remainder of their life intact rather than submit to radical procedures that cause major changes in body appearance or function. After providing all available information, the health care team must respect the desires of the patient in planning the treatment.

PURPOSES OF SURGERY

The role of surgery in diagnosis, staging, and planning for further treatment or palliation is explained in this section. Reconstruction, rehabilitation, and implantation of devices are also discussed.

Diagnosis

Cancer surgery is performed for a number of reasons. A surgical procedure may be the only way to obtain a positive diagnosis of cancer or to rule out cancer when a tumor is present. Surgery may be a way to diagnose and treat cancer at the same time. This is done by means of an excisional biopsy, which involves removing the entire tumor and examining it for disease. This may be all the treatment that is needed if the area around the tumor is free of cancer cells.

An incisional biopsy, the removal of a small portion of tissue for histologic examination, may be done when the tumor is large or very invasive and cannot be removed completely, or when definitive treatment involves extensive resection. If the physician suspects that the tumor is a melanoma, for example, definitive diagnosis is essential before wide excision of the tumor area is performed. The pathology report on the tissue obtained by this method determines the future course of treatment.

Aspiration biopsy, also used to obtain cytologic diagnosis, is performed by inserting a hollow needle into the tumor and aspirating material with a syringe. This technique is often used for breast tumors. Needle biopsy uses a needle designed to actually remove a core of tissue from a target organ like the prostate or the liver. These techniques are sometimes used with radiographic or ultrasonographic visualization to achieve precise localization and needle placement.

Tissue biopsy specimens are also obtained via endoscopy—by excising small pieces of tissue, scraping with a brush or sponge, or collecting washings of the area.

Staging

Surgery is sometimes used to stage disease. Staging determines the progression of the disease and helps to determine the future course of treatment. The term "staging procedure" is most often associated with Hodgkin's disease. A staging procedure includes splenectomy, liver biopsy, lymph node biopsy, and sometimes bone marrow biopsy. The surgeon also places clips to mark areas to be targeted in future radiation therapy. Another type of staging is the examination of lymph node chains to determine the progress of the disease and see whether or not it would be beneficial to perform a more radical procedure. For example, pelvic lymph node biopsies are performed before proceeding with radical cystectomy.

Second-Look Procedures

A second-look procedure is another type of staging procedure used in connection with ovarian cancer, which at the time of diagnosis is usually disseminated throughout the pelvic cavity. At the initial surgery, all visible tumor material larger than 2 cm is removed. Surgeons know that this is not a curative process; they are applying the concept of cytoreduction. The objective of cytoreduction is to reduce the number of cancer cells that remain in the body and will later have to be destroyed by chemotherapy. The second-look procedure is a laparotomy performed to determine the response to the chemotherapy by gross and microscopic examination of the pelvic cavity, including biopsies, washings of the pelvis, and Pap smears of the diaphragm.

Treatment of Cancer

Treatment of cancer is another purpose of surgical intervention. Excision of the primary tumor is the most frequent initial approach to curing the disease. Localized lesions such as basal cell carcinomas can be treated easily and effectively with surgery alone. Metastatic lesions can also be treated by surgical removal. It is well known that certain types of cancer tend to metastasize to certain organs: lung cancer to the brain, prostate cancer to the vertebrae, colon cancer to the liver, bone cancer to the lung.

These patterns of metastasis can be explained by circulatory patterns and by tumor biology. Isolated metastatic lesions can be treated easily and effectively by surgical excision.

Even when it is known from the outset that a large and invasive tumor cannot be completely excised, a debulking surgical procedure can reduce the burden of tumor cells remaining in the body. This gives the adjuvant therapy fewer tumor cells to attack, and thus increases the effectiveness of the treatment.

Bone Marrow Transplants

Certain types of cancer are now being treated by bone marrow transplants. Such treatment is most frequently used for leukemias and lymphomas, but sometimes also for other types of malignancies. The treatment involves destroying the bone marrow of the patient using very large doses of chemotherapy or radiation, and then transplanting marrow that has been harvested from the patient (autologous) or from a compatible donor (allogenic).

The perioperative nurse becomes involved in the procedure at the time of bone marrow harvest, which is performed with the patient under either general or spinal anesthesia. The usual site for aspiration of the bone marrow is the posterior iliac crests. The patient is positioned prone and is prepped from the middle back to the upper thighs. The bone marrow is aspirated by performing multiple punctures into the posterior iliac crests using special bone marrow needles (Fig. 20-4).

The marrow is drawn into syringes that are rinsed with saline and a heparin solution before being used. The marrow is then transferred into a blood collection bag that has also been prepared with a heparin solution. The bags are sent to the laboratory as soon as they are filled, so that a cell count can be obtained. The number of cells in the aspirate determines the volume of marrow that must be withdrawn. If an inadequate amount of cells is provided from the posterior iliac crests, it may be necessary to turn the patient supine to aspirate from the anterior iliac crests and the sternum.

Special activities required of the scrub person during the procedure are preparation of the collection bags and syringes and transferring the aspirate into the collection bags. The circulating nurse must ensure that blood has been cross-matched for the patient, as a volume of blood equal to the number of units of marrow withdrawn is always administered intraoperatively. The circulator must also be prepared to turn the patient if that becomes necessary. If a spare operating room bed is available, it is easiest to turn the patient onto that bed, remove the used bed, and then proceed to reprep and redrape the patient.

Prevention

Prevention of cancer is another reason that surgery may be performed. Certain conditions or diseases—and sometimes family history—predispose some persons to develop cancer. Surgery can be performed to eliminate that possi-

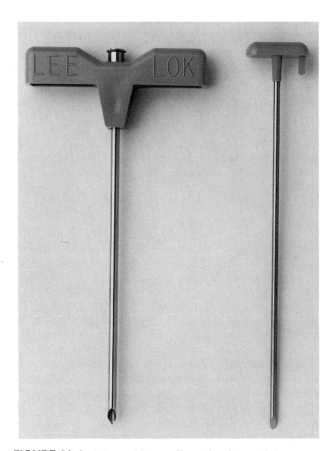

FIGURE 20-4 Disposable needle and stylet used for harvesting bone marrow. (Courtesy of Lee Medical, Ltd.)

bility. Because cryptorchidism can increase the possibility of testicular cancer, orchiopexy is performed. Persons who have multiple polyposis of the colon have a 50% chance of developing cancer by age 40 years and almost a 100% chance by 70 years. Such persons should have colectomy before age 20, to prevent the cancer (Rosenberg, 1989). Family history of breast or ovarian cancer may also be an indication for prophylactic removal of those organs.

Palliation

Normally, cancer surgery is performed with the objective of cure. To subject an individual to radical procedures that may have a profound effect on appearance or function cannot be justified unless there is a significant chance of eradicating the cancer. Palliative procedures do not help to cure the patient; they are performed to alleviate pain and to reestablish function when tumor bulk is causing obstruction. Pressure from tumors on nearby organs and nerves can be very painful. If the bulk of the tumor can be reduced, the patient's quality of life may improve.

Patients with inoperable bronchial tumors with impending airway obstruction may be relieved by laser ablation of the encroaching tumor using the flexible bronchoscope. Large masses in the neck that cause airway obstruction may require tracheostomy for palliation.

Obstructions of the gastrointestinal tract may be removed or bypassed to restore function. Patients who have received radiation to the abdomen or pelvis may have multiple adhesions in that area that can cause obstruction. Lysis of the adhesions, or in severe cases bypassing the area entirely with gastrostomy, jejunostomy, or colostomy, will facilitate nutrition and elimination. Pelvic radiation can also cause fistulae between bladder and vagina or bladder and rectum. An ileal conduit or colostomy can help the patient manage these problems.

Reconstruction and Rehabilitation

Reconstructive procedures are a fairly new aspect of oncologic surgery. In past decades it was thought that there was no point to performing reconstructive surgery on a cancer patient. Deficits in appearance and function were addressed by using external prostheses. In many instances this is still the case, but as surgeons become more skilled—and patients more aware of the options available to them—reconstructive cancer surgery is becoming a growing field. The available technology involved in microsurgery has allowed transfer of free flaps from one part of the body to another. Free myocutaneous flaps are often used in reconstructive procedures of the head and neck. Defects in this area can be devastating to the patient because they are so obvious. Many such patients hesitate to go out in public because of the manner in which these defects affect their appearance and their function. (Imagine not being able to close your mouth, to swallow your saliva, to close your eye. Imagine having no nose. Persons who have undergone extensive cancer surgery often have problems like these.) Even such a simple reconstructive procedure as creation of a tracheoesophageal fistula can make a great difference by enabling a postlaryngectomy patient to speak.

Women who undergo mastectomy for cancer can now be assured before that disfiguring procedure that reconstruction can be performed. Some women can even have reconstruction at the time of the mastectomy using surgical implants. If there is inadequate tissue to provide coverage for the implant, a tissue expander can be inserted at the time of mastectomy, and implant surgery performed when adequate tissue expansion has occurred. In addition to surgical implants, myocutaneous flaps from the latissimus dorsi and the rectus abdominis muscles can be used to create a new breast. The nipple-areola complex is formed later using skin grafts and tattooing. The psychological benefits that these procedures afford women with breast cancer are significant and help the patient accept the surgical treatment option more easily.

Previously, diagnosis of a primary bone tumor almost always meant amputation. Unfortunately, osteosarcomas most often affect young persons. Limb salvage techniques, using wide tumor resection and replacing bone with metal implants and frozen allogenic bone grafts, have proven successful and obviate amputation. Use of limb salvage rather than amputation in selected cases does not alter survival rates (Piasecki, 1990).

Emergency Procedures

Although cancer surgery is rarely performed on an emergency basis, certain conditions do require immediate intervention. Tumors that erode into blood vessels or through the walls of hollow organs require rapid repair. Obstruction in the urinary or respiratory tract calls for quick intervention. Spinal or brain tumors that cause rapid deterioration of neurological status are treated with emergency surgical intervention. Cancer patients with bone metastases sustain pathological fractures that require fixation.

Implantation of Devices

Many cancer patients who otherwise would not require surgery come to the operating room for implantation of devices that afford venous or arterial access to provide nutrition or long-term drug administration for pain control, antibiotics, or chemotherapy.

Central venous catheters are implanted for purposes of nutrition by hyperalimentation, drug therapy, or blood sampling. Central venous catheters are not usually implanted in the operating room, unless the patient requires anesthesia for the procedure.

Another form of vascular access, implantable vascular access devices, have metal ports with a Silastic injection area. They are implanted subcutaneously and are attached to a catheter that terminates in a blood vessel. The port is accessed percutaneously using a special, non-coring-type of needle to penetrate the Silastic membrane. Ports may also be implanted to give access to the central nervous system by placing the catheter in the epidural space and the port in the flank area. This allows administration of chemotherapeutic agents that do not cross the blood-brain barrier and can also be used for systemic pain control with intrathecal morphine.

Patients with tumors of the central nervous system can benefit from implantation of an Ommaya reservoir (Fig. 20-5), a small hollow dome made of Silastic that is connected to a short catheter. The reservoir is implanted under the scalp, and the catheter enters the lateral ventricle via a small burr hole in the skull. Drugs are injected into the reservoir percutaneously and are delivered to the ventricle by depressing the reservoir. Medications for chemotherapy and for pain control are administered by this method.

Implantable pumps such as the Infusaid are also used to provide continuous infusion of medications. Such pumps are entirely self-contained and are implanted into the body. The pump is attached to a catheter that terminates in a blood vessel. Drugs are injected into the pump percutaneously and are then delivered to the patient over a predetermined time. This type of device is sometimes implanted in the abdominal cavity with the catheter in the hepatic artery for treatment of liver cancer.

Patients who need to be fed by bypassing upper sections of the gastrointestinal tract come to the operating room for placement of a gastrostomy tube or a feeding jejunostomy.

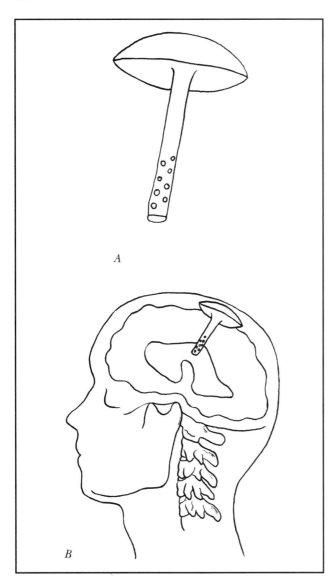

FIGURE 20-5 *A,* Ommaya reservoir. *B,* Ommaya reservoir in lateral ventricle.

Implantation of radiotherapeutic materials is also performed in the operating room. Insertion of tandem and ovoids was described previously. Iridium needles are used to treat cancer of the vulva and the breast. Numerous special hollow needles are placed into affected tissue. After proper placement has been verified by radiography, the radioactive sources are placed into the needles. Delayed placement of the radioactive material is done to protect the health care team from excessive exposure to the radiation. Endobronchial radiation is delivered by catheters containing radioactive material. These catheters are placed via bronchoscope in the operating room. Seeds or grains of radioactive gold or iodine may be placed in body cavities. Head and neck cancers are sometimes treated by using radium needles or wires. Safe handling of radioactive materials in the operating room is discussed later in this chapter.

UNIQUE ASPECTS

There are several unique aspects of cancer surgery that distinguish it from other types of surgery. Tumors are unpredictable in their size, location, and invasiveness of other organs. Despite the impressive tumor visualization provided by magnetic resonance imaging and computed tomography, the exact extent of a tumor is not always known without direct intraoperative observation. Routine operative techniques to deal with these tumors are not described in the textbooks. The surgeon must make numerous decisions as tissue dissection is performed in the area of the tumor. The perioperative nurse must be constantly alert to the anatomy in the area and to the changing conditions in the area of dissection. The tumor may involve organs and areas not previously expected. Obtaining a set of vascular instruments or chest instruments or having a tracheostomy tray nearby may be indicated. Bone instruments may be required to gain access to unanticipated areas. It may be necessary to change the position of the patient intraoperatively.

Surgical procedures are often complex and lengthy. Sometimes, planned procedures may not be performed because of the extent and unresectability of the tumor, tissue friability, or difficulty of access. A palliative or supportive procedure may be done that is different from the planned one.

The perioperative nurse caring for cancer patients must be attentive, knowledgeable, and flexible, and must be able to adapt to constantly changing situations. Because some procedures are very lengthy, a change in the nursing staff often occurs while the procedure is in progress. It is important to accomplish such a change as smoothly as possible, so as to not interrupt the care of the patient. Careful reporting about the condition of the patient, progress of the procedure, status of specimens sent, and the availability of blood and blood products is essential before the departing nurses can leave the patient.

Cancer surgeons generally make large incisions when exploring a body cavity. This affords easy access to the tumor, but also permits obligatory assessment of all the organs in that body cavity for evidence of spread of the cancer from the primary site. Tumors may be removed en bloc to include the affected organ as well as the surrounding lymph nodes.

Since it is impossible to grossly visualize a cancer cell, the surgeon may not be certain of the exact margins of the tumor. The margins must be assessed in terms of depth as well as width and length. Determinations of tumor margins are made in consultation with the surgical pathologist. The specimen is marked with a suture or a clip and identified in terms like *superior, inferior, lateral,* or *medial,* to describe its relation to other body structures. The pathologist then performs frozen section examinations on the edges of the tumor indicated by the surgeon, to determine if these margins are free of cancer cells. It is essential that these specimens be identified meticulously by the perioperative nurse, and that good communication with the pathologist be maintained. The nurse should notify the pathologist in advance that a series of specimens will be arriving for frozen section examination, so that the pathologist can be prepared. Sometimes small pieces of tissue from the margin areas are sent for serial examinations. There may be large numbers of these specimens, and they are often removed very rapidly. Accurate recording is essential for proper diagnosis. If the tissue is being removed so rapidly that the circulating nurse cannot keep up with the labeling, the scrub person can assist by labeling specimens not yet handed off the field using a glove wrapper and a skin marker. When dealing with the very tiny specimens, it is important that they not be allowed to dry out, and that they can be easily dropped into the specimen container. This can be accomplished by placing the tissue on small pieces of wet Telfa. The circulating nurse must also keep in the operating room a list of what specimens are sent, so that the results of the examinations can be recorded as they are reported back by the pathologist.

Many cancer procedures are done in two stages, the first diagnostic (breast biopsy, laryngoscopy with biopsy) and the second therapeutic (mastectomy, laryngectomy). In the past, when the second procedure was indicated, it was performed immediately, the rationale being that the patient would have only one hospitalization and one anesthesia and spread of cancer cells caused by disturbing the tumor would be avoided. Today, it is unusual to perform a radical procedure without first informing the patient about the definitive diagnosis and all available treatment options. Most often, the diagnostic procedure is performed on an outpatient basis, the treatment plan is agreed upon, and the patient returns for the extensive surgery better prepared for the surgical experience and the outcome.

NURSING CARE

The perioperative nursing care of the patient with cancer is unique in several ways. Many cancer patients are quite ill. Most will be categorized by the American Society of Anesthesiologists (ASA) as physical status Class III or IV. All will be, at minimum, ASA Class II, owing to the presence of the disease. Though these patients are quite ill, since most cancer surgery is not performed on an emergency basis, the patient can be prepared properly and the surgery delayed until the patient is in optimal condition.

Psychosocial Implications

For many people the psychosocial implications of the diagnosis of cancer and the need for surgery are devastating. The nurse must be sensitive to the psychosocial aspects of care, for the patient and for the family during the perioperative period. Although cancer is most common in older adults, it can occur at any age. The developmental stage of the patient determines how the nurse addresses the psychosocial aspects of care. When the patient is a child, the parents may require most of the support, though children exhibit surprising depth of understanding about their condition. There is still a certain stigma connected with the diagnosis of cancer, and the nurse must be aware of this while encouraging patients and their families to deal openly and honestly with the diagnosis and treatment plan.

Preoperative Assessment

The trend for as many patients as possible to be treated on an ambulatory or same-day admission basis necessarily limits the amount of time the nurse has to spend with the patient and family preoperatively. It is not realistic to expect that the nurse will be able to address all of the psychosocial aspects of cancer surgery with the patient and family during that time. This does not mean that psychosocial care can be ignored. The nurse must always be sensitive to the feelings of the patient.

Individuals facing surgery for cancer may go into the procedure very uncertain about the outcome. Perhaps the diagnosis or the extent of the tumor is to be established by the procedure, so the prognosis is unknown. The patient may be going into the operating room facing loss of function or an alteration in appearance that will cause a great change in lifestyle. Will the patient's role in the family change? A man who has been supporting his family may be facing loss of job and income. Who will take care of his family while they are taking care of him? Will there be a lot of pain postoperatively? What is the prognosis? Is death imminent? Will the patient be able to eat, eliminate waste, walk, talk, see? These stresses affect the patient and the family, and each displays a variety of coping mechanisms. The nurse can help by listening, touching when appropriate, reassuring, and providing information. Compassion, as demonstrated by modifying hospital routines to accommodate patients' needs, is appreciated. Patients who wear glasses, facial prosthetics, or hearing aids or use speech assistive devices should be permitted to retain these items until the last possible moment. Families of patients who are having cancer surgery often have to spend many hours in the waiting room. The nurse should see that they receive periodic progress reports during the procedure.

When performing the preoperative assessment of the cancer patient to plan care, in addition to the normal assessment standards the nurse should be alert for certain conditions and situations that are often present in cancer patients. Patients who have had cancer for a long time may be cachectic, with poor nutritional status and poor tissue condition. If they have been immobile, their range of motion may be diminished. There may be changes in function due to prior surgeries. The following points should be assessed:

1. Presence of concomitant diseases
2. Purpose of the surgery
3. Primary tumor or metastatic disease?
4. Nutritional status
5. Tissue condition
6. Presence of ostomies, prostheses, catheters, implants, or other devices

7. Use of speech, visual, or hearing devices
8. Dates of prior surgery, radiation, or chemotherapy
9. Date of last menstrual period
10. Name and relationship of primary support person

Results of this assessment will be used when formulating the expected outcomes, nursing diagnoses, and the intraoperative care plan for the patient.

Intraoperative Considerations

Intraoperatively, unique needs of oncology patients must be considered as the nurse plans, implements, and evaluates the nursing care provided.

Impaired host defense

Persons with cancer have impaired host defense mechanisms. Immunosuppression, part of the disease process, may be exacerbated by radiation or chemotherapy. Any surgery impairs host defenses just by virtue of the surgical wound and the effects of general anesthesia, but cancer patients are especially susceptible to infection. The nurse ensures the use of meticulous aseptic technique by all members of the health care team.

Tissue friability

Prior radiation of the surgical site causes adhesions and increased friability of the tissue, which can result in increased bleeding and can much prolong the surgical procedure with tedious dissection of the tissue. The nurse must be prepared to offer additional instrumentation and hemostatic agents when tissue of this type is encountered.

Changing situations

Tumors may invade or surround major blood vessels or nerves. Again, meticulous dissection may be involved, and additional instrumentation may be required. As the anatomical structures are exposed, the nurse should prepare to provide vascular instruments, a nerve stimulator, or blood replacement. For head and neck procedures, inadvertent pressure on the carotid artery may cause cardiac arrhythmias. The nurse should be alert for these changes and for the need to provide emergency resuscitation equipment.

Bone metastasis

Bone metastasis causes softening of the bones that may lead to fractures from the slightest stress. The long bones, spine, and ribs are most susceptible to pathological fractures. The nurse must ensure careful positioning and moving of the patient to avoid damage to the skeleton.

Positioning

The length of some oncologic procedures requires that special attention be given to patient positioning, maintenance of temperature, and adequacy of circulation. Since cancer patients may have been ill for some time prior to surgery, they are often malnourished. This means that their tissue may be in inferior condition. Minimizing tissue damage for a poorly nourished patient undergoing a lengthy procedure is a real challenge for the perioperative nurse, and one that can make a significant contribution to the patient's care. Implementation of the following measures helps prevent or minimize tissue damage:

- Add additional padding to the operating room bed: "egg crate" foam, air, or gel mattress.
- Use foam protectors on pressure points: knees, heels, elbows, occiput.
- Ensure adequate numbers of personnel to position the patient.
- Avoid shearing of tissue caused by pulling or sliding.
- Maintain body alignment.
- Support extremities when moving the patient.
- Assess peripheral pulses before and after positioning.
- Stay at the patient's side during anesthesia induction and emergence, to control unexpected movement.
- Provide appropriate restraint devices and apply them properly.
- Place a bolster at the soles of the feet to prevent foot drop.
- Avoid pooling of fluids under the patient.
- Provide mechanisms for continued functioning of drainage devices and ostomies.
- Avoid tissue compression by instruments, equipment, or personnel.
- Ensure that arms are secured to padded armboards or are padded and tucked securely at the patient's sides.
- Assist anesthesia providers to reposition the patient's head at intervals if possible.
- Provide protection for the eyes with padding, shields, or goggles.
- Apply the dispersive electrode over intact skin and remove carefully.
- Ensure that all jewelry, hairpins, and other items that could cause injury have been removed.

Despite all of these measures, tissue damage sometimes occurs. Careful documentation and follow-up are important in such cases. Further research may provide answers to this unsolved problem facing perioperative oncologic nurses.

Circulation

During long procedures the patient's circulation can be enhanced by the application of elastic hose or wraps or the use of sequential compression devices. Proper positioning, use of pneumatic tourniquets according to protocol, and assessment of peripheral pulses before and after positioning also ensure optimal circulation.

Hypothermia

The patient can become hypothermic because of the length of the procedure or because large body cavities are open and internal organs exposed. Hypothermia can be avoided by the use, under and over the patient, of warming blankets, of heat lamps, and of warm air devices. Core temperature should be monitored continuously. Parenteral and irrigation fluids should be warmed before use. Exposure of body parts is minimized. If the head and arms are not involved in the procedure, they may be kept warm with blankets or plastic coverings.

Preventing the spread of cancer

Several techniques can be used to reduce the number of cancer cells that are spread as a result of the surgical procedure. The system of strict "cancer technique," in which clamps are never reused and a new set of instruments is used for closure, is considered passé. The only time clamps need to be discarded is if they have been used to grasp gross tumor tissue. In that case, it is best to pass them off with the specimen. When a procedure involves two surgical sites, instruments used in an area containing cancer should not be reused in an area that is free of it. For example, if a skin graft is to be performed to cover an area where a tumor has been excised, it is ideal to harvest the graft at the beginning of the procedure. If this is not feasible, a set of instruments that will be used to take the graft should be isolated at the beginning of the procedure. The team members harvesting the graft should change gloves before proceeding if they have been working in the area of tumor. For a breast biopsy followed by mastectomy, a separate Mayo tray of instruments should be set up for the biopsy. Following the biopsy, team members should change gloves and proceed with the mastectomy using "fresh" instruments. This principle can be applied to other circumstances when it is desirable to isolate tumor cells from other body tissues.

Airway maintenance

If the patient has a tumor near the upper airway, intubation can sometimes be a problem. While the use of flexible laryngoscopes has facilitated difficult intubation, sometimes the procedure proves impossible to do. When the patient has already received medication and the airway is not controlled, emergency tracheostomy may be necessary. The scrub person and the circulating nurse should always be prepared for this situation in a head and neck procedure, as the need is immediate. Nurses must observe the intubation carefully and not be occupied with other tasks at that time. The nurse should also ensure that a surgeon capable of performing the tracheostomy is in the room at the time of induction.

Specimens

Proper handling of specimens removed from cancer patients is another very important nursing activity. Future treatment of the patient may depend on the results of the pathological analysis. Correct labeling of the specimen is essential to identify margins of the tumor and the site from which the tissue was removed. When multiple lymph nodes are removed, they must also be identified carefully. Routine preservation of the specimen should not be done if special studies are to be performed on the tissue. Fro-

zen section specimens must be delivered to the laboratory immediately and without preservatives. Special studies such as flow cytometry require that specimens be delivered to the laboratory sterile. Estrogen and progesterone receptors cannot be identified if the specimen has been preserved in formalin, so the specimen should be sent to the laboratory immediately.

Radioactive materials

Safe handling of radioactive materials in the operating room is always a concern. As with any other type of radiation, the staff should be concerned with exposure time, distance, and shielding. The radioactive materials should not be transported to the operating room from the laboratory until just before they are to be used, and then in a lead container on a cart with a long handle. If the material is sterilized in the operating room, a radiation symbol is placed on the autoclave to alert personnel (Fig. 20-6). All entrances to the operating room where the material is

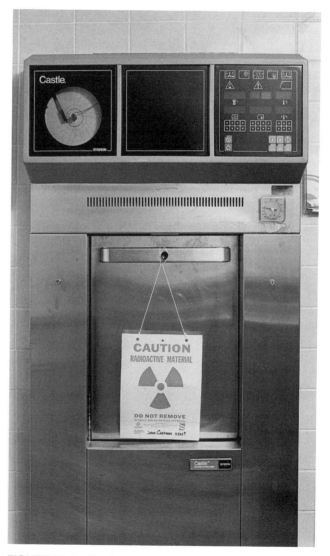

FIGURE 20-6 Caution sign on autoclave where radioactive materials are being sterilized. (*Courtesy of the University of Texas M.D. Anderson Cancer Center, Houston, TX.*)

in use must also be labeled with a radiation symbol so that no one enters inadvertently. Personnel preparing the radioactive material use lead shields between themselves and the source. Lead aprons are not adequate protection from this type of source and therefore should not be used. The lead shields can be draped and placed between the team members and the surgical site. Distance is increased by using a long ring forceps to handle the radioactive source. Exposure to active sources should be rotated among operating room staff, and doses received should be monitored by devices recommended by the facility's radiation safety officer.

SUMMARY

This chapter has discussed the many treatments available for oncologic patients—surgery accompanied by adjuvant therapies. The decision-making process that precedes the treatments is also discussed, along with the crucial role of the patient and family members in choosing specific forms of therapy.

Care of cancer patients presents many unique challenges to the perioperative nurse. Use of the nursing process ensures care that is individualized, state-of-the-art, and comprehensive. The procedures are varied and interesting, and each patient presents new opportunities for creative nursing activities. Perioperative nurses find their rewards by contributing to a positive outcome for these patients.

REFERENCES

Dachowski, L. J., & DeLaney, T. F. (1992). Photodynamic therapy: The NCI experience and its nursing implications. *Oncology Nursing Forum, 19*, 63–67.

Mayer, D. K., (1989). Dimensions in biological response modifiers. *Dimensions in Oncology Nursing, 3*, 6–8.

Piasecki, P. A. (1990). Bone cancer. In S. L. Groenwald, M. H. Frogge, M. Goodman, & C. H. Yarbro. (Eds.). *Cancer nursing, principles and practice* (2nd ed.). Boston: Jones and Bartlett.

Rieger, P. T. (1991). Biotherapy. In S. Otto (Ed.). *Oncology Nursing*. St. Louis: Mosby–Year Book.

Rosenberg, S. A. (1989). Principles of surgical oncology. In V. T. DeVita, S. Hellman, & S. A. Rosenberg (Eds.). *Cancer: Principles and practice of oncology*. Philadelphia: J. B. Lippincott.

Agency for Health Care Policy and Research (AHCPR)
AHCPR Publications Clearinghouse
P. O. Box 8547
Silver Spring, MD 20907
(800) 358-9295

American Academy of Ambulatory Care Nursing
East Holly Avenue
Box 56
Pitman, NJ 08071-0056
(609) 256-2350

American Academy of Orthopedic Surgery (AAOS)
222 S. Prospect Avenue
Park Ridge, IL 60068-4057
(708) 823-7118

American Academy of Pediatrics (AAP)
141 Northwest Point Road
P. O. Box 927
Elk Grove Village, IL 60009-0927
(708) 228-5005

American Association for Respiratory Care (AARC)
11030 Ables Lane
Dallas, TX 75229
(214) 243-2272

American Association for Retired Persons (AARP)
1909 K Street
Washington, DC 20049
(202) 331-2200

American Association of Occupational Health Nurses
   (AAOHN)
50 Lenox Pointe
Atlanta, GA 30324
(404) 262-1162

American Association of Diabetes Educators
500 Michigan Avenue, Suite 1400
Chicago, IL 60611
(312) 993-0043

American Association of Gynecologic Laparoscopists
13021 E. Florence Avenue
Santa Fe Springs, CA 90670
(213) 946-8774

American Association of Critical-Care Nurses (AACN)
101 Columbia
Aliso Viejo, CA 92656
(714) 362-2400

American Association of Blood Banks
8101 Glenbrook Road
Bethesda, MD 20814-2749
(301) 907-6977

American Association of Nurse Anesthetists (AANA)
222 South Prospect Avenue
Park Ridge, IL 60068-4001
(708) 692-7050

American Association of Tissue Banks
1350 Beverly Road, Suite 220-A
McLean, VA 22101
(703) 827-9582

American Bar Association
1800 M Street, NW
Washington, DC 20036
(202) 331-2200

American Cancer Society
1599 Clifton Road, NE
Atlanta, GA 30329
(404) 320-3333

American College of Emergency Physicians
P. O. Box 61991
Dallas, TX 75261-9911

American College of Nurse Midwives
1522 K Street, NW, Suite 1100
Washington, DC 20005
(202) 289-0171

American College of Obstetricians and Gynecologists
   (ACOG)
409 12th Street, SW
Washington, DC 20024
(202) 638-5577

American College of Occupational and Environmental
   Medicine (ACOEM)
55 W. Seegers Road
Arlington Heights, IL 60005
(708) 228-6850

American College of Surgeons (ACS)
55 E. Erie Street
Chicago, IL 60611-2797
(312) 664-4050

American Dental Association
Division of Scientific Affairs
211 E. Chicago Avenue
Chicago, IL 60611
(312) 440-2500

American Dietetic Association (ADA)
216 W. Jackson Blvd., Suite 800
Chicago, IL 60606-6995
(312) 889-0040

American Federation for Clinical Research
1350 Connecticut Avenue, NW
Suite 1100
Washington, DC 20036
(202) 223-2477

American Fertility Society (AFS)
2140 11th Avenue South, Suite 200
Birmingham, AL 35205-2800
(205) 933-8494

American Heart Association
7272 Greenville Avenue
Dallas, Texas 75231-4596
(214) 373-6300

American Hospital Association (AHA)
1 N. Franklin
Chicago, IL 60606
(312) 422-3000

American Institute of Architects (AIA)
1735 New York Avenue, NW
Washington, DC 20006
(202) 626-7300

American Medical Association (AMA)
515 N. State Street
Chicago, IL 60610
(312) 464-4818

American National Standards Institute (ANSI)
11 W. 42nd Street
New York, NY 10036
(212) 642-4900

American Nephrology Nurses Association (ANNA)
East Holly Avenue
Box 56
Pitman, NJ 08071-0056
(609) 256-2320

American Nurses Association (ANA)
American Academy of Nursing (AAN)
American Nurses Foundation (ANF)
600 Maryland Avenue, SW
Suite 100 West
Washington, DC 20024
(202) 554-4444

American Organization of Nurse Executives (AONE)
1 N. Franklin
Chicago, IL 60606
(312) 422-2800

American Public Health Association (APHA)
1015 Fifteenth Street, NW
Washington, DC 20005
(202) 789-5600

American Red Cross
17th and D Streets, NW
Washington, DC 20006
(202) 789-8300

American Society for Gastrointestinal Endoscopy (ASGE)
13 Elm Street
P. O. Box 1565
Manchester, MA 01944
(508) 526-8330

American Society for Healthcare Central Service Personnel of the American Hospital Association (ASHCSP)
1 N. Franklin
Chicago, IL 60606
(312) 422-3750

American Society for Healthcare Environmental Services Personnel (ASHESP)
1 N. Franklin
Chicago, IL 60606
(312) 422-3860

American Society for Hospital Engineering (ASHE)
1 N. Franklin
Chicago, IL 60606
(312) 422-3800

American Society for Hospital Materials Management of the American Hospital Association
1 N. Franklin
Chicago, IL 60606
(312) 422-3840

American Society for Laser Medicine and Surgery, Inc.
813 Second Street, Suite 200
Wausau, WI 54401
(715) 845-9283

American Society for Microbiology (ASM)
1325 Massachusetts Avenue, NW
Washington, DC 20005-4171
(202) 737-3600

American Society for Parenteral and Enteral Nutrition (ASPEN)
8630 Fenton Street, Suite 412
Silver Spring, MD 20910-3805
(301) 587-6315

American Society for Testing Materials (ASTM)
1916 Race Street
Philadelphia, PA 19103
(215) 299-5400

American Society of Hospital Pharmacists (ASHP)
4630 Montgomery Avenue
Bethesda, MD 20814
(301) 657-3000

American Society of Law and Medicine
765 Commonwealth Avenue
Boston, MA 02215
(617) 262-4990

American Society of Ophthalmic Registered Nurses (ASORN)
P. O. Box 193030
San Francisco, CA 94119
(415) 561-8513

American Society of Plastic and Reconstructive Surgical Nurses
East Holly Avenue
Box 56
Pitman, NJ 08071-0056
(609) 589-6247

American Society of Post Anesthesia Nurses (ASPAN)
11512 Allecingie Parkway
Richmond, VA 23235
(804) 379-5516

American Society of Testing Materials (ASTM)
1916 Race Street
Philadelphia, PA 19103-1187
(215) 977-9679

American Urological Association, Allied, Inc.
11512 Allecingie Parkway
Richmond, VA 23235
(804) 379-1306

Association for Professionals in Infection Control and
   Epidemiology (APIC)
1016 Sixteenth Street, NW, 6th Floor
Washington, DC 20036
(202) 296-2724

Association for the Advancement of Medical
   Instrumentation (AAMI)
3330 Washington Blvd., Suite 400
Arlington, VA 22201-4598
(703) 525-4890

Association for the Care of Children's Health (ACCH)
7910 Woodmont Avenue, Suite 300
Bethesda, MD 20814-3015
(301) 654-6549

Association of Hospital Employee Health Professionals
   (AHEHP)
1809 19th Street, 1st Floor
Sacramento, CA 95814

Association of Operating Room Nurses (AORN)
AORN Foundation
2170 S. Parker Road, Suite 300
Denver, CO 80231-5711
(303) 755-6300

Association of Surgical Technologists
7108 C. S. Alton Way
Englewood, CO 80112
(303) 694-9130

Association of Women's Health, Obstetric, and Neonatal
   Nurses (AWHONN)
409 12th Street, SW, Suite 300
Washington, DC 20024-2137

Australian Confederation of Operating Room Nurses
   (ACORN)
P. O. Box 1021
Hobart, Tasmania 7001
Australia
(002) 209262

Centers for Disease Control and Prevention (CDC)
Hospital Infections Program
1600 Clifton Road
Atlanta, GA 30333
(404) 639-1550

College of American Pathologists (CAP)
325 Waukegan Road
Northfield, IL 60093-2750
(708) 446-8800

Dermatology Nurses Association
East Holly Ave.
Box 56
Pitman, NJ 08071
(609) 256-2330

Emergency Care Research Institute (ECRI)
5200 Butler Pike
Plymouth Meeting, PA 19462
(610) 825-6000

Emergency Nurses Association
216 Higgins Road
Park Ridge, IL 60068
(708) 698-9400

Encyclopedia of Associations
   National Organizations of the U.S.
(27th ed., 1993)
Gale Research, Inc.
835 Penobscot Building
Detroit, MI 48226-4094

Federated Ambulatory Surgery Association (FASA)
700 N. Fairfax Street, Suite 520
Alexandria, VA 22314
(703) 836-8808

Government Printing Office (GPO)
Superintendent of Documents
Washington, DC 20402
(202) 523-5240

Health Care Material Management Society (HCMMS)
13223 Black Mountain Road #1-432
San Diego, CA 92129-2699
(619) 538-0863;   (800) 543-5885

Health Industry Distributors Association (HIDA)
225 Reinekers Lane
Suite 650
Alexandria, VA 22314-2875
(703) 549-4432

Health Industry Manufacturers Association (HIMA)
1030 15th Street, NW
Suite 1100
Washington, DC 20005
(202) 452-8240

Infection Control Society of South Africa
P. O. Box 12
Pretoria, 0001
South Africa

Institute for Healthcare Management
One Exeter Plaza
Ninth Floor
Boston, MA 02116

International Association of Healthcare Central Service
   Materiel Management
213 W. Institute Place, Suite 412
Chicago, IL 60610

International Council of Nurses and Florence
Nightingale International Foundation
3, Place Jean-Marteau
1201 Geneva,
Switzerland

International Society of Technology Assessment in
Health Care (ISTAHC)
1101 Fourteenth Street, NW, Suite 1100
Washington, DC 20005
(202) 371-1887

Intravenous Nurses Society (INS)
Two Brighton Street
Belmont, MA 02178
(617) 489-5205

Joint Commission on Accreditation of Healthcare
Organizations (JCAHO)
One Renaissance Boulevard
Oakbrook, IL 60181
(708) 916-5600

Joint Committee on Health Care Laundry Guidelines
c/o International Association for Hospital Textile
Management
P. O. Box 1283
Hallandale, FL 33009
(305) 457-7555

Midwest Bioethics Center
410 Archibald, Suite 106
Kansas City, MO 64111
(816) 756-2713

National Association for Homecare
519 C Street, NE
Stanton Park
Washington, DC 20002-5809
(202) 547-7424

National Association of Emergency Medical Technicians
9140 Ward Parkway
Kansas City, MO 64114
(816) 444-3500

National Association of Orthopedic Nurses (NAON)
East Holly Avenue
Box 56
Pitman, NJ 08071-0056
(609) 582-0111

National Association of Pediatric Nurse Associates and
Practitioners (NAPNAP)
1101 Kings Highway North, Suite 206
Cherry Hill, NJ 08034
(609) 667-1773

National Association of Quality Assurance Professionals
Association Management Center
5700 Old Orchard Road
Skokie, IL 60077
(708) 965-2776

National Institute for Nursing Research
9000 Rockville Pike
HIH Bldg. 31
Rm. 5B03
Bethesda, MD 20892
(301) 496-8230

National Committee for Clinical Laboratory Standards
(NCCLS)
711 East Lancaster Avenue
Villanova, PA 19085
(215) 525-2435

National Federation of Specialty Nursing Organizations
875 Kings Highway
West Deptford, NJ 08096
(919) 781-0411

National Fire Protection Association (NFPA)
1 Batterymarch Park
Quincy, MA 02269-9101
(617) 770-3000

National Gerontological Nursing Association
7250 Parkway Drive
Suite 510
Hanover, MD 21076
(800) 723-0560

National Institute of Occupational Safety and Health
(NIOSH)
Robert A. Taft Laboratories
4676 Columbia Parkway
Cincinnati, OH 45226

National Institutes of Health
9000 Rockville Pike
Clinical Center Bldg. 10
Room 2C206
Bethesda, MD 20892
(301) 496-0441

National Reference Center for Bioethics Literature
Kennedy Institute of Ethics
Georgetown University
Washington, DC 20057
(800) MED-ETHX
(202) 687-3885

National Safety Council
1121 Spring Lake Drive
Itasca, IL 60143-3201
(708) 285-1121

National Student Nurses' Association (NSNA)
555 W. 57th Street
New York, NY 10019
(212) 581-2211

National Technical Information Service (NTIS)
U.S. Department of Commerce
Springfield, VA 22161
(800) 336-4700

Occupational Safety and Health Administration (OSHA)
Department of Labor
200 Constitution Avenue, NW
Washington, DC 20210
(202) 513-7075

Oncology Nursing Society (ONS)
501 Holiday Drive
Pittsburgh, PA 15220
(412) 921-7373

Operating Room Nurses' Association of Canada
(ORNAC)
2864 W. 3rd Avenue
Vancouver, BC
Canada V6K 1M7

Pacific Center for Health Policy and Ethics
University of Southern California
Los Angeles, CA 90089-0071
(213) 740-2541

Sigma Theta Tau International
550 W. Worth Street
Indianapolis, IN 46202
(317) 634-8171

Society for Health and Human Values
6728 Old McLean Village Drive
McLean, VA 22101
(703) 556-9222

Society for Healthcare Epidemiology of America (SHEA)
875 Kings Highway, Suite 200
Woodbury, NJ 08096
(609) 845-1636

Society of Gastrointestinal Nurses and Associates, Inc.
  (SGNA)
1070 Sibley Tower
Rochester, NY 14604-1072
(800) 245-SGNA

Society of Otorhinolaryngology and Head/Neck Nurses
439 North Causeway
New Smyrna Beach, FL 32169
(904) 428-1695

South African Nurses Association
P. O. Box 12
Pretoria, 0001
South Africa

South African Theatre Sisters Association (SATS)
P. O. Box 231
Panorama, 7506
South Africa

The Hastings Center
255 Elm Road
Briarcliff Manor, NY 10510
(914) 762-8500

The Kennedy Institute of Ethics
Georgetown University
Washington, DC 20057
(202) 625-2383

U.S. Department of Health and Human Services
U.S. Public Health Service (USPHS)
Rockville, MD 20857

U.S. Environmental Protection Agency (EPA)
401 M Street, SW
Washington, DC 20460
(800) 858-7377

U.S. Food and Drug Administration (FDA)
8787 Georgia Avenue
Silver Spring, MD 29010

Visiting Nurse Associations of America
3801 E. Florida Avenue
Suite 900
Denver, CO 80210
(303) 753-0218

World Health Organization
Avenue Appia
1211 Geneva,
Switzerland

World Research Foundation
15300 Ventura Boulevard, Suite 405
Sherman Oaks, CA 91403
(818) 907-5483

Wound Ostomy and Continence Nurses Society
  (WOCN)
2755 Bristol Street
Suite 110
Costa Mesa, CA 92626
(714) 476-0268

Index